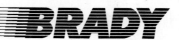

SIXTH EDITION

FIRST RESPONDER

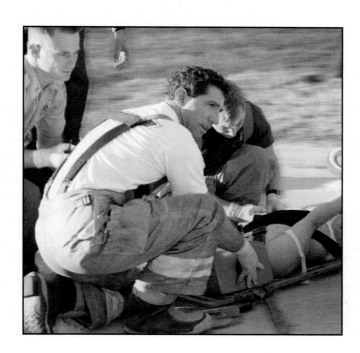

J. David Bergeron
Gloria Bizjak

Medical Reviewers
Frank T. Barranco, Sr., M.D.
Howard A. Werman, M.D.

Prentice
Hall

Upper Saddle River, New Jersey 07458

Library of Congress Cataloging-in-Publication Data

Bergeron, J. David, 1944—
    First responder/J. David Bergeron, Gloria Bizjak ; medical
reviewers, Frank Barranco, Howard A. Werman.—6th ed.
        p.; cm.
    Includes index.
    ISBN 0-13-030726-2 (pbk. : alk. paper)
    1. Medical emergencies. 2. Emergency medical technicians.
    I. Bizjak, Gloria. II. Title.
    [DNLM: 1. Emergency Medical Services. 2. Emergencies. 3.
Emergency Medical Technicians. 4. Emergency Treatment. WX 215
B496f 2001]
    RC86.7.B47 2001
    616.02'5—dc21   00-045416
                                                          CIP

Publisher: Julie Alexander
Executive Editor: Greg Vis
Managing Development Editor: Lois Berlowitz
Development Editor: John Joerschke
Director of Manufacturing & Production: Bruce Johnson
Managing Editor: Patrick Walsh
Production Editor: Navta Associates, Inc.
Production Liason: Cathy O'Connell
Manufacturing Manager: Ilene Sanford
Director of Marketing: Leslie Cavaliere
Marketing Manager: Tiffany Price
Photographers: Stephen Bell, George Dodson,
    Michael Gallitelli, Michal Heron, Richard Logan
Creative Director: Marianne Frasco
Cover Design: Joe David Smith
Interior Design: Rosemarie Votta
Composition: Navta Associates, Inc.
Printing and Binding: Banta-Menasha.

Prentice-Hall International (UK) Limited, *London*
Prentice-Hall of Australia Pty. Limited, *Sydney*
Prentice-Hall Canada Inc., *Toronto*
Prentice-Hall Hispanoamericana, S.A., *Mexico*
Prentice-Hall of India Private Limited, *New Delhi*
Prentice-Hall of Japan, Inc., *Tokyo*
Prentice-Hall Singapore Pte. Ltd.
Editora Prentice-Hall do Brasil, Ltda., *Rio de Janeiro*

NOTICE ON CARE PROCEDURES

It is the intent of the authors and publisher that this textbook be used as part of a formal First Responder education program taught by qualified instructors and supervised by a licensed physician. The procedures described in this textbook are based upon consultation with First Responder and medical authorities. The authors and publisher have taken care to make certain that these procedures reflect currently accepted clinical practice; however, they cannot be considered absolute recommendations.

The material in this textbook contains the most current information available at the time of publication. However, federal, state, and local guidelines concerning clinical practices, including, without limitation, those governing infection control and universal precautions, change rapidly. The reader should note, therefore, that new regulations may require changes in some procedures.

It is the responsibility of the reader to familiarize himself or herself with the policies and procedures set by federal, state, and local agencies as well as the institution or agency where the reader is employed. The authors and the publisher of this textbook and the supplements written to accompany it disclaim any liability, loss, or risk resulting directly or indirectly from the suggested procedures and theory, from any undetected errors, or from the reader's responsibility to stay informed of any new changes or recommendations made by any federal, state, and local agency as well as by his or her employing institution or agency.

NOTICE ON GENDER USAGE

The English language has historically given preference to the male gender. Among many words, the pronouns, "he" and "his" are commonly used to describe both genders. Society evolves faster than language, and the male pronouns still predominate our speech. The authors have made great effort to treat the two genders equally, recognizing that a significant percentage of First Responders are female. However, in some instances, male pronouns may be used to describe both males and females solely for the purpose of brevity. This is not intended to offend any readers of the female gender.

Photo credits: We wish to thank the following companies for their cooperation in providing photographs of helmets that appear in Chapter 12: AFX North American, Inc.; Giro Sports Design; International Riding Helmets, Inc.; Schutt Sports.

10 9 8 7 6 5 4 3

ISBN 0-13-030726-2

CONTENTS

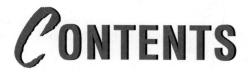

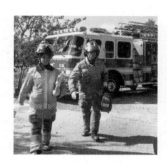
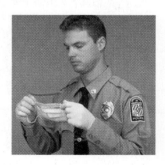

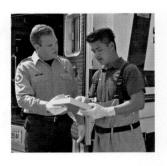

CHAPTER 3

LEGAL AND ETHICAL ISSUES   31

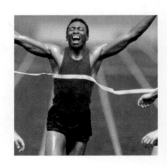

CHAPTER 4

THE HUMAN BODY   45

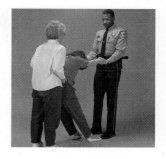
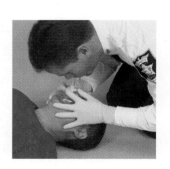

UNIT 3 PATIENT ASSESSMENT

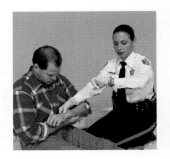

UNIT 4 CIRCULATION

CHAPTER 8

*C*ARDIOPULMONARY RESUSCITATION (CPR) 183

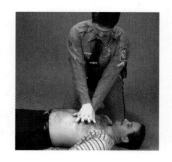

CHAPTER 9

*T*WO-RESCUER CPR 227

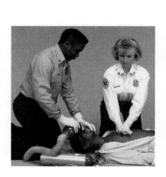

UNIT 5 ILLNESS AND INJURY

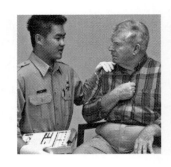

CHAPTER 12

*M*USCLE AND BONE INJURIES **369**

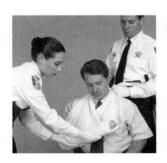

UNIT 6 CHILDBIRTH AND CHILDREN

CHAPTER 13

CHILDBIRTH 449

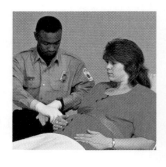

CHAPTER 14

INFANTS AND CHILDREN 479

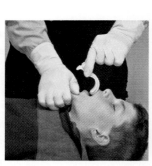

UNIT 7   EMS OPERATIONS

CHAPTER 15   *G*AINING ACCESS AND TRIAGE   521

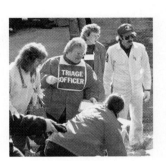

APPENDICES

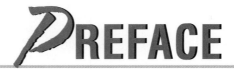

PREFACE

THE FIRST RESPONDER PROGRAM

The July/August 1994 issue of *RESCUE-EMS Magazine* described the plans of the National EMS Education and Practice Blueprint Project Task Force. This Blueprint provided outlines of the EMS system programs, including one for First Responder. The National Association of EMS Educators (NAEMSE) has studied the strengths and weaknesses in the National Standard Curriculum since EMS systems have initiated the Blueprint programs. The winter 1999 newsletter *Domain* explains the latest projections for EMS programs. These projections have been incorporated into this First Responder text and the supplemental instructor and student materials. The text also follows the guidelines set by the U.S. Department of Transportation (DOT) National Standard Curriculum.

Using these projections and guidelines, physicians, curriculum designers, instructors, and emergency care providers have designed First Responder courses to meet training needs in their communities. While all First Responder courses meet the same National Standard Curriculum objectives, jurisdictions may present additional prerequisites or require that some prerequisites be met before enrolling in the course. Emergency care procedures, for the most part, remain the same from EMS system to EMS system. However, many EMS programs may require completion of American Heart Association (AHA) CPR, or basic life support, before entering a First Responder program. While CPR guidelines are undergoing changes for the *layperson*, this textbook includes the most recent AHA guidelines for the *emergency care provider* at the time of printing. This new edition has removed the AED procedures from the appendix and has included them in the CPR chapters. AED has become an important part of basic life support, and many public facilities are beginning to place them on the premises and train their personnel in their use.

The other appendices, including *Determining Blood Pressure, Breathing Aids and Oxygen Therapy, Pharmacology, Swimming and Diving Accidents,* and *Stress Management* are there to meet the varying needs of jurisdictions throughout the country. A new appendix, *First Responder Roles and Responsibilities*, defines the roles and responsibilities of each level of emergency care: First Responder, EMT-Basic, and EMT-Paramedic. The chart shows the overlapping roles of the care providers as they respond with actions and interact with each other through the phases of an emergency and carry out their roles in the EMS system.

One of the most critical advances in emergency care is the use of personal protection, or barrier devices, against infectious diseases. More effective barrier devices have been designed, and it is important that First Responders understand their protective abilities and use them appropriately. The incidence of infection from infectious diseases, such as hepatitis, tuberculosis, and the HIV virus, remains low in emergency care providers, but it can only continue to be minimal if emergency care providers continue to use barrier devices consistently and correctly.

THE LEARNING PACKAGE

Instructors will want to use instructional methods and students will want to be aware of learning techniques that enable learning. The First Responder textbook, the CD-ROM, the Workbook, and the Instructor's Resource Manual provide ideas for instruction and information and activities for learning. These ideas and activities are based on the experiences and suggestions of emergency care instructors and providers, EMS system committees, curriculum designers with backgrounds in emergency care, physicians and other medical personnel, and industry and the military involved in safety training. The Instructor's Resource Manual includes the DOT objectives and unit outlines that correlate with the textbook; the Student Workbook includes thought-provoking questions and activities that relate to real-life field experiences.

Additional features in this edition are the database flow diagrams and the injury or medical mini-flow assessment and care charts. These diagrams condense printed information into easy-to-follow visual diagrams that provide an instant review of material. The flow charts guide the First Responder student through the steps of assessment, care, and decision making. While many flow diagrams are provided, not all emergency scenarios are represented by them. Students will find that by using the basic design of the mini-flow assessment and care charts, they can design their own flow diagrams for other emergencies, use them for review, and apply the steps quickly as they practice skills procedures during training and use them on actual emergency care situations. The database flow diagrams are an excellent review resource.

Though many First Responder classes are taught in the traditional classroom by one instructor, many training programs are implementing major changes in teaching and learning, such as:

✓ Using telecommunications and technology

✓ Using multiple instructors and team-teaching techniques

✓ Moving training from "seat-time" to competency, or outcomes

✓ Making traditional academic calendars (semesters) or forms of synchronous delivery obsolete

✓ Implementing instructional roles that reflect new modes of course development and delivery

Regardless of the mode of delivery, First Responder instructors and students can anticipate an exciting and interesting training course that provides all the necessary preparation for caring and care-giving field providers. Take full advantage of all the materials provided, try different teaching and learning methods, and participate in the suggested activities for a new adventure in learning.

J. David Bergeron and Gloria Bizjak

ACKNOWLEDGMENTS

MEDICAL REVIEWERS

Our special thanks to *Dr. Frank T. Barranco, Sr.,* Emeritus Assistant Professor of Orthopedic Surgery, Johns Hopkins; Fire Surgeon, Baltimore County Fire Department; Retired Chief Physician, Baltimore City Police and Fire Departments, and to *Dr. Howard A. Werman,* Associate Professor, Department of Emergency Medicine, The Ohio State University College of Medicine and Public Health, Columbus, Ohio. The reviews from Dr. Barranco and Dr. Werman were carefully prepared, and we appreciate the thoughtful advice and keen insight offered. We are also grateful for the review of the Fifth Edition material offered by *Dr. M.S. Bogucki,* Assistant Professor, Section of Emergency Medicine, Yale University School of Medicine, New Haven, CT; Medical Director, Connecticut Fire Academy; EMS Medical Advisor, Branford, Guilford, and New Haven Fire Departments; Fire Surgeon, Branford Fire Department.

CONTRIBUTORS

Warren D. Bowman, M.D., FACP
National Medical Director Emeritus for the National Ski Patrol; Past President of the Wilderness Medical Society; Clinical Associate Professor of Medicine Emeritus at the University of Washington in Seattle.

Ed Gjoldstad
BMW Quality Control Manager, Tischer Auto Park, Silver Spring, MD

David M. Habben, NREMT-P
EMS Instructor/Consultant, Boise, ID.

Eric W. Heckerson, R.N., B.S.N., M.A. NREMT-P
EMS Specialist, Mesa Fire Department, Mesa, AZ. Active in EMS program coordination at local, regional, and state levels. Adjunct faculty member of Mesa Community College's EMT/Fire Science Department.

Jo Anne Schultz, B.A., NREMT-P
Paramedic, Lifestar Ambulance, Inc., Salisbury, MD; Level II instructor, Maryland Fire and Rescue Institute, University of Maryland; Paramedic instructor, Maryland Institute of Emergency Medical Services Systems, University of Maryland; ACLS, BTLS, and PALS instructor.

We wish to thank **George Wm. "Bill" Krause,** MT (ASCP), MS, MBA, an independent instructional materials developer from Owings Mills, Maryland, and educator of physics and forensic sciences in Baltimore County. Bill's involvement with this textbook began in 1998 with extensive reviews of the Fourth Edition and recommendations for change based on the latest course requirements at that time and 1999 as cited by the U.S. Department of Transportation.

Content decisions for the Fifth Edition and this new Sixth Edition flowed more smoothly thanks to guidelines Bill helped construct with the authors. For this edition, Bill helped develop the flow diagrams found throughout the text. His ideas have carried over into development of the Workbook and new technologies for the instruction of emergency care providers.

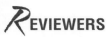EVIEWERS

We wish to thank the following EMS professionals who reviewed material for the Sixth Edition of *First Responder*. The quality of their reviews has been outstanding, and their assistance is deeply appreciated.

Doug Lawson
Devil Lake, ND

Jon F. Levine
Medical Director
Boston Emergency Medical Services
Boston, MA

Geoffrey T. Miller
Assistant Professor
Institute of Public Safety
Santa Fe Community College
Gainseville, FL

James E. Walker
Special Projects Coordinator
Northeastern University
Burlington, MA

Jeff Zuckernick
EMS Department
Kapiolani Community College
Honolulu, HI

We also wish to express appreciation to the following EMS professionals who reviewed earlier editions of *First Responder*. Their suggestions and insights helped to make this program a successful teaching tool.

Chad D. Andrews, BA, EMT-P, EMS-I
Program Director of Emergency Medical Services
Kirkwood Community College
Cedar Rapids, IA

Sgt. Charles Angello
Essex County Police Academy
Cedar Grove, NJ

John L. Beckman, FF/EMT-P
Firefighter/Paramedic
Affiliated with Addison Fire Protection District
Highland Park Hospital
Highland Park, IL

Kenneth O. Bradford, EMT-P
Santa Rosa Jr. College
Emergency Medical Care Programs
Petaluma, CA

Steven M. Carlo, BS, FNAEMD, EMT-I, EMD
Erie Community College—North
Emergency Medical Technology Dept
Williamsville, NY

Patricia A. Ciara, B.S., EMT-P
Assistant Deputy Chief Paramedic
EMS/CME Supervisor
Chicago Fire Department
Chicago, IL

Jo Ann Cobble, M.A., NREMT-P, R.N.
Chair, Dept EMS
University of Arkansas for Medical Sciences
Little Rock, AR

Captain Dale A. Crutchley, NREMT-P
EMS Administrator/Training Coordinator
Annapolis Fire Department
Annapolis, MD

Jeff Daleske, NREMT-P
Program Coordinator
Mercy School of EMS
Des Moines, IA

Gary Dean
Education Coordinator
East Texas Medical Center EMS
Tyler, TX

Garry L. DeJong, NREMT-P
EMS Training Coordinator
Captain, Albuquerque Fire Department
Albuquerque, NM

Jerry Domaschk, NREMT-P
Instructor
Louisiana Technical Colleges
Schriever, LA

TJ Feldman, MA, EMT-B
West Hartford, CT

Alejandro Garcia, EMT-P
EMS Coordinator
Wichita Falls Fire Department
Wichita Falls, TX

Donald Graesser
Bergen County EMS Training Center
Paramus, NJ
Jaime S. Greene, BA, EMT-B
EMT Education Program Director
Palm Beach County Schools
West Palm Beach, FL

Steve Harrell, EMT-P
Associate Professor
Daytona Beach Community College
Daytona Beach, FL

Glenn R. Henry, NREMT-P
Transport Coordinator-Rainbow Response
Egleston Children's Hospital
Atlanta, GA

Sgt. David M. Johnson, NREMT-P
Emergency Services Unit
Montville Twp Police
Montville, NJ

Jerry W. Jones, MPA, BA, EMT-IV
Paramedic Program
Columbia State Community College
Shelbyville, TN

Kathleen M. King, BA, MS, EMT-B
Instructor
Northampton County EMS Training Institute
Northampton Community College
Bethlehem, PA

Barbara L. Klingensmith, MS, NREMT-P
Director, Public Services Programs
Edison Community College
Fort Myers, FL

Tom LeGros, NREMT
Fire District 12
St. Tammany, LA

John A, Lewin, EMT-P
EMS Coordinator
Illinois State Police Academy
Springfield, IL

Glenn H. Luedtke, NREMT-P
Director
Cape & Islands Emergency Medical Services System
Cape Cod, MA

Sergeant David M. Magnino, EMT-P
Paramedic: California Highway Patrol Academy
Emergency Medical Services
West Sacramento, CA

William D. McElhiney
Massachusetts State Police
Medical Unit
New Braintree, MA

Ronold Morton
EMS Coordinator
Marshall Fire/EMS
Marshall, TX

Ronald A. Olson
Milwaukee Police Department Training Bureau
Milwaukee, WI

Ham Robbins
Rent-A-Medic
Eastport, ME

Bryan Scyphers
Chairperson, Public Safety Services
Davidson County Community College
Winston-Salem, NC

Mark Slettum
North EMS Education
Division of North Memorial Health Care
Robbinsdale, MN

E.A. Sowinski, BSN, RN, NREMT-B
Delaware State Fire School
Dover, DE

Michael Strong, FF/EMT-P
Public Safety Training Associates
Paw Paw, MI

Jack L. Taylor, BA, EMT-P, I/C
EMS Program Director
Kalamazoo Valley Community College
Kalamazoo, MI
Tim Taylor, NREMT-P
Captain, Department of Fire and Rescue
Prince William County
Woodbridge, VA

Ronald C. Thomas, Jr.
Training and Research Manager
Florida State Fire College
Ocala, FL

Pat D. Trevathan M.S., EMT-Instructor/Coordinator
KY Tech Fire/Rescue Training
West KY State Technical Institute
Paducah, KY

Holly Weber, NREMT-B, I/C
Stonehearth Open Learning Opportunities, Inc. (SOLO)
Conway, NH

𝒫HOTO ACKNOWLEDGMENTS

Photo Credit Chapter Opener 4—The Stock Market, DiMaggio/Kalish

Companies We wish to thank the following companies for their cooperation in providing us with photos: Laerdal Medical; Nellcor; Puritan; Bennett, Inc.

Organizations We wish to thank the following organizations for their assistance in creating the photo program for this book:

William Nesmith, Assistant Chief, Hillsborough County Fire Department, Tampa, FL; from the Hillsborough Sheriff's Office: Sheriff Cal Henderson, Lt. Rocky Rodriguez, Sergeant Ray Lawton, Corporal Tony Roper, and Debbie Carter, Public Information Specialist; from LifeFleet Ambulance Service, Largo, FL: Nestor Berrios-Torres, Supervisor Hillsborough Office; Herman Cortez, Acting Operations Manager; Tom Maiolo, Area Service Manager; and Ted Rogers, NREMT-P Field Training Officer. Steven T. Edwards, Director Maryland Fire & Rescue, University of Maryland.

The publisher wishes to make special mention of the extraordinary commitment of many weeks of personnel services and equipment provided by the Sarasota County Fire Department, Sarasota, FL. Our appreciation to Sarasota County Government, County Administration James L. Ley; Sarasota County Fire Department, Fire Chief John Albritton; Deputy Fire Chief Julius Halas, Division Chief Brian Gorsky, Lt. Paul Dezzi

Appreciation also is extended to: Sheriff Geoffrey Monge, Sarasota County Sheriff's Department; Lt. Harry Mofield, Florida Highway Patrol; Mesa Fire Department, Mesa, AZ.

Technical Advisors Thanks to the following people for providing technical support during the photo shoots: Lt. Paul Dezzi, Debbie Peace, Sarasota County Fire Department; Barbara Klingensmith, MS, FF/NREMT-P, Director of Public Services Program, Edison Community College, Ft. Myers, FL.

INTRODUCTION

LEARNING TO BE A FIRST RESPONDER

First Responder programs were developed to provide highly trained individuals with the skills necessary to begin assessing and caring for patients at the scene of injury or illness. In many areas of the nation, First Responders now are able to reach patients in less than ten minutes from the onset of the emergency. This quick response and the quality care rendered save thousands of lives each year.

First Responder programs are growing in number and complexity each year. This commitment to the First Responder concept has allowed the First Responder to become an important part of emergency services in the United States. Other nations also are developing similar programs.

The first five editions of this textbook and the third edition update were used by several hundred thousand students as part of their training. This new edition maintains what was found to be successful in these editions and also includes some new topics and concepts that have recently become a part of most First Responder courses. This text also bases its format on the U.S. DOT First Responder National Standard curriculum as well as the recent projections made by the National Association of EMS Educators (NAEMSE), who has studied the strengths and weaknesses since EMS systems began using the National Standard Curriculum.

You are about to begin your training to become a First Responder. Most likely, your training will take place in a course that follows the guidelines set by your local Emergency Medical Services (EMS) system. Your course might be a state- or company-designed course. These courses are probably based on the guidelines originally developed as the 40-hour First Responder Course by the U.S. Department of Transportation (DOT).

The National EMS Education and Practice Blueprint Project Task Force (see Preface) describes a First Responder as a rescuer who ". . . uses a limited amount of equipment to perform initial assessment and intervention and is trained to assist other EMS providers. The Sixth Edition of this textbook continues to take into account the "Blueprint" curricula, follows DOT guidelines for First Responder, includes EMT-Basic national program terminology and assessment and care procedures, uses current American Heart Association guidelines, and adds Automated External Defibrillation (AED) procedures to the CPR chapters. Changes occur because medicine and the EMS system are dynamic, technology improves, and different care procedures evolve as new techniques are found to be effective. This textbook responds to these changes and meets the needs of the patients, the emergency care provider, and the EMS system.

Because each jurisdiction has somewhat different requirements, First Responder students should check with their instructor, who is the authority for their course. With frequent medical discoveries and changing procedures, it is not always possible for jurisdictions and publishers to keep every protocol or publication 100 percent current on a daily basis. However, your instructor will learn of protocol and procedure changes and inform you of new requirements and responsibilities. If your course uses several references (textbooks, protocols, certification requirements), or if this text and other references take different approaches to emergency care procedures, your instructor will tell you what guidelines, policies, and procedures to follow for your jurisdiction.

REMEMBER: As a First Responder, you are part of the EMS system. The care you provide must follow your state and local guidelines.

Using this Textbook

OBJECTIVES

Each chapter begins with a list of Objectives, which tell you what you should be able to do by the end of the chapter. These Objectives are taken from the U.S. DOT First Responder National Standard Curriculum. They are called behavioral or performance objectives because they state specific behaviors that you are expected to be able to show or perform as a result of learning. They direct you to learn or change behavior and show that change through some type of performance. The three kinds of Objectives listed are knowledge (cognitive), in which you are asked to learn information; attitude (affective), in which you are asked to change a value, belief, or feeling about something; and showing (psychomotor), in which you are asked to apply or demonstrate some knowledge or skill that you have learned.

LEARNING TASKS

Following the list of objectives is an additional list of items called Learning Tasks. By completing these tasks, you will take further steps in learning and skill areas that will prepare you for performing the many duties expected of a First Responder. In most cases, these Learning Tasks go beyond what is explicitly stated in the DOT Objectives, but cover areas required of First Responders by their departments, jurisdictions, and Medical Director.

CHAPTER STRUCTURE

The first steps of becoming a First Responder are included in the first four chapters of this text. Chapter 1 defines the roles and responsibilities that you must learn in order to become a First Responder. Important components of First Responder responsibilities are personal safety and scene size-up to ensure safety, which is described in Chapter 2. In addition, First Responders must be familiar with legal and ethical aspects of emergency care, discussed in Chapter 3. In Chapter 4, the First Responder will learn the parts of the human body, which will help in assessing and recognizing signs and symptoms of injuries and illnesses through a simple head-to-toe approach. By thoroughly studying these first four chapters, you will be working toward fulfilling the role of a First Responder. You will also be well prepared to study and understand the units that follow on Airway Management Patient Assessment, Circulation, Illness and Injury, Childbirth and Children, and EMS Operations.

As you study each chapter in this book, you should:

1. Go over the list of Objectives found at the beginning of the chapter.
2. Make sure that you understand all the Objectives before reading the chapter.
3. Read the list of Learning Tasks at the beginning of each chapter. As your instructor guides you through the lesson's discussion and activities to complete the Objectives, you will also find you cover many of the Learning Tasks. If you do not cover them all in class, talk and work with your classmates or personnel at your station to be sure you understand and can perform these tasks.
4. Read the chapter, keeping the list of Objectives and Learning Tasks in mind.
5. Give special consideration to illustrations, charts, and lists emphasized in the text.

6. After reading the chapter, go back over the list of Objectives and Learning Tasks to see if you can accomplish each of those listed.

7. Go back over the sections of the chapter that deal with the Objectives and Learning Tasks you could not meet.

UNIT SKILLS

The DOT curriculum provides time for review, practice, and evaluation at the end of each module or unit. The First Responder course you are taking also includes time for review and practice. This text provides Skill Check Lists at the end of each unit that review the skills learned in each unit. These skills lists also review and relate the skills learned in previous units that you will continue to perform throughout the course. Supplements to the textbook, such as the CD-ROM and the Student Workbook, also provide self-tests and exercises that will reinforce textbook information and activities and relate learned material to real-life situations. The self-tests and exercises will help you review important material that was covered in the unit and allow you to assess what you have learned and what you still need to study. Many of the exercises are designed for you to work with fellow students or personnel at your agency. You will find that learning with others who are learning and asking questions, too, and working with those who have experience will help you grasp information easily and more quickly than working on your own. Your instructor will also provide class time to practice skills and will coach you while you learn, giving you feedback or evaluating you on how well you are doing or in what areas you need to continue to practice.

You will find that the lists of Objectives and the Learning Tasks will also act as a self-test when you finish reading the chapters. Review them and see which ones you can answer and perform. Review and continue to practice the information and skills for the Objectives and Learning Tasks that you cannot answer or perform.

MEDICAL TERMS AND PRONUNCIATION

As you read through this text, you will note various types of terms. The first type will be common, everyday terms, such as *chest*. You will also see terms from medicine and anatomy, such as *thoracic*. When a medical term is used for the first time, a pronunciation guide may be given in the margin definition; for example, thoracic (tho-RAS-ik). Capitalized letters indicate the portion of the word that is accented. Practice saying these words and try to use them in conversations with your instructor and fellow students.

Having a large vocabulary of medical terms is not very important for First Responders. In fact, most new programs have reduced the number of medical terms presented to the First Responder student. In emergency situations, telling the emergency squad that the patient has chest pains is as meaningful as saying the patient has pains in the thorax. Telling an emergency medical technician (EMT) that the patient may have a fractured right thigh bone will have as much meaning as saying a fractured right femur. There are some terms that you must learn and use. These will be noted in each chapter.

It is important, however, that you can recognize and define many terms taken from medicine and anatomy. Even though you will not use these terms yourself, other members of the emergency care team may use them when conversing with you. In addition, as part of your continuing education as a First Responder, you will run into these terms in articles and reports. For these reasons, you should not ignore anatomical and medical terms.

FLOW-OF-CARE DIAGRAMS

There are many strategies you can use with your instructor, classmates, or when working alone that allow you to have a battery of teaching tools to help you learn. We each learn a little differently from the other and in large categories, some people will find that they are usually visual learners, or sometimes do best hearing words. Finding your own combination of learning tools is part of getting off to a good start in any course.

Flow diagrams are learning tools. They help you to learn an assessment or a care procedure. The keyword here is "helps." Not every step is shown every time. The flow diagram does not stand alone. In this text, it works along with PHOTO SCANS and lists to help you learn portions of a part of specific instructions in a chapter. *Do not* try to memorize flow diagrams or spend so much time learning how to make the diagram that you do not have time to evaluate what you have learned and note how it fits in with other things you have studied or are studying in the course.

The flow diagrams used in this book do have portions that ask you to make yes or no decisions or to see which assessment procedures should work best for the patient being described or the care procedures that your medical director has approved for the assessment results you are obtaining. Again, do not memorize flow diagrams; however, do compare them with lists and SCANS. Thus, the SCAN and the flow diagram do come together as two tools that have far more impact than just reading. You are **interacting** with the teaching tools to produce results you can measure in terms of your understanding a section within a chapter.

Unless your instructor gives you specific directions to create flow diagrams, you may choose to develop your own here, using what is done in the textbook and the workbook. A very good book to help those of you who really enjoy utilizing flow diagrams is *Essentials of Flowcharting*, Fifth Edition by Boillot, Gleason, and Horn, published by Irwin/McGraw-Hill (ISBN 0-697-25418-6).

REMEMBER: Flow diagrams are learning tools, NOT complete protocols or lists of every step in assessment and care for every situation seen in First Responder-level emergency care.

LEVELS OF LEARNING

All First Responders need the same knowledge and skills. However, while you are learning, it might be useful for you to know what is considered to be basic information and techniques. A *First* has been placed next to all basic information and skills when they are presented in this text. This is not all you need to learn. It is important that you pay attention to the Objectives for each chapter.

The Objectives for each chapter include a list of psychomotor skills. Knowing the steps to a certain procedure will be part of the chapter. Selected psychomotor skills are also included in each Unit Review. However, being able to do the procedure will not come from studying this text or listening to lectures. Laboratory practice sessions and field sessions will be needed to perfect these skills.

HOW TO STUDY

Every person is unique. Since you are a little different from every other student, how you study will be a very personal thing. There are some standard recommendations that you might find helpful. First of all, you must follow directions given by your instructor and the directions given in this text. If you take off on your own, you could spend too much time on minor points and not enough time on what is critical knowledge for a First Responder.

Be sure to take notes during your training. You should have class notes, reading notes, and notes from any practical situations that are part of your First Responder course.

If possible, have your own place to study, removed from other activities. This will keep away distraction and help prevent some poor past habits of studying that waste time. Study by yourself until you are able to meet all the chapter Objectives and Learning Tasks.

If you do not understand something presented in class or in this text, see your instructor. Your fellow students may not understand any more than you do. They also lack the experience your instructor will have.

After you have studied and feel that you can meet all the Objectives, then do meet with fellow students. Studies have shown that people remember things for a longer period of time if they have the opportunity to talk about their studies. If you have found that reading is not your best way of learning, then these meetings will be very important. You will soon see that being able to communicate with others is an important part of the task of a First Responder. Even if you have been trained in dealing with the public, you will still need practice in communicating the new information you will be using in this course.

When you study from this textbook, you should:

1. Take notes on the statements that apply to the chapter Objectives.
2. Keep a list of page numbers to go with Objectives.
3. If you are allowed to keep your text, mark important items in your book.
4. After finishing your reading and before checking back on the list of Objectives, be sure to go back over all illustrations, charts, and lists in the chapter.

NEW MULTIMEDIA PROGRAM

Our new Multimedia Program features two key items:

■ **Companion Website** (www.prenhall.com/bergeron): Tied chapter-by-chapter to the text, this *free* site includes an online study guide that provides you with immediate feedback as well as links to other EMS-related sites.

■ **Student CD-ROM:** This CD-ROM, packaged *free* with your text, contains vocabulary building puzzles and word games, lecture notes, an audio-glossary, and web links.

RESPONSIBILITY

It has been said that the responsibility for teaching is the teacher's and the responsibility for learning is the student's. It is your responsibility to learn what your instructor teaches. As a First Responder, it will be your responsibility to know all local and state requirements and regulations related to First Responders and the services that they perform.

In addition to the above responsibilities, as a First Responder, you will be expected to stay up-to-date in both information and skills. After completing your training, it is recommended that you set aside 30 minutes to an hour each week to review part of a chapter in this text, some of your lecture notes, or some other source of First Responder information. Your local or state emergency services director will be able to tell you what you will need in terms of updated bulletins and continuing education.

It is doubtful that you would be taking this course unless you had the attitude of a professional, so nothing need be said about motivation and your responsibilities to those who are providing you with this First Responder course. All that remains to be said in this introduction is good luck and enjoy your entry into the world of emergency care services.

WELCOME TO THE SIXTH EDITION OF

FIRST RESPONDER

J. David Bergeron
Gloria Bizjak

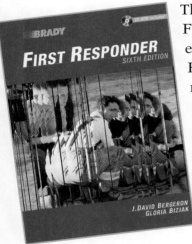

The leader in the field, this easy-to-understand text provides clear First Responder-level training for fire service, emergency, law enforcement, military, civil, and industrial personnel. The Sixth Edition of *FIRST RESPONDER* retains the hallmark that has made it the best-selling First Responder book on the market—solid, thorough coverage of the U.S. DOT First Responder National Standard Curriculum. New features, including *Flow-of-Care* diagrams, new appendices, and a state-of-the-art multimedia support package further clarify and illustrate important points, allowing students to better *understand, practice and master* the skills and concepts they need in order to become effective First Responders.

FULL TEACHING AND LEARNING PACKAGE

Setting the standard for instructor resources! *FIRST RESPONDER* has a comprehensive **Teaching/Learning Package** that includes:

- **Companion Website** (www.prenhall.com/bergeron) Contains chapter-by-chapter interactive review quizzes with immediate scoring and feedback and annotated links to appropriate EMS resources. In addition to resources for the student, you will find our Syllabus Manager feature, which allows you to create your own online syllabus.

- **First Responder PowerPoint Slides** (0-13-015875-5) Provide you with everything you need for a dynamic presentation. This set contains 700 easy to use PowerPoint slides that follow the U.S. DOT curriculum.

- **Instructor's Resource Manual** (0-13-032482-5) Contains lecture outlines, suggested lesson plans, additional classroom activities, and assignments.

- **Custom Test Manager** (Win 0-13-032485-X) This computerized test manager contains approx. 500 text-specific questions on disk in a customizable format that contains an electronic gradebook and allows for online testing using a LAN.

- **Certificates of Completion** (0-8359-5268-1) Call your Brady representative for more details.

THE CONTENT YOU TRUST

You have always relied on *FIRST RESPONDER* to provide the content you need in a manner that students can easily understand.

NEW TO THIS EDITION

- **Flow-of-Care Diagrams,** new to this edition, provide students with visual schematics to help them learn and apply patient assessment and other skills critical to First Responder training.

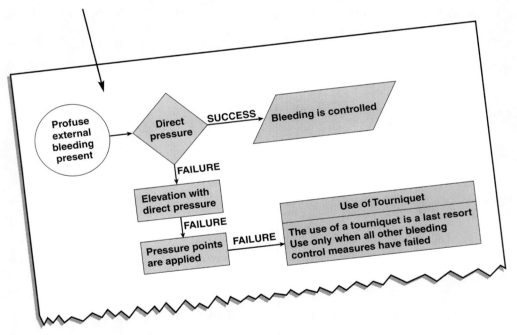

- **Updated Content** including: updated Skills Lists and information on ski boot fractures and helmet removal.

- **New Appendix on Roles and Responsibilities** helps First Responder students understand their role within the overall EMS team.

NEW TECHNOLOGY TO MEET THE NEEDS OF TODAY'S STUDENTS

In today's fast-paced learning environment, training takes place beyond the printed page. *FIRST RESPONDER'S* rich multimedia package expands upon the book content to provide interactive learning opportunities.

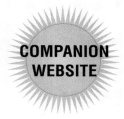

COMPANION WEBSITE

www.prenhall.com/bergeron

This *free* text-specific website provides students with additional online resources to aid in their learning.

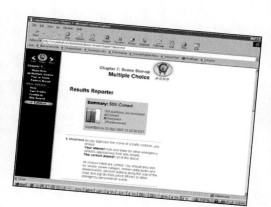

Anatomy Matching Exercises — Covering all the major body systems, these exercises help students learn important anatomy and physiology.

Audio-glossary — Students can hear the pronunciation of difficult EMS terms they need to learn.

Interactive Student Quizzes provide chapter-by-chapter questions with immediate feedback to help students master the necessary concepts to be an effective EMT.

Links — Annotated links to useful EMS sites.

Syllabus Manager — Online aid for instructors who wish to post course syllabi and assignments on the web for easy student access.

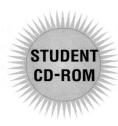

STUDENT CD-ROM

This useful multimedia tool brings an added dimension to your students' learning experience with quizzes and games, lecture notes, an audio-glossary and links to EMS-related web sites for further study.

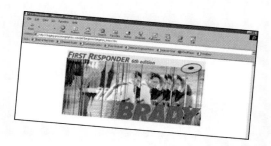

Browser-based Interface — Allows students to access the CD using familiar commands and programs, such as Netscape or Internet Explorer.

Vocabulary Games — Engaging crossword puzzles are a fun way for students to practice their mastery of EMS language.

ADDITIONAL STUDENT RESOURCES

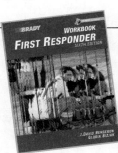

Student Workbook (0-13-032487-6) Additional multiple choice, labeling, and fill-in-the-blank questions help students practice and master the concepts they need to know to become effective First Responders.

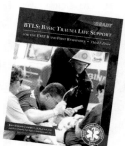
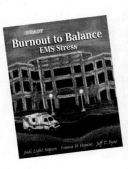
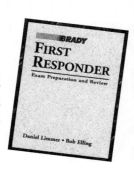
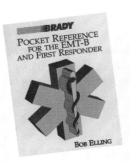

CHAPTER 1

/NTRODUCING THE EMS SYSTEM

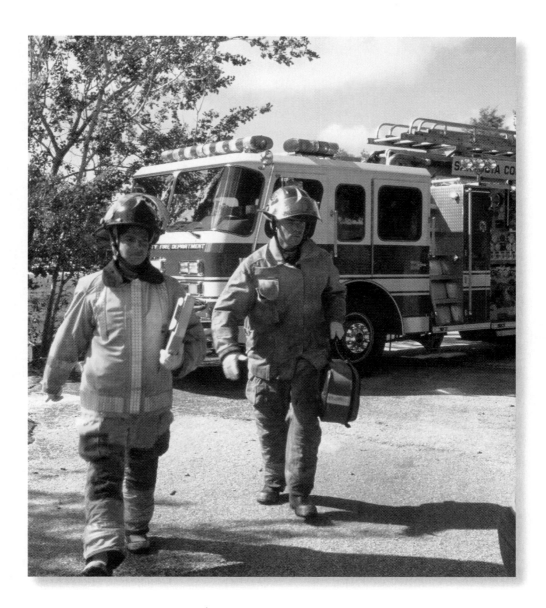

*T*housands of people become ill or are injured every day. Realizing that one of these ill or injured persons is depending on you to provide assistance often causes feelings of inadequacy. You can learn the steps for providing appropriate care by participating in a training program that teaches basic emergency care skills. This chapter will introduce you to the Emergency Medical Services system and to the roles and responsibilities of the First Responder.

National Standard Objectives

This chapter focuses on the objectives of Module 1, Lesson 1–1 of the U.S. DOT First Responder National Standard Curriculum and serves as an instructional aid to help you meet any specific objectives added to the course by your local EMS system.

By the end of this chapter, you will be able to:
(from cognitive or knowledge information) . . .

1–1.1	Define the components of Emergency Medical Services (EMS) systems. (pp. 3–4)
1–1.2	Differentiate the roles and responsibilities of the First Responder from other out-of-hospital care providers. (pp. 3, 6–11)
1–1.3	Define medical oversight and discuss the First Responder's role in the process. (pp. 5–6)
1–1.4	Discuss the types of medical oversight that may affect the medical care of a First Responder. (pp. 5–6)
1–1.5	State the specific statutes and regulations in your state regarding the EMS system. (pp. 6, 14)

Feel comfortable enough to
(by changing attitudes, values, and beliefs) . . .

1–1.6	Accept and uphold the responsibilities of a First Responder in accordance with the standards of an EMS professional. (pp. 6–8)
1–1.7	Explain the rationale for maintaining a professional appearance when on duty or when responding to calls. (p. 10)
1–1.8	Describe why it is inappropriate to judge a patient based on a cultural, gender, age, or socioeconomic model, and to vary the standard of care rendered as a result of that judgement. (p. 9)

LEARNING TASKS

It is very important that you understand just what is expected of you as a First Responder. When you do, you can act more quickly and provide better emergency care. As you participate in this program and practice your skills, think about the four major duties of First Responders and be able to:

✓ Apply these duties directly to patients.

It is also important to know exactly what your responsibilities are as a First Responder when responding to an emergency scene. There are specific responsibilities for each level of certification, and being aware of those pertaining to your level means there will be less duplication of services. Be able to:

✓ Perform those activities that fall under the heading of First Responder responsibilities.

THE EMS SYSTEM

Medical care saves millions of lives each year. The advances made in medicine during the last 50 years are startling. Highly trained health care teams use accurate methods of detecting illness, complex medical procedures, elaborate equipment, and new wonder drugs to provide the best of care for patients. Before the twentieth century, most patients who entered hospitals did so to die. Today, we fully expect the vast majority of hospitalized patients to recover and lead normal lives.

COMPONENTS OF THE EMS SYSTEM

If hospitals stood by themselves, waiting for patients to come to them, many individuals would die before reaching medical care. Fortunately, it is possible to extend care out to the patient through a chain of human resources known as the **Emergency Medical Services (EMS) system** (Scan 1-1). Once this system is activated, care begins at the emergency scene and continues during transport to the medical facility. After transport, an orderly transfer to the emergency department staff at the medical facility ensures continued care.

ACTIVATING THE EMS SYSTEM

Once an emergency occurs and it is recognized, the EMS system must be activated. Most citizens activate it by way of a 911 phone call to an emergency dispatcher, who then sends available responders—**First Responders,** EMT-Basics, and advanced life support providers (EMT-Intermediates and EMT-Paramedics) to the scene. Refer to Table 1-1 to differentiate the roles and responsibilities of these four types of responders.

Some systems may not have a 911 activation system, and the caller may need to seek initial help through fire, police, or rescue personnel. The most desirable EMS activation is the *enhanced* 911 service that allows for caller

emergency medical services system
the chain of human resources and services linked together to provide continuous emergency care from the prehospital scene, through transport, and at the medical facility.

first responder
a member of the EMS system who has been trained to render first care for a patient and to help EMTs at the emergency scene.

TABLE 1-1: LEVELS OF EMS TRAINING

There are four levels of EMS training. These levels of training are based on the U.S. Department of Transportation's National Standard Curriculum but vary slightly from state to state. Your instructor will explain variations that exist in your area.

■ **First Responder**—This level of training is designed specifically for the person who is often first to arrive at the scene. Many police officers, firefighters, and industrial workers are certified as First Responders. This training emphasizes activating the EMS system and providing immediate care for life-threatening injuries and illnesses, controlling the scene, and preparing for the arrival of the ambulance.

■ **EMT-Basic**—In most areas, EMT-B is considered the minimum level of certification for ambulance personnel. The training emphasis is on assessment and care of the ill or injured patient.

■ **EMT-Intermediate**—An EMT-I is a basic level EMT who has passed specific additional training programs in order to provide some level of advanced life support. Some of the additional skills an EMT-I may be able to perform are the initiation of IV (intravenous) lines, advanced airway techniques, and administration of medications beyond those the EMT-B is permitted to administer.

■ **EMT-Paramedic**—Paramedics can generally perform relatively invasive field care, including insertion of endotracheal (ET) tubes, initiation of IV lines, administration of medications, interpretation of electrocardiograms, and cardiac defibrillation.

The EMS System

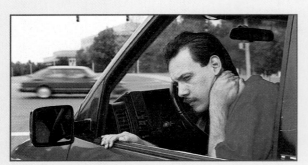

1. Emergency scene.

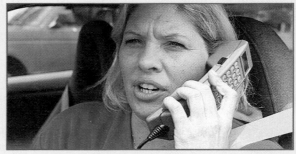

2. Recognition of accident and activation of EMS.

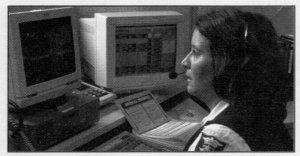

3. EMS dispatch.

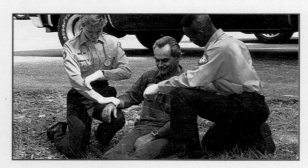

4. Arrival of First Responders.

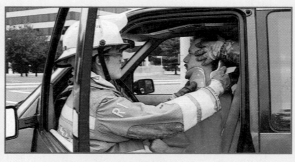

5. Care given at the scene.

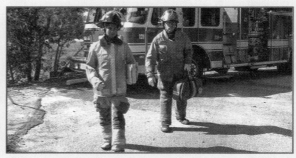

6. Arrival of additional EMS.

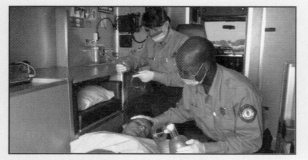

7. Care during transport.

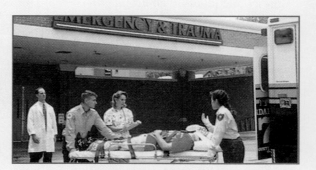

8. Transfer to hospital emergency department.

information (for example, phone number and address) to be received electronically. In an enhanced 911 service, the dispatcher is trained to help and instruct bystanders to do no harm, protect the patient, and initiate certain aspects of emergency care.

No matter which way the system is activated, after responders arrive at the scene and provide emergency care, the patient is transported to the medical facility.

THE IN-HOSPITAL CARE SYSTEM

From the ambulance, the emergency department receives the patient. Here, the patient receives laboratory tests, diagnosis, and further treatment. The emergency department is the gateway to the rest of the services offered by the hospital. If a patient has serious injuries, the emergency department gives care to stabilize the patient, and the operating room is readied to provide further life-saving measures. Some hospitals handle all routine and emergency cases but have a specialty that sets them apart from other hospitals. One specialty hospital is the trauma center, in which surgery teams are available 24 hours a day. Some hospitals have centers that specialize in the care of certain conditions and patients, such as burn centers, pediatric centers, perinatal centers, and poison control centers. There are many key members of the hospital portion of the EMS system, including physicians, nurses, physician assistants, respiratory and physical therapists, technicians, aides, and more.

MEDICAL OVERSIGHT

First | Each EMS system has a Medical Director, a physician who assumes the ultimate responsibility for medical direction, or oversight of the patient care aspects of the EMS system (Figure 1.1). The Medical Director also oversees training and develops protocols (lists of steps, such as assessment and care steps and interventions to be performed in different situations). EMTs at basic or advanced levels act as designated agents of the physician. This means that their authority to give medications and provide emergency care is actually an extension of the Medical Director's license to practice medicine.

The physician obviously cannot physically be present at every emergency, so the EMS system develops standing orders. These standing orders are in the form of protocols that authorize rescuers to perform particular skills in certain situations without actually speaking to the Medical Director. This kind of "behind the scenes" medical direction is called **off-line medical direction.** Procedures

off-line medical direction protocols developed by an EMS system that authorize rescuers to perform particular skills in certain situations without actually speaking to the Medical Director.

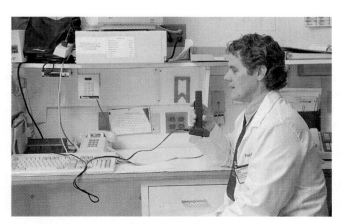

FIGURE 1.1 Medical direction given by on-line orders.

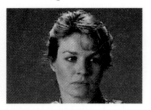

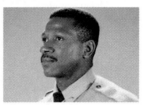

on-line medical direction orders to perform a skill or administer care from the on-duty physician given by radio or phone to a rescuer.

scope of practice set of responsibilities and ethical considerations that define the extent or limits of the care provider.

FIGURE 1.2
First Responders.

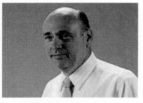

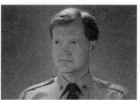

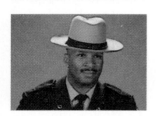

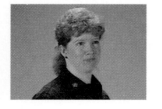

not covered by standing orders or protocols require the rescuer to contact the on-duty physician by radio or telephone prior to performing a skill or administering care. Orders from the on-duty physician given in this manner—by radio or phone—are called **on-line medical direction.**

As a First Responder, you will have little access to the Medical Director in the event of an emergency. It will be necessary for you to adhere to the training you receive or to follow the orders of providers with a higher level of certification if they are present at the scene. All personnel, however, must provide care only within their **scope of practice.** Your instructor will inform you of your local policies. Always follow your local protocols. There are specific statutes and regulations regarding EMS in every state and in some local jurisdictions. Your instructor will also inform you of these.

THE FIRST RESPONDER

The lack of people with enough training to provide care before more highly skilled EMS providers arrive at a scene is the weakest link in the chain of the EMS system. It is believed that the training of First Responders will help correct this problem.

First | First Responders are trained to reach patients, find out what is wrong, provide emergency care, and only when necessary, move patients without causing further injury. These individuals are usually the first trained personnel to reach the patient. A First Responder may be a law enforcement officer, a member of the fire service, a coworker, or a private citizen who arrives first at the scene (Figure 1.2). In all cases, a First Responder is trained and has successfully completed a First Responder course. All police officers and firefighters should be trained to the First Responder level. Industry needs to have many of its employees trained as well. Truck drivers, known for their willingness to help at the scene of highway accidents, could save many lives if they were trained to the First Responder level. Of course, the more private citizens who are willing to be trained as First Responders, the stronger the EMS system will become.

Since the beginning of First Responder training programs, hundreds of thousands of people have completed formal courses, with many of these people going on to provide essential care. In most areas of the United States, First Responders are now an important part of the EMS system. The care they provide reduces suffering, prevents additional injuries, and saves many lives.

ROLES AND RESPONSIBILITIES

Personal Safety

First | Your primary concern as a First Responder at an emergency scene is *personal safety*. The desire to help those who are in need of care may tempt you to ignore the hazards at the scene. You must make certain that you can safely reach the patient and that you will remain safe while providing care.

Part of a First Responder's concern for personal safety must include the proper protection from infectious diseases. As a First Responder assessing or providing care for patients, you must avoid direct contact with patient blood or other body fluids, membranes, wounds, and burns. Personal protection from possible contact with infectious agents may require the use of:

- Approved latex or vinyl gloves
- Pocket face masks with one-way valves and special filters for rescue-breathing procedures
- Protective eyewear such as goggles or face shields to avoid contact with droplets expelled during certain care procedures (for example, assisting with childbirth)
- Face masks to avoid contact with airborne microorganisms
- Gowns or aprons to avoid being splashed by blood or other body fluids or having direct contact with contaminated items

Typically, you will need no more than latex or vinyl gloves in most care situations; however, all the items listed above should be on hand for the rendering of safe care. More will be said about infectious diseases and personal protection in Chapter 2.

First Responders who are in law enforcement or the fire service may find that they are required to carry out certain duties before attempting to provide patient care. If this applies to you, always follow your department's standard operating procedures.

First | The EMS system responds to an emergency scene to provide care for the patient. Remember, **as a First Responder, you are part of the EMS system.** Your activities at the scene and the care you provide until more highly trained personnel arrive will help to save lives, prevent additional injury, and give comfort to patients.

Patient-Related Duties

Before care begins for someone, that person is a victim. Once you start to carry out your duties as a First Responder, the victim becomes a patient. Your presence at the scene means that the EMS system has begun its first phase of care. True, the patient may need a physician at the hospital to survive, but the patient's chances of reaching the hospital alive are greatly improved because a First Responder has initiated emergency care.

First | As a First Responder, you have four main patient-related duties to carry out at the emergency scene (Figure 1.3). These duties are:

1. **Safely gain access to the patient, using simple hand tools when necessary.** You must gain access to patients, whether they are surrounded by a crowd, trapped in a vehicle, or inside a building. You must control an accident scene in order to protect yourself and the patients and to prevent additional accidents. At the same time, you ensure that the EMS system dispatcher is alerted so more highly trained personnel can be sent to the scene. Should the police, fire department, rescue squad, power company, or others be needed at the scene, you must assure that the dispatcher is aware of this need. If your system trains dispatchers in emergency medical dispatch procedures, they may provide assistance or directions by phone or radio until more highly trained personnel arrive.

2. **Find out what is wrong with the patient and provide emergency care using a minimum amount of equipment.** You find out what is wrong with the patient by gathering information from the scene, bystanders, and the patient, and by examining and assessing the patient. To the best of your ability, you then provide **emergency care** to the level of your training. Remember, emergency care deals with both illness and injury. Emergency care can be as simple as providing emotional support to someone who is frightened because of an accident. Or it can be more complex,

emergency care the prehospital assessment and basic care for the sick or injured patient. The physical and emotional needs of the patient are considered and attended to during care.

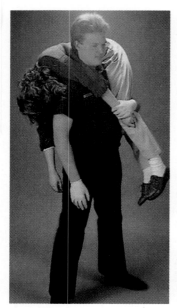
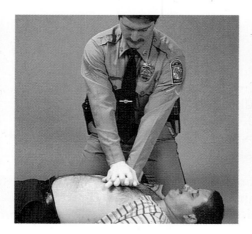
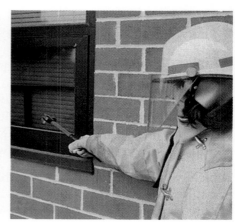
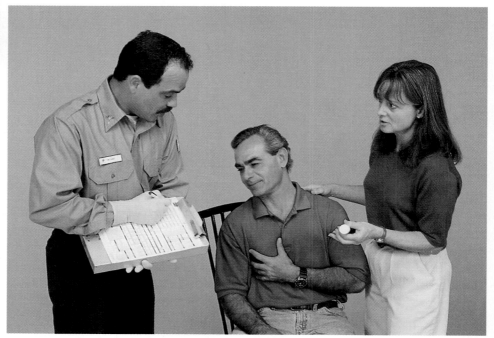

FIGURE 1.3
First Responders at the emergency scene.

requiring you to deal with life-threatening emergencies, such as starting basic life-support measures for a heart attack victim. In later chapters, you will learn how emotional support and physical care skills can be combined to help the patient until more highly trained personnel arrive.

3. **Lift or move the patient only when required and do so without causing additional injury.** You need to judge when safety or care requires you to move or reposition patients and do so using techniques that minimize causing additional injury.

4. **Transfer the patient and patient information to more highly trained personnel when they arrive at the scene.** You must provide for an orderly transfer of patients and patient information to more highly trained personnel when they arrive at the scene. You may also be asked to assist them and work under their direction.

TRAITS

To be a First Responder, you must be willing to take on additional duties and responsibilities. It takes hard work and study to be a First Responder. This

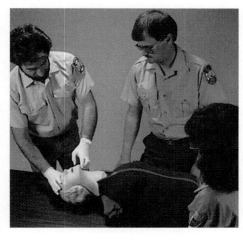

FIGURE 1.4
As a First Responder, you must focus on keeping your skills sharp and current.

effort does not end with your course, since you must keep your emergency care skills sharp and current (Figure 1.4). You also may be required to be recertified periodically.

If you want to be a First Responder, you have to be willing to deal with people. Individuals who are sick or injured are not at their best. You must be able to overlook rude behavior and unreasonable demands, realizing that patients may act this way because of illness or injury. Dealing with people is one of the hardest things we do. To do so in a professional manner is sometimes very difficult.

First | All patients have the same right to the very best of care. Your respect for others and your acceptance of their rights are an essential part of your total patient care as a First Responder. You cannot modify the care you provide according to your view of religious beliefs, cultural expression, age, gender, social behavior, socioeconomic background, or geographical origin. Likewise, you must take a realistic view; not all care can be *identical*, independent of patient age (for example, assessment of the severity of burns to a child or to a patient who is over 35 years of age). Nor can you ignore the fact that the poor often have a history of inadequate health care and improper diet. ***Every patient is unique*** and deserves to have his or her needs met and cared for as specifically as standard care procedures will permit.

To be a First Responder, you must be honest and realistic. When helping patients, you cannot tell them they are OK if they are sick or hurt. You cannot tell them that everything is all right, when they know that something is wrong. Telling someone not to worry is foolish. When an emergency occurs, there is truly something to worry about. Your conversations with patients can help them to relax if you are honest. By telling patients that you are trained in emergency care and that you will help them, you ease their fears and gain their confidence. Letting patients know that additional help is on the way also will help them to relax.

There are limits to what you can say to a patient. Telling a patient that her child is dead or a loved one is seriously injured will not help the patient. When rendering emergency care, more tact may be necessary. By saying that someone is taking care of the loved ones, you may be able to set the patient at ease. Remember, people under the stress of illness or injury often cannot tolerate any additional stress.

Being a First Responder requires that you control your own feelings at the emergency scene. You must learn to become involved with caring for patients, while controlling your emotional reactions to injury or serious illness. Patients do not need sympathy and tears. They need your professional care.

Providing First Responder-level care requires you to admit that accidents and other emergency scenes will affect you. You may have to speak with other EMS care providers or a specialist within the EMS system to resolve the stress and emotional problems caused by providing care. (Chapter 2 deals with stress management.)

As a First Responder, you have to be a highly disciplined professional at the emergency scene. Watch your language in front of patients and bystanders. Do not make comments about patients and the horror of an accident. Concentrate on patients and avoid unnecessary distractions. Something as simple as smoking a cigarette at the scene shows that you are not willing to discipline yourself to the level required.

No one can demand that you change your lifestyle to be a First Responder; however, since you may be called on to provide care almost anywhere anytime, you should consider these few things. Your appearance relates to gaining patient confidence. Putting on a clean shirt before running out to the store may not seem to be a reasonable request. Having one less drink at a party may sound unimportant. Yet the significance of such actions may be very important if you have to provide care at an accident.

To be a First Responder, you must keep yourself in reasonably good physical condition. If you are unable to provide needed care because you cannot bend over or catch your breath, then all your training is worthless.

When you complete your training and become a First Responder, you are someone special, filling a very important need in your community.

$\mathcal{S}$KILLS

In addition to learning facts and information, you will be required to perform certain skills as part of your First Responder training. These skills vary from course to course. The list below is an example of the skills learned by the typical First Responder. You are not expected to memorize this list. Read the list and check off each skill as you learn it in your course. As a First Responder, you should be able to:

❑ Assess and control the scene of a simple accident
❑ Gain access to patients in vehicles by way of doors and windows
❑ Gain access to patients in buildings by way of doors and windows
❑ Evaluate a scene in terms of safety and possible cause of an accident
❑ Gather information from patients and bystanders
❑ Properly use all items of personal safety
❑ Conduct a patient assessment
❑ Determine vital signs (pulse, breathing, relative skin temperature)
❑ Determine assessment signs
❑ Relate signs and symptoms to illnesses and injuries
❑ Open a patient's airway, provide airway care, and perform pulmonary resuscitation for adults, infants, children, and patients who breathe through surgical openings in their necks (neck breathers)
❑ Utilize a pocket face mask with one-way valve and HEPA filter to provide ventilations
❑ Detect cardiac arrest and perform one- and two-rescuer cardiopulmonary resuscitation (CPR)
❑ Control bleeding by using direct pressure, direct pressure and elevation, pressure dressings, pressure points, and tourniquets

- Detect shock (including allergy shock) and care for patients who develop shock
- Detect and provide care for closed injuries and open injuries, including face and scalp wounds, nosebleeds, eye injuries, neck wounds, chest injuries (including rib fractures, flail chest, and penetrating chest wounds), abdominal injuries, and injuries to the genitalia
- Carry out basic dressing and bandaging techniques
- Detect and care for painful, swollen, deformed extremities, including possible fractures, dislocations, sprains, and strains, using soft splints and/or commercial and noncommercial rigid splints
- Detect and care for possible injuries to the cranium and face (skull)
- Detect and care for possible injuries to the neck and spine
- Detect and care for possible heart attacks, strokes, congestive heart failure, seizures, and emergencies related to diabetes
- Care for cases of poisoning
- Classify and provide care for burns
- Detect and care for smoke inhalation
- Detect and care for heat and cold emergencies, including possible heat exhaustion, heat stroke, heat cramps, frostnip, frostbite, freezing, and hypothermia
- Assist a mother in delivering her baby
- Provide initial care for the newborn
- Detect and care for drug abuse and alcohol abuse patients
- Perform nonemergency and emergency patient moves when required
- Perform triage at a multiple-patient emergency scene
- Work under the direction of EMTs to help them provide patient care, doing what you have been trained to do

In some systems that have very special needs, all or any of the following may be required:
- Provide for the patient's airway
- Determine blood pressure
- Use a bag-valve-mask resuscitator (ventilator)
- Deliver oxygen when appropriate, modifying techniques when the patient has a chronic obstructive pulmonary disease (COPD)
- Apply or assist in the application of a traction splint
- Apply or assist in the application of a rigid cervical or extrication collar
- Assist in securing a patient to a long spine board or other device used to immobilize the patient's spine

*E*QUIPMENT, TOOLS, AND SUPPLIES

Most First Responders carry very little in the way of equipment, tools, and supplies. Even if you are provided with an emergency care kit, you may find yourself providing care when you do not have the kit. The typical First Responder course includes how to use items found at the emergency scene and how to make items for emergency use.

The DOT has recommended that First Responders know how to use, and have available whenever possible, the following items (Figure 1.5):

- Triangular bandages
- Roller-type bandages
- Universal dressings/gauze pads
- Occlusive dressings (for airtight seals)

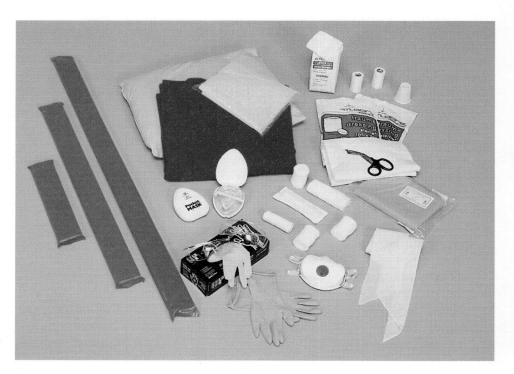

FIGURE 1.5
Emergency medical care equipment and supplies.

- Adhesive tape
- Bandage shears
- Eye protector (paper cup or cone)
- Stick (for tourniquet)
- Blanket and pillow
- Upper and lower extremity splint sets

In some localities, First Responders are expected to take blood pressure. In these areas, the kit would include a blood pressure cuff and stethoscope. A few areas of the country have First Responders provide oxygen and/or suction the patient's mouth and nose when appropriate. The First Responders in these areas are provided with oxygen delivery systems. In some cases, they also carry suctioning devices.

Equipment and supplies for personal protection should be carried to help protect the rescuer from disease-causing agents (contagious diseases). Typically, the First Responder should have:

- Latex or vinyl gloves
- Eye protection (goggles or face shields)
- Masks and barrier devices for ventilating patients, including high efficiency particulate air (HEPA) masks and respirators (see Chapters 2 and 6).
- Gowns

You may be required to know how to use or make and use other items because you may have to improvise. Your instructor may add to the above list, including those items needed for personal safety (see Chapter 2).

The DOT has suggested that all First Responders should be able to use the following tools and equipment for gaining access to patients. Your course may include other items.

- Jack and jack handle
- Pliers, screwdriver, hammer, and knife
- Rope

Summary

The **Emergency Medical Services (EMS) system** is a chain of human services established to provide care to the patient at the scene and during transport to the hospital emergency department. There are four levels of EMS training: First Responder, EMT-Basic, EMT-Intermediate, and EMT-Paramedic.

Each EMS system has a Medical Director, a physician who assumes the ultimate responsibility for **medical direction,** or oversight of the patient care aspects of the EMS system. Medical direction can be **off-line** (including protocols established by the Medical Director that authorize rescuers to perform particular skills in certain situations without actually speaking to the Medical Director) or **on-line** (radio or phone contact with the on-duty physician prior to performing a skill or administering care).

The weakest link in the EMS chain is the care provided by untrained individuals who arrive before the EMTs. It is believed that First Responders will help solve this problem.

First Responders are an important part of the EMS system and are usually the first trained personnel to arrive at the emergency scene. The EMS system's primary goal is personal safety, which must begin with that of the care providers themselves. Patient assessment and care cannot begin unless the scene and the rescuers are safe.

First Responders' four main duties are gaining access to the patient, finding out what is wrong with the patient and providing emergency care, moving patients (when necessary), and transferring the patient and patient information when more highly trained personnel arrive at the scene. Encompassed in these are responsibilities such as controlling the scene, calling the EMS system dispatcher, obtaining help from bystanders, and assisting more highly trained personnel upon their arrival.

First Responder emergency care deals with both injury and illness. Care can range from emotional support to basic life support measures. First Responders have to maintain skills, keep up-to-date, and deal with people. They must also know what they should and should not say to patients and their families. Performing as professionals is important for First Responders.

Remember and Consider...

The decision to become a First Responder is an important one. Full consideration should be given to all aspects before taking this step. Once you have decided, however, you will find it to be very rewarding.

✓ Remember the components of the EMS system and the level of care each can perform. When you turn over care of a patient to another member of the EMS system, be sure he or she is certified and able to provide adequate care for that patient. If someone tells you he or she is an EMT-B, you have the right, even the responsibility, to request proof of certification if the person is unknown to you.

✓ Keep the roles and responsibilities as well as the traits of the First Responder in mind. Go over a mental checklist occasionally to make sure you are maintaining the necessary level of competency.

✓ Think about the qualities you would like to see in a First Responder who renders care to you or your loved ones. Do you have those qualities? If not, think about how you can come closer to being that kind of First Responder. If possible, talk to someone who is a First Responder or EMT to get additional insight.

Investigate...

✓ Determine the locations of medical facilities in your area and the level of care they are able to make available. Also find out where specialty centers are located and how patients are transported to them if they are not in the immediate area.

✓ Learn what you must do to refresh your knowledge and maintain your certification. Find and attend continuing education classes whenever possible.

✓ Investigate the specific statutes and regulations in your state regarding the EMS system.

CHAPTER 2

THE WELL-BEING OF THE FIRST RESPONDER

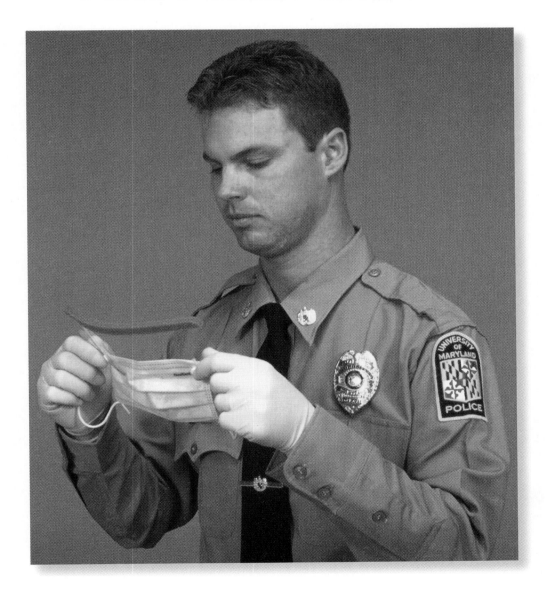

Learning how to take care of yourself in emergency situations is critical. If you do not take care of your own safety first, you will likely become a part of the problem, further stressing the EMS system. First Responders face challenges—emotional and physical—when acting as part of the EMS team. Knowing about these dangers beforehand can help prepare you to handle them when they arise. This chapter helps you to learn what to expect and describes how you can assist yourself, the patient, the patient's family, your own family, and other First Responders in dealing with stress. Aspects of personal safety, including how you can protect yourself from infectious diseases, are presented.

National Standard Objectives

This chapter focuses on the objectives of Module 1, Lesson 1–2 of the U.S. DOT First Responder National Standard Curriculum and serves as an instructional aid to help you meet any specific objectives added to the course by your local EMS system.

By the end of this chapter, you will know how to: (from cognitive or knowledge information) . . .

1–2.1 List possible emotional reactions that the First Responder may experience when faced with trauma, illness, death, and dying. (pp. 18–19)

1–2.2 Discuss the possible reactions that a family member may exhibit when confronted with death and dying. (pp. 18–19)

1–2.3 State the steps in the First Responder's approach to the family confronted with death and dying. (p. 19)

1–2.4 State the possible reactions that the family of the First Responder may exhibit. (p. 19)

1–2.5 Recognize the signs and symptoms of critical incident stress. (pp. 19–20))

1–2.6 State possible steps that the First Responder may take to help reduce/alleviate stress. (pp. 19–21)

1–2.7 Explain the need to determine scene safety. (pp. 27–28)

1–2.8 Discuss the importance of body substance isolation (BSI). (pp. 21–22)

1–2.9 Describe the steps the First Responder should take for personal protection from airborne and bloodborne pathogens. (pp. 22–27)

1–2.10 List the personal protective equipment necessary for each of the following situations: (pp. 22–28; Appendix 4)

- Hazardous materials
- Rescue operations
- Violent scenes
- Crime scenes
- Electricity
- Water and ice
- Exposure to bloodborne pathogens
- Exposure to airborne pathogens

LEARNING TASKS

Many states have a crisis intervention team in place to help prehospital care providers, in-hospital care providers, and police agencies deal with stress from a difficult emergency. These teams can be critical in assisting emergency workers to be able to return to providing services. Talk with your agency and find out about crisis intervention resources. Be able to:

✓ Identify the crisis intervention team in your state and determine how to access its services.

Feel comfortable enough to (by changing attitudes, values, and beliefs) . . .	**1–2.11**	Explain the importance for serving as an advocate for the use of appropriate protective equipment. (pp. 26–27)
	1–2.12	Explain the importance of understanding the response to death and dying and communicating effectively with the patient's family. (pp. 18–19)
	1–2.13	Demonstrate a caring attitude toward any patient with illness or injury who requests emergency medical services. (pp. 19, 27)
	1–2.14	Show compassion when caring for the physical and mental needs of patients. (pp. 18, 19, 27)
	1–2.15	Participate willingly in the care of all patients. (pp. 18, 19, 27)
	1–2.16	Communicate with empathy to patients being cared for, as well as with family members and friends of the patient. (pp. 18, 19)
Show how to (through psychomotor skills) . . .	**1–2.17**	Given a scenario with potential infectious exposure, the First Responder will use appropriate personal protective equipment. At the completion of the scenario, the First Responder will properly remove and discard the protective garments. (pp. 21–24)
	1–2.18	Given the above scenario, the First Responder will complete disinfection/cleaning and all reporting documentation. (pp. 23–27)

Protecting yourself and your patients from infectious diseases is very important. You must wear protective equipment when responding to emergencies, and you should use special disinfectants to clean equipment. As a First Responder, you must be able to:

✓ Put on all personal protective equipment and use it in appropriate situations.

✓ Take off and appropriately discard or dispose of all personal protective equipment.

✓ Disinfect or clean all equipment used in patient care that is not disposable.

✓ Dispose of all disposable equipment used in patient care.

One of your most important jobs is to stay safe, both physically and emotionally. If you become a victim, you will be of little or no use to a patient, and you may actually put other rescuers in danger as well. Safeguard yourself by doing the following:

✓ Learn about stressors and understand how to deal with them, especially those that accompany critical incidents.
✓ Ensure scene safety always.
✓ Before treating a patient, always use universal precautions (gloves—minimum; mask, goggles, gown—as necessary).

EMOTIONAL ASPECTS OF EMERGENCY MEDICAL CARE

CAUSES OF STRESS

Emergencies are stressful. While most emergencies will be considered "routine," some have a potential for causing excess stress on EMS providers. Some stressful situations are:

- *Mass casualties*—A mass casualty is a single incident that involves multiple patients. Such an incident can range from a motor vehicle accident in which two drivers and a passenger are injured to a hurricane that causes the injury of hundreds of people.
- *Pediatric patients*—Emergencies involving infants or children are considered some of the most stressful that health-care providers are required to handle. They may range from simple injuries to serious trauma to sudden infant death syndrome (SIDS).
- *Death*—It is sometimes difficult for a health-care provider to deal with the death of a patient, but even more so if the patient is young or known to the provider.
- *Violence*—Not only is it difficult for the First Responder to witness violence against others, it is also a dangerous situation for the First Responder. It is important to take steps to protect yourself when responding to a violent situation.
- *Abuse and neglect*—Cases of abuse and neglect occur in all social and economic levels of society. You may be called upon to treat infant, child, adult, or elderly victims.
- *Death or injury of a coworker*—Bonds are formed between members of emergency medical services. The death or injury of another provider, even if you do not personally know that person, can cause a stress response.

Remember that as a First Responder, you will experience personal stress and also encounter patients and bystanders who are in stressful situations.

DEATH AND DYING

As a First Responder, you will at some time have to deal with patients who are suffering from terminal illnesses. Patients, and their families, will have many different reactions to these terminal illnesses. A basic understanding of what they are going through will help you to deal with both their stress and your own.

When a patient finds out that he is dying, he will go through several stages, each varying in duration and magnitude. Sometimes these stages will not be in the same order, and sometimes they will overlap each other. Whatever the length or order of these stages, they all affect both the patient and his or her family. The stages include the following:

- *Denial, or "not me"*—The patient denies that he is dying and puts off having to deal with the situation.
- *Anger, or "why me?"*—The patient is angry with the situation. This anger is often vented upon family members or even EMS personnel.
- *Bargaining, or "OK, but first let me . . . "*—The patient feels that making bargains will postpone the inevitable.
- *Depression, or "OK, but I haven't . . . "*—The patient becomes sad and depressed and often mourns things that he has not accomplished. He then usually retreats into his own little world and becomes unwilling to communicate with others.
- *Acceptance, or "OK, I'm not afraid"*—The patient works through all the stages and finally is able to accept death, even though he may not welcome it. Frequently the patient will reach this stage before family members do, in which case he may find himself comforting them.

First Responders may also encounter sudden, unexpected death, in which case family members are likely to react with a wide range of emotions.

You may use several approaches when dealing with a patient or family members who are confronted with death or dying. Most patients just want someone to listen to them as they express their feelings. First Responders may simply offer these patients the following courtesies:

- *Recognize the patients' needs.* Treat them with respect and do whatever is possible to preserve their dignity and sense of control. Speak directly to the patients and avoid talking about them to family members or friends in their presence. Try to respond to their choices about how to handle the situation. Allow patients to talk about their feelings, although it may make you feel uncomfortable, but respect their privacy if they do not want to express personal feelings.
- *Be tolerant of angry reactions from the patients or family members.* Sometimes they will direct their anger at you, but do not take it personally. The patient and family need a chance to vent, and they will often choose whoever is there as a target.
- *Listen empathetically.* Try to understand the feelings of the patient or family member. There is seldom anything you can do to "fix" the situation, but sometimes just listening is very helpful.
- *Do not give false hope or reassurance.* Avoid saying things like "everything will be all right" or "there must be some good reason for this to happen." The family knows things will not be all right, and they do not want to try to justify what is happening. A simple "I'm sorry" is sufficient.
- Offer comfort. Let both the patient and the family know that you will do everything you can to help or that you will help them to find assistance from other sources if needed. Remember, a gentle tone of voice and possibly a reassuring touch can be very helpful.

*S*IGNS AND SYMPTOMS OF STRESS

The way you handle stress can affect both your emotional health and the way you respond to emergencies, so it is important to recognize the signs and symptoms of stress when they appear. These signs and symptoms include irritability with family, friends, and coworkers; inability to concentrate; changes in daily activities, such as difficulty sleeping or nightmares, loss of appetite, and loss of interest in sexual activity; anxiety; indecisiveness; guilt; isolation; and loss of interest in work or poor performance. In addition, you might experience constipation, diarrhea, headache, nausea, and hypertension.

DEALING WITH STRESS

Stress may be caused by a single event, or it may result from the combined effects of several incidents. It is important to remember that any incident may cause different reactions in different health-care providers.

Stress may also be caused from a combination of factors, including personal problems, such as friends and family members who just do not understand the job. It is frequently necessary for health-care providers to work on holidays, weekends, and during important family events. This is often frustrating to these friends and family members, which may cause stress in the provider. It can also be difficult when family and friends do not understand the strong emotions that may be caused by responding to a serious incident.

There are several ways in which a First Responder can deal with stress. It is often difficult to make changes in the habits or lifestyles you have developed, but it is essential to consider the effects that current conditions are having on your well-being. Remember that your health and well-being are of primary importance. Look carefully at your life habits and consider making adjustments.

Lifestyle Changes

First | There are several ways you can change your lifestyle when trying to deal with stress. They include the following (see also Appendix 4):

- Develop more healthful and positive dietary habits. Avoid fatty foods and increase your carbohydrate intake. Also reduce your consumption of alcohol, sugar, and caffeine, which can negatively affect sleep patterns and cause irritability.
- Exercise. Properly performed exercise helps to "burn off" stress. It also can help you to deal with the physical aspects of your responsibilities such as carrying equipment and performing other physically demanding emergency procedures.
- Devote time to relaxing. Consider trying relaxation techniques, which include deep-breathing exercises and meditation.
- If possible, request a change in your work environment or shifts, allowing more time to relax with family or friends or ask for a rotation to a less stressful assignment for a brief time.
- Seek professional help from a mental health professional, a social worker, or a member of the clergy.

Critical Incident Stress Debriefing (CISD)

critical incident stress debriefing (CISD) process in which teams of professional and peer counselors provide emotional and psychological support to EMS personnel who are or have been involved in a critical (highly stressful) incident.

First | A **critical incident stress debriefing (CISD)** is a process in which teams of trained peer counselors and mental health professionals meet with rescuers and health-care providers who have been involved in a major incident. These meetings are usually held within 24 to 72 hours after the incident, and the goal is to assist the providers in dealing with the stress related to that incident (Figure 2.1).

Participation in a CISD is strictly voluntary. No one should ever be forced or coerced to attend. Participants are encouraged to talk about their fears or their reactions to the incident. This is NOT a critique, and all participants should be made aware that whatever is said during this debriefing will be held in the strictest confidence, both by the participants themselves and the debriefing team.

These debriefings are usually very helpful in assisting the emergency services team members to better understand their reactions and feelings both during and after the incident. They usually also come to understand that other members of the team were very likely experiencing similar reactions.

After the open discussion, during which everyone is encouraged to share but not forced to do so, the CISD teams offer suggestions on how to deal with and prevent further stress. It is important to realize that stress after a major incident is both normal and to be expected. The CISD process can be very helpful in speeding up the recovery process.

Your instructor will inform you of situations in which CISD should be requested and how to access the local system.

BODY SUBSTANCE ISOLATION (BSI)

FIRST RESPONDERS AT RISK

First | Because First Responders deal with medical emergencies and unpredictable situations, they need to protect themselves against exposure to infectious diseases. In order to protect themselves, they need to take **body substance isolation (BSI)** precautions, which are a form of infection control based on the presumption that all body fluids are infectious. BSI calls for always using appropriate barriers to infection at the emergency scene, such as gloves, masks, gowns, and protective eyewear.

Consider the following situations:

1. A police officer puts handcuffs on a suspect who has a minor laceration on his hand.

2. A firefighter finds his leather gloves soaked with blood after extricating a patient from a wrecked car.

> **WARNING:**
> Liquid or droplet exposure to skin, hair, gloves, clothing, and equipment requires seeking recommendations from medical direction as to how to proceed. Washing with soap may not be enough. Contact with any unknown microbe or a potential pathogen may require being seen by a physician.

body substance isolation (BSI) a form of infection control based on the presumption that all body fluids are infectious.

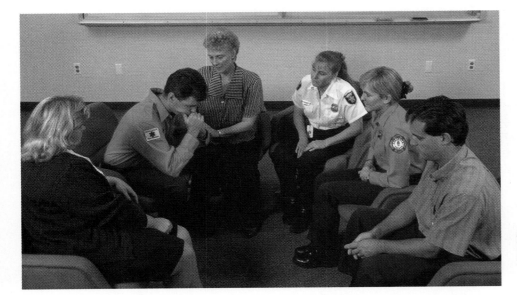

FIGURE 2.1
First Responders at a critical incident stress debriefing.

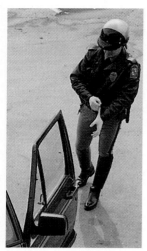

FIGURE 2.2
Law enforcement officers need to take precautions when dealing with injured individuals in unknown situations.

3. A corrections officer touches dried blood in a prison cell.

4. A sheriff's deputy is searching the front seat of a suspect's car and is stuck by a needle that a suspect dropped the night before.

5. A firefighter checking the equipment on his truck handles a tool covered with blood from an earlier call.

6. The firefighters who arrive first at the shopping center to care for a patient who has suddenly become ill are exposed to the patient's heavy coughing spells.

In each situation, the First Responder may be at risk of exposure to an infectious disease. What BSI precautions could be taken in each case?

1. At the start of each shift, the police officer should check his hands for breaks in the skin and cover areas that are not intact (Figure 2.2). If his hands come into contact with blood or other body fluids, he should promptly wash them with soap and water or a commercially produced antiseptic hand cleanser.

2. Similarly, the firefighter should check his hands for broken skin before each shift. He can wear latex gloves under the leather gloves, but not in an actual fire situation (Figure 2.3). In either case, he should promptly wash his hands with soap and water. The blood-soaked gloves should be placed in a designated container, then decontaminated or disposed of according to OSHA (the U.S. Occupational Safety and Health Administration) guidelines.

3. The corrections officer should be trained to recognize that even dried blood is potentially infectious, and she should wash her hands with soap and water.

4. The sheriff's deputy should use a flashlight, mirror, or a probe to search the car and don protective gloves before putting her hand where she cannot see (Figure 2.4).

5. Fire crews should carefully clean all equipment after each run; the firefighter could wear latex gloves while carrying out the check of EMS-related gear.

6. First response crews should wear gloves, masks, and eye protection when working on any patient who is bleeding or spraying airborne droplets to protect against both bloodborne and airborne pathogens.

These are just a few of the many situations that could put First Responders at risk of exposure to infectious diseases. OSHA points out that "emergency responders frequently face unpredictable, uncontrollable, dangerous, and life-threatening circumstances. Anything can happen in an emergency." Making an arrest, helping a heart-attack victim, carrying a child from a burning building, stopping a brawl, helping deliver a baby—each situation has the potential to expose a First Responder to infectious diseases.

In emergency situations, First Responders need to use good judgment and follow OSHA and department procedures. In the next section, you will learn about the four diseases of most concern to First Responders and how employers and employees can minimize the risk of exposure to these diseases.

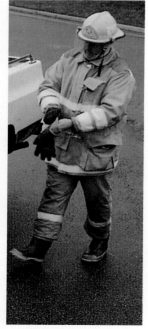

FIGURE 2.3
In nonfire situations involving injuries, firefighters should use latex gloves under their leather gloves.

DEALING WITH RISK

First Responders are familiar with handling risk. Yet some emergency personnel worry more about getting AIDS than they do about going into a burning building.

The fact is that the disease feared most—AIDS—is the one a First Responder is least likely to get. As an emergency worker, your chances of being infected with HIV, the virus that causes AIDS, are very slight, even if you come in direct contact with infected blood or body fluids. The First Responder is at a much greater risk of contracting hepatitis B (HBV). An estimated 250 health-care workers die each year from HBV or its complications, more than from any other infectious disease.

Regardless of the risk of infection, all EMS personnel must follow the rules for their own safety and the safety of others. Keep in mind that an organism that can cause disease may not always do so and that it may affect different people in different ways. An organism that you transfer from one patient to another may cause disease in the second patient, but not the first. In other words, the way disease is spread and develops is a subject that is so complicated that its study is a specialty unto itself. Do not guess at which precautions are necessary or assume that you can easily determine on your own how to prevent disease. We are about to present a very specific set of rules on *personal protection*. You have entered this course prepared to help care for illness and injury. You can begin by not becoming a patient at the scene and by not spreading infections.

Infections are caused by organisms such as viruses (which cause illnesses such as colds, flu, HIV, and hepatitis) and bacteria (which cause sore throats, food poisoning, rheumatic fever, gonorrhea, Legionnaire's disease, and tuberculosis [TB] to name a few). There are both viral and bacterial forms of pneumonia and meningitis. These organisms are also called **pathogens.** The term *pathogen* means to generate suffering (patho-, suffering; -gen, create or form). Pathogens are spread by exposure to body fluids such as blood and semen and exposure to airborne droplets such as those that come from coughing, sneezing, spitting, or even breathing close to someone's face.

First Responders should learn about infectious diseases in order to prevent the spread of both disease and misinformation. Misplaced fears, especially about AIDS, can make First Responders careless about other dangers. Knowledge is the best protection.

Infectious diseases are a real danger to First Responders; however, if you learn and follow safety procedures and use the personal protective equipment (PPE) provided by your agency, the risks can be minimized.

First | OSHA has issued strict guidelines about the precautions to take to reduce exposure to infectious disease. You can transmit pathogens to the patient and the patient can transmit them to you unless you use **personal protective equipment (PPE)** (Figures 2.5 and 2.6):

- *Gloves*—latex, vinyl, or other synthetic. Inspect your hands before donning and cover any broken skin. Don (put on) your gloves before contact with the patient. Put on a second pair of gloves (double glove) if you are working around sharp objects such as broken glass and metal edges at an accident scene. If the outer gloves are torn, the gloves underneath still provide a layer of protection. Change between patients and always wash hands after use. OSHA has stated that handwashing is one of the most important steps to take for infection control.
- *Face shields or masks*—for blood or fluid splatter, wear surgical-type masks; for fine particles of airborne droplets (coughing), wear a high-efficiency particulate air (HEPA) mask (Figure 2.7); a surgical-type mask may be placed on the patient as well if he or she is alert and cooperates (monitor respirations).
- *Eye protection*—the mucous membranes of your eyes can absorb fluids and are a route for infection. Use eyewear that protects from both the front and sides.

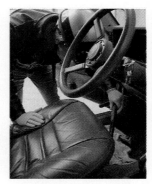

FIGURE 2.4
To avoid an accidental needle stick or other injury, a police officer can use a probe to search beneath a car seat.

pathogens the organisms that cause infection, such as viruses and bacteria.

personal protective equipment (PPE) equipment such as eyewear, mask, gloves, gown, or turnout gear or helmet that protect the EMS worker from infection and/or from exposure to hazardous materials and the dangers of rescue operations.

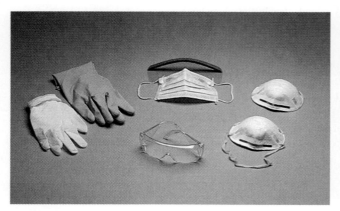

FIGURE 2.5
Personal protective equipment (PPE).

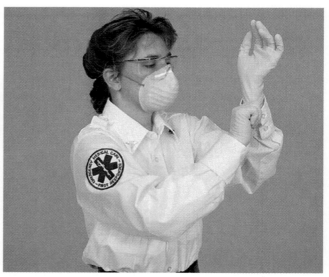

FIGURE 2.6
Always wear the appropriate personal protective equipment (PPE) to prevent exposure to infectious diseases.

■ *Gowns*—protect clothing and bare skin when there is arterial or spurting bleeding, childbirth, or multiple injuries with heavy bleeding.
Dispose of all used personal protective equipment (PPE) appropriately. Do not leave personal protective equipment (PPE) lying around the scene.

Since you cannot tell if patients have infectious diseases just by looking at them and you do not know you are carrying a pathogen until you begin to see the signs and feel the symptoms, it is important to wear personal protective equipment (PPE) for all patient contact situations. This includes wearing gloves at all times plus face shields and eye protection whenever you may be exposed to splattering fluids or airborne droplets. This protection builds a barrier between you and the patient.

ℬLOODBORNE AND AIRBORNE PATHOGENS

Infectious diseases range from such generally mild conditions as influenza to life-threatening diseases like tuberculosis. The four diseases of most concern to First Responders are HIV, hepatitis, tuberculosis, and meningitis (Table 2–1).

HIV, or human immunodeficiency virus, is the pathogen that causes AIDS. As yet, there is no cure for HIV, but there are newly developed medications that help reduce the patient's symptoms. New medical developments, however, should not prevent a First Responder from using personal protective equipment while caring for every patient.

First Responders should keep in mind several facts about HIV. First, HIV does not survive well outside the body. It also is not as concentrated in body fluids as the hepatitis B virus (HBV). As a result, HIV is much more difficult to transmit than HBV. The routes of exposure are limited to direct contact with unintact (open) skin or mucous membranes and with blood, semen, or other body fluids. Thus, it is very unlikely that a rescuer taking BSI precautions will get the disease on the job. Even accidental needlesticks transmit the disease in fewer than 1% of cases, according to OSHA.

In contrast to HIV, hepatitis B (HBV) is a very tough virus. It can survive on clothing, newspaper, or other objects days after infected blood has dried. First Responders should recognize that even dried body fluids are potentially

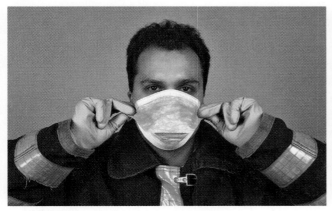

FIGURE 2.7A
High-efficiency particulate air
(HEPA) mask.

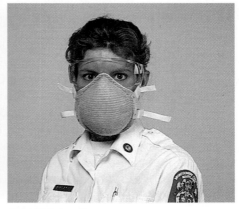

FIGURE 2.7B
Wear a HEPA mask when you suspect
a patient may have tuberculosis (TB).

infectious and that they should take the appropriate measures to prevent contact. HBV causes permanent liver damage in many cases and can be fatal. Several other forms of the disease, including hepatitis C and non-A and non-B hepatitis, are less common than HBV but still present a risk to First Responders.

Tuberculosis (TB), a lung infection, can also be fatal. Thought to have been nearly eradicated as recently as 1985, TB has had a recent resurgence. Even worse, new strains of the disease are resistant to treatment with traditional medication. Unlike HIV and HBV, TB is spread by aerosolized droplets in the air, usually the result of coughing and sneezing. Thus, TB can be contracted even without direct physical contact with a carrier. Use of one-way air masks for rescue breathing and HEPA (high-efficiency particulate air) masks when TB is suspected greatly reduces the risk of exposure to this airborne disease.

Meningitis, an inflammation of the lining of the brain and spinal cord, is also a serious disease, especially for children. The most infectious varieties of meningitis are caused by bacteria. Meningitis is transmitted by respiratory droplets, like TB, but is far easier to contract. The disease may have a rapid onset (several hours to a few days) and needs quick treatment with antibiotics. First Responders should make sure that EMS and hospital staffs inform them if they have been in contact with a patient infected with meningitis or a scene that may be contaminated with the organism that causes the disease. Antibiotics taken after exposure to bacterial meningitis may prevent acquiring the disease.

TABLE 2-1: *D*ISEASES OF CONCERN TO FIRST RESPONDERS

DISEASE	HOW TRANSMITTED	VACCINE
AIDS/HIV (Acquired Immune Deficiency Syndrome)	Needlesticks, blood splash on mucous membranes (eye, mouth), or blood contact with open skin	No
Hepatitis B Virus (HBV)	Needlesticks, blood splash on mucous membranes (eye, mouth), or blood contact with open skin; some risk during mouth-to-mouth CPR	Yes
Tuberculosis (TB)	Airborne aerosolized droplets	No
Meningitis	Respiratory secretions or saliva	Yes, for one strain

(Table shows routes of transmission in emergency situations—other means of transmission are possible.) Adapted from *U.S. Fire Administration Guide to Developing and Managing an Emergency Service Infection Control Program.*

PROTECTING FIRST RESPONDERS

Today, governments at the local, state, and federal levels are taking steps to protect First Responders from exposure to infectious diseases. Several years ago, the Centers for Disease Control and Prevention (CDC) called for workers to practice universal precautions with certain body fluids that were considered infectious. Now the stricter BSI standard is recommended. BSI assumes that all body fluids are potentially hazardous and treats all patients with the same precautions. This is very important, since the vast majority of HIV-infected individuals are unaware of their status. The main point of BSI precautions is that First Responders should approach all patients as if they carried an infectious disease.

In 1992, OSHA issued guidelines for employers whose workers run a risk of occupational exposure to bloodborne diseases. All such agencies are required to implement plans to meet the OSHA standards.

The following list summarizes the main features of an OSHA-mandated infectious disease program.

1. Provide a free hepatitis B vaccination—a safe, routine procedure that protects against HBV infection.

2. Educate employees about bloodborne diseases and train employees in safe work practices, including use of personal protective equipment. Training should include questions and answers about individual work sites, hands-on practice with protective gear, and information on reporting exposures.

3. Establish safe workplace procedures, including appropriate personal protective equipment, changes of uniform, and safe facilities for cleaning or disposing of contaminated gear (sometimes through local hospitals).

4. Supply personal protective equipment such as gloves, gowns, masks, eyeshields of the correct fit, and resuscitation equipment and pocket masks with one-way valves.

5. Set up engineering controls, such as special containers for needles, alternative handwashing when soap and water are unavailable, and labels for containers with contaminated items.

6. Provide an equipment cleaning site separate from food preparation areas where contaminated tools, handcuffs, and so on can be cleaned.

7. Ensure proper waste disposal according to local regulations, so that used latex gloves and dressings are not left at emergency scenes or around agency facilities.

8. Implement postexposure follow-up to determine the significance of an exposure incident, document the event, and test the employee.

This outline of exposure-control procedures is not comprehensive. Actual programs vary by state, jurisdiction, and agency. Your employer is required to make infection-control procedures a part of job training. Do not hesitate to suggest changes or improvements that you feel are necessary.

Your instructor will show you how to properly put on, or don, and use your protective equipment so that you maintain its sterility or cleanliness where it will contact you or your patient. You will also learn how and where to properly dispose of all used materials, what containers are for soiled linens, and how they are labeled. In addition, it is important that all reusable equipment is cleaned or disinfected with soap and water and/or a bleach solution. You must learn, understand the need for, and practice these infection-control procedures to reduce your risk. These procedures are based on guidelines from OSHA and the Centers for Disease Control and Prevention, and practicing them is a part of your responsibility as a First Responder.

EMPLOYEE RESPONSIBILITIES

An infection-control program will only work if First Responders learn and follow correct procedures. First Responders have an obligation to adhere to safe work practices in order to protect themselves, their families, and the public. Washing hands regularly, using gloves and other personal protective equipment, and making safe work practices a habit are good ways to start. Following infection-control procedures will help you do your job safely. As a First Responder, you may not withhold emergency care from a patient that you think may have an infectious disease. With the proper precautions, however, you can provide emergency care to persons infected with HIV or HBV without putting yourself at risk. To date, there are no known cases of emergency workers contracting HIV or HBV during routine patient care using gloves and appropriate personal protective equipment. First Responders who practice infection control should feel confident that they are not risking their lives.

SCENE SAFETY

Assuring scene safety starts before First Responders actually arrive at the scene. En route to the scene, it is important to get information from dispatch about the incident. The nature of the call, which dispatch can generally describe, helps First Responders to determine what type of body substance isolation and equipment may be needed and what type of approach precautions to take. Dispatchers will not always have complete or accurate details about the incident. Often, those who call in emergencies are excited, nervous, confused, in pain, or hysterical. They may even hang up before they finish giving all the details. First Responders must become familiar with their response areas and the types of calls typical to those areas, so they can be prepared for the expected as well as the unusual and so they can take all precautions.

When approaching the scene, look around for hazards and listen for noises in the area. Is it quiet, and is that normal for this area? Is there yelling, screaming, gunshots, dogs barking? Decide where to place the vehicle: before the scene to provide lighting; beyond it to provide quick and easy supply access and patient loading; on the street to block traffic and protect the scene, or off the street to protect EMS personnel. When deciding where to position the vehicle, consider that placement must provide for access to equipment, efficient loading of the patient, and continued traffic flow where possible or at least rerouting of traffic around the scene. As a part of approaching the scene and deciding where to place the vehicle, you will also be surveying the scene for a variety of hazards that range from inconvenient to critically dangerous.

It is important that you do a scene size-up before approaching the patient to assure the safety of not only the patient and yourself but bystanders as well. There may be hazardous materials, toxic substances, downed power lines and broken poles, or unstable vehicles at the scene. Environmental conditions such as icy and slippery roads, steep grades, rocky terrain, or heavy traffic and a crowd of onlookers must all be considered in your approach and placement of your vehicle and care of your patient. Violent domestic or social situations may involve weapons—not just guns but knives or bats, boards, chains, and other striking items. All of these can be used to harm you as they did the victim. You may also be responding to a crime scene where you *do* want to be aware of the

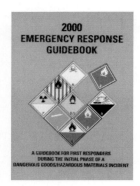

FIGURE 2.8
North American Emergency Response Guidebook.

hazardous materials incident the release of a harmful substance into the environment.

potential for violence, where you *do not* want to approach until it is clear, and where you *do not* want to disturb evidence any more than you must while caring for the patient. Similarly, you may be approaching any type of hazardous or environmentally unsafe scene where you *do* want to be aware of the need for safety precautions, where you *do not* want to approach until it is safe to do so, and where you *do not* want to cause further hazards or harm yourself, the patient, or bystanders and onlookers who are merely curious about the scene events or who are trying to help you. When necessary, notify dispatch that you need assistance for crowd control and police officers for protection and scene security.

Keeping yourself safe is your first responsibility. Once you can assure your own safety, approach and take care of the patient. Following are specific types of unsafe incidents where First Responders must take special precautions.

HAZARDOUS MATERIALS INCIDENTS

Some chemicals can cause death or health complications, even if you only briefly come into contact with them or inhale them. Some of these types of dangerous chemicals are being transported by truck or rail, and some may be stored in warehouses or used in local industries. If there is an accident in which transported chemicals are spilled or if stored containers begin to leak, the spilled chemicals are likely to be considered a hazard to the community and to responding EMS personnel.

First Responders should maintain a safe distance from the source of the hazard and treat it as a **hazardous materials incident.** Placards may help with identifying materials in motor vehicle accidents. These placards use coded colors and identification numbers that are listed in the *North American Emergency Response Guidebook* (Figure 2.8) published by the U.S. Department of Transportation (DOT). This book should be placed in every emergency response vehicle. It can provide important information about a hazardous substance, as well as information on safe distances, emergency care, and suggested procedures in the event of spills or fire.

It is always wise to carry a pair of binoculars in your vehicle. This way, you can identify hazardous materials placards from a safe distance, thus ensuring your own safety.

As a First Responder, your most important duty in a hazardous materials incident is to recognize potential problems and take action to preserve your own safety and that of others. (See Chapter 15 for a lengthier discussion of the First Responder's responsibilities at a hazardous materials incident.) You should also make sure an appropriately trained hazardous materials response team is notified. These teams have special training and equipment to handle these incidents, so it is important that you not take any action other than protecting yourself, patients, and bystanders at the scene. An inappropriate action could cause a larger problem than the already existing one.

Many emergency response departments require hazardous materials training at the awareness level. Your instructor can inform you of the requirements in your area.

RESCUE OPERATIONS

First Responders may be first on the scene or be assisting with motor vehicle crashes ranging from fender benders to major incidents involving several vehicles, which often cause dangers to the patient as well as the rescuer. Rescue scenes may include dangers from electricity, fire, explosion, hazardous materials, traffic, or water or ice emergencies. It is important to evaluate each situation and request the appropriate department to assist in handling these incidents. You may need the police, fire department, power company, or other specialized personnel. Never perform acts that you are not properly trained to do. Secure the scene to the best of your ability; then wait for the help you have requested to arrive. Remember that whenever you are working at a rescue operation, you must use personal protective equipment that may include turnout gear, protective eyewear, helmet, and puncture-proof gloves as well as latex or vinyl gloves.

VIOLENT AND CRIME SCENES

First Responders may also respond to scenes to assist patients who are victims of violence or crimes. Your first priority, even before patient care, is to be certain the scene is safe. Dangerous persons or pets, people with weapons, intoxicated people, and others may present problems you are not prepared to handle. It is important to recognize these situations and request the necessary help. Wait until help arrives to secure the scene and make it safe for you to perform your duties. Remember that your first consideration is your own safety and personal protection. Always don appropriate personal protective equipment. In some areas, emergency care providers are issued bulletproof vests for their protection.

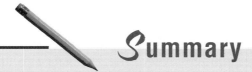

Summary

Safeguarding your well-being is critical. One way to do this is to make lifestyle changes that help to reduce the stress associated with responding to emergency situations.

Many situations put the First Responder at risk of exposure to infectious disease. It is important that the First Responder be familiar with and follow OSHA guidelines for infection control.

Learning about infectious diseases not only helps to reduce their spread but also reduces misinformation and misplaced fears when working with patients. To protect yourself from pathogens, use **personal protective equipment** such as gloves (always), and face shields or masks, eye protection, and gowns where necessary. This protection between you and the patient is called **body substance isolation.** Dispose of personal protective equipment items appropriately.

Four **pathogens** present especially significant risks to First Responders. They are HIV and hepatitis (typically bloodborne) and tuberculosis and meningitis (typically airborne). Do not limit your thinking to just these four, and do not believe that an outbreak must be reported for there to be a danger.

BSI precautions consider that all body fluids are potentially infectious and all patients are treated with the same precautions. This is important since both you and the patient may be carrying a pathogen without knowing it. A summary of the OSHA mandated infectious disease program states that vaccinations, education, and personal protective equipment must be provided for personnel; safe workplace procedures must be established; waste disposal, cleaning sites, and engineering controls must be provided; post-exposure follow-up, documentation, and testing are also important parts of the guidelines.

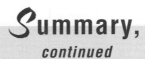

It is the responsibility of the First Responder to learn, understand, and practice these procedures and to provide emergency care to all patients regardless of their real or potential level of infection. Ensure your personal safety by being alert to the potential for danger at every emergency call.

Remember and Consider...

Remember that your safety has to come first. In order for you to help others, you must first take care of yourself. Keep in mind that your emotional safety is also important in order to prevent "burn out," which often causes a loss of personnel to emergency response services.

✔ Think about a network of family or friends who may be able to assist you in handling stress.

✔ Make sure you have the necessary personal protective equipment available whenever you may be responding to an emergency. Use that personal protective equipment every time, on every call. If you do this, you will never have to wonder if your were protected on "that" call.

Investigate...

✔ Learn how to access the CISD in your local area. Be sure your department is aware of CISD availability and knows when to notify CISD counselors.

✔ Practice putting on personal protective equipment and determine what equipment is necessary for different types of emergency responses. Learn how to properly dispose of items after use.

✔ Learn what types of specialized assistance are available in your area and how to establish contact in case of an emergency.

CHAPTER 3

LEGAL AND ETHICAL ISSUES

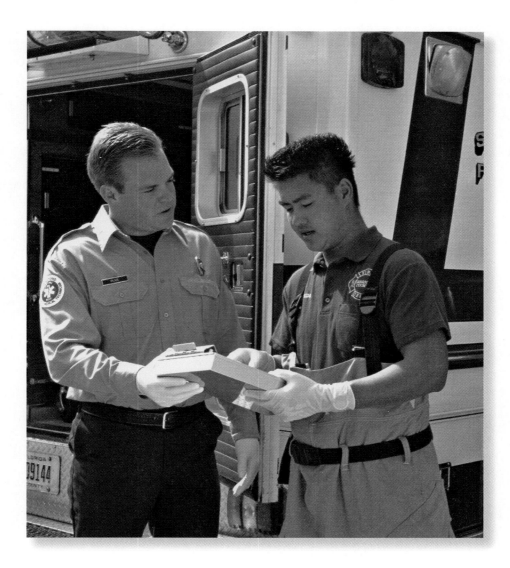

Legal and ethical issues are important to the First Responder. There are decisions that must be made in relation to patient care, and understanding the legalities and ethics of the situation will aid in making these decisions. Should the First Responder stop to aid victims of an automobile crash when off duty? Should the First Responder release patient information to an attorney on the telephone? Can a child with a broken arm be treated, even if a parent is not present? Can a child-care provider give permission for a child to be treated? This chapter provides you with information and guidance that will be of assistance to you when these decisions must be made.

National Standard Objectives

This chapter focuses on the objectives of Module 1, Lesson 1–3 of the U.S. DOT First Responder National Standard Curriculum and serves as an instructional aid to help you meet any specific objectives added to the course by your local EMS system.

By the end of this chapter, you will know how to:
(from cognitive or knowledge information) . . .

1–3.1	Define the First Responder scope of care. (p. 33)
1–3.2	Discuss the importance of Do Not Resuscitate [DNR] (advance directives) and local or state provisions regarding EMS application. (pp. 36–37)
1–3.3	Define consent and discuss the methods of obtaining consent. (pp. 34–36)
1–3.4	Differentiate between expressed and implied consent. (pp. 35–36)
1–3.5	Explain the role of consent of minors in providing care. (pp. 35–36)
1–3.6	Discuss the implications for the First Responder in patient refusal of transport. (pp. 34–35)
1–3.7	Discuss the issues of abandonment, negligence, and battery and their implications to the First Responder. (pp. 34, 37–39)
1–3.8	State the conditions necessary for the First Responder to have a duty to act. (pp. 37–38)
1–3.9	Explain the importance, necessity, and legality of patient confidentiality. (pp. 39–40)
1–3.10	List the actions that a First Responder should take to assist in the preservation of a crime scene. (p. 41)
1–3.11	State the conditions that require a First Responder to notify local law enforcement officials. (pp. 40, 41)
1–3.12	Discuss issues concerning the fundamental components of documentation. (p. 42)

Feel comfortable enough to
(by changing attitudes, values, and beliefs) . . .

1–3.13	Explain the rationale for the needs, benefits, and usage of advance directives. (pp. 36–37)
1–3.14	Explain the rationale for the concept of varying degrees of DNR. (pp. 36–37)

*L*EARNING TASKS

Good Samaritan laws have been developed in most states to protect individuals who help people needing emergency care.

✔ Find out if your state has a Good Samaritan law.

✔ Find out how the Good Samaritan law relates to you when you provide patient care in an emergency situation when you are on duty and when you are off duty.

Do Not Resuscitate (DNR) orders are different for each state. It is necessary for the First Responder to become familiar with the legal DNR orders for his or her region or state and the laws and rules governing their implementation. These situations are always stressful for both the family members and the EMS personnel, and the window of time for making a resuscitation decision is very small.

✔ Become familiar with the forms and policies pertaining to DNR orders in your state.

*S*COPE OF CARE

*L*EGAL DUTIES

First | Most of us have heard about people being sued because they stopped to help someone. Successful suits of this type are not very common. Each state has established guidelines to allow emergency care to be given without the provider having to worry about being sued. These laws require that a certain **standard of care** be provided.

standard of care the care expected based on the provider's training and experience, taking into account the conditions under which the care is rendered.

What is considered to be the standard of care is based on laws, administrative orders, and guidelines published by the EMS system and other emergency care organizations and societies. This standard of care allows you to be judged based on what is expected of someone with your training and experience, working under similar conditions.

Your First Responder course follows guidelines proposed by the U.S. Department of Transportation (DOT) or another authority that has studied what is needed to provide the standard of care required at the First Responder level. You will be trained so that you can provide this standard of care. If the care you provide is not up to this standard, you may be sued and held liable for your actions.

There may also be medical oversight available in your locality. You may be required to communicate with your Medical Director by telephone or radio or there may be approved standing orders or protocols for you to follow.

Keep written notes of what you do at the emergency scene, especially if a crime has occurred. You may be called on to provide this information at a later date. If your EMS system requires you to complete forms, submit reports, or sign patient transfer papers, do so at the proper time. You must be able to show that you provided the standard of care.

ETHICAL RESPONSIBILITIES

There are also ethical responsibilities that the First Responder must be aware of. The primary ethical consideration is to make the physical and emotional needs of the patient a priority. An example would be turning up the heat if the patient feels cold, even if you are feeling overheated. Another ethical responsibility is maintaining your skills and knowledge. This includes practicing until you have obtained confidence and mastery of the skills. You must also attend continuing education and refresher programs. Every patient deserves the best care possible, and it is necessary to keep yourself ready to provide that level of care at all times. It is also important that you be honest in reporting care that was provided to a patient, even if a mistake was made. While all EMS providers should attempt at all times to provide the correct care, mistakes do happen. This should be reported accurately and completely so any corrective procedures necessary may be instituted as soon as possible.

CONSENT

COMPETENCE

Competence is the patient's ability to understand the questions of the First Responder and to understand the implications of decisions made. In order for a First Responder to receive consent or refusal of care, the First Responder should determine competency. The patient is not competent to make medical decisions in certain cases, such as intoxication, drug ingestion, serious injury, or mental incompetence. In order to determine competency, the First Responder may ask questions that a competent adult should be able to answer, such as where the patient is at the time, what season of the year it is, and so on. Answering these questions, however, does not always establish competence, as in suicidal patients.

REFUSAL OF CARE

First Adults, when conscious and competent, have the right to refuse your care (refusal of service). Their reasons may be based on religious grounds. They may base their decision on a lack of trust. In fact, they may have reasons that you find senseless. For whatever reason, competent adults may refuse care. You cannot force care on them, nor can you legally restrain them until EMTs arrive. (You could be charged with assault and battery.) Your only course of action is to try to gain their confidence through conversation. The courts recognize implied refusal of care. In other words, the patient does not have to speak to refuse your care. If the patient shakes his head to signal "no," or if he holds up his hand to signal you to stop, the patient has refused your help. Should the patient pull away from you, this may be viewed as refusal of care.

When your services are refused:
- Do *not* argue with patients.
- Do *not* question their reasons if they are based on religious beliefs.
- Do *not* touch patients. If you do, this could be considered to be assault and battery or a violation of their civil rights.
- Stay calm and professional. Any added stress to patients because of your actions could cause serious complications.

- Make certain that dispatch is alerted, even if patients have stated they do not want anyone's help.
- Talk with the patients. Let them know that you are concerned. Tell them that you respect their right to refuse care, but that you think they should reconsider your offer to help.
- When possible, have a neutral witness to your offer of help, your explanation of your level of training, why you think care is needed, and the patient's refusal to accept your care. If your EMS system provides you with release forms, ask the patient to please read and sign the form. Make certain that you ask patients if they understand what they have read before signing the form. Have a witness to any signing of forms.

A parent or legal guardian can refuse to let you care for a child. If the reason is fear or lack of confidence, simple conversation may change the individual's mind. In cases involving children, if the adult takes the child from the scene before EMTs arrive, you *must* report the incident to the EMTs or to the police. Some states have special laws protecting the welfare of children. In these states, such information may have to be passed on to the courts in order to find out if the child eventually received needed care.

EXPRESSED CONSENT

First | An adult patient of legal age, when conscious and competent, can give you **expressed consent** to provide care. In First Responder care, this consent is usually oral. To qualify as expressed consent, the patient must be making an informed decision (Figure 3.1). You need to tell the patient that you are a First Responder, trained in emergency care.

expressed consent informed consent by a rational adult patient, usually in oral form, to accept emergency care.

You also must tell the patient:
- Your level of training
- Why you think care may be necessary
- What you are going to do
- If there is any risk to the care you offer or risk related to refusing care

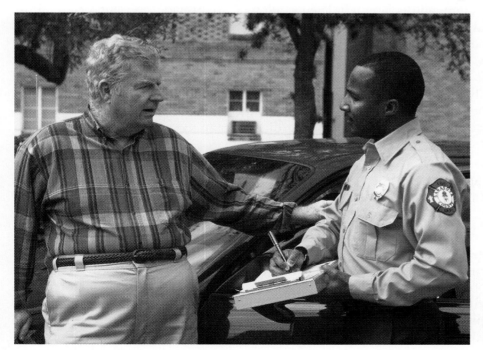

FIGURE 3.1
Obtaining consent from an adult patient.

FIGURE 3.2
Minor's consent.

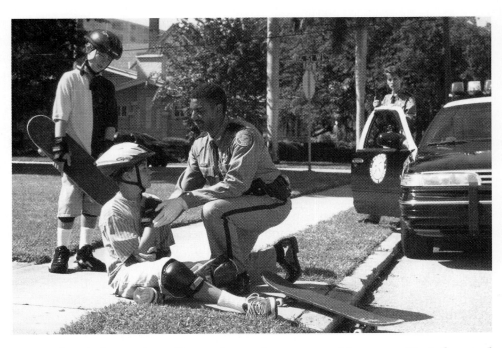

informed consent
expressed consent
given by a rational
adult patient after
being informed of the
provider's training and
what care procedures
are to be done. Risks
and options may have
to be discussed.

implied consent a
legal position that
assumes that an
unconscious or badly
injured adult patient
would consent to
receiving emergency
care. This form of
consent may apply to
other types of patients
(for example, mentally
ill).

minor's consent a
form of implied
consent used when a
minor is seriously ill
or injured and the
parents or guardians
cannot be reached
quickly.

Having this information allows the patient to provide you with **informed consent.**

There are occasions when a child refuses care, but a parent or guardian consents to your providing care. Legally, you have received expressed consent to care for this patient. Of course, gaining the child's confidence and easing any fears should be part of your care.

IMPLIED CONSENT

In emergency situations in which a patient is unconscious, confused, or so severely injured that a clear decision cannot be made, you have the right to provide care based on **implied consent.** The law assumes that the patient, if able to do so, would want to receive care and treatment. Since children and mentally incompetent adults are not legally allowed to provide consent or to refuse medical care, a form of implied consent is used in most states when a minor is involved and the parents or guardians are not on the scene and cannot be reached quickly. The law assumes that they would want care to be provided for their child. This is called **minor's consent** (Figure 3.2). The same holds true in cases of mentally ill persons who are hallucinating or having homicidal or suicidal thoughts or in cases of emotionally disturbed or retarded individuals. It is assumed that their parents, legal guardians, or family would give consent.

DO NOT RESUSCITATE (DNR) ORDERS

First | At some time, you will come upon a patient who has a Do Not Resuscitate (DNR) order. This is a legal document, usually signed by the patient and his or her physician, which states that the patient has a terminal illness and does not wish to prolong life through resuscitative efforts. A DNR order is called an "advance directive" because it is written and signed in advance of any event where resuscitation might be undertaken. It is more than the expressed wishes of the patient or family; it is an actual document. In some cases, the patient will be wearing a DNR bracelet. This should not be mistaken for a Medic Alert bracelet, which gives information about medical conditions and/or allergies.

There are varying degrees of DNR orders, expressed through a variety of detailed instructions that may be part of the order. Such an instruction might stipulate, for example, that resuscitation be attempted only if cardiac or respiratory arrest is observed, but not attempted if the patient is found already in arrest (to avoid the possibility of resuscitating a patient who may already have sustained brain damage). Many states also have laws governing living wills, statements signed by the patient, usually regarding use of long-term life-support and comfort measures such as respirators, intravenous feedings, and pain medications.

If the patient herself refuses care, then becomes unconscious, implied consent usually takes over and care begins. It is a legal and ethical dilemma that is usually best resolved by providing care. It is better to be criticized or sued for saving a life than for letting a patient die. A legal DNR order prevents these unwanted resuscitation efforts and other awkward situations. In most cases, the oral requests of a family member are not reason to withhold care.

*N*EGLIGENCE

First | The basis for most lawsuits involving prehospital emergency care is **negligence.** This is a term often used to indicate either that you did not do what was expected or that you did something carelessly. From a legal standpoint, negligence is a more complicated concept. As a First Responder, you could be sued for negligence if all the following occurred while you were providing care:

- You (the First Responder) had a *duty to provide care* or decided for yourself to assume the responsibility to provide care.
- Care for the patient was not provided to the *standard of care*.
- The patient was injured in some way as a result of this *improper care*.

First Responders in the police and paid fire service have a **duty to act.** This means that they are required, at least while on duty, to provide care according to their department's standard operating procedures. In some localities, this duty to act may also apply to paid First Responders when they are off duty.

The duty to act is not so clear in the case of volunteer First Responders. While on duty, these volunteers also may have a duty to act when at an emergency scene. What is expected when they are off duty is unclear because many states do not have specific laws concerning First Responders. Most laws provide direction for physicians and nurses only, while some legislation deals with allied health specialists and EMTs. Several states are now in the process of considering more specific laws for their EMS systems.

Since the laws governing the duty to act vary from state to state, and what is implied in laws that cover the emergency services also varies, your instructor or local EMS system will tell you the specifics as to when you are required to respond and provide care. Your duties will be spelled out, considering your level of training and your safety at the emergency scene.

A First Responder is part of the EMS system and might be considered to have a duty to act once help is offered to a patient. If care is offered and then accepted by the patient, it could be assumed that the First Responder has

negligence at the First Responder level, negligence usually is a failure to provide the expected standard of care, leading to additional injury of the patient.

duty to act requirement that First Responders in the police and paid fire service, at least while on duty, must provide care according to their department's standard operating procedures.

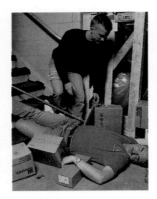

FIGURE 3.3
Duty to Act. Some First Responders have a duty to help victims of an emergency.

accepted a duty to act. A court might decide that this meets the first requirement for negligence in cases where the standard of care was not met and the patient suffered injury due to this improper care (Figure 3.3).

The second condition for negligence would be applicable if the care was substandard for the First Responder's level of training and experience under the conditions of the emergency scene. The same would apply if the care rendered was above the level of training. In either case, the care provided was not the standard of care.

Finally, if the first two points are established, the suit for negligence may be successful if the patient was injured (damaged) in some way due directly to the inappropriate actions of the First Responder. This is a complex legal problem, made more difficult by the fact that the damage can be physical, emotional, or psychological.

Physical damage is the easiest to understand. For example, if a First Responder moved a patient's fractured leg before applying a splint and the standard of care states that the First Responder should have suspected a fracture and splinted the limb, then the First Responder may be negligent if this action worsened the existing injury.

The same case becomes much more involved when the patient claims that the First Responder's inappropriate action caused emotional or psychological problems. The court could decide that the patient has been damaged and establish the third requirement for negligence.

Inappropriate care does not always involve splinting, bandaging, or some other physical skill. If you tell an injured or ill patient that he or she does not need to be seen by EMTs or other more highly trained personnel, you could be negligent if:

- You had a duty to act.
- The patient accepted your care.
- The standard of care stated that you should have alerted or had someone alert the EMS dispatcher and request an EMT response.
- The delay in care caused complications that led to additional injury.

As a general rule, you should always advise the patient to seek treatment by EMTs and to go to the hospital.

First A requirement for the proof of negligence is the failure of the First Responder to provide care to the recognized standard of care. There is no guarantee that you will not be sued, but a successful suit is unlikely if you provide care to this standard.

If your state has a **Good Samaritan law**, you will be granted immunity (protection from civil liability) if you act in good faith to provide care to the level of your training and to the best of your ability. You will be trained to deliver the standard of care expected of First Responders. Your instructor will explain any differences in the laws of your state.

The other factor you must consider is how the Good Samaritan laws of your state affect your immunity if you are a paid provider of emergency care. In some states, special laws apply to paid providers, while the Good Samaritan laws apply only to volunteers. Again, your instructor or local EMS system can provide you with the needed information.

REMEMBER:

A requirement for proof of negligence is the First Responder's failure to provide the recognized standard of care.

good samaritan laws a series of state laws designed to protect certain care providers if they deliver the standard of care in good faith, to the level of their training, and to the best of their abilities.

ABANDONMENT

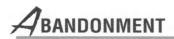

First | Once you stop to help someone who is sick or injured, you have legally begun care. Once care is begun, you have a duty to continue to provide care until you turn over patient care to someone more qualified (EMT, doctor), and you are obligated by the standard of care—that which governs all First Responder actions. If you leave the scene before more highly trained personnel arrive, you have *abandoned* the patient and are subject to legal action under specific laws of **abandonment** (Figure 3.4). Since you are not trained in medical diagnosis or how to predict the stability of a patient, you should not leave the patient if someone with training equal to your own arrives at the scene. The patient may develop more serious problems that would be better handled by two First Responders. Some legal authorities consider abandonment to include the failure to turn over patient information during the transfer of the patient to more highly trained personnel. You must inform these providers of the facts that you gathered, the assessment made, and the care rendered.

abandonment to leave a sick or injured patient before equal or more highly trained personnel can assume responsibility for care.

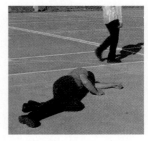

FIGURE 3.4 Abandonment. Once care is initiated, the rescuer assumes responsibility until relieved by equally or more highly trained personnel.

CONFIDENTIALITY

You should not provide care for patients and then speak to your friends, family, and other members of the public (including the press and media) about the details of your care. You should not name the individuals who received your care. If you speak of the accident, you should not relate specifics about what a

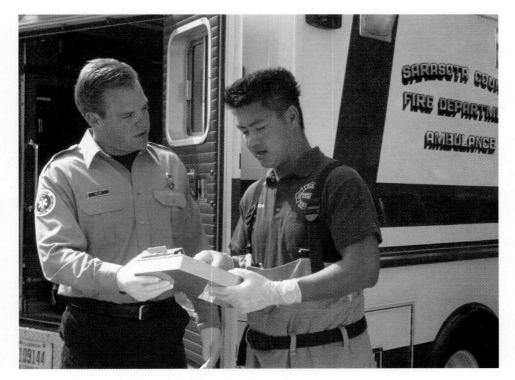

FIGURE 3.5 Maintain patient confidentiality. Discuss care only when turning over the patient to persons providing a higher level of care.

patient may have said, any unusual aspects of behavior, or any descriptions of personal appearance. To do so invades the privacy of the patient. Your state may not have specific laws stating the above, but most individuals in emergency care feel very strongly about protecting the patient's right to privacy, and this information should only be released if the patient has authorized you to do so in writing.

A signed release form is not required for you to pass on information that is pertinent to the care of the patient to EMT-Bs or Paramedics who may arrive to transport and continue care for the patient (Figure 3.5). This pertinent information may also be passed on to emergency department personnel who will be caring for the patient.

REPORTABLE EVENTS

First Responders cannot limit their activities to assessment and care for patients, turn them over to the EMT-Bs and Paramedics, assist in transport and continued care, and deliver the patient to the hospital. Some additional activities are required specific to state guidelines or industrial or military protocols; others are required universally. For example, all First Responders must report certain events or conditions that they know or suspect have occurred. In fact, federal and state agencies require that certain events be reported. These events include exposures to blood and other body fluids and certain infectious diseases, vehicle accidents, drug-related injuries, and crimes that result in knife or gunshot wounds, child and elder abuse, domestic violence, and rape. Check with your chief officer or EMS division or with state and federal agencies to learn which incidents are reportable in your area and to whom or which agency you report these incidents. Crimes, vehicle accidents, and drug injuries are reported to the police; exposures are usually first reported to your employing or volunteer agency.

SPECIAL SITUATIONS

ORGAN DONORS

You may respond to a call where a critically injured patient is near death and is an organ donor. An organ donor is a patient who has completed a legal document that allows for donation of organs and tissues in the event of his or her death. A family member may give you this information, or you may find an organ donor card in the person's personal effects. Sometimes this information is indicated on the patient's drivers license. Ideally, a family member or police officer should go through the person's effects, but you can look for this document without consent of the patient or his or her family.

Emergency care for a patient who is an organ donor must not differ in any way from the care for a patient who is not a donor. All emergency care measures must be taken, including performing CPR on a patient you might not normally resuscitate due to the extent of fatal injuries. The oxygen delivered to body cells by CPR will help preserve the organs until they can be harvested for implantation in another person.

MEDICAL IDENTIFICATION DEVICES

Another special situation involves the patient who wears a medical identification device (Figure 3.6). This device is worn to alert EMS personnel that the patient has a particular medical condition, such as heart conditions, allergies, diabetes, or epilepsy. If the patient is unconscious or unable to answer questions, this device may provide important medical information. The medical identification device may be worn as a necklace, bracelet, or ankle bracelet. It may also be on a card carried by the patient.

CRIME SCENES

A crime scene is defined as the location where a crime has been committed or any place evidence relating to a crime may be found. Many crime scenes involve crimes against people, which may cause injuries that are serious. Once the scene has been made safe by police, providing patient care is a priority.

When the First Responder is providing care at a crime scene, certain actions should be taken to preserve evidence. Make as little impact on the scene as possible, moving only items that prevent patient care. Remember the position of the patient and preserve any clothing you may remove or damage. Try not to cut through holes in clothing from gunshot wounds or stabbing. Remember and report any items you move or touch. If you arrived at the scene before the police, remember if doors were ajar or windows open. These signs indicate danger for you as well. If you have any reason to suspect that the scene is not safe, you should go no farther until police say it is safe to do so.

It is important that EMS personnel and police work together. Sometimes the police may be unfamiliar with EMS procedures and request that you delay patient care so they may take pictures or interview the patient. It does not help if tempers are allowed to flare in situations such as this. Explain to the officers as calmly and quickly as possible that delay may cause serious problems in this case and continue your care. It is not appropriate for either of you to engage in an argument while patient care is being performed. This is best handled after the event, perhaps at a joint critique of the incident. As you become familiar with the police officials in your community, and they with you, knowledge of and respect for your respective jobs will grow between you, making you a more effective team in emergency situations. It may be a good idea to establish in advance how these situations will be handled so that there are no conflicts on scene.

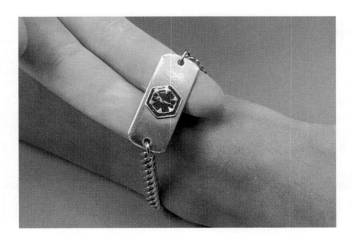

FIGURE 3.6
Medic Alert bracelet.

DOCUMENTATION

Documentation is an important part of the patient care process and may last long after the call is over. Some states may not require First Responders to complete specific types of documentation, but you would be wise to keep records of all calls to which you respond, in case they are needed in the event of subpoena or lawsuit. Your instructor will inform you of legal requirements in your area.

You may be required by law to make written or verbal reports in special situations such as child, elder, or spouse abuse; wounds sustained or potentially sustained by violent crime; sexual assault; or infectious-disease exposure. Again, your instructor will inform you of requirements in your area.

Summary

First Responders have to learn and maintain their skills and knowledge to a level where they can perform patient care to the expected standard. In many states, specific laws have been written to allow you to provide emergency care to patients without fear of successful civil legal action being taken against you. Good Samaritan laws may provide most First Responders with immunity. You are protected if you act in good faith, providing the First Responder **standard of care** to your level of training and to the best of your abilities.

A patient may refuse your care. You must have **expressed consent** from a conscious, competent adult patient. This consent is usually oral. It must be **informed consent,** with the patient knowing your level of training and what you are going to do. In cases in which the patient is unable to give consent, you may care for the patient under the law of **implied consent.** Implied consent also applies to children (**minor's consent**) and emotionally or mentally disturbed or retarded patients when their parents or legal guardians are not present.

A First Responder might be found **negligent** if he or she has a duty to provide care, does not provide care to the standard of care, and the inappropriate care causes injury (damage) to the patient. When you stop to provide care, you are responsible for the patient until someone more highly trained takes over. If you start to care for a patient and then leave the scene, you can be charged with **abandonment.**

Patients have a right to privacy. First Responders must respect patient confidentiality. Remember that care for organ donors should not differ from care given to any other patient. Always keep in mind that medical identification devices worn or carried by a patient can provide important medical information. Take care to preserve evidence when caring for a patient at a crime scene. Documentation is part of the patient care process. Keep records!

Remember and Consider...

Every time you respond to a call, you will be faced with some aspect of legal or ethical issues. It may be as simple as making sure the patient is willing to accept your help or as complex as a terminally ill patient who refuses your care. You may have to decide whether or not to stop and help even though you are off duty. You may worry about being sued.

✔ Make sure you are aware of legal requirements and are comfortable with ethical decisions in order to reduce your stress in these situations.

Investigate...

Knowledge is your best protection. Each state enacts laws that protect citizens, and the laws of each state may vary. Be sure you are familiar with the laws of your state that guide the actions of First Responders. Check with your department's legal office or with your supervising officers on the legal details of patient consent and care in various situations such as competent and incompetent adult and emancipated child, consent and refusals, and crime scenes.

✔ Find out what types of consent forms and run sheets for documentation are used in your jurisdiction.

✔ Obtain and review a sample DNR order from the library or a lawyer. Find out if DNR bracelets are used in your jurisdiction.

✔ Learn the different types of evidence and ways you may help to preserve them at a crime scene.

CHAPTER 4

THE HUMAN BODY

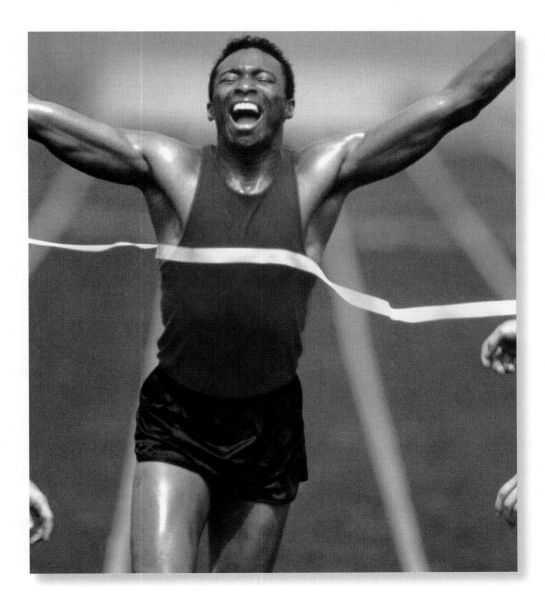

A First Responder will not be able to provide care for an ill or injured patient unless he or she first has an idea of where the problem lies. This requires a patient assessment. To perform an adequate patient assessment, the First Responder must be familiar with the normal anatomy of the human body and topographical terminology. This chapter provides information about the anatomy and function of the human body as well as terminology that will assist in reporting information gained during patient assessment.

National Standard Objectives

This chapter focuses on the objectives of Module 1, Lesson 1–4 of the U.S. DOT First Responder National Standard Curriculum and serves as an instructional aid to help you meet any specific objectives added to the course by your local EMS system.

By the end of this chapter, you will know how to (from cognitive knowledge information) . . .

1–4.1 Describe the anatomy and function of the respiratory system. (p. 52; also see Chapter 6, pp. 89–93)

1–4.2 Describe the anatomy and function of the circulatory system. (p. 52; also see Chapter 8, pp. 187, 212–213 and Chapter 11, pp. 299–301)

1–4.3 Describe the anatomy and function of the musculoskeletal system. (p. 53; also see Chapter 12, pp. 373–377, 411–414)

1–4.4 Describe the components and function of the nervous system. (p. 53; also see Chapter 12, pp. 412–414)

LEARNING TASKS

A basic understanding of the normal anatomy and function of the human body will help the First Responder to know when something is wrong with a patient. Your instructor will help you be able to:

✔ Learn ways in which First Responders may be able to apply their knowledge of anatomy.

Topographical and directional terms aid in reporting patient problems more accurately. Learning these terms will make it possible to give an accurate patient report, even over the telephone or radio. Practice using these terms and be able to:

✔ Describe the anatomical position.
✔ Define and properly apply the terms *anterior, posterior, midline, medial, lateral, proximal, distal, superior, inferior, patient's right,* and *patient's left*.

It is also helpful to know the five major regions of the body and the contents of the four major body cavities when you assess a patient and relay patient information. Be sure you are able to:

✔ Use common terminology to list the five major regions of the body and the subdivisions of each region.
✔ Name and locate the four major body cavities.
✔ Name and locate the organs contained in each of the body cavities.
✔ Identify the four abdominal quadrants.
✔ Name two types of structures that are found in every location in the body.

First Responders may find anatomy and function of the human body to be intimidating, but once you become familiar with a few basic terms, you will find it is not as difficult as you believed. You should practice applying the knowledge gained in this chapter until you can look at another person's body and mentally determine the position of the major organs of the chest and abdomen. You should also be able to begin at the head and name the major bones of the body.

OVERVIEW OF THE HUMAN BODY

THE HEAD-TO-TOE APPROACH

Students beginning training in First Responder and emergency care courses are often a little worried about having to learn human **anatomy.** Relax. You will not be learning very many new terms or structures. You might be a little surprised to find where some structures are located, since few of us have an accurate idea of the exact location of all of our body structures. As a First Responder, you will not need to be as precise as medical personnel are when they consider the human body. However, you will need to know the basic body structures and their locations. No one will be asking you to take a stethoscope and outline the borders of the heart. You know, generally, where the heart is located in the chest. We will show you some quick ways to be more specific about the location of the heart when we study CPR, or cardiopulmonary resuscitation (KAR-de-o-PUL-mo-ner-e re-SUS-si-TAY-shun).

anatomy the study of body structure.

You probably know the general location of the lungs. You may be a little off in locating the stomach and the liver. Odds are you will be less accurate in locating the uterus (womb), and even less accurate in locating the ovaries. The main thing to keep in mind as you begin your studies is that you know all these structures exist and you have a general idea of where they are located.

Do not become too concerned with trying to learn a lot of medical terminology. A head is still a head and feet are still feet. Most of the terms relating to human anatomy are so important to us that they have been a part of our vocabulary for years. Brain, eyes, ears, teeth, heart, lungs, liver, stomach, bladder, and spinal cord are all valid terms in emergency medicine.

You will learn a few new terms. You will also take a few terms that you may have heard before (such as *carotid artery*) and make them as much a part of your vocabulary as heart and lung.

First To be a First Responder, you must be able to look at a person's body and know the major internal structures and the general location of these structures. Your concern is not how the body looks dissected or how the body looks on an anatomical wall chart. You must be concerned with living bodies and knowing where things are located as you look from the outside.

You know about blood vessels and nerves. As you look at any region of the body, remember:

■ For our purposes, blood vessels go everywhere in the body, to every structure.
■ For our purposes, nerves go everywhere in the body, to every structure.

When you look at an arm, you must see something that is alive and part of a living organism. You know that an arm is made of muscles, bones, blood vessels, nerves, and other tissues. When you assess injuries, *never* forget that there could be internal bleeding and that damaged nerves may be causing pain, loss of feeling, or even loss of function.

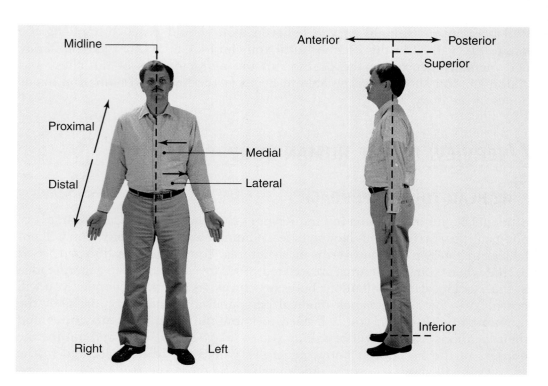

FIGURE 4.1
Directional terms.

DIRECTIONAL TERMS

The following is a set of very basic terms to use when referring to the human body (Figure 4.1):

- *Anatomical position*—Consider the human body, standing erect, facing you. The arms are down at the sides, and the palms of the hands are forward. References to all body structures describe the body in the **anatomical position.** This is very important when considering the bones and blood vessels in the arm.

- *Right and left*—Always refer to the **patient's right** and **patient's left.** Even though you may think this is very simple, many students find it difficult. Practice until you can use these terms correctly every time.

- *Anterior and posterior*—**Anterior** refers to the front of the body, and **posterior** indicates the back of the body. For the head, the face is considered anterior, while all the remaining structures are posterior. The rest of the body can be easily divided into anterior and posterior by following the side seams of your clothing.

- *Midline*—An imaginary vertical line can be used to divide the body into right and left halves. Anything toward the **midline** is said to be **medial,** while anything away from the midline is said to be **lateral.** Remember the anatomical position, which places the thumb on the lateral side of the hand and the little finger on the medial side.

There are other directional terms that can be useful. **Superior** means toward the top of the head, as in "the eyes are superior to the nose." **Inferior** means toward the feet, as in "the mouth is inferior to the nose." You cannot say something is superior or inferior unless you are comparing at least two structures. The heart is not superior, it is superior to the stomach. Since you are using the anatomical position for all your references to the body, any medical professional

anatomical (AN-ah-TOM-i-kal) position the standard reference position for the body in the study of anatomy. The body is standing erect, facing the observer. The arms are down at the sides, and the palms of the hands face forward.

anterior the front of the body or body part.

posterior the back of the body or body part.

medial toward the midline of the body.

lateral to the side, away from the midline of the body.

superior toward the head (for example, the chest is superior to the abdomen).

inferior away from the head; usually compared with another structure that is closer to the head (for example, the lips are inferior to the nose).

will know what you mean when you say a wound is just above the eye. For this reason, superior and inferior may be optional terms in your course.

Proximal and **distal** also may be optional terms in your course. These two terms are often used incorrectly and should be avoided unless you are certain of their correct usage. If we limit our discussion to the anatomy a First Responder must know, most medical professionals only use *proximal* and *distal* in reference to the arms and legs. To use proximal and distal, there must be a point of reference and two structures to be compared. The structure closest to the point of reference is said to be proximal, while the structure farthest away is distal. It helps to think that the close structure is the *proxim*ity of the reference, while the far structure is some *dist*ance away.

The most commonly used points of reference are the shoulder joint and the hip joint. Thus, the elbow is said to be proximal when compared to the wrist, which is distal. The knee is proximal when compared to the ankle. Trying to remember all this in an emergency situation could lead to some confusion.

Most First Responders do not deal with accidents and medical emergencies on a daily basis. Unless they review and use the terms, they find the terminology becoming less useful with time. Be aware that medical and rescue personnel are trained to take your information. They will not be confused if you say front, back, above, and below. Do not let terminology stand in the way of clear communication with EMT-Bs, Paramedics, doctors, and other medical professionals.

proximal closer to the torso.

distal farther away from the torso.

*B*ODY REGIONS

First | The human body can be divided into five regions (Figure 4.2). These regions have the common, everyday names of head, neck, trunk, upper extremities (shoulders, arms, and hands), and lower extremities (hip joint, legs, and feet). Later in this text, you will be asked to study some specific areas within each of these regions. For example, you will have to understand the pelvic girdle and how the legs join the trunk of the body so that you can relate certain injuries to specific types of accidents. For now, in order to begin your new approach in viewing the body, start with the simplest of subdivisions:

*N*ote

In an emergency, if you are not certain about the correct usage of a medical term, use the common term. You may damage your credibility by using the wrong medical term, or you may delay the EMTs as they try to determine the actual meaning of what you have said.

Head
Cranium—housing the brain
Face
Mandible (MAN-di-bl)—the
    lower jaw

Neck

Trunk
Chest—known as the thorax
    (THO-raks)
Abdomen—extending from the
    lower ribs to the pelvic girdle
Pelvis—protected by the bones
    of the pelvic girdle

Upper Extremities
Shoulder joint
Arm
Elbow
Forearm
Wrist
Hand

Lower Extremities
Hip joint
Thigh
Knee
Leg
Ankle
Foot

The terms *cranium*, *thorax*, and *mandible* may not be used in most daily conversations, but all the other terms are already part of your vocabulary. The significant thing is to begin looking for these simple subdivisions each time you

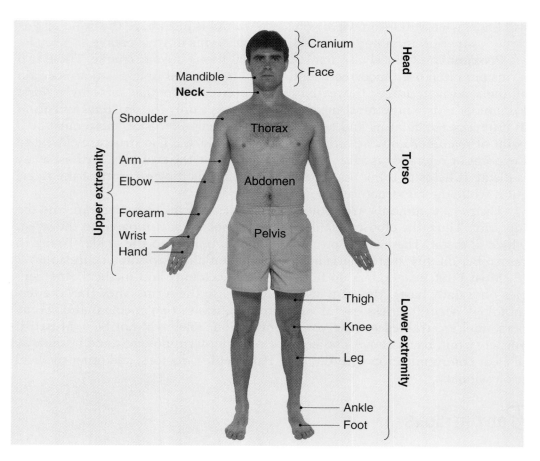

FIGURE 4.2
Body regions.

consider possible diseases and injuries. As stated earlier, more specifics will be covered throughout this text.

BODY CAVITIES

First | There are four major body cavities, two anterior and two posterior (Figure 4.3). Housed in these cavities are the vital organs, glands, blood vessels, and nerves.

FIGURE 4.3
Body cavities.

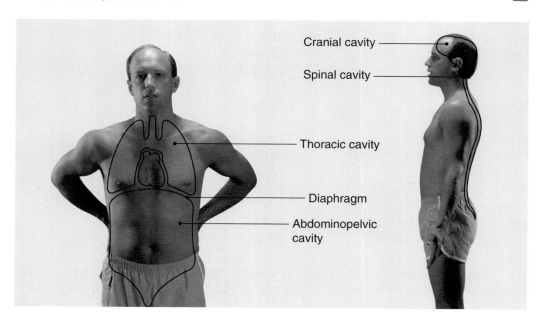

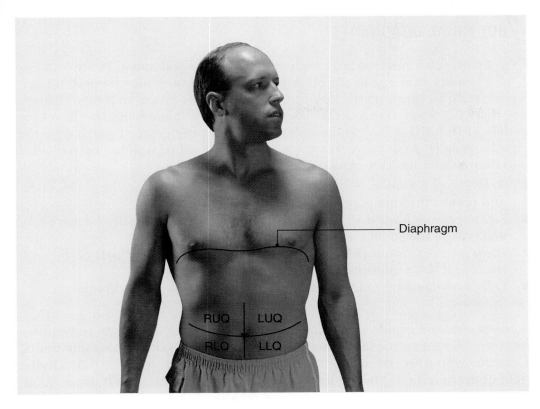

FIGURE 4.4
Location of diaphragm
and abdominal
quadrants.

Anterior Cavities

- *Chest cavity*—Also known as the **thoracic cavity.** It is enclosed by the rib cage, protecting the lungs, heart, great blood vessels, part of the windpipe (trachea), and part of the esophagus (e-SOF-ah-gus), which is the tube leading from the throat to the stomach. The lower border of the chest cavity is the **diaphragm,** a dome-shaped muscle used in breathing. The diaphragm separates the thoracic cavity from the abdominopelvic (ab-DOM-i-no-PEL-vik) cavity. It is important to know the location of the diaphragm (Figure 4.4).

- *Abdominopelvic cavity*—The anterior body cavity below the diaphragm. If you study more anatomy on your own, you will see this term, but most people use the terms **abdominal cavity** and **pelvic cavity** to describe the two portions of the abdominopelvic cavity.

  - *Abdominal cavity*—The abdominal cavity lies between the thorax and the pelvis and is separated from the thoracic cavity by the diaphragm. The stomach, liver, gallbladder, pancreas, spleen, small intestine, and most of the large intestine can be found in this cavity. The abdominal cavity, unlike the other body cavities, is not surrounded by bones. If you consider all the organs in this cavity and the lack of this bony protection, it is easy to see why blows to the abdomen can cause severe injury.

  - *Pelvic cavity*—Protected by the bones of the pelvic girdle, this cavity houses the urinary bladder, portions of the large intestine, and the internal reproductive organs.

Posterior Cavities

- *Cranial cavity*—This is the braincase of the skull, housing the brain and its specialized membranes.

- *Spinal cavity*—This cavity runs through the center of the backbone, protecting the spinal cord and its specialized membranes.

thoracic (tho-RAS-ik) cavity the anterior body cavity that is above (superior to) the diaphragm. The *thorax* (THO-raks).

diaphragm (DI-uh-fram) the muscular structure that divides the chest cavity from the abdominal cavity.

abdominal cavity the anterior body cavity that extends from the diaphragm to the region protected by the pelvic bones.

pelvic cavity the anterior body cavity surrounded by the bones of the pelvis

ABDOMINAL QUADRANTS

First | The abdomen is a large body region, and the abdominal cavity contains many vital organs. In other body regions, bones may be used for reference, such as counting the ribs or using a bump or notch on a bone. This is not the case when trying to be specific about the abdomen. The navel, or *umbilicus* (um-BIL-i-kus), is the only quick point of reference available for the First Responder. To improve this situation, the abdominal wall has been divided into four quadrants (Figure 4–4). These quadrants are:

- *Right upper quadrant* (RUQ)—containing most of the liver, the gallbladder, and part of the small and large intestine.
- *Left upper quadrant* (LUQ)—containing most of the stomach, the spleen, and part of the small and large intestine.
- *Right lower quadrant* (RLQ)—containing the appendix and part of the small and large intestine.
- *Left lower quadrant* (LLQ)—containing part of the small and large intestine.

Some organs and glands are located in more than one quadrant. As you can see from the above list, the large intestine is found, in part, in all four quadrants. The same is true for the small intestine. Part of the stomach can be found in the right upper quadrant. The left lobe of the liver extends into the left upper quadrant. Pelvic organs are included in these quadrants, with the urinary bladder being assigned to both lower quadrants.

The kidneys are a special case. They are not part of the abdominal cavity, since they are located behind the cavity's membrane lining. Consider one kidney to be RUQ and the other to be LUQ. However, do not let this abdominal classification make you think that the kidneys are in the abdominal cavity. The location of the kidneys makes them subject to injury from blows to the midback. Any pain or ache in the back may involve the kidneys. The pancreas and the aorta are also located behind the abdominal cavity membrane. The pancreas is mostly in the right upper quadrant, and the aorta lies just in front of the spinal column.

BODY SYSTEMS

Knowing the body systems and their functions can prove to be of value to the First Responder. However, most training courses do not have the time to go into great detail in terms of anatomy and physiology. Throughout this text, specific anatomy and some basic functions will be covered as they apply to injury, disease, illness, and the First Responder-level care.

Remembering the different body functions can be useful when trying to determine the extent of injury or the nature of an illness. The following is a list of the major body systems and their primary functions:

- *Circulatory system*—moving blood, carrying oxygen and nutrients to the body's cells, and removing wastes and carbon dioxide from these cells. It includes the heart, blood vessels, and blood (see also Chapter 11).
- *Respiratory system*—exchanging air to bring in oxygen and expel carbon dioxide. Oxygen is placed into the bloodstream while carbon dioxide is being removed. The respiratory system includes the nose, mouth, structures in the throat, lungs, and associated muscles (see also Chapters 6 and 10).

- *Digestive system*—digesting and absorbing food and removing certain wastes (Scan 4-1; see also Chapter 10).
- *Urinary system*—removing chemical wastes from the blood and helping to balance water and salt levels of the blood (see also Chapter 11).
- *Reproductive system*—producing all structures and hormones needed for sexual reproduction. Sometimes classified with the urinary system as the genitourinary (jen-e-to-U-re-NER-e) system (see also Chapter 11).
- *Nervous system*—controlling movement, interpreting sensations, regulating body activities, and generating memory and thought. It includes the brain, spinal cord, and nerves (see also Chapter 11).
- *Endocrine* (EN-do-krin) *system*—producing the chemicals called hormones that help regulate most body activities and functions.
- *Musculoskeletal* (MUS-kyu-lo-SKEL-et-l) *system*—providing protection and support for the body and internal organs and permitting body movement. It is made up of bones and skeletal muscles, tendons, and ligaments (see also Chapter 12).
- *Special senses*—providing sight, hearing, taste, smell, and the sensations of pain, cold, heat, and tactile responses, such as smoothness, roughness, softness, and the like (see Chapter 11).
- *Skin*—protecting the body from heat, cold, and pollution of the environment; bacteria; and other foreign organisms. It is the largest organ of the body, which covers and protects the body's many tissues, organs, and systems. It regulates body temperature and senses heat, cold, touch, pain, and pressure. It also regulates body fluids and chemical balance. (see also Chapters 10 and 11).

In addition to the above, there is a system to protect the body from disease-causing organisms (*immune system*).

RELATING STRUCTURES TO THE BODY

First | In this section, we will use a series of illustrations to show what you should be able to do as a First Responder considering the human body. Your problem is a complex one, requiring much thought and practice before you will be comfortable with your new knowledge. As we stated earlier, your task is to know the general location of structures as you view the external body. On many of these illustrations, you will see a line representing the diaphragm. Being able to visualize the position of the diaphragm will greatly help you understand how the various organs and glands fit into the body.

Begin with Figure 4.5. Note the position of the heart in the chest cavity. As a quick point of reference, use your fingers to find a small, hard spot just below your breastbone (sternum). This is the **xiphoid process,** a major body landmark. You can find a point directly over the inferior (lower) border of the heart by measuring two finger-widths up from this point. Look at yourself in a mirror and find this point. Each time you look in the mirror during your training, try to visualize where your heart is located.

   Figure 4.6 shows the position of the lungs in the chest cavity. The lungs are protected by the rib cage. By studying this figure, you will have a good idea of the size, shape, and position of the lungs.

xiphoid (ZI-foid) process the inferior portion of the sternum.

FIGURE 4.5
Position of the heart.

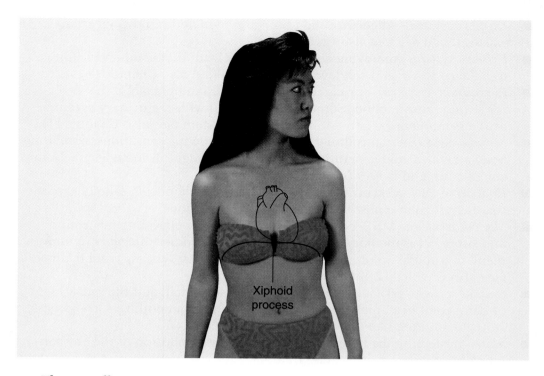

The two illustrations in Figure 4.7 show the position of the stomach, liver, and the first portion of the small intestine (called the *duodenum* [du-o-DE-num]). The lower ribs protect the stomach and liver (Scan 4–1). The level of the xiphoid process is where the esophagus enters the stomach, immediately after passing through the diaphragm. If this makes sense to you, then you are gaining a firm grasp of human anatomy. If it does not, then you need to set aside time to review the first part of this chapter.

The first portion of the small intestine is important in emergency medicine because it is held in a more rigid position than the rest of the small intestine. Forceful blows to the abdomen, often received in automobile accidents, may injure the first portion of the small intestine without causing any significant damage to the rest of the intestine.

FIGURE 4.6
Position of the lungs.

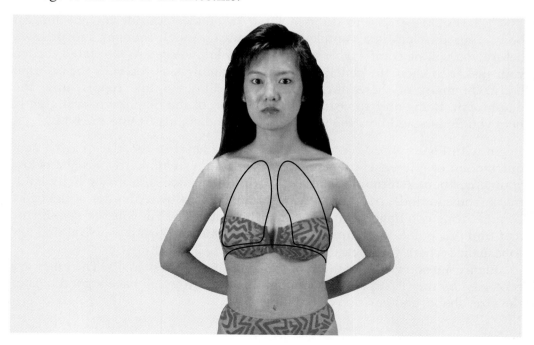

Major Body Organs

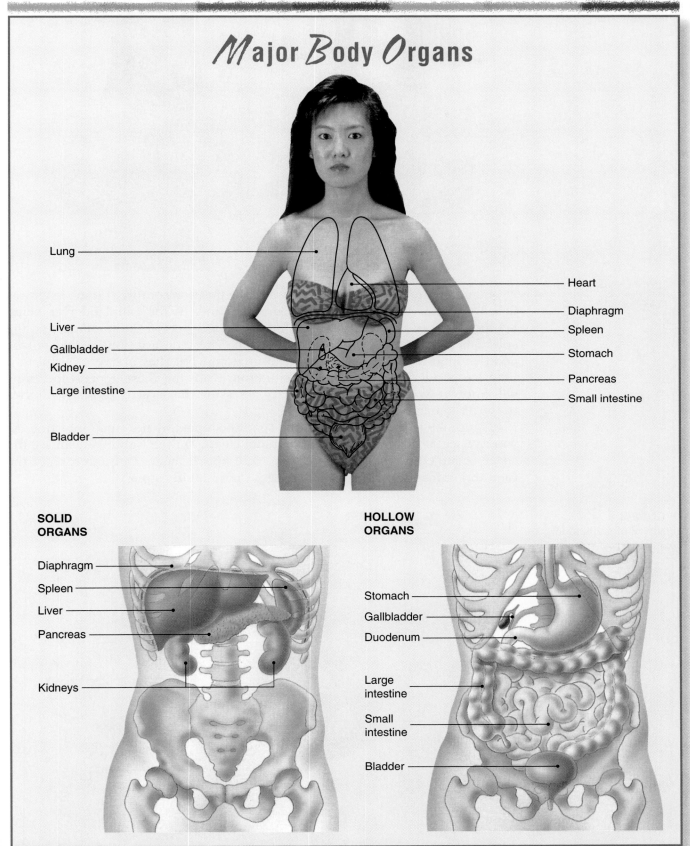

SOLID ORGANS

Diaphragm
Spleen
Liver
Pancreas

Kidneys

HOLLOW ORGANS

Stomach
Gallbladder
Duodenum

Large intestine

Small intestine

Bladder

Lung

Heart
Diaphragm
Spleen
Stomach
Pancreas
Small intestine

Liver
Gallbladder
Kidney
Large intestine

Bladder

FIGURE 4.7
Position of the
stomach, liver, and
duodenum.

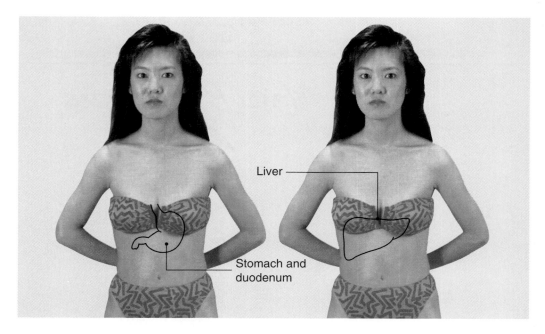

Using Figure 4.8, you can quickly add the positions of three other structures based on what you have already learned. Think of the gallbladder as being behind the liver, the pancreas as behind the lower part of the stomach, and the spleen behind the left side of the stomach. These descriptions would not be good enough if you were a student of anatomy, but they are very useful to a First Responder in an emergency situation. Knowing these general locations will improve your chances of correctly assessing the severity of many injuries to the abdomen.

Figure 4.9 shows, on the left, the space occupied by the small intestine. As you can see, it fills most of the abdominal cavity. On the right, you can see the space occupied by the large intestine. Note how it passes through each of the four abdominal quadrants as it "frames" the small intestine.

FIGURE 4.8
Position of gallbladder,
pancreas, and spleen.

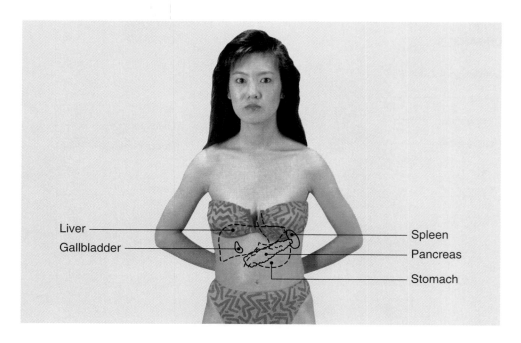

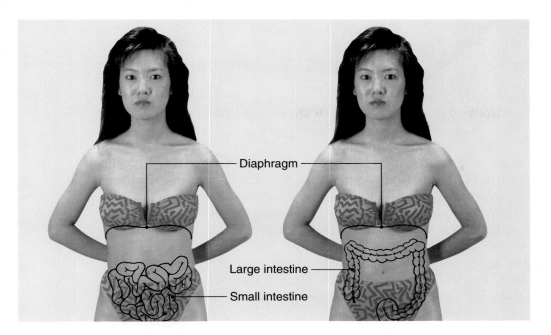

FIGURE 4.9
Position of the small
and large intestine.

Diaphragm

Large intestine

Small intestine

The kidneys and the urinary bladder are shown in Figure 4.10. Remember, the kidneys are behind the abdominal cavity, and the bladder is in the pelvic cavity. Although they appear well protected, injuries to these structures are common in motor vehicle accidents. This is particularly true when occupants not wearing seat belts are thrown about in the passenger compartment. Internal organs may also be injured by gunshots, stabbings, severe blows to the abdomen or back, and forces or weights that cause crushing.

We have spent a good deal of time and effort on the illustrations dealing with anterior cavities and their structures. Scan 4–1 sums up this material with an internal view, a view of the hollow organs, and a view of the solid organs. This shows you all that you have covered so far. Study these drawings and spend the time to relate the positions of these organs to the body's exterior.

FIGURE 4.10
Position of the urinary
system.

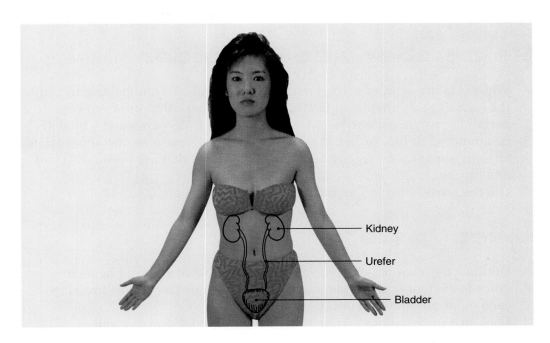

Kidney

Urefer

Bladder

Summary

A knowledge of the body's basic anatomy and general functions helps First Responders assess patients and communicate with other emergency care providers.

Care providers refer to the **patient's right** and the **patient's left,** with the body in the **anatomical position.** An imaginary vertical line, the **midline,** divides the body into halves. Toward the midline is **medial;** away from the midline is **lateral. Superior** is toward the top of the head, and **inferior** is toward the feet. The terms **proximal** and **distal** refer to the arms and legs. Proximal is toward the torso; distal is away from the torso.

The body is divided into five regions: the head, the neck, the trunk, the upper extremities, and the lower extremities. It has four cavities, two anterior (the **thoracic cavity** and the **abdominopelvic cavity,** separated by the **diaphragm**) and two posterior (the **cranial cavity** and the **spinal cavity**). The abdomen is divided into **four quadrants,** centered around the navel: the **right upper quadrant,** the **left upper quadrant,** the **right lower quadrant,** and the **left lower quadrant.**

The ten **body systems** include the **circulatory system** (heart, blood vessels, blood), the **respiratory system** (nose, mouth, throat structures, lungs, muscles), the **digestive system** (stomach, intestines, liver, gallbladder), the **urinary system** (kidneys, ureters, bladder, urethra), the **reproductive system** (uterus, ovaries, fallopian tubes, testicles), the **nervous system** (brain, spinal cord, nerves), the **endocrine system** (adrenal, thyroid, and other special glands and cells), the **musculoskeletal system** (bones, skeletal muscles, tendons and ligaments), the **skin** (skin, hair, sweat glands), and the **special senses** (eyes, ears, nose, mouth).

Remember and Consider

✔ While it is important for the First Responder to learn and be able to use the terms in this chapter, it is even more important that information pertaining to the patient be passed on to other EMS personnel who will be attending to him or her. If you are unable to remember the appropriate term to use in an emergency situation, use terms that are familiar to you and others.

✔ Use the terms *anterior, posterior, medial,* and *lateral.*

Investigate

✔ Outline your own major body cavities and list what is found in each.

✔ Point to each of your abdominal quadrants. Name the organs found in each quadrant and find out their functions.

✔ Look in a mirror. Locate your heart, lungs, xiphoid process, and diaphragm.

✔ Locate your bladder and kidneys.

CHAPTER 5

LIFTING AND MOVING PATIENTS

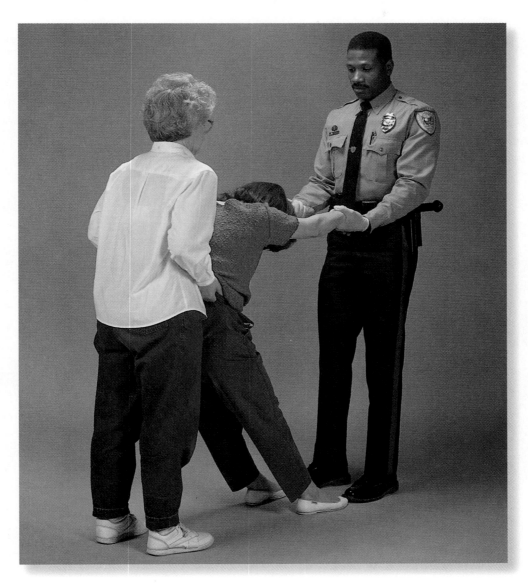

*M*any First Responders are injured every year because they attempt to lift or move patients improperly. One of the most important things you can do for yourself, your coworkers, and any patients you may help is to learn how to lift and move patients in a manner that will not cause injury to anyone. It is also important to know when and how to move patients from where they are found before the EMS crew arrives. Learning these simple techniques will make it possible for you to be an effective First Responder for many years to come.

This chapter focuses on the objectives of Module 1, Lesson 1–5 of the U.S. DOT First Responder National Standard Curriculum and serves as an instructional aid to help you meet any specific objectives added to the course by your local EMS system.

By the end of this chapter, you will know how to (from cognitive or knowledge information) . . .

1–5.1	Define body mechanics. (p. 61)
1–5.2	Discuss the guidelines and safety precautions that need to be followed when lifting a patient. (p. 61)
1–5.3	Describe the indications for an emergency move. (p. 62)
1–5.4	Describe the indications for assisting in nonemergency moves. (p. 66)
1–5.5	Discuss the various devices associated with moving a patient in the out-of-hospital arena. (pp. 73–77)

Feel comfortable enough to (by changing attitudes, values, and beliefs) . . .

1–5.6	Explain the rationale for properly lifting and moving patients. (p. 61)
1–5.7	Explain the rationale for an emergency move. (p. 62)

Show how to (through psychomotor skills) . . .

1–5.8	Demonstrate an emergency move. (pp. 62–65)
1–5.9	Demonstrate a nonemergency move. (pp. 66–69)
1–5.10	Demonstrate the use of equipment utilized to move patients in the out-of-hospital arena. (pp. 73–80)

*L*EARNING TASKS

In an emergency situation, it is important to know how to safely move a patient in the most expedient way.

✔ Learn the most common emergency moves to be used by First Responders and be able to demonstrate them.

There will also be situations where a patient needs to be moved, but in which you have more time and can use different methods that require equipment and/or additional people.

✔ Learn the most common nonemergency moves to be used by First Responders and be able to demonstrate them.

PRINCIPLES OF MOVING PATIENTS

ROLE OF THE FIRST RESPONDER

Whenever possible, you should not move a patient. First Responders should care for a patient, try to keep the patient stable, and wait for the EMTs to respond. This holds true even when the patient appears to be able to move about. Keeping the patient at rest is your best course of action. Remember, you may have missed the signs of an injury or a medical problem during your assessment of the patient. Also, not all patients are honest in answering your questions during an interview. Some patients will deny injury or illness.

WHEN TO MOVE A PATIENT

First There will be times when you must move patients, perhaps in order to remove them from immediate danger or in order to prevent further injury. You may also be called upon to assist other EMS responders in lifting and moving patients. With the proper techniques, this can be done safely. Remember, proper lifting and moving must be practiced on every call.

BODY MECHANICS AND LIFTING TECHNIQUES

First **Body mechanics** is the proper use of your body to facilitate lifting and moving. There are important things that must be done to lift efficiently and prevent injury.

body mechanics the proper use of the body to facilitate lifting and moving and prevent injury.

Planning is important before lifting a patient or an object. Know the weight of the patient or object and request additional help if it is needed. It is also important to consider any physical limitations that may make lifting difficult or unsafe for you. Whenever possible, lift with a partner whose strength and height are similar to yours. Communicate with your partner and with the patient when you are ready to lift and continue to communicate throughout the process.

When you are ready to lift, follow these rules to prevent injury:

- *Position your feet properly*—They should be on a firm, level surface and positioned shoulder-width apart.
- *Use your legs, not your back, to do the lifting*—Keep your back straight and bend your knees.
- *Never twist or attempt to make any moves other than the lift*—Attempts to turn or twist while you are lifting are a major cause of injury.
- *When lifting with one hand, do not compensate*—Avoid leaning to either side. Keep your back straight and locked.
- *Keep the weight as close to your body as possible*—This is part of good body mechanics and allows you to use your legs rather than your back while lifting. The farther the weight is from your body, the greater your chance of injury.
- *When carrying a patient on stairs, use a stair chair instead of a stretcher whenever possible*—Keep your back straight. Flex your knees and lean forward from the hips, not the waist. If you are walking backwards down stairs, ask a helper to steady your back.

Moving and Positioning Patients

Emergency Moves

There are times when a patient must be moved immediately. These situations call for **emergency moves.** An emergency move should take place when:

emergency move
a patient move that is carried out quickly when the scene is hazardous, care of the patient requires repositioning, or you must reach another patient needing lifesaving care.

- **There is immediate danger to the patient if not moved**—Uncontrolled traffic, fire or threat of fire, possible explosions, impending structural collapse, possible electrical hazards, toxic gases, and other such dangers may make it necessary to move a patient quickly in order to protect both you and the patient.
- **Lifesaving care cannot be given because of the patient's location or position**—You may have to move a patient to a hard, flat surface to provide CPR, or you may have to move a patient in order to reach a profusely bleeding wound.
- **You are unable to gain access to other patients who need lifesaving care**—You may have to quickly move a patient with no neck or spinal injuries in order to reach another patient needing lifesaving care. This is seen most often in motor vehicle accidents.

Emergency moves rarely provide any protection to patient injuries, and they may cause great pain for the patient. This is justified because of the reasons listed above for emergency moves—the situation is too dangerous for you and the patient, or lifesaving care cannot be provided unless the patient is moved quickly.

The greatest danger in moving a patient quickly is the possibility of making a spinal injury worse. It is impossible to remove a patient from a vehicle quickly and at the same time provide much protection to the spine. But if the patient is on the floor or ground, it is important to make every effort to pull the patient in the direction of the long axis of the body to provide as much protection to the spine as possible. The long axis of the body is the line that runs down the center of the body from the top of the head and along the spine.

Drags

There are several rapid moves called drags. In this type of move, the patient is dragged by the clothes, the feet, the shoulders, or a blanket (Scan 5-1). These moves are reserved for emergencies because they do not provide protection for the neck and spine. Most commonly, a long-axis drag is made from the area of the shoulders. Dragging from the shoulder area causes the remainder of the body to fall into its natural anatomical position, with the spine and all limbs in normal alignment. *Never* drag a patient sideways. *Always* drag in the direction of the length, or long axis, of the body. Imagine dragging a patient from one side and the twisting and aggravation of injuries that could result. When you are using a drag method and you have to take the patient down stairs or an incline, you should go first and use a shoulder drag to pull the patient headfirst by lifting at the armpits.

Other Emergency Moves

There are many other techniques that can be used to move a patient quickly. Some require only one rescuer (Scan 5-2); others require two rescuers (Scan 5-3). Remember that any emergency move must be justified and that it should be carried out as quickly as possible.

Emergency Moves—One-Rescuer Drags

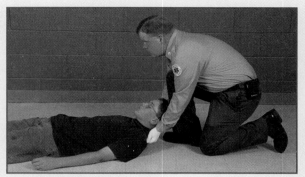

CLOTHES DRAG.

CAUTION: Always pull in the direction of the long axis of patient's body. Do not pull patient sideways. Avoid bending or twisting trunk.

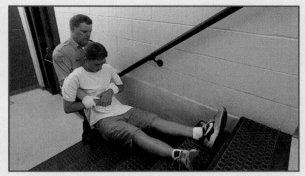

INCLINE DRAG. Always headfirst.

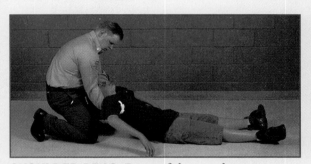

SHOULDER DRAG. Be careful not to bump patient's head.

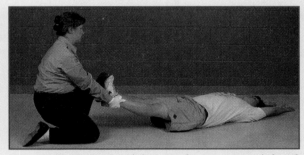

FOOT DRAG. Be careful not to bump patient's head.

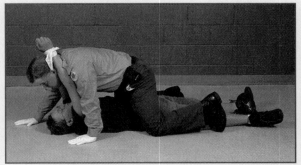

FIREFIGHTER'S DRAG. Place patient on his back and tie hands together. Straddle patient, facing his head; crouch and pass your head through his trussed arms and raise your body. Crawl on your hands and knees. Keep patient's head as low as possible.

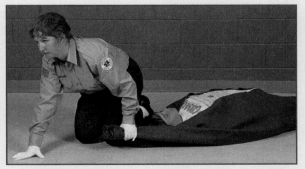

BLANKET DRAG. Gather half of the blanket material up against patient's side. Roll patient toward your knees so that you can place the blanket under him. Gently roll patient back onto the blanket. During the drag, keep patient's head as low as possible.

Emergency Moves—One Rescuer

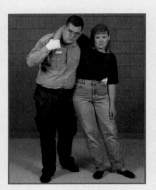

ONE-RESCUER ASSIST. Place patient's arm around your neck, grasping her hand in yours. Place your other arm around patient's waist. Help patient walk to safety. Be prepared to change movement technique if level of danger increases. Be sure to communicate with patient about obstacles, uneven terrain, and so on.

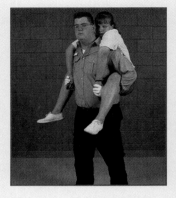

CRADLE CARRY. Place one arm across patient's back with your hand under her arm. Place your other arm under her knees and lift. If patient is conscious, have her place her near arm over your shoulder.

NOTE: This carry places a lot of weight on the carrier's back. It is usually appropriate only for very light patients.

PIGGY BACK CARRY. Assist patient to stand. Place her arms over your shoulder so they cross your chest. Bend over and lift patient. While she holds on with her arms, crouch and grasp each thigh. Use a lifting motion to move her onto your back. Pass your forearms under her knees and grasp her wrists.

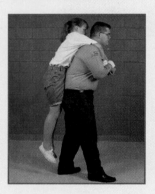

PACK STRAP CARRY. Have patient stand. Turn your back to her, bringing her arms over your shoulders to cross your chest. Keep her arms as straight as possible, her armpits over your shoulders. Hold patient's wrists, bend, and pull her onto your back.

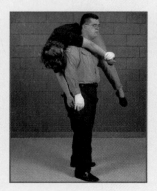

FIREFIGHTER'S CARRY. Place your feet against patient's feet and pull her toward you. Bend at waist and flex knees. Duck and pull her across your shoulders, keeping hold of one of her wrists. Use your free arm to reach between her legs and grasp her thigh. Allow weight of patient to fall onto your shoulders. Stand up. Transfer your grip on thigh to patient's wrist.

Emergency Moves—Two Rescuers

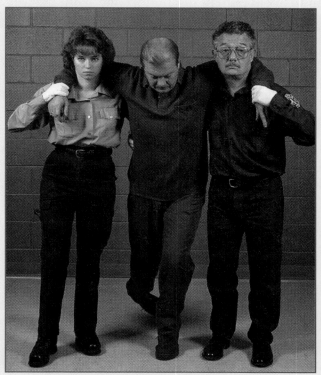

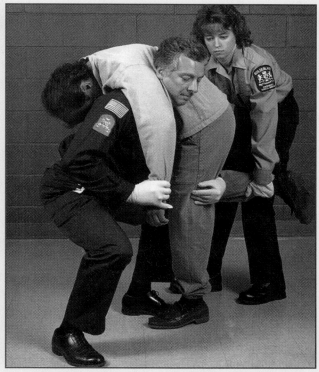

TWO-RESCUER ASSIST. Patient's arms are placed around shoulders of both rescuers. Each rescuer grips one of patient's hands, places free arm around patient's waist, and helps patient walk to safety.

FIREFIGHTER'S CARRY WITH ASSIST. The rescuer lifting patient conducts steps for firefighter's carry. The second rescuer helps to position patient.

NONEMERGENCY MOVES

nonemergency move a patient move that is carried out if there are other factors at the scene causing the patient to decline, you must reach other patients, part of the care required forces you to move the patient, or the patient insists on being moved.

First | **Nonemergency moves** are used when there is no immediate threat to life. Unless you are alone, all nonemergency moves should be carried out with the help of other trained personnel or bystanders. More often than not, you will have to make emergency moves by yourself. Nonemergency moves should be carried out in such a way as to prevent additional injury to the patient. Care should be taken to avoid patient discomfort and pain.

Follow these rules for a nonemergency move:

- The patient should be conscious.
- The initial assessment should be completed.
- Pulse and breathing rates and character should be stable and within normal ranges.
- There should be no uncontrolled external bleeding or any indications of internal bleeding.
- There must be absolutely no signs of neck or spinal injury, and the mechanism of injury should not point to possible neck or spinal injury.
- All possible fractures and extremity injuries must be immobilized or splinted.

Even though there is no immediate danger to yourself or to the patient, a nonemergency move could be justified because:

- **Factors at the scene cause patient decline**—If a patient's condition is rapidly declining due to heat or cold, moving may be necessary. If the patient is reacting strongly to something at the scene and may go into anaphylactic (allergy) shock, you may have to move the patient. These situations rarely call for emergency moves.
- **You must reach other patients**—When there are other patients at the scene, you may need to move the first patient in order to reach them and provide care.
- **Care requires moving the patient**—This is usually seen in cases where there are no injuries or severe medical problems. Problems due to extreme heat or cold, such as heat cramps, heat exhaustion, hypothermia, and local cold injuries (frostbite and freezing) are good examples. Reaching a source of water for washing in cases of serious chemical burns may be a reason to move a patient.
- **The patient insists on being moved**—You are not allowed to restrain patients. If they will not listen to the reasons why they should not be moved and are trying to move on their own, you may have to assist them. Sometimes a patient becomes so upset that stress worsens the condition. If this type of patient can be moved, and the move is short, you may have to make it in order to keep the patient stable.

If one of these situations exists, you may consider using one of the following nonemergency moves.

The Direct Ground Lift

First | The direct ground lift (three-rescuer lift) is a nonemergency move and is *not* recommended for use on patients with possible neck or spinal injuries. While this procedure can be carried out by two people, at least three are recommended. Additional rescuers can be used for the move by having them position themselves opposite the three main participants in the move.

To perform a direct ground lift (Figure 5.1), the patient should be lying face up and the arms should be placed on the chest. You and your helpers should line up on one side of the patient. You should be at the patient's head. One helper should be positioned at the patient's midsection and the other helper at the patient's lower legs. Each of you should drop to one knee. This should be the knee closest to the patient's feet.

Place one arm under the patient's neck and grasp the far shoulder so you will be able to cradle the head. Your other arm should be placed under the patient's back, just above the waist. Your helper at the patient's midsection should place one arm above and one arm below the patient's buttocks. The helper at the patient's lower legs should place one arm under the patient's knees and the other arm under the patient's ankles.

First, on your signal, everyone should lift the patient up to the level of their knees.

Second, on your signal, everyone should roll the patient toward their chests.

Third, on your signal, everyone should stand while holding the patient. You can now move the patient, reversing the process when it is time to stop the move and place the patient back into a lying position.

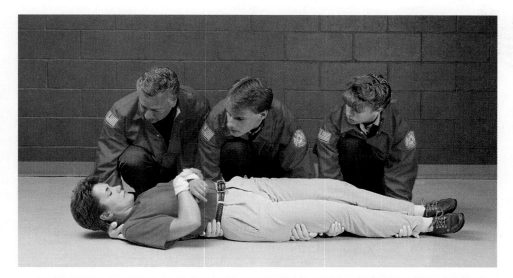

FIGURE 5.1A
Direct ground lift, step 1.

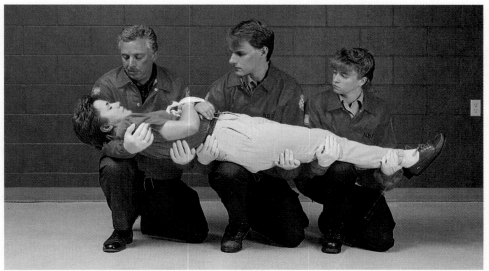

FIGURE 5.1B
Direct ground lift, step 2.

FIGURE 5.1C
Direct ground lift, step 3.

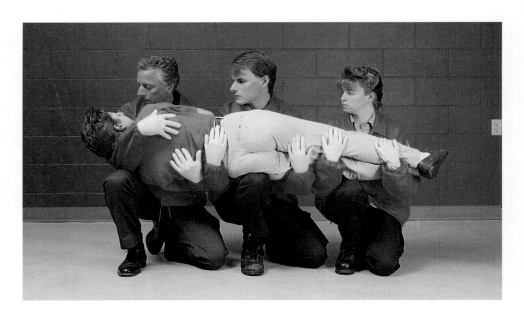

FIGURE 5.1D
Direct ground lift, step 4.

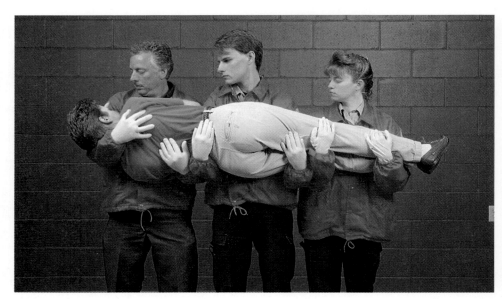

Note

It is poor practice to use a two-rescuer ground lift. This procedure does not allow enough support for the patient and control during the move. If you must use this move and have only one helper, position this helper at the patient's thigh so one arm can be placed on the patient's back above the patient's buttocks and one arm under the patient's knees.

The Extremity Lift

First An extremity lift requires two people (Figure 5.2). This lift should not be performed if there is any possibility of head, neck, spine, shoulder, hip, or knee injuries, or any possible fractures or other painful, swollen, deformed injuries to the upper or lower extremities that have not been immobilized. Ideally, the patient should not have any possible fractures or the painful, swollen, deformed extremities should be splinted. The patient should be conscious; if not, you may have incorrectly assessed neck and spinal injuries.

The patient should be placed face up, with knees flexed. You should kneel at the head of the patient, placing your hands under the patient's shoulders. Have your helper stand at the patient's feet and grasp the patient's wrists. Direct your helper to pull the patient into a sitting position, while you push the patient from

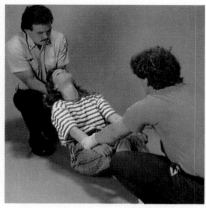

FIGURE 5.2A
Extremity lift, step 1. When possible, protect skin surfaces including your arms.

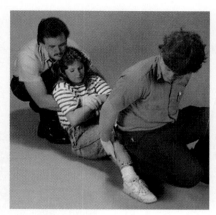

FIGURE 5.2B
Extremity lift, step 2.

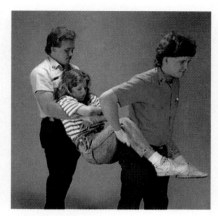

FIGURE 5.2C
Extremity lift, step 3.

the shoulders. (Do not have your helper pull the patient by the arms if there are any signs of painful, swollen, deformed extremity injuries.) Slip your arms under the patient's armpits and grasp the wrists. Once the patient is in a semi-sitting position, have your helper turn his back to the patient, crouch down, and grasp the patient's legs behind the knees.

Direct your helper so that you both stand at the same time ("Ready? . . . lift"), and move as a unit when carrying the patient. Try to walk out of step with your partner to avoid swinging the patient. Direct your helper as to when to stop the carry and when to place the patient down into a lying or seated position.

TRANSFER OF PATIENT FROM BED TO STRETCHER

Once EMS arrives at the scene, they may require your assistance in moving the patient from a bed to a stretcher. This may be accomplished using either the direct carry or the draw sheet method.

Direct Carry Method

The direct carry is performed in order to move a patient with *no suspected spine injury* from a bed or from a bed-level position to a stretcher (Scan 5-4). Position the stretcher perpendicular to the bed with the head end of the stretcher at the foot of the bed and prepare it by unbuckling straps and removing other items. Two rescuers stand between the bed and the stretcher, facing the patient. The first rescuer slides an arm under the patient's neck and cups the patient's shoulder while the second rescuer slides a hand under the patient's hip and lifts slightly. The first rescuer then slides his other arm under the patient's back while the second rescuer places his arms underneath the patient's hips and calves. Both rescuers slide the patient to the edge of the bed, lift/curl the patient towards their chests, and then rotate and place the patient gently onto the stretcher.

Direct Carry

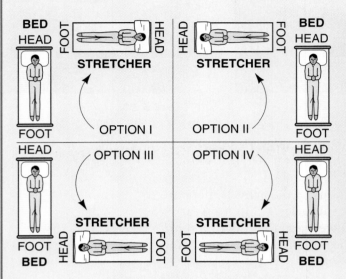

Stretcher is placed at 90° angle to bed, depending on room configuration. Prepare stretcher by lowering rails, unbuckling straps, and removing other items. Both First Responders stand between stretcher and bed, facing patient.

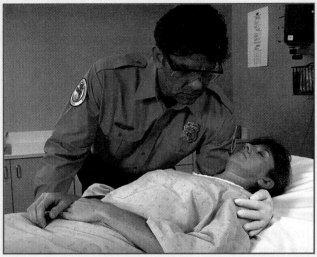

1. The head-end First Responder cradles patient's head and neck by sliding one arm under patient's neck to grasp shoulder.

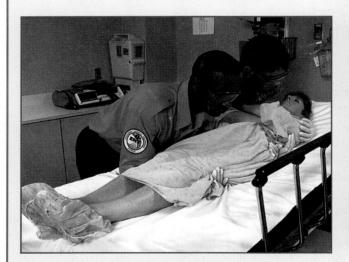

2. Foot-end First Responder slides hand under patient's hips and lifts slightly. Head-end First Responder slides other arm under patient's back. Foot-end First Responder places arms under hips and calves.

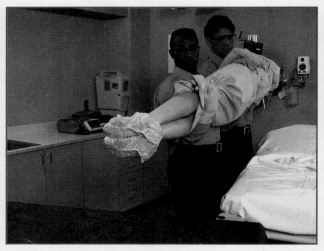

3. First Responders slide patient to edge of bed and bend toward her with their knees slightly bent. They lift and curl patient to their chests and return to a standing position. They rotate and slide patient gently onto stretcher.

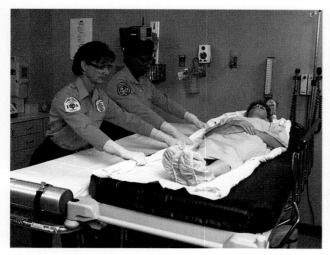

FIGURE 5.3A
Draw sheet method, step 1.

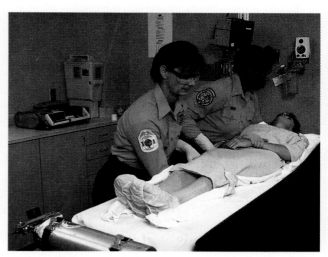

FIGURE 5.3B
Draw sheet method, step 2.

Draw Sheet Method

The other method of moving a patient with no suspected spine injury from a bed to a stretcher is the draw sheet method (Figure 5.3). Loosen the bottom sheet of the bed, then position the stretcher next to the bed. Adjust the height of the stretcher, lower rails, and unbuckle the straps. Both rescuers reach across the stretcher and grasp the sheet firmly at the patient's head, chest, hips, and knees, then slide the patient gently onto the cot.

*P*ATIENT POSITIONING

The Recovery Position

Positioning the patient is also a very important part of your care. Unresponsive patients without suspected spinal injury should be placed in the recovery position, which helps them to maintain an open and clear airway. Place patients on their left side to aid drainage of fluids and vomitus. Remember that patients with trauma or suspected spinal injury should not be moved until additional EMS resources arrive to evaluate and stabilize these patients. To place an unresponsive but uninjured patient in the recovery position (Figure 5.4), perform the following steps:

1. Raise the patient's left arm above the head. (A variation is to leave the patient's arm at the side and roll the patient so the arm is just behind him or her when positioned on the side.)

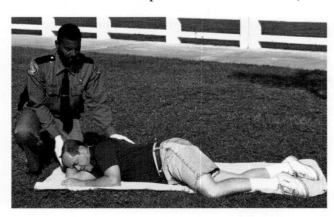

FIGURE 5.4
Placing the patient in recovery position.

2. Cross the patient's right arm over the chest and the right leg over the left leg.

3. Grasp the patient's right shoulder and hip and roll the patient toward you. The patient's head will rest on the raised left arm (or on the patient's forearm if the left arm positioned at the patient's side for the roll is now behind the patient). The head should be as close to the midline position of the body as possible.

4. Position the patient's right forearm on the floor/ground/cot (or under the patient's face if the left arm is at the side of and behind the patient) and place the right hand under the side of the face. The arm will support the patient in this position; the hand will cushion the face and allow the head to angle slightly downward for airway drainage.

5. Bend the patient's right knee so it touches the ground and helps support the patient in this position.

Later chapters will provide incidents and situations where you will use the recovery position. Refer to Chapter 8 (Figure 8.26), Chapter 10 (Scan 10-3), and Chapter 12 (Figure 12.41)

Many patients who do not have suspected spinal injuries may be placed in a position of comfort. This includes many patients with medical complaints such as chest pain, nausea, or difficulty breathing. In this situation, allow the patient to choose a position he feels comfortable in. Breathing is often aided by placing the patient in a semi-sitting, or Fowler's, position. This position of comfort must be used cautiously in case the patient vomits. Always position yourself appropriately to manage the patient's airway and monitor his level of consciousness. Place the patient into the recovery position at the first sign of a decreased level of consciousness.

The Log Roll

When an unresponsive patient is face down (prone), you must assess breathing differently. Place your hand in front of the patient's mouth and nose to feel for breathing. If you feel breath on your hand, the patient has an airway and is breathing. The patient's condition may worsen, however, and ideally, you want him on his back (supine) for further assessment, proper airway maintenance and care, and basic life-support steps if they become necessary. To move a prone patient to a supine position and assure stability of the head and spine where a trauma injury is suspected, perform a log roll. This patient-moving method can be done with two rescuers, but three and four rescuers can minimize twisting of the patient's spine during the procedure. Perform the following steps:

1. One First Responder will kneel at the patient's head and hold or stabilize the patient's head and neck in a neutral or anatomical position in-line with the patient's spine.

2. A second rescuer kneels at the patient's side and positions the patient's arms. (Note: There are two methods of arm positioning; each has a specific advantage. One method is to raise and extend the patient's arm above his head. This allows for easy rolling to that side and provides support for the head during the roll, which is helpful if you must do the log roll alone. A second method is to place the patient's arm along his side. The patient's arm will help splint, support, and maintain alignment of the spine during the move. The second method may work better when there are multiple rescuers.

The First Responder at the patient's head must maintain head alignment during the log roll, regardless of the patient's arm positioning. Check with your instructor for the preferred method in your jurisdiction.)

3. The second rescuer will kneel between the patient's shoulders and hips. If other rescuers are available, all of them will kneel along the side of the patient from shoulders to knees.

4. The rescuer(s) will grasp the patient's shoulders, hips, knees, and ankles. If only one rescuer is available to roll the patient, grasp the heavy parts of the torso—the shoulders and hips.

5. The First Responder at the patient's head will signal and give directions: On three, roll: one, two, three, roll together. All rescuers will slowly roll the patient in a coordinated move and carefully keep the patient's spine in neutral, in-line position during the entire move and until the patient is supine.

Sometimes the patient is supine but must be placed on a blanket or spine board. Begin with steps 1 through 5 above. Maintain control of the patient when she is rolled onto her side. Without removing your hands, continue with the following:

1. The First Responder at the patient's head will continue stabilization of the cervical spine until rescuers position a blanket or spine board behind the patient.

2. In a coordinated move, the rescuers will slowly roll the patient onto the blanket or spine board at the signal and directions of the First Responder at the patient's head.

3. Assure that the patient is positioned on the center of the spine board. If you must adjust the patient's position, be sure to keep her head and spine in neutral alignment.

EQUIPMENT FAMILIARITY

Remember that the First Responder will often be asked to assist EMS with packaging and loading the patient into the ambulance. It is necessary for the First Responder to be familiar with the various carrying and packaging devices that may be used. Some typical equipment that may be used is included in Scan 5-5. Many First Responder courses do not include information and practice on immobilization devices. Your instructor will teach you the procedures if First Responders are expected to perform them in your jurisdiction. Do not try to learn the procedures on your own. When you package a patient on an immobilization device, you must also stabilize the head and neck first by placing the correct type and size of cervical collar on the patient (Scans 5-6 and 5-7). These collars, also called extrication collars, are rigid supports that help maintain head and neck stability and alignment with the body in patients who have suspected neck and spinal injuries (Scans 5-8 and 5-9). Again, do not try to learn the steps of placing a collar on a trauma patient without proper instruction. Your instructor will teach you the steps if First Responders are required to use collars in your jurisdiction. (Refer to Chapter 12 for information and for care of patients with spinal injuries.)

Patient Carrying Devices

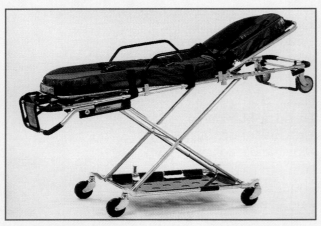

WHEELED STRETCHER—Head can be elevated to benefit some patients

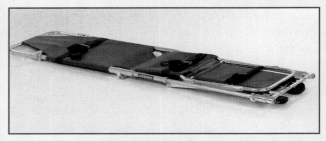

PORTABLE STRETCHER—Beneficial in multiple-casualty incidents

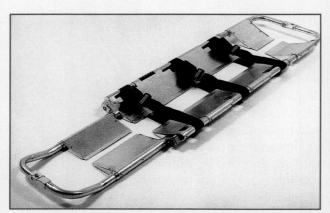

SCOOP (ORTHOPEDIC) STRETCHER—Allows quick immobilization of hip injuries or multiple injuries and patient transfer. New devices are sturdier and support spinal injuries.

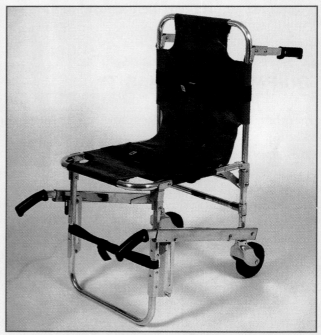

STAIR CHAIR—For use on stairs or tight places

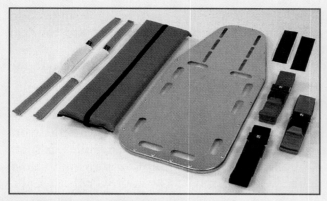

SHORT SPINE BOARD—Used to remove patients from vehicles

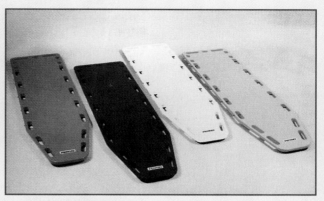

LONG SPINE BOARD—Used for patients found lying down or standing

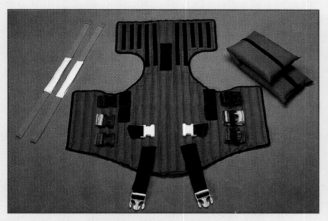

VEST-TYPE EXTRICATION DEVICE—Wraps help stabilize the patient's head, neck, and spine

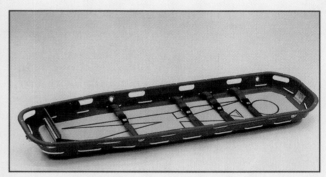

BASKET STRETCHER—Used to transport over rough terrain

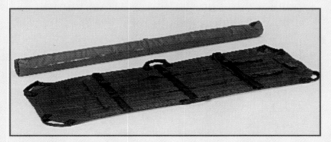

FLEXIBLE STRETCHER—Used in restricted areas or narrow hallways

Some typical equipment that may be used for packaging and loading the patient includes:

- *Wheeled Stretcher*—This device is commonly referred to simply as "the stretcher" or "the cot." It is the device that is in the back of all ambulances. The many brands and types of wheeled stretchers are all used to transport a patient in a reclining position. The head of this stretcher can be elevated, which will be beneficial for some patients.

- *Portable Stretcher*—Portable or folding stretchers may be beneficial in multiple-casualty incidents (incidents with many patients). The stretchers may be canvas, aluminum, or heavy plastic and usually fold or collapse.

- *Stair Chair*—The stair chair has many benefits for moving patients from the scene to the stretcher. The first benefit, as the name implies, is that it is excellent for use on stairs. It may also be useful for moving through tight places where a stretcher will not fit. It has a set of wheels that allow rescuers to roll it over flat surfaces like a wheelchair.

- *Scoop (Orthopedic) Stretcher*—This device is called the scoop stretcher because it splits into two pieces vertically and can be used to "scoop" the patient up. Newer models are sturdier and more inflexible than older ones and provide spinal support. Follow your local protocols on the use of this device. It is very useful for moving patients with hip injuries or multiple injuries or for transferring patients from a bed or the floor to a wheeled stretcher, as well as from the wheeled stretcher to the hospital bed.

- *Spine Board*—There are two types of spine boards, or backboards: long and short. The long spine board is used for patients who are found lying down or standing and must be immobilized. Short spine boards are used primarily for removing patients from vehicles when it is suspected that they have neck or spinal injuries. Once secured to the short spine board, the patient can be moved from a sitting position in the vehicle to a supine position on a long spine board. Often, a vest-type extrication device is used in place of a short spine board.

- *Vest-Type Extrication Device*—This commercially made immobilization vest wraps around the patient's torso to stabilize the spine. It has an extended section above the vest with side flaps for stabilizing the patient's head and neck. Straps and padding are provided to secure the head, and straps are attached to the vest to secure the chest and legs. It also has handles that will aid in lifting the patient onto a long spine board.

- *Basket Stretcher*—A basket stretcher can be used to move a patient from one level to another or over rough terrain. The basket should be lined with a blanket before positioning the patient.

- *Flexible Stretcher*—A flexible stretcher is made of canvas, rubberized, or other flexible material, often with wooden slats sewn into pockets and three carrying handles on each side. Because of its flexibility, it can be useful in restricted areas or narrow hallways.

Cervical Spine Immobilization Collars

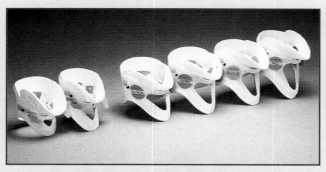

STIFF NECK CERVICAL SPINE IMMOBILIZATION COLLARS *(Laerdal Medical Corporation)*

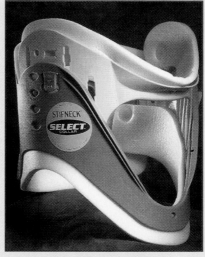

THE STIFNECK® SELECT™ COLLAR—Can be adjusted to fit all sizes *(Laerdal Medical Corporation/John Hill Photography)*

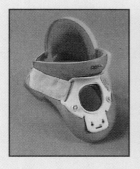

PHILADELPHIA CERVICAL COLLARS—Assembled and disassembled *(Philadelphia® Cervical Collar Co.)*

Sizing a Cervical Spine Immobilization Collar

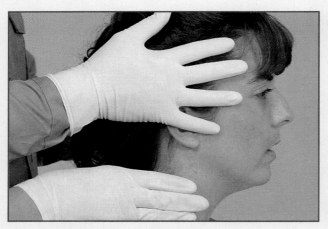

1. To size a cervical spine immobilization collar, first draw an imaginary line across the top of the shoulders and the bottom of the chin. Use your fingers to measure the distance from the shoulder to the chin.

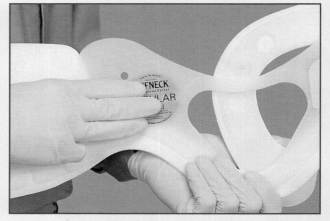

2. Check the collar you select. The distance between the sizing post (black fastener) and lower edge of the rigid plastic should match that of the number of stacked fingers previously measured against the patient's neck.

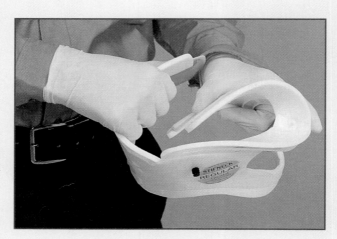

3. Assemble and preform the collar.

Applying a Cervical Spine Immobilization Collar to a Sitting Patient

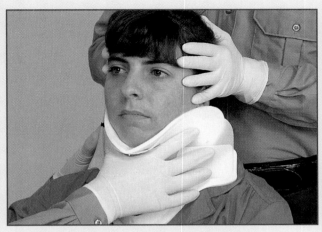

1. After selecting the proper size, slide the cervical spine immobilization collar up the chest wall. The chin must cover the central fastener in the chin piece.

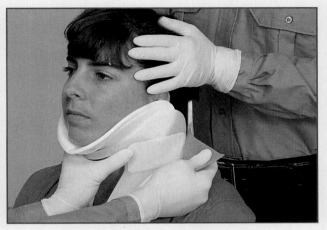

2. Bring the collar around the neck and secure the Velcro. Recheck the position of the patient's head and collar for proper alignment. Make sure the patient's chin covers the central fastener of the chin piece.

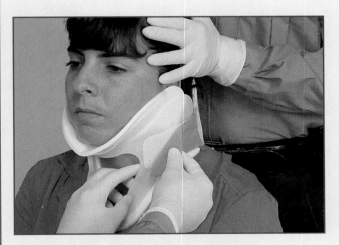

3. If the chin is not covering the fastener of the chin piece, readjust the collar by tightening the Velcro until a proper sizing is obtained. If further tightening will cause hyperextension of the patient's head, then select the next smaller size.

NOTE: With the collar alone in place, there can still be movement of the lower cervical region. Maintain the patient's head in a neutral position.

Applying a Cervical Spine Immobilization Collar to a Supine Patient

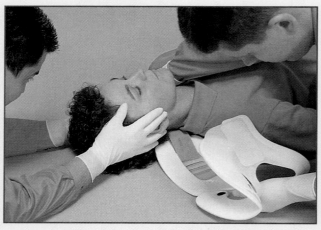

1. Slide the back portion of the cervical spine immobilization collar behind the patient's neck. Fold the loop Velcro inward on the foam padding.

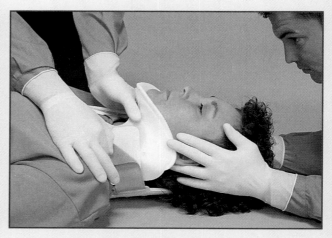

2. Position the collar so that the chin fits properly. Secure the collar by attaching the Velcro.

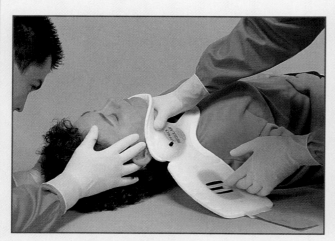

3. An alternative method of applying the collar to a supine patient is to start by positioning the chin piece and then sliding the back portion of the collar behind the patient's neck.

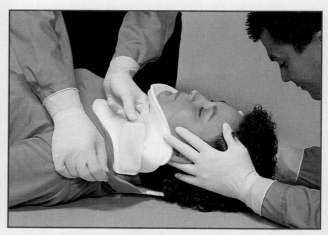

4. Hold the collar in place by grasping the trachea hole. Attach the loop Velcro so it mates with (and is parallel to) the hook Velcro.

Summary

Whenever possible, you should not move a patient. However, if you find it necessary to move a patient, you should use the proper **body mechanics.** This includes positioning your feet properly; using your legs, not your back, to lift; avoiding turns or twists as you lift; keeping your back straight and locked; keeping the weight you are lifting close to your body; and using a stair chair when carrying a patient down the stairs.

Emergency moves are carried out quickly when the scene is hazardous, care of the patient requires repositioning, or you must reach another patient needing lifesaving care. A heavy patient or one who is unconscious or unable to move alone can be removed by using one of the drag methods. Always drag the patient in the direction of the length of the body, keeping the patient's head as low as possible. The use of a drag may also be appropriate where there are possible spinal injuries.

Nonemergency moves can be carried out if factors at the scene are causing the patient to decline, you must reach other patients, part of the care required forces you to move the patient, or the patient insists on being moved and tries to do so alone. Nonemergency moves should be carried out only on conscious patients. You should have completed the initial assessment. The patient should be stable, with normal rates and character for breathing and pulse. There should be no serious bleeding and no signs of spinal injuries. All possible fractures and other painful, swollen, deformed extremity injuries must be immobilized or splinted.

The direct ground lift is a nonemergency move that can be used for patients with no neck or spinal injuries. You should have two, three, or more people to help. The patient must be supported by the head, neck, back, and knees. A helper should control and support the patient above and below the buttocks. Another helper should support the patient's knees and ankles. When moving the patient, you should keep the patient rolled toward your chest.

The extremity lift is a good nonemergency move. This move should not be used if the patient has possible head, neck, or spinal injuries, is unconscious, or has injuries to the upper or lower extremities (including the shoulder and hip). This lift requires two rescuers, with you lifting the patient at the shoulders and your helper lifting the patient at the knees.

Properly position patients depending on their injuries. An unresponsive patient *without* suspected spinal injury should be placed in the recovery position. Conscious patients *without* suspected spinal injuries, such as those with chest pain, nausea, or difficulty breathing, may be placed in a position of comfort, usually a semi-sitting position.

Various devices are available to EMS for use with packaging and loading a patient into the ambulance. These include wheeled, portable, scoop (orthopedic), basket, and flexible stretchers, as well as the stair chair and long and short spinal immobilization devices.

Remember and Consider...

Using poor body mechanics is dangerous not only to you, but to the patient and to your coworkers as well.

✔ Learn and practice proper methods of lifting and moving patients until you are able to perform them effortlessly.

Remember that it is also dangerous to push yourself past your physical limits.

✔ Never hesitate to ask for assistance from other EMS providers if a patient or equipment is too heavy for you to lift alone.

Investigate...

Each EMS system has various types of equipment for packaging and carrying patients.

✔ Find out what kinds of patient carrying devices are used on the ambulances in your community and become proficient in using them.

Study the following scenarios. Place check marks in the columns below as appropriate to indicate the skills you would perform for each scenario. Discuss answers with other students and your instructor.

SCENARIO 1: You are first on the scene of a bicycle accident. A 7-year-old boy, learning to ride his two-wheeler, lost control and crashed into a parked car. He fell to the ground and is being comforted by his mother when you arrive. His mother has removed his helmet, and there are no injuries to his head. The boy is sitting on the curb near his bike and the car, crying and holding his knee, which is bleeding and dripping blood down his leg. He squirms and kicks at you as you try to move his hand so you can see his wound.

SCENARIO 2: Your unit arrives first at the home of Mrs. Maloney, who is an 87-year-old woman with severe arthritis. Her neighbor called 911 because she found Mrs. Maloney still in bed at 10:00 A.M. when she checked on her. Mrs. Maloney is awake and alert, but says her arthritis is really bothering her today and she just doesn't feel like getting up. You notice she is also coughing heavily and is having trouble breathing, but she says she doesn't smoke.

Instructors will demonstrate all skills and will give you time to practice them while they coach you.

NOTE: Demonstrate all lifting and moving skills with a patient and partner of appropriate size to prevent injury to yourself during practice.

Skills	Scenarios	
	#1	**#2**
Body substance isolation (see Chapter 2):		
1. Demonstrate how to put on gloves, using sterile techniques		
2. Demonstrate safe techniques for taking off and disposing of gloves		
3. Demonstrate or describe how and when to use eye/face protection		
Lifting and moving patients (see Chapter 5):		
4. Stabilize a patient's head and spine (sitting, supine, standing)		
5. Partner measures and applies extrication collar (sitting, supine, standing)		
6. Switch positions and perform #4 and #5 above		
See Scan 5-1 for the following skills:		
7. Demonstrate a clothes drag		
8. Demonstrate an incline drag (headfirst)		
9. Demonstrate a shoulder drag		

Skills	Scenarios	
	#1	**#2**
10. Demonstrate a foot drag		
11. Demonstrate a firefighter's drag		
12. Demonstrate a blanket drag		
See Scan 5-2 for the following skills:		
13. Demonstrate a one-rescuer assist		
14. Demonstrate a cradle carry		
15. Demonstrate a pack strap carry		
16. Demonstrate a firefighter's carry		
17. Demonstrate a piggy back carry		
See Scan 5-3 for the following skills:		
18. Demonstrate a two-rescuer assist		
19. Demonstrate a firefighter's carry with assist		
With an appropriate number of partners:		
20. Demonstrate a direct ground carry (Figures 5.1A through 5.1D)		
21. Demonstrate an extremity lift (Figures 5.2A through 5.2C)		
The following moves will require a cot, stretcher, or bed:		
22. Demonstrate a direct carry with a partner (Scan 5-4)		
23. Demonstrate the draw sheet method of a moving a patient (Figures 5.3A and 5.3B)		
24. Log-roll a patient		
25. Place a patient in the recovery position (Figure 5.4)		
The following skills will require a wheeled stretcher:		
26. Demonstrate how to strap and secure a patient		
27. Demonstrate how to raise and collapse the cot		
28. Demonstrate safe methods of patient loading and unloading		

Work with a group of classmates to create scenarios that will use listed skills. Exchange them with other class groups to check your knowledge and to practice your decision-making skills.

AIRWAY MANAGEMENT

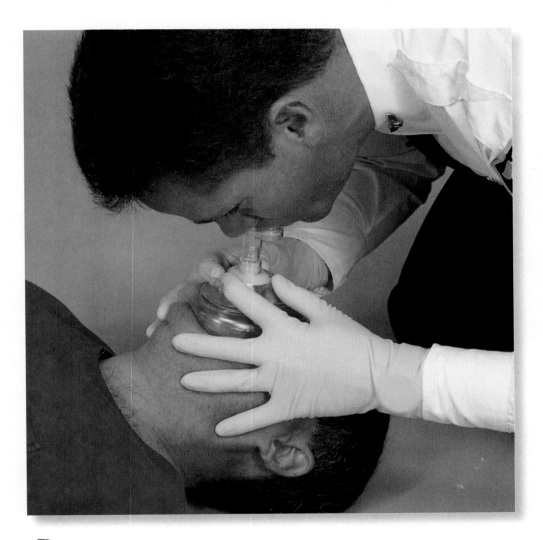

*B*reathing is life, and we take in each life-giving breath through simple passages—our mouth and nose and windpipe. These few important parts of our bodies begin the airway to our lungs. The lungs take in oxygen when we inhale and get rid of waste gases, such as carbon dioxide, when we exhale. Blood that circulates to the lungs from the heart drops off carbon dioxide and picks up oxygen. The heart then pumps this oxygen to the rest of the body. Blood returns to the heart with waste gases, which are pumped to the lungs for exchange with oxygen. This continuous function of breathing and gas exchange is a simple process and something we don't think about—until we can't do it. This chapter will explain the process of breathing and the steps to take for patients who are not breathing or who are having difficulty breathing because of airway obstructions.

National Standard Objectives

This chapter focuses on the objectives of Module 2, Lesson 2–1 of the U.S. DOT First Responder National Standard Curriculum and serves as an instructional aid to help you meet any specific objectives added to the course by your local EMS system.

NOTE: Not all First Responder programs teach the use of breathing aids. This chapter will cover basic techniques for assisted ventilations and for the use of airway adjuncts and suctioning equipment.

By the end of this chapter, you will know how to: (from cognitive or knowledge information) . . .

2–1.1   Name and label the major structures of the respiratory system on a diagram. (p. 92)

2–1.2   List the signs of inadequate breathing. (p. 93)

2–1.3   Describe the steps in the head-tilt, chin-lift. (p. 94)

2–1.4   Relate mechanism of injury to opening the airway. (pp. 94–95, 103–104)

2–1.5   Describe the steps in the jaw thrust. (pp. 94–95)

2–1.6   State the importance of having a suction unit ready for immediate use when providing emergency medical care. (pp. 111–112, 115–116, 120, 125)

2–1.7   Describe the techniques of suctioning. (p. 121)

2–1.8   Describe how to ventilate a patient with a (pocket) resuscitation mask or barrier device. (pp. 96–98)

2–1.9   Describe how ventilating an infant or a child is different from an adult. (pp. 100–101)

2–1.10 List the steps in providing mouth-to-mouth and mouth-to-stoma ventilation. (pp. 98–99, 102–103)

2–1.11 Describe how to measure and insert an oropharyngeal (oral) airway. (pp. 115–117, 118)

2–1.12 Describe how to measure and insert a nasopharyngeal (nasal) airway. (pp. 117, 119)

2–1.13 Describe how to clear a foreign body airway obstruction in a responsive adult. (pp. 107–108, 111)

2–1.14 Describe how to clear a foreign body airway obstruction in a responsive child with complete obstruction or partial airway obstruction and poor air exchange. (pp. 107–109, 111)

2–1.15 Describe how to clear a foreign body airway obstruction in a responsive infant with complete obstruction or partial airway obstruction and poor air exchange. (pp. 106–107, 109–110, 112–113)

2–1.16 Describe how to clear a foreign body airway obstruction in an unresponsive adult. (pp. 107–109, 111–112)

2–1.17 Describe how to clear a foreign body airway obstruction in an unresponsive child. (pp. 107–109, 111–112)

2–1.18 Describe how to clear a foreign body airway obstruction in an unresponsive infant. (pp. 106–107, 109–110, 113–114)

Feel comfortable enough to (by changing attitudes, values, and beliefs) . . .	2–1.19	Explain why basic life-support ventilation and airway protective skills take priority over most other basic life support skills. (pp. 88, 104, 124)
	2–1.20	Demonstrate a caring attitude towards patients with airway problems who request emergency medical services. (pp. 101–104, 106, 111)
	2–1.21	Place the interests of the patient with airway problems as the foremost consideration when making any and all patient care decisions. (pp. 88–89, 94, 100–101, 106)
	2–1.22	Communicate with empathy to patients with airway problems, as well as with family members and friends of the patient. (pp. 101–102, 106)

Show how to (through psychomotor skills) . . .	2–1.23	Demonstrate the steps in the head-tilt, chin-lift. (pp. 94–95)
	2–1.24	Demonstrate the steps in the jaw thrust. (pp. 94–95)
	2–1.25	Demonstrate the techniques of suctioning. (p. 121)
	2–1.26	Demonstrate the steps in mouth-to-mouth ventilation with body substance isolation (barrier shields). (pp. 96–98)
	2–1.27	Demonstrate how to use a (pocket) resuscitation mask to ventilate a patient. (pp. 96–98)
	2–1.28	Demonstrate how to ventilate a patient with a stoma. (pp. 102–103)
	2–1.29	Demonstrate how to measure and insert an oropharyngeal (oral) airway. (pp. 115–117, 118)
	2–1.30	Demonstrate how to measure and insert a nasopharyngeal (nasal) airway. (pp. 117–119)
	2–1.31	Demonstrate how to ventilate infant and child patients. (pp. 100–101)
	2–1.32	Demonstrate how to clear a foreign body airway obstruction in a responsive adult. (pp. 107, 111)
	2–1.33	Demonstrate how to clear a foreign body airway obstruction in a responsive child. (pp. 107, 111)
	2–1.34	Demonstrate how to clear a foreign body airway obstruction in a responsive infant. (pp. 106–107, 112–113)
	2–1.35	Demonstrate how to clear a foreign body airway obstruction in an unresponsive adult. (pp. 107–108, 111–112)
	2–1.36	Demonstrate how to clear a foreign body airway obstruction in an unresponsive child. (pp. 107–108, 111–112)
	2–1.37	Demonstrate how to clear a foreign body airway obstruction in an unresponsive infant. (pp. 106–107, 109–110, 113–114)

⊿EARNING TASKS

Chapter 6 explains the functions of the airway and breathing. As you work through this chapter, you will need to understand why airway and breathing/ventilation is the first and most important step you take in patient care and be able to:

✔ State three reasons why we must breathe to stay alive.

When patients stop breathing, a First Responder only has a few minutes to assist them in starting the breathing process again. But if the delay is too long between no breathing and breathing again, patients will die. Those few minutes are critical, and you need to understand what happens in those few minutes. Be able to:

✔ Explain the difference between clinical death and biological death and the approximate times for each before brain cells begin to die if the patient does not receive oxygen.

When we breathe, pressure inside the lungs changes so that air flows in and out. Breathing in is an active process that requires muscle contractions, but breathing out is a passive process that works as muscles relax. The lungs function by pressure changes similar to blowing up a balloon and allowing it to deflate. Think about that process and be able to:

✔ Relate, in a very general way, changes in volume and pressure in the lungs to the process of breathing.

When First Responders must assist a patient in breathing, sometimes they ventilate with too much pressure and too frequently, so that the exhalation phase is not complete. When this happens, the lungs get overfilled and the extra air has to go somewhere—to the stomach. If that happens, you must notice and know what to do about it:

gastric distention
inflation of the stomach.

✔ State two things to do when air gets in the patient's stomach (**gastric distention**) from assisted ventilations.

As long as we breathe normally, we do not think about it. Sometimes, events or actions cause our airway to become blocked, and it becomes difficult or impossible to breathe. What are the causes? How can you tell if someone is having a problem? What can First Responders do to help? You must be able to:

✔ List five factors that may cause airway obstruction.

✔ List three signs of partial airway obstruction.

✔ State when you should care for a partial airway obstruction as if it were a complete airway obstruction.

✔ Describe two things you will commonly notice about a conscious patient with a complete airway obstruction.

First Responders have enough to remember, think about, and do if someone is not breathing or has an airway obstruction. With practice, all of these steps become automatic and you will perform them with little thought. But in some incidents, you will have to take one more step or precaution to help someone who is not breathing. For trauma incidents, always consider a possible spinal injury and stabilize the head while opening the airway so you do not cause further spinal damage. Be able to explain why and:

✔ Demonstrate the techniques used for patients with possible neck or spinal injuries.

The Occupational Safety and Health Administration (OSHA) and the Centers for Disease Control and Prevention (CDC) guidelines state that EMS personnel can reduce the risk of contracting infectious diseases by using pocket face masks with one-way valves and high-efficiency particulate air (HEPA) filter inserts when ventilating patients. Also wear latex or vinyl gloves during assessment and care of all patients.

BREATHING

WHY WE BREATHE

To maintain life, we breathe. The act of breathing is called **respiration.** During the breathing process, oxygen is brought into the body and carbon dioxide is expelled. The body's cells, tissues, and organs need oxygen for life and energy, and all life processes require energy. The body uses oxygen to produce energy to contract muscles, send nerve impulses, digest food, and build new tissues.

In addition to supplying the cells with oxygen, breathing also removes carbon dioxide from cells. As the body uses oxygen to produce energy, carbon dioxide is given off as a waste product. The process of breathing keeps up a constant exchange of carbon dioxide and oxygen. If breathing is not adequate or if it stops, carbon dioxide accumulates in the body's cells and becomes a deadly poison. An increase in carbon dioxide shows up in certain signs and symptoms: the person will start panting to try to rid the body of the excess carbon dioxide; the person becomes drowsy as brain cells react to excess carbon dioxide; as brain cells start to die, the person may start to hallucinate and lose the ability to make breathing efforts. The individual will become unconscious and, if someone does not assist ventilations, will go into a coma and die.

By regulating the blood and tissue levels of carbon dioxide, the respiratory system plays a key role in keeping a normal acid-base balance. This is measured using the pH scale. A low pH indicates too much acid and may be caused by a buildup of carbon dioxide, as may be seen in respiratory failure. Cells live and function within a very narrow range of pH. If breathing is not adequate or if it fails, this balancing function stops. If our blood pH level goes too far one way or the other on the scale, cells stop functioning and die. The brain is also very sensitive to improper levels of pH balance. Without proper pH, brain functions quickly cease, including those that control breathing.

When breathing stops, the heart will also stop shortly after. This is because the heart is made of muscle cells that require a continuous supply of oxygen to contract. The moment when both heartbeat and respirations have stopped is called **clinical death.** Over the next 4 to 6 minutes, oxygen is depleted and cells begin to die. This is the period when it is critical for the patient to receive oxygen and assisted ventilations. If the patient's cells do not receive oxygen within 10 minutes, they quickly die. The organ affected first, and the most critical one, is the brain. **Biological death** occurs during this 6- to 10-minute time frame (Figure 6.1). A patient is biologically dead when the brain cells die. Clinical death can be reversed. Biological death is irreversible.

respiration the act of breathing; the exchange of oxygen and carbon dioxide that takes place in the lungs.

Note

The process of biological death may be delayed by cold temperatures, especially in cold-water drowning situations. This is because the oxygen-requiring cell functions are profoundly slowed by the cooling of the body. Always perform resuscitation procedures on cold-water drowning victims, even if they have been in the water longer than 10 minutes.

clinical death the moment that breathing and heart actions stop.

biological death when the brain cells die. This is usually within 10 minutes of respiratory arrest.

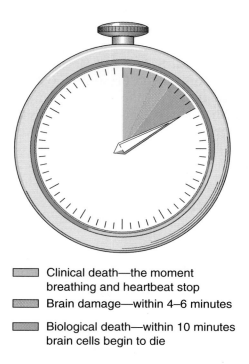

FIGURE 6.1
Without oxygen, brain cells begin to die within 10 minutes. Cell death may begin in as little as 4 minutes..

▭ Clinical death—the moment breathing and heartbeat stop
▭ Brain damage—within 4–6 minutes
▭ Biological death—within 10 minutes brain cells begin to die

How WE BREATHE

Breathing is automatic. Even though you can control depth and rate sometimes, that control is short-term and is soon taken over by involuntary orders from the respiratory centers of the brain. If you try to hold your breath, these centers will urge you to breathe, then take over and force you to breathe. If you try to breathe slow, shallow breaths while running, these centers will automatically adjust the rate and depth of breathing to suit the needs of the body cells. Asleep, or even unconscious, if there is no damage to these respiratory centers and the heart continues to circulate oxygenated blood to the brain, breathing will be an involuntary, automatic function. The needs of your cells, not your will, are the determining factors in the control of breathing.

The lungs are very elastic and expandable. This expansion is limited by the size of the chest cavity and the pressure within the cavity pushing back on the lungs. To inhale air (**inspire**), the size of the chest cavity must increase and the pressure inside the cavity must be reduced. A simple law governs respiration: **as volume increases, pressure decreases** (Figure 6.2).

If you take the air out of a small balloon and place this same amount of air into a larger balloon, the final pressure inside the large balloon will not be as great as it was in the smaller one. Why? The larger balloon has a greater volume to be filled. The air from the small balloon will produce less pressure inside the large one.

First The volume of the chest cavity is increased by muscle contraction. This may sound backwards because contractions usually make things smaller. However, as the muscles between the ribs contract, they pull the front of the ribs upward and force them outward. When the **diaphragm** muscle contracts, it flattens downward and increases the size of the chest cavity above it. These muscle actions make the chest cavity larger and increase its volume. With each inspiration, the volume in the chest cavity increases and causes a decrease in the pressure within the lungs. Figure 6.3 illustrates the breathing process.

When the volume of the chest cavity increases and the pressure within the chest cavity decreases, the lungs will expand automatically. As the lungs

inspire to inhale air.
inspiration the process of breathing in.

diaphragm the dome-shaped muscle that separates the chest and abdominal cavities. It is the major muscle used in breathing.

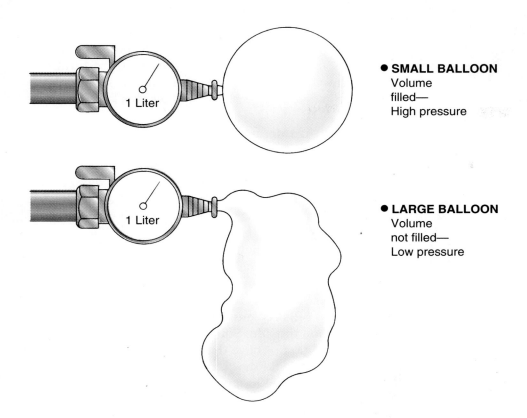

FIGURE 6.2
An equal amount of air delivered to each balloon will not produce the same pressure. An increase in volume means a decrease in pressure.

- **SMALL BALLOON**
  Volume filled—
  High pressure

- **LARGE BALLOON**
  Volume not filled—
  Low pressure

expand, the volume inside each lung increases. This means that the pressure inside each lung will decrease. Air moves from high pressure (atmosphere) to low pressure (lungs). Therefore, when the pressure inside the lungs becomes less than the pressure in the atmosphere, air will rush into the lungs. (A punctured automobile tire demonstrates this fact.) Air will move into the lungs until the air pressure in the lungs equals the air pressure in the atmosphere. Inspiration is an *active* process. Rib and diaphragm muscles contract, causing expansion of the chest cavity.

To exhale air (**expire**), the process is reversed. The diaphragm and the muscles between the ribs relax, which reduces the volume in the chest cavity. In the smaller cavity, pressure builds in the lungs until it becomes greater than the pressure in the atmosphere and we must exhale. Air flows from high pressure (full lungs) to low pressure (atmosphere). Expiration is a *passive* process. Muscles do not have to work to relax and allow air to leave the lungs and return to the atmosphere.

expire to exhale air.
expiration the passive process of breathing out.

INSPIRATIONS AND EXPIRATIONS

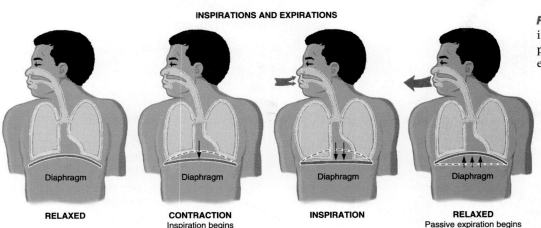

| RELAXED | CONTRACTION Inspiration begins | INSPIRATION | RELAXED Passive expiration begins |

FIGURE 6.3 Changes in volume and pressure produce inspiration and expiration.

Respiratory System Anatomy

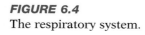 Several important parts of the respiratory system have been discussed: the respiratory centers in the brain and the muscles of respiration, including the diaphragm and those between the ribs. Other major structures of the respiratory system include the following structures of what is known as the upper and lower airway (Figure 6.4):

- *Nose*—the primary path for air to enter and leave the system.
- *Mouth*—the secondary path for air to enter and leave the system.
- *Throat*—an air and food passage, also called **pharynx.**
- *Larynx*—an air passage at the top of the windpipe, also called *voice box*.
- *Bronchial tree*—tubes that branch from the windpipe and take air to the lungs. Its two main branches are the primary bronchi, one for each lung. These branch into secondary bronchi in the lobes of the lungs. The secondary bronchi then branch into bronchioles, many of which have alveoli, microscopic air sacs where the exchange of gases actually takes place.
- *Lungs*—elastic organs containing the bronchioles, small branching air passages in the lungs, and alveoli. These are the small air sacs at the end of the bronchioles where blood cells replenish their oxygen supply and release their accumulated carbon dioxide. Some of the bronchioles are called terminal bronchioles and do not have these microscopic air sacs. They are blind tubes, coming to an end that is closed off. As air enters these terminal bronchioles, it helps the lungs to expand and ensure that the lungs expand their pathways wide enough to allow air to enter deeply into the lungs. This is important since some diseases will harden or close off these terminal bronchioles and reduce the ease of required breathing.
- *Trachea*—an air passage to the lungs below the larynx, also called the *windpipe*.
- *Epiglottis*—a leaf-shaped structure that covers the larynx when we swallow food and fluids and prevents them from entering the windpipe.

pharynx (FAR-inks) the throat.

larynx (LAR-inks) the airway between the throat and the windpipe. It contains the voice box.

trachea (TRAY-ke-ah) the windpipe.

epiglottis (EP-i-GLOT-is) a flap of cartilage and other tissues that is located above the voice box. It helps to close off the airway when a person swallows.

FIGURE 6.4
The respiratory system.

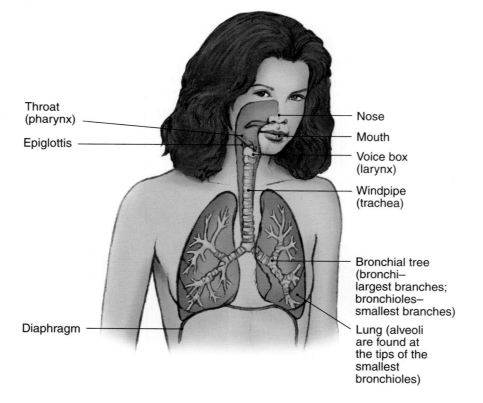

Throat (pharynx)
Epiglottis
Nose
Mouth
Voice box (larynx)
Windpipe (trachea)
Bronchial tree (bronchi–largest branches; bronchioles–smallest branches)
Diaphragm
Lung (alveoli are found at the tips of the smallest bronchioles)

When foreign objects lodge in any part of the airway, or when excess saliva or respiratory secretions accumulate in the mouth and interfere with breathing, they cause an airway obstruction.

The Respiratory Cycle

When our breathing muscles (the diaphragm and those between the ribs) contract and enlarge the chest cavity, oxygen flows through the mouth and nose, into the throat, past the open epiglottis, and into the trachea. Oxygen then flows into the left and right branches of the bronchi, then through the smaller bronchioles to the clusters of alveoli. The alveoli are surrounded by tiny blood vessels called capillaries. Gases—oxygen and carbon dioxide—can easily pass through the thin capillary membranes. Oxygen passes through alveoli to the blood, which delivers it to all body cells. Carbon dioxide passes from the blood cells in the capillaries back to the alveoli and out through the bronchial tree to the mouth or nose.

ASSESSMENT

Signs of Normal Breathing

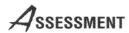 In the initial patient assessment, you approach a patient and form a general impression. (See Chapter 7.) You will find that you can quickly determine if someone is comfortable and breathing normally or if someone is distressed and having trouble breathing. As you approach and when you begin the rest of your initial assessment, you will perform the following steps:

■ **Look** for the even and effortless rise and fall of the chest associated with breathing.
■ **Listen** for air entering and leaving the nose or mouth. The sounds should be quiet like a soft breeze (no gurgling, gasping, wheezing, or other unusual sounds).
■ **Feel** for air moving into and out of the nose or mouth.
■ **Observe** skin color. While every person's skin is a different color, the skin should not be tinted blue, gray, or ashen. Look for signs of these tints especially around the lips and eyes and in the nail beds. These tints will be obvious in these places, regardless of the skin color, if the patient is not ventilating properly.

Signs of Inadequate Breathing

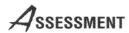 A patient who has **inadequate breathing** will have the following signs and symptoms:

■ No chest movements, or uneven chest movements
■ No air heard or felt at the nose or mouth
■ Noisy breathing or gasping sounds
■ Breathing that is irregular, too rapid, or too slow
■ Breathing that is too shallow or deep and labored, or appears to be an effort, especially in infants and children
■ Breathing that uses muscles in the upper chest and around the neck
■ Nostrils that flare when breathing, especially in children
■ Skin that is tinted blue, gray, or ashen
■ Sitting or leaning forward in a tripod position to make breathing easier

> **Note**
>
> The rate and depth of breathing should be in the normal range while sitting quietly or "at rest": For the adult—12 to 20 breaths per minute; for the child—15 to 30 breaths per minute; for the infant—25 to 50 breaths per minute.

PULMONARY RESUSCITATION

Pulmonary refers to the lungs. *Resuscitation* is any effort to revive or to restore normal breathing function. When you perform **pulmonary resuscitation,** you are providing artificial or *assisted ventilations* to the patient in an attempt to restore the normal delivery of oxygen into the blood and removal of carbon dioxide.

Since you may be providing air to the patient's lungs that has already been in your lungs, you may wonder if you are providing enough oxygen to the patient. The air you exhale still contains oxygen. The atmosphere contains about 21% oxygen. The air exhaled from your lungs into the patient contains almost 16% oxygen. This is more than enough oxygen to keep most patients biologically alive until they can receive supplemental oxygen and care at a hospital.

OPENING THE AIRWAY

As part of the initial assessment, you will make certain that the patient has an open airway and adequate breathing. The simple process of opening the airway will often relieve many problems of partial airway obstruction caused by the tongue. In an unconscious patient, the muscles begin to relax and the tongue, a muscle, will drop into the back of the throat and obstruct the airway (which, by the way, causes snoring when sleeping if the airway is only partially obstructed). If a patient is conscious and is showing signs of obstruction (panicked look and movement and hands at the throat), immediately begin the steps to relieve airway obstructions (discussed later in this chapter).

Repositioning the Head

WARNING:

This procedure is *not* to be used on any patient who has possible injuries to the neck or spine.

First | Simply repositioning the head may be enough to open the airway. If the patient is lying down with his head on several pillows or up against some object and the head is flexed forward, tilt the head back slightly by removing pillows or repositioning him so that the head is not flexed forward. Patients under the influence of alcohol or drugs often have trouble holding a head position that will keep the airway open.

There are two methods of opening the airway. The first, the head-tilt, chin-lift, is used for ill or injured patients with no possibility of spinal injury. The second, the jaw thrust, is used for patients who have a mechanism of injury that indicates possible spinal injury.

Head-tilt, chin-lift Maneuver To perform the head-tilt, chin-lift maneuver, place one hand on the patient's forehead and tilt it back slightly. At the same time, place the fingertips of the other hand under the bony parts of the chin. (Be careful not to compress the soft tissues under the jaw.) Lift up the patient's chin so the lower teeth are almost touching the upper teeth (Figure 6.5). This head-tilt, chin-lift maneuver will move the tongue out of the back of the throat and allow air to flow freely as the patient breathes. This maneuver will also move the neck, which you do not want to do if the patient has a possible spinal injury. In cases in which there may be a spinal injury, use the next maneuver, the jaw thrust.

Jaw-thrust Maneuver This maneuver is the only recommended manual procedure for patients with possible neck or spinal injuries (Figure 6.6). Position yourself at the top of the patient's head. Reach forward and place one hand on

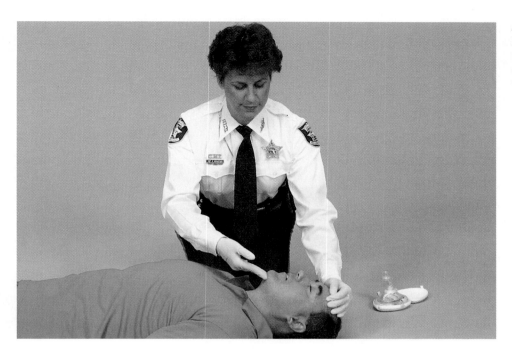

FIGURE 6.5
If there are no spinal injuries, use the head-tilt, chin-lift maneuver to open the airway.

each side of the chin behind the jaw just below the ears. You may press your thumbs against the cheekbones for leverage. Push the jaw forward. Do not tilt or rotate the patient's head.

RESCUE BREATHING

When First Responders perform rescue breathing, they can come into direct contact with the patient's body fluids, such as respiratory secretions and saliva droplets, blood, or vomitus. Take all steps necessary to ensure protection from infectious diseases. Use personal protective equipment and face shields or barrier devices (face masks). The mouth-to-mask method of assisting ventilations prevents the transmission of infectious agents. Your course may include the use of approved face shields and barrier devices that will provide effective assisted ventilations and will prevent direct patient contact.

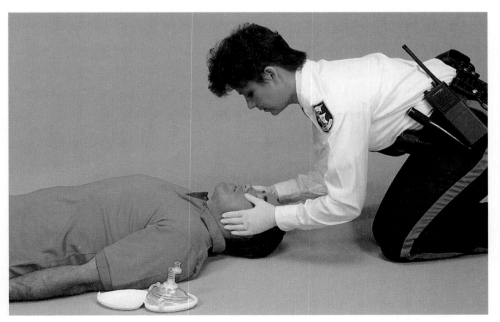

FIGURE 6.6
Use the jaw-thrust maneuver if there are possible neck or spinal injuries.

The mouth-to-mouth and mouth-to-nose methods are also included in this chapter. Citizens learn these methods because they do not normally carry barrier devices, and they would usually perform assisted ventilations on family members. Emergency services personnel would not use these techniques. Remember that gloves should be worn throughout any patient encounters.

Mouth-to-Mask Ventilation

The mouth-to-mask technique is recommended for rescue personnel. A **pocket face mask** or similar barrier device allows you to provide ventilations without direct contact with the patient's mouth and nose. The mask has a one-way valve in the stem so the patient's body fluids cannot reach the rescuer. A disposable filter called a high-efficiency particulate air (HEPA) filter is also available (Figure 6.7). It snaps inside the pocket face mask and traps air droplets and secretions such as those from meningitis and tuberculosis.

The pocket face mask is made of soft plastic materials that can be folded and carried in your pocket. It is available with or without an oxygen inlet. You provide mouth-to-mask ventilations through a chimney on the mask (Figure 6.8). If the mask has a second port for oxygen, you can simultaneously ventilate the patient with air from your own lungs and with additional oxygen from an oxygen source (Figure 6.9).

Another advantage of the pocket face mask is that it allows you to use both hands to maintain the proper head tilt or jaw thrust and still hold the mask firmly in place. It is relatively easy to keep a good seal between the face mask and the patient's face with this device.

The pocket face mask can be used with or without an oropharyngeal or nasopharyngeal airway in place (discussed later in this chapter), but these airway adjuncts (aids) can help First Responders maintain the patient's airway.

First | Use the following steps when you provide mouth-to-mask ventilations (Figure 6.10):

1. Determine if the patient is unresponsive. If you are alone with an adult patient, alert the EMS dispatcher immediately. For a child or an infant, provide one minute of resuscitation first, then call 911.

2. Put on gloves. Position the patient, then position yourself at the patient's head and open the patient's airway.

3. Check for breathing:

   –**Look** for chest movements. Does the chest rise and fall evenly?

   –**Listen** for air flow from the mouth or nose. Are there unusual sounds (gurgling, crowing, snoring)?

   –**Feel** for air exchange against your cheek at the patient's mouth and nose.

   –**Observe** skin color, such as blue, gray, or ashen tints.

   Take at least 3 to 5 seconds to determine if the patient is breathing.

pocket face mask
a device used to help provide mouth-to-mask ventilations. It has a chimney to allow the rescuer to provide breaths without touching the patient. A one-way valve is present in most models to prevent rescuer contact with the patient's blood and body fluids. A HEPA filter can also be inserted to prevent transmission of airborne pathogens. Some masks have an inlet for supplemental oxygen.

FIGURE 6.7
A Pocket face mask parts: one-way valve, mask, HEPA filter.
B Assembled pocket face mask.

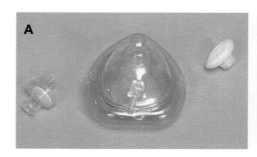
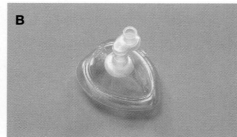

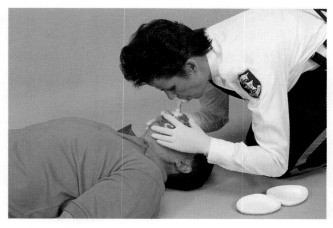

FIGURE 6.8
Mouth-to-mask ventilation through the chimney with a one-way valve.

4. Position the mask on the patient's face so that the apex (upper tip of the triangle) is over the bridge of the patient's nose and the base is between the lower lip and the projection of the chin.

5. Firmly hold the mask in place while keeping the airway open:
    –Place both thumbs and the index fingers on the dome of the mask above and below and close to the chimney. Apply even pressure on both sides of the mask.
    –Place the third and fourth fingers of each hand under each jaw. Lift the jaw forward.

6. Take a deep breath and exhale into the port of the one-way valve attachment on the mask chimney (1.5 to 2.0 seconds for adults; 1.0 to 1.5 seconds for infants and children with a properly sized mask). Watch for the patient's chest to rise.

7. Remove your mouth from the port and allow the patient to exhale. Continue this cycle of providing a breath every 5 seconds for an adult and every 3 seconds for a child or an infant.

If air does not enter on the initial breath, reposition the patient's head, replace the mask, and try again. If air still does not enter, perform the steps for an obstructed airway (explained later).

Dentures can cause an airway obstruction and interfere with your efforts to ventilate a patient. If dentures are secure, leave them in. If they are loose, remove them. It may be difficult to get a good mask-to-face seal when dentures are removed. You will have to make sure you place the mask properly and open the airway appropriately.

> **Note**
> Some guidelines allow adult masks to be inverted for use on children. Make certain that this procedure is approved by your state EMS Medical Directors and that the mask you are using has been approved for this procedure by the manufacturer. Pediatric-sized masks can be used to assist ventilations on patients with stomas.

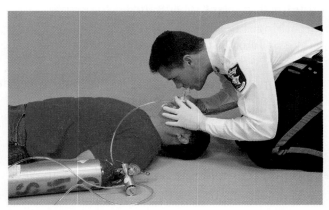

FIGURE 6.9
Providing supplemental oxygen to the patient through the oxygen inlet on the pocket face mask.

FIGURE 6.10
Mouth-to-mask ventilation:
A open the airway; **B** look,
listen, and feel for air
exchange; **C** ventilate as you
watch for the chest to rise;
D allow passive expiration
as you watch for the chest
to fall.

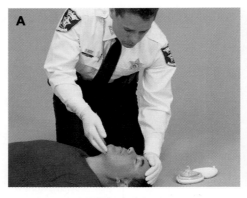

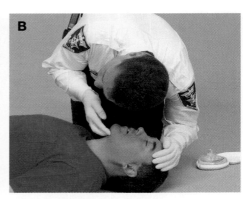

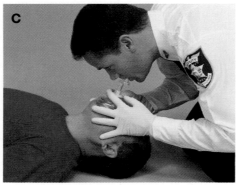

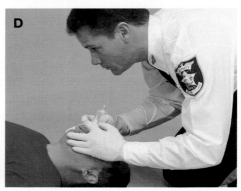

You are providing adequate ventilations to the patient when you:
- See the chest rise and fall with each ventilation.
- Ventilate twelve times a minute for adults and twenty times a minute for infants and children.

Your efforts are inadequate and you must make adjustments when:
- The chest does not rise and fall with each ventilation.
- Your rate is too slow or too fast.
- An inadequate seal is maintained on the mask or air leaks around the mask.

Mouth-to-Mouth Ventilation

Mouth-to-mouth ventilation is a very efficient method of assisting ventilations. It can be done without any special equipment but may expose the rescuer to potentially infectious body fluids.

When performing mouth-to-mouth ventilation, you should:

1. Determine that the patient is unresponsive. Alert the EMS dispatcher before starting resuscitation on an adult patient.

2. Properly position the patient and yourself. Then open the airway with the head-tilt, chin-lift maneuver or jaw-thrust maneuver.

3. Check for breathing: Look, listen, and feel for air exchange and observe skin color. Take **at least 3 to 5 seconds** to determine if the patient is breathing.

4. Keep the airway open as you pinch the nose closed with the thumb and forefinger of the hand on the patient's forehead. (You can use your thumbs or your cheek to seal the nose when performing the jaw-thrust maneuver.)

5. Open your mouth wide and take a deep breath.

6. Place your mouth around the patient's mouth and make a **tight seal** with your lips against the patient's face.

7. Exhale slowly into the patient's airway until you see the chest rise and feel resistance to the flow of your breath. If this first attempt to provide a breath fails, reposition the patient's head or reopen the airway with the jaw-thrust maneuver and try again.

8. Break contact with the mouth to allow the patient to exhale. Quickly take in another deep breath and ventilate the patient again. You will give two initial ventilations.

9. If the patient does not begin breathing again, check for a pulse. If the patient has a pulse but is not breathing, continue with the following steps:

   –Take a deep breath.

   –Seal your mouth around the patient's mouth and ventilate the patient, until you observe the chest rise.

   –Break contact with the mouth and release the pinch on the nose to let the patient exhale while you . . .

   –Turn your head to watch the patient's chest fall and . . .

   –Take a deep breath to begin the cycle again.

Note

If First Responders use automated external defibrilllators (AEDs) in your jurisdiction, prepare the equipment, analyze the patient, and shock if indicated. Follow your local protocol.

Deliver breaths to the adult patient at **one breath every 5 seconds** or at a rate of twelve breaths per minute; to a child or an infant patient at **one breath every 3 seconds** or at a rate of twenty breaths per minute. (Neonatal resuscitation is covered in the CPR chapters.) Every few minutes, stop and check for a carotid pulse. If there is no pulse, begin CPR. If the patient has a pulse, continue pulmonary resuscitation until the patient begins to breathe unaided, until someone trained in mouth-to-mouth techniques can replace you, or until you are too exhausted to continue.

If you are following the correct procedures, and the patient's airway is not obstructed, you should be able to **feel** resistance to your ventilations as the patient's lungs expand, **see** the chest rise and fall, **hear** air leaving the patient's airway as the chest falls, and **feel** air leaving the patient's mouth as the lungs deflate. Monitor the patient to determine if he has begun to breathe unassisted.

IMPORTANT:

Deliver one breath every 5 seconds to adults, one breath every 3 seconds to children and infants.

The most common problems with the mouth-to-mouth technique are:

- Failure to form a tight seal over the patient's mouth (often caused by pushing too hard in an effort to form a tight seal).
- Failure to pinch the nose completely closed.
- Failure to tilt the head back far enough to open the airway.
- Failure to open the patient's mouth wide enough to receive ventilations.
- Failure to deliver enough air during a ventilation.
- Providing breaths too quickly (less than 1.5 to 2.0 seconds per breath for adults and 1.0 to 1.5 seconds for infants and children).
- Failure to clear the airway of obstructions.

Two additional problems, air into the patient's stomach and vomiting, will be covered later in this chapter.

Mouth-to-Nose Ventilation

Patients may have injuries to the mouth and jaw, missing teeth or dentures, and airway obstructions that will make mouth-to-mouth techniques ineffective. For these patients, you will have to use the mouth-to-nose technique. (Depending on the location of the obstruction, mouth-to-nose ventilation may not work if mouth-to-mouth has failed, but it *should* be tried.) Like mouth-to-mouth ventilation, mouth-to-nose ventilation exposes the rescuer to potentially infectious body fluids.

Note

You may use the jaw-thrust maneuver with the mouth-to-nose technique. Seal the patient's mouth with your cheek.

Most of this procedure is the same as mouth-to-mouth: use the head-tilt, chin-lift maneuver or jaw-thrust maneuver to open the airway; give the first two ventilations; give two breaths at the same rates as done for mouth-to-mouth ventilation.

The differences in the mouth-to-nose procedure are that you will:

- Use your thumb to seal the mouth shut. Do *not* pinch the nose.
- Seal your mouth around the patient's nose.
- Deliver ventilations through the nose and be sure to keep the patient's mouth closed.
- Break contact with the nose and open the mouth slightly to allow the patient to exhale. Keep your hand on the patient's forehead to keep the airway open.

Special Patients

Until now, we have been considering adult patients without spinal injuries. As a First Responder, you may have to assist ventilations on other types of patients, including infants and children, elderly patients, neck breathers, and accident victims (some with possible neck and spinal injuries). Some of these conditions are discussed on the following pages.

Infants (Birth to 1 Year) and Children (1 to 8 Years) The airways of infants and children have several physical characteristics that are different from adults. In the infant and child:

- The mouth and nose are much smaller and more easily obstructed than in an adult.
- The tongue takes up more space in the mouth and throat.
- The windpipe is smaller and more easily obstructed by swelling.
- The windpipe is also softer and more flexible and is easily obstructed by opening the airway too far (hyperextension).
- The chest muscles are not as well developed, and the infant and child depend more on the diaphragm for breathing.
- The chest cavity and lung volumes are smaller, so gastric distention occurs more commonly.

It is important to know that respiratory distress and failure lead to cardiac arrest with little chance of survival. The First Responder must recognize and aggressively treat airway and respiratory problems.

 When assisting ventilations for an **infant** (Figure 6.11) or **small child,** you should:

1. Determine if the patient is unresponsive. Make sure you have gloves on. Open airway and check breathing. If the patient is not breathing, give two breaths. If air enters, check pulse. If no pulse, start CPR. If there is a pulse, ventilate for one full minute. Then alert the EMS dispatcher or have someone else call 911. If air does not enter on the initial breath, reposition the head and try again. If air still does not enter, perform the steps for an obstructed airway.

2. Lay the patient on a hard surface.

3. Open the airway with a slight head-tilt, chin-lift maneuver and check for breathing. Keep the infant's airway open by placing the head in the neutral position and the child's airway open by placing the head in the "sniffing position" (tilted slightly back, as when a person sniffs). Use the jaw-thrust maneuver with neck stabilization if you suspect spinal injury.

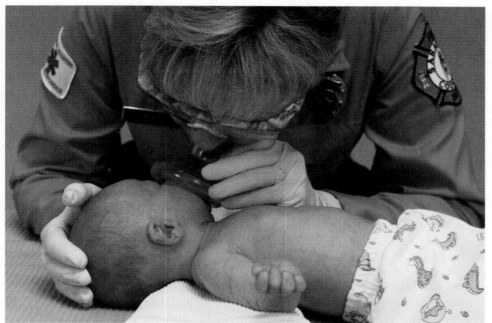

FIGURE 6.11
Ventilating an infant.

4. Position a face mask or other device over the face. If you are not using a barrier device, use the mouth-to-mouth technique for large children and the mouth-to-mouth-and-nose technique (cover both the mouth and nose with your mouth) for infants and small children.

5. Assist ventilations with gentle but adequate breaths. The volume of breath for the infant or child is determined by ventilating until you *see the chest rise*. Be aware of resistance to your breaths and watch for the chest to rise.

6. Break contact to allow the patient to exhale or allow the patient to exhale through the one-way valve of the face mask.

7. Give ventilations at a rate of **one breath every 3 seconds** for infants and children. Take 1.0 to 1.5 seconds per breath.

Terminally Ill Patients Many more terminally ill patients are choosing to spend their remaining time at home with family and friends. Many of these patients enter a hospice program, which supports and advises the patient and family, or make arrangements for advance directives (Do Not Resuscitate, or DNR, orders) with their doctors. For guidelines on how to care for hospice or DNR patients, check your jurisdiction for training programs and follow your local protocols.

Elderly Patients Elderly patients may also require special care because of changes in their bodies that are normal for aging. First, the lungs may have lost some elasticity, and the rib cage may be more rigid and harder for you to expand when assisting ventilations. The jaw joints and neck may be arthritic, which may make it harder to open the airway, but you will be able to get sufficient air in the patient with the usual maneuvers. In the mouth-to-mask method, air will still enter the nose, even if the mouth will not open, but your ventilations may have to be a little more forceful (Figure 6.12). If you are not using a barrier device, you may have to use the mouth-to-nose method instead of mouth-to-mouth to assist ventilations. Patients who have lost their teeth and have not been using dentures have receding chins and sunken cheeks that make the mouth-to-mouth seal impossible. Always be aware of resistance to your ventilations and the rise and fall of the chest.

FIGURE 6.12
Ventilating an elderly
patient.

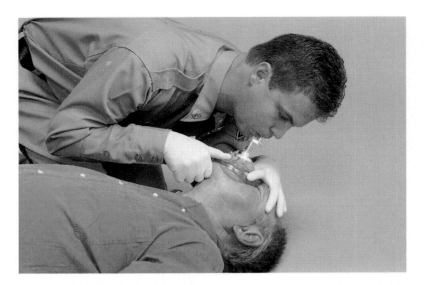

Second, realize that the elderly patient's bones may be more brittle than younger patients. If elderly patients have fallen, they are more likely to suffer spinal injury. When such injuries are possible or when you are in doubt, use the jaw-thrust maneuver in place of the head-tilt, chin-lift maneuver.

Finally, you may be faced with bystanders who say such things as, "He's so old. Let him die in peace." It is not their right to make that decision. You are charged with the responsibility to attempt to assist all patients needing such care, unless direct orders stating otherwise have been given to you by a physician. What bystanders tell you may not be what the patient wants. Any time there is conflict in care priorities, medical direction should be contacted, and the assistance of a physician obtained.

Neck Breathers Some people have had a surgical procedure called a *laryngectomy* to remove part or all of their larynx (voice box). An opening is made outside the throat to the windpipe (trachea) so there is an adequate airway for breathing. These patients now breathe through this opening in the neck (Figure 6.13). This opening, not the mouth or nose, is now the beginning of their airway.

FIGURE 6.13
The neck breather's
airway has been
changed by surgery.

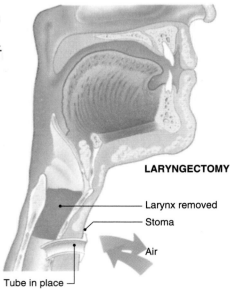

LARYNGECTOMY

Larynx removed

Stoma

Air

Tube in place

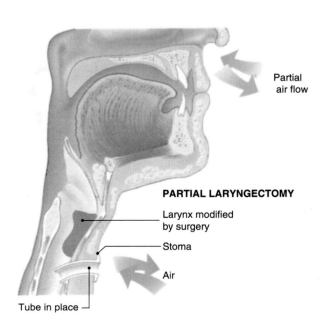

Partial
air flow

PARTIAL LARYNGECTOMY

Larynx modified
by surgery

Stoma

Air

Tube in place

First | The opening in the neck is called a **stoma.** It is usually in the front of the neck, but it may be in the side. Since the patient no longer takes air into the lungs by way of the nose and mouth, you will have to use the mouth-to-mask-to-stoma technique to assist ventilations. Always look to see if there is a stoma. If so, provide artificial ventilation with a face mask or shield. Currently, there is no specific mask for ventilating these patients, but a pediatric (infant's) mask often fits and works well to establish a seal around the stoma. You may also assist ventilations by attaching the bag-valve resuscitator directly to the patient's stoma tube if one is in place in the stoma opening. Protective barrier shields may be used when you assist ventilations by the mouth-to-stoma method. Follow the protocols of your jurisdiction. Remember, direct contact increases the risk of infection.

stoma (STO-mah)
any permanent opening that has been surgically made. The opening in the neck of a neck breather.

When ventilating a stoma patient (Figure 6.14), you should wear gloves and:

1. Keep the patient's head in a neutral or normal position. Do *not* tilt the head.

2. Clean away mucus or encrusted matter from around the neck opening or breathing tube. Do *not* remove the breathing tube.

3. Use the same procedures as you would for mouth-to-mouth or mouth-to-mask resuscitation, except:

    – Do *not* pinch the patient's nose closed.

    – Place the mask or barrier device on the neck over the stoma and breathe through the chimney or one-way valve, or

    – Place your mouth directly over the patient's stoma.

If the chest does not rise, the patient may be a partial neck breather. This means that the patient takes in and expels some air through the mouth and nose. In such cases, you will have to pinch the nose closed, seal the mouth with the palm of your hand, and ventilate through the stoma.

Accident Victims Opening the airway and assisting ventilations are easier for you to perform when the patient is lying down. This means that accident victims who are still in their vehicles must be repositioned. You know that you risk causing further spinal injury if you move them, but you must be realistic. If you wait for other EMS personnel to arrive, or if you take time to put on a rigid cervical collar and secure the patient to a spineboard, the patient will be biologically dead from lack of oxygen to the brain. Airway and breathing are always the first priorities.

Without risking your own safety, reach the victim as quickly as possible. Look, listen, and feel for breathing before moving the patient, even to open the airway. If the patient is breathing, the airway is open and you do not have to move the patient. If you believe the mechanism of injury may have caused damage to the spine or neck and the patient is not breathing, stabilize the head and open the airway with the jaw-thrust maneuver and check for breathing. If

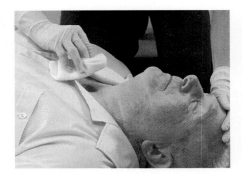
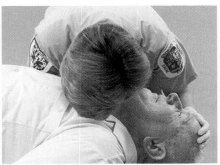

FIGURE 6.14
Use a pediatric-sized pocket face mask for mask-to-stoma ventilations.

the patient is now breathing, keep the airway open maintaining in-line C-spine immobilization and monitor breathing until assistance arrives. If the patient is not breathing and he is in a position where you cannot maintain an airway while you assist ventilations, you will have to reposition him. Your instructor will show you methods to practice so you can reposition a patient with maximum head stabilization and as little spinal movement as possible. One method is to cradle the patient with his neck on your upper arm by wrapping one arm around the top of the head and holding the chin in your hand. Then slide the patient onto his back. If you have help, hold the patient's head and neck in line with the rest of the spine with both of your hands and forearms and work swiftly with your helpers to lay the patient flat.

Air in the Stomach and Vomiting

A common problem of assisted ventilations is that overinflating the lungs will force air into the patient's stomach. Remember to carefully watch the chest rise as you ventilate. It will only rise so far. Don't keep ventilating when it no longer rises any farther. When the chest rises completely, allow the patient to exhale. Forcing more air than the lungs can hold during ventilation may cause or worsen inflation of the stomach. Air in the stomach will cause it to bulge, or distend. This condition is called gastric distention. Watch for distention as you are performing artificial ventilation. Excessive distention will force the patient's diaphragm upward into the chest cavity, which will reduce lung capacity. Reduced chest capacity restricts ventilations and reduces oxygen flow to the body. Gastric distention will cause extra pressure in the stomach, which may cause the patient to vomit. Do not worry about slight bulging, but you will have to make adjustments if you notice extensive bulging. In cases of air in the stomach where you see a noticeable bulge, reduce the force of your ventilations and:

■ Reposition the patient's head to provide a better airway.
■ Be prepared for vomiting. If the patient begins to vomit, turn the patient (not just the head) to one side so the vomitus will flow out of the airway and not back into it. (The vomitus will obstruct the airway and damage the lungs.) Have suction equipment on hand if you carry it on your unit.
■ Stabilize the head and move the patient as a unit if you suspect spinal or neck injuries. If the patient is an unresponsive medical patient with no indication of trauma, place the patient in the recovery position. (Refer to Chapter 5, Figure 5.4; Chapter 8, Figure 8.26; Chapter 10, Scan 10-3; and Chapter 12, Figure 12.41.)
■ Do *not* push in on the stomach to release the air. This may cause vomiting, which may block the airway or enter the lungs. Even if the patient is on his side when he vomits, the vomitus will not simply flow out. Clear the mouth with gauze and finger sweeps with your gloved hand, and/or through suctioning.

AIRWAY OBSTRUCTION

CAUSES OF AIRWAY OBSTRUCTION

First | Many factors can cause the airway to become partially or fully obstructed. In the following list, the first three are upper airway obstructions that you will be able to relieve (Figure 6.15):
■ **Obstruction by the tongue**—the tongue falls back in the throat to block the airway.

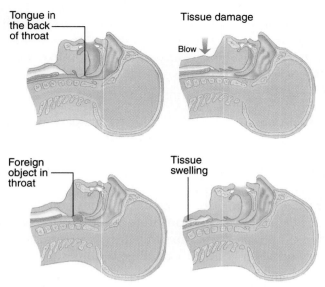

FIGURE 6.15
Four possible causes of airway obstruction.

- **Obstruction by the epiglottis**—the patient attempts to force inspirations when he is having difficulty breathing. This effort may create a negative pressure that can force the epiglottis and perhaps the tongue to block the airway.
- **Foreign objects** (also called mechanical obstruction)—objects and other matter, such as pieces of food, ice, toys, dentures, vomitus, and liquids pooling in the back of the throat, can block the airway.

The following obstructions may be impossible for you to relieve, but you will still attempt to assist ventilations.

- **Tissue damage**—accident-related tissue damage can be caused by punctures to the neck, crush wounds to the neck and face, upper-airway burns from breathing hot air (as in fires), poisons, and severe blows to the neck. The tissues of the throat and windpipe become swollen and make it difficult for air to flow through the airway.
- **Infections**—pharyngeal and epiglottic infections can produce airway obstruction.

A patient who is having difficulty breathing may have only a partial obstruction and may still be able to move some air. Your impulse may be to assist this patient, but in some cases, you will not interfere.

Signs of Partial Airway Obstruction

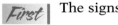 The signs of partial airway obstruction include the following:

- Unusual breathing sounds, such as:
  - *Snoring*—usually caused by the tongue partially or intermittently obstructing the back of the throat.
  - *Gurgling*—usually caused by fluids or blood in the airway or by a foreign object in the windpipe that will stimulate excess fluids in order to try and dislodge it.
  - *Crowing*—usually caused by spasms of the larynx (voice box).
  - *Wheezing*—usually due to swelling or spasms along the lower airway but does not always mean there is an airway problem; wheezing may sound serious but is not usually associated with airway obstruction.
  - *Stridor*—usually caused by a blockage in the throat or larynx (voice box) and typically heard when the patient inhales.

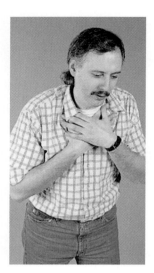

FIGURE 6.16
A distress signal for choking.

■ Breathing is present, but skin is blue, gray, or ashen at the lips, earlobes, fingernail beds, or tongue. The usual presentation in an awake patient is fear and panic. Nothing invokes terror in a person like a threatened airway or the inability to breathe.

■ Breathing keeps changing from normal to labored.

If a conscious patient has some air exchange with a partial airway obstruction, encourage the patient to cough. A forceful cough indicates that enough air is being exchanged. Encourage the patient to continue coughing so that any foreign materials may be dislodged and expelled. Do not interfere with the patient's efforts to clear the airway.

If the patient has poor air exchange and cannot cough or can only cough weakly, begin care as if there is a **complete airway obstruction.** (Care steps will follow later in the chapter.) Do the same if the patient has poor air exchange at first assessment or when good air exchange becomes poor air exchange.

Signs of Complete Airway Obstruction

When the airway is completely obstructed, the conscious patient will try to speak and cough but will not be able to. The patient will often grasp the neck and open the mouth widely, which is a universal sign that indicates an inability to breathe (Figure 6.16). The unconscious patient will not have any of the typical chest movements or the other signs of good air exchange.

CORRECTING UPPER AIRWAY OBSTRUCTION—FOREIGN BODY

When a patient shows the universal sign of airway obstruction, move swiftly to clear the airway. When the patient is unconscious, quickly take appropriate actions to determine if there is an airway obstruction and clear the airway. Since so many cases of airway obstruction are caused by relaxation of the tongue, always make certain that the airway is open using manual maneuvers. Once this has been done, move on to the recommended maneuvers to clear obstructions from the airway. Perform the following steps for the patients listed:

Back Blows for Infants

Back blows create a pressure in the chest that helps to dislodge an obstruction. Use backblows only on infants.

First | For an infant with a complete airway obstruction, you will:

1. Support the infant, face down, on your forearm (Figure 6.17). Use your hand to support the infant's jaw and chest. You can assure better patient support if you are seated or kneeling and resting your forearm on your thighs. Keep the infant's head lower than the chest.

WARNING:

Back blows are recommended for infants who have complete airway obstructions. Do not use this procedure on children and adults.

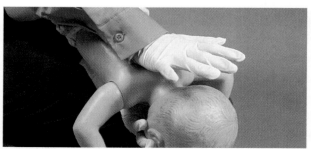

FIGURE 6.17
Support the infant, face down, on your forearm.

2. Use the heel of your other hand to deliver five sharp rapid blows to the midline of the infant's back between the shoulder blades.

Do *not* place the infant or very small child into this head-down position if he has a partial airway obstruction and you observe that he is breathing adequately or coughing to clear the airway.

Abdominal Thrusts for Adults and Children

To perform abdominal thrusts, press into the abdomen just below the rib cage with your fists. This forceful thrust will create a pressure that causes an artificial cough. The cough pushes trapped air in the lungs upward through the airway, which can dislodge the obstruction.

If the patient with an airway obstruction is **conscious** and is standing or sitting:

1. Position yourself behind the patient.

2. Slide your arms under the patient's armpits and wrap them around the patient's waist (Figure 6.18).

3. Make a fist and place the thumb side against the midline of the abdomen, just above the navel. Keep your fist below the rib cage and avoid the area just below the breastbone (sternum) at the level of the xiphoid process.

4. Grasp your fist with your free hand and apply pressure as an inward and upward thrust. Deliver separate rapid inward and upward thrusts. Repeat them until the airway is cleared or the patient becomes unconscious.

If the patient with an airway obstruction is **unconscious** or **becomes unconscious,** you will (Scan 6-1):

1. Place the patient on his back.

2. Kneel and straddle the patient's hips. This position helps you deliver effective, abdominal thrusts.

3. Place the heel of one hand on the abdomen at the midline between the navel and the rib cage. Your fingers should point toward the patient's chest. Keep your hand below the patient's rib cage and avoid the area just below the breastbone.

4. Place your free hand over the positioned hand.

5. Press your hands inward and upward toward the diaphragm. Deliver **five rapid abdominal thrusts.**

> **WARNING:**
> Do *not* practice abdominal thrusts on your classmates or any other person. While this procedure must be practiced so you learn to perform the important steps, it can be dangerous when performed on a conscious, healthy person. Practice only on the manikins that are provided by your instructor.

> *N*ote
> If the patient is very large or if you are small, you can deliver effective thrusts if you straddle one leg of the patient. For the child patient (under 8 years), you may kneel at the child's feet or place the child on a table and stand at his feet.

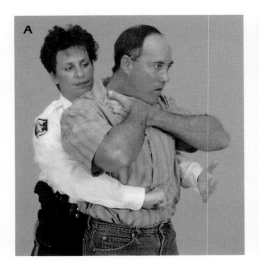
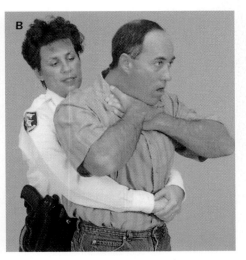

FIGURE 6.18
Correct positioning is important for delivering abdominal thrusts.

Clearing the Airway—
Unconscious Adults and Children

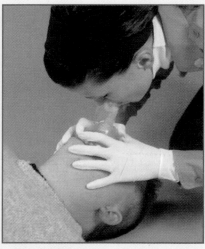

1. Open the airway. Look, listen, and feel for breathing. Attempt to ventilate.

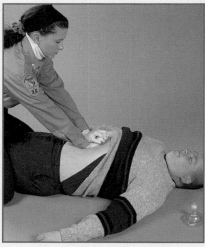

2. If ventilations are unsuccessful, reposition the head and attempt to ventilate again. If there is an obstruction, deliver abdominal thrusts.

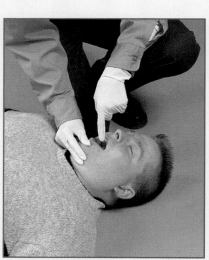

3. Open the mouth and look for foreign bodies. If you see an object, use a finger sweep to clear the mouth.

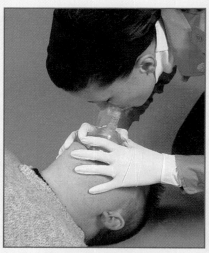

4. Attempt ventilations again and, if necessary, repeat the sequence of abdominal thrusts, finger sweeps, and ventilations.

Do *not* use this procedure on infants and very small children. Internal organs can be damaged if abdominal thrusts are used on infants or very small children. This technique may rupture or lacerate the liver, lungs, and heart, or internally damage the heart. It may also break ribs. The American Heart Association (AHA) does not recommend abdominal thrusts for infants.

Chest Thrusts for Special Patients

Chest thrusts also create a pressure or artificial cough in the chest that can dislodge an obstruction. Use the chest-thrust technique in place of abdominal thrusts when the patient is an infant, a very small child, or pregnant. You may also use it on patients who are so large that you cannot wrap your arms around the waist.

To use the chest thrust technique on an adult patient or a pregnant patient who is standing or seated (Figure 6.19), you will:

1. Position yourself behind the patient and slide your arms under the armpits so that you can encircle the chest with your arms.
2. Form a fist with one hand and place the thumb side on the breastbone about two or three finger-widths above the lower tip.
3. Grasp your fist with your free hand and deliver **distinct thrusts** directly *backward* until the object is expelled or the patient loses consciousness. Do not deliver thrusts in an upward or downward direction or off to one side.

First | If you must perform chest thrusts on a very large adult or a pregnant patient who is lying down (Figure 6.20) and you cannot straddle the hips or one leg, you should:
1. Kneel beside the patient's chest.
2. Place the heel of one hand on the midline of the breastbone, two to three finger-widths from the lower tip. Lift and spread your fingers so that they will not apply pressure on the ribs.
3. Place your free hand on top of this hand.
4. Lean forward until your shoulders are directly over the midline of the patient's chest.
5. Deliver **distinct thrusts** in a downward direction, applying enough force to compress the chest cavity. Continue until the object is expelled or the patient loses consciousness.

If you perform chest thrusts on an infant (Figure 6.21), you will:
1. Support the infant, face down and head lower than body, on your forearm and deliver five back blows.
2. Sandwich the infant between your arms and then turn the infant over to

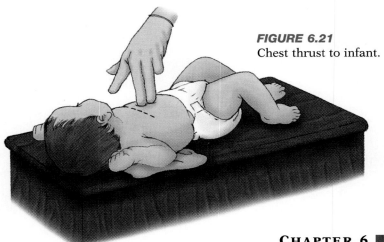

FIGURE 6.21
Chest thrust to infant.

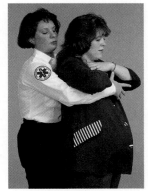

FIGURE 6.19
Chest thrust to an obese or pregnant patient.

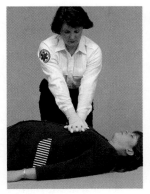

FIGURE 6.20
Chest thrust to a supine obese or pregnant patient.

> **WARNING:**
> Do *not* use abdominal thrusts on infants or very small children.

> ***N*ote**
> If the chest thrust is done on a child, use one hand to apply the compressions while kneeling at the child's side.

*N*ote

Finger sweeps may dislodge dentures. If this happens, remove them from the patient's mouth; don't attempt to replace them.

a face-up position on your thigh. Support the head as you turn the infant. Keep the head lower than the trunk and apply **five slow distinct** chest thrusts, using the tips of two or three fingers. Press along the midline of the breastbone, one finger-width below an imaginary line drawn directly between the nipples.

Finger Sweeps

The finger sweep is the next step in clearing the airway. You will only perform finger sweeps if you can see the object in the mouth.

You can use your fingers to remove a foreign object from a patient's airway once the object is dislodged or partially dislodged (Figure 6.22). Be sure you do not force the object back down the patient's throat when you use the finger sweep. When you use finger sweeps to clear an object from the patient's airway, you will:

1. Place the patient on his back.
2. Use one hand to steady the forehead and tilt it back slightly. This should open the mouth just far enough for you to place the thumb of the other hand against the patient's lower teeth and the index finger against the upper teeth.
3. Open the patient's mouth by crossing your thumb and index finger (crossed-finger technique). Once the mouth is open, grasp the lower jaw and tongue and lift it slightly. This is known as the "tongue-jaw lift" (Figure 6.23).
4. Look into the mouth. If you see the object, use your finger to sweep any foreign materials that you see from the mouth. You may have to turn the patient's head to one side to help clear the mouth. *When you use this technique on infants and children, use your little finger.* Remember, their airways are smaller and their tissues more delicate. Do not attempt to sweep the mouth if you do not see an object. Sweeping without first looking is called "blind" finger sweeps. If you do not see an object, there is nothing to sweep.

A conscious person has a gag reflex. Probing the mouth with your finger may cause vomiting. The patient may vomit and inhale this vomitus into the lungs. *Use the finger sweep technique only on unconscious patients.*

FIGURE 6.22
A Open the mouth with the crossed-finger technique.
B Then use a finger sweep to remove foreign objects.

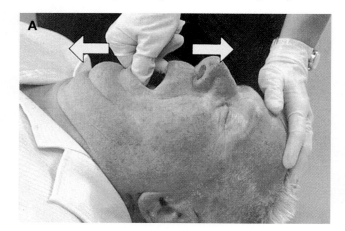
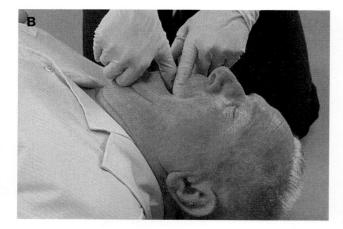

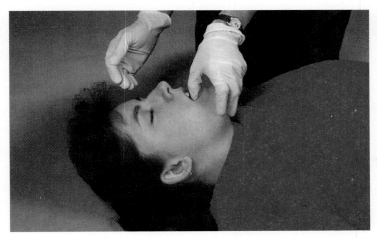

FIGURE 6.23
Tongue-jaw lift.

CORRECTING AIRWAY OBSTRUCTIONS—COMBINED PROCEDURES

The American Heart Association (AHA) has researched the proper techniques to be used in cases of partial and full airway obstruction. As part of their Basic Cardiac Life Support Program, the AHA has shown that a specific sequence of actions will provide the rescuer with the greatest chance of clearing the patient's airway. EMS systems recognize the procedures set by the AHA and recommend the same **combined procedure sequence.**

Procedures used to clear the airway are considered effective if any of the following happens:

- The patient shows good air exchange or spontaneous breathing.
- The patient regains consciousness.
- Skin color improves.
- The foreign object is expelled from the mouth.
- The foreign object is expelled into the mouth where it is visible to the rescuer and can be removed.

First | ADULT OR CHILD—CONSCIOUS

1. Determine that there is **complete obstruction** or a partial obstruction with poor air exchange. Ask, "Are you choking?" or "Can you speak?" Look and listen for signs of complete obstruction or poor air exchange. Tell the patient you will help.
2. Position yourself to give up to five abdominal thrusts in rapid succession (or chest thrusts on a pregnant or obese patient, infant, or very small child). If the patient's airway remains obstructed . . .
3. Repeat the thrusts until the airway is cleared or until the patient loses consciousness.

First | ADULT OR CHILD—LOSES CONSCIOUSNESS

1. Help the patient to the ground to prevent injury from falling and position him on his back. Make sure your gloves are on.
2. Quickly alert EMS dispatch at once if the patient is an adult. If the patient is a child or an infant, alert dispatch after giving one minute of ventilation if the obstruction is cleared quickly; or call EMS if the obstruction is not cleared and attempts to ventilate are not successful.

3. Use the tongue-jaw lift to open the mouth. Look for the object and perform finger sweeps only if you see the object.

4. Open the patient's airway by the head-tilt, chin-lift maneuver for the adult. Use a slight head-tilt with chin-lift for the child.

5. Attempt to give **two ventilations**. If your attempt to ventilate fails, reposition the head and attempt to ventilate again. If this fails . . .

6. Perform **five abdominal thrusts** in rapid succession.

7. Check the mouth for foreign bodies and finger sweep. If you cannot find and remove the obstruction . . .

8. Open the airway and repeat your attempt to ventilate the patient. If this fails . . .

9. Repeat the sequence of:
   – Repositioning and attempting ventilations
   – Providing abdominal thrusts
   – Looking for objects and performing finger sweeps
   – Attempting to ventilate

Continue these efforts until the obstruction is cleared. Even if you can do no more than partially dislodge the obstruction, you will be able to provide some air exchange.

First | *A*DULT OR CHILD—UNCONSCIOUS

1. Check to see if the patient is unresponsive. Make sure your gloves are on. Alert EMS dispatch at once for an adult patient. If the patient is a child, alert EMS after giving one minute of ventilation if the obstruction is cleared quickly, or call EMS if the obstruction is not cleared and attempts to ventilate are not successful.

2. Open the airway.

3. Attempt to give the patient **two adequate ventilations.** If you are not successful . . .

4. Reposition the patient's head and repeat your attempt to ventilate the patient. If you are not successful . . .

5. Deliver **five abdominal thrusts,** then check the mouth for the object. Finger sweep if you see the object. If these procedures fail . . .

6. Attempt to ventilate and repeat the sequence: reposition and attempt ventilations, provide abdominal thrusts, perform finger sweeps, and attempt to ventilate until successful.

Chest thrusts must be used for infants, obese patients, and women in the later stages of pregnancy.

First | *I*NFANT—CONSCIOUS

1. Assess the breathing to make certain that the problem is due to an airway obstruction. If you are working alone, call for help.

2. Support the infant's head as you place the infant face down on your forearm. Use your thigh to support your forearm. Remember to keep the infant's head lower than the trunk.

3. Rapidly deliver **five back blows.** If this fails . . .

4. Support the infant's head and sandwich him between your arms. Turn the infant over onto his back and keep the head lower than the trunk. Use your thigh to support your forearm.

REMEMBER:

Chest thrusts must be used for infants, obese patients, and women in the later stages of pregnancy.

5. Deliver **five chest thrusts** with the tips of two or three fingers along the midline of the breastbone. Place the index finger one finger-width below an imaginary line between the nipples and the middle finger below it on the sternum.

6. Continue with the sequence of back blows and chest thrusts until the object is expelled or the infant loses consciousness. ◢

First | **I**NFANT—LOSES CONSCIOUSNESS (SCAN 6-2)

1. Make sure your gloves are on. Give one minute of ventilations if the obstruction is quickly cleared, then alert the EMS dispatcher. Call dispatch if the obstruction is not cleared quickly and attempts to ventilate are not successful.

2. Place the infant on his back and open the mouth with the tongue-jaw lift. Look in the mouth. If you see the object, use your little finger to sweep the mouth.

3. Open the airway and attempt to ventilate. If this fails, reposition the head and attempt to ventilate again. If unsuccessful . . .

4. Deliver **five back blows.** If this fails . . .

5. Deliver **five chest thrusts.**

6. Use the tongue-jaw lift and look for and remove any visible foreign objects.

7. Reattempt to ventilate. If this fails . . .

8. Continue the sequence of back blows, chest thrusts, finger sweep of visible foreign object, and attempts to ventilate; reposition and attempt to ventilate again until you are successful. ◢

First | **I**NFANT—UNCONSCIOUS

1. Establish unresponsiveness by tapping or shaking the infant's foot. Make sure your gloves are on. When working alone, give one minute of ventilation, then alert the EMS dispatcher.

2. Position the infant on his back on a flat surface or on your forearm. Be sure to support the infant's head.

3. Open the airway.

4. Attempt to ventilate. If this fails . . .

5. Reposition the infant's head and attempt to ventilate again. If this fails . . .

6. Support the infant's head and place him face down on your forearm. Support your forearm with your thigh and keep the infant's head lower than his trunk. Deliver **five back blows.** If this fails . . .

7. Sandwich the patient between your arms, and place him in a face-up position on your thigh. Deliver **five chest thrusts.** If this fails . . .

8. Use the tongue-jaw lift and remove any visible foreign objects.

9. Open the airway and attempt to ventilate. If this fails, reposition the head and attempt to ventilate again. If this fails . . .

10. Repeat the sequence of:
    – Five back blows
    – Five chest thrusts
    – Looking for and removing visible foreign objects and
    – Attempt to ventilate, reposition, and attempt to ventilate again until you are successful. ◢

If the infant is in respiratory arrest and you have cleared the airway enough to provide adequate ventilations, deliver two breaths and check for heart action to see if CPR must be started (see Chapter 8).

Clearing the Airway—Unconscious Infants

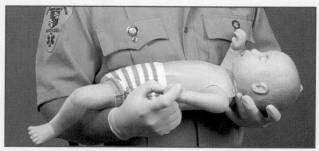

1. Determine unresponsiveness. Position the patient.

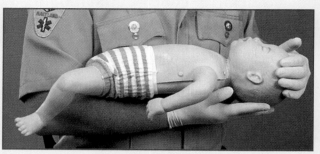

2. Open the airway. Establish breathlessness.

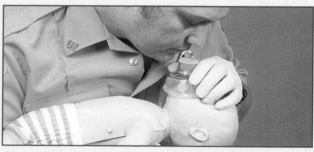

3. Attempt to ventilate. If this fails, reposition the patient's head and try again.

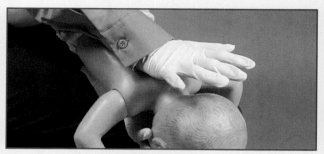

4. Deliver five back blows.

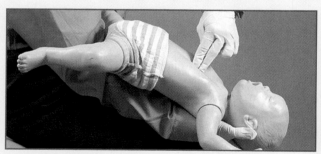

5. Deliver five chest thrusts.

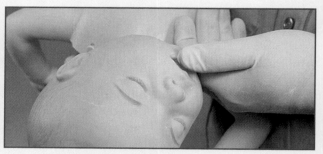

6. Look for and remove visible objects with a finger sweep.

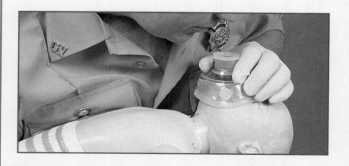

7. Attempt to ventilate again and, if necessary, repeat the sequence of back blows, abdominal thrusts, removing visible objects, and ventilations.

AIDS TO RESUSCITATION

Note

EMS personnel use many types of equipment and special techniques to care for patients with airway and breathing problems. *All of this equipment and these techniques require special supervised training and practice to learn and maintain these skills.*

Some jurisdictions and agencies do not require First Responders to use special equipment for breathing and circulation. This section is provided for First Responders who must learn such skills to meet the requirements of their EMS agency. These skills must be learned and practiced on manikins under your instructor's supervision. The pocket face mask with one-way valve and HEPA filter were covered earlier in this chapter. Students who are training to use the bag-valve-mask ventilator and provide oxygen therapy should refer to Appendix 2.

INTRODUCTION

The use of rather simple but special adjunct equipment can help First Responders provide more effective respiratory and circulatory resuscitation. The EMS system uses a variety of respiratory and circulatory support equipment, much of which is considered to be part of advanced life support and is beyond the scope of First Responder training courses. But three pieces of adjunct equipment are commonly taught in First Responder programs. These devices are the two types of airways—the **oropharyngeal airway,** and the **nasopharyngeal airway**—and the pocket face mask discussed earlier in this chapter.

The advantages of using these pieces of adjunct equipment include:
- They help the rescuer maintain an open airway for the patient.
- They allow the rescuer to deliver more effective ventilations.
- The pocket face mask is an important piece of personal protective equipment that acts as a barrier device for infection control.

One disadvantage of all adjunct equipment is that it can delay the beginning of resuscitation if it is not readily available. *Never* delay the start of ventilations or cardiopulmonary resuscitation while you try to find, retrieve, or set up adjunct airway equipment. Your pocket face mask, even airways, should always be as handy as your latex or rubber gloves.

Another disadvantage of some adjunct equipment is that it must be maintained and kept in working order. Unless cared for properly, adjunct devices can fail to function. Always dispose of nonreusable patient care items or thoroughly disinfect all reusable adjunct equipment after each use.

oropharyngeal (or-o-fah-RIN-je-al) airway a curved breathing tube inserted into the patient's mouth. It will hold the base of the tongue forward.

nasopharyngeal (na-zo-fah-RIN-je-al) airway a flexible plastic tube that is lubricated and then inserted into a patient's nose down to the level of the nasopharynx (back of the throat) to allow for an open upper airway. Supplemental oxygen may be delivered through this tube.

OROPHARYNGEAL AIRWAYS

"Oro" refers to the mouth. "Pharyngeo" refers to the throat. An oropharyngeal airway is a device, usually made of plastic, that can be inserted into the patient's mouth and into the back of the throat. It helps to maintain an open airway for breathing or resuscitation.

Once a patient's airway is open, an oropharyngeal airway can be inserted to help keep it open. The device has a flange that fits against the patient's lips. The rest of the airway holds down the patient's tongue and curves back into the throat.

Use oropharyngeal airways only on **unconscious** patients who do not have a gag reflex. These devices can stimulate the gag reflex and cause vomiting in patients who are not unconscious. If the patient vomits, he can aspirate or breathe the vomitus back into the lungs, a serious complication. Oropharyngeal airways also can cause spasms along the airway of a conscious or semiconscious patient. If the patient is responsive, even if disoriented or confused,

WARNING:

Do *not* use oropharyngeal airways on conscious patients or on unconscious patients who have a gag reflex.

do *not* insert an oropharyngeal airway. Do not continue to insert or leave the airway in the patient's mouth if you meet any resistance or if the patient begins to gag as you insert it.

If you carry a suction unit and are trained to use it, have it ready for any patient who is unconscious and may need an airway. *Follow your local guidelines for using airways.*

Rules for Using the Oropharyngeal Airway

1. Open the patient's airway first. Insertion of an oropharyngeal airway does not replace this step.

2. Use only on unconscious patients with no gag reflex. If the patient gags, do not use the airway.

3. When inserting the airway, take care not to push the patient's tongue back into the throat.

4. While inserting the airway, listen for gagging. Remove the device immediately if the patient begins to gag.

5. Once the airway is in place, continue to monitor the patient's airway. If the patient regains consciousness, he may attempt to remove, displace, or cough up the airway; you must be ready to assist or remove it. Continue to monitor respiration.

Measuring the Oropharyngeal Airway

There are numerous standardized sizes of oropharyngeal airways designed to fit infants, children, and adults (Figure 6.24). To use this device effectively, you must be able to select the correct size for the patient. An airway that is the proper size will extend from the center of the patient's mouth to the angle of the jaw bone (mandible). Before using an airway, hold the device against the patient's face and measure to see if it extends from the center of the mouth to the angle of the lower jaw (Scan 6-3-1). The airway also may be sized by holding it at the corner of the patient's mouth and seeing if it will extend to the tip of the earlobe on the same side of the face. If the airway is not the correct size, do not use it on the patient; select another airway and remeasure to check correct size before inserting.

Sometimes it is difficult to find the correct size oropharyngeal airway for a patient. If the airway is too long, it might become displaced by muscular action and block the airway. If the device is too short, it will curve into the tongue instead of into the back of the throat, and it may also block the airway. The device must be the correct size to be used.

FIGURE 6.24
Various sizes of oropharyngeal airways.

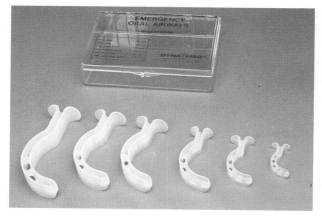

Inserting the Oropharyngeal Airway

See Scan 6-3 for the steps for measuring and inserting an oropharyngeal airway. To insert an oropharyngeal airway, you should:

1. Have mask ready and don latex or vinyl gloves.
2. Remove dentures or partial plates if present.
3. Place the patient on his back, and open the airway manually; measure an airway.
4. Cross your thumb and forefinger and then scissor open the patient's mouth at the corner; or pull down on the chin with your thumb.
5. Position the airway so that its tip is pointing toward the roof of the patient's mouth.
6. Insert the airway and slide it along the roof of the patient's mouth, past the uvula (the soft tissue hanging down at the back of the mouth). Be certain not to push the tongue back into the throat.
7. Rotate the airway 180 degrees (one-half turn) until the tip is pointing down the patient's throat.
8. Keep the airway open. Check to see that the flange of the airway is against the patient's lips. If the airway is too long, it will keep slipping out of the mouth and the flange will not rest on the patient's lips; if the airway is too short, the patient's mouth may remain slightly open in an awkward position. Remove and replace a too-long or too-short airway with one of the correct size.
9. Ventilate the patient with the mouth-to-mask technique.

To insert the oropharyngeal airway in an infant or a child, alter the above steps slightly. *For infants and children, grasp the tongue gently and pull it forward before inserting the airway. Then, insert the oropharyngeal airway with the tip pointing toward the tongue and throat, in the same position it will be in after insertion* (Figure 6.25), *rather than upside down.* The airway is inserted in this way because the infant's and child's mouth is smaller and the upper portion of the oral cavity is more easily injured than the adult's. Turning the airway may damage the mouth tissues.

The oropharyngeal airway is an adjunct; head position still must be maintained.

NASOPHARYNGEAL AIRWAYS

The nasopharyngeal airway is being used more frequently because it is easy to insert, it does not stimulate a gag reflex, it does not have to be removed if the patient becomes conscious or starts breathing, and it is more comfortable for the patient. It is a soft, flexible tube that is inserted through the nose rather than in the mouth. It is easy to insert because you do not have to reposition the patient's head and pry open the mouth. If there is any injury to the mouth, teeth, or oral cavity, the nasopharyngeal device will still allow you to provide an open airway for the patient. The only precaution is for patients with possible skull or facial fracture. If there is any indication of head or mid-face (including nasal) injury or the mechanism of injury suggests either or both, do not insert the nasopharyngeal airway.

Inserting the Nasopharyngeal Airway

To insert a nasopharyngeal airway, you should (Figure 6.26):

1. Don gloves and have mask ready.

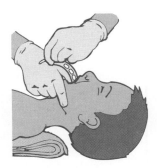

FIGURE 6.25
Unlike insertion for adults, the oropharyngeal airway for infants and children is inserted in the same position it will be in after insertion.

Inserting an Oropharyngeal Airway

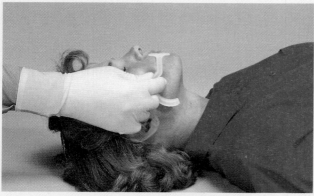

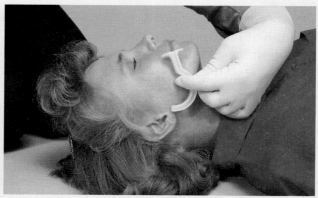

1. Select an oropharyngeal airway. One way to measure is from the center of the mouth to the angle of the lower jaw.

2. Another way to measure is from the corner of the mouth to the tip of the earlobe.

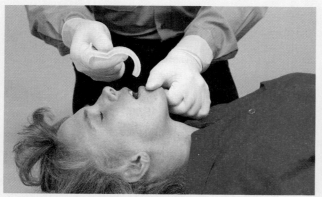

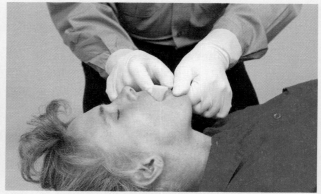

3. Insert the airway, with the tip pointing to the roof of the patient's mouth.

4. Rotate the airway into position.
NOTE: Never practice the use of airways on anyone. Manikins should be used for developing airway skills.

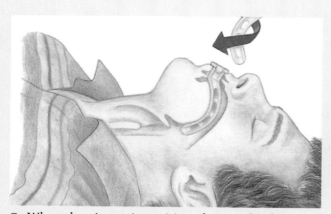

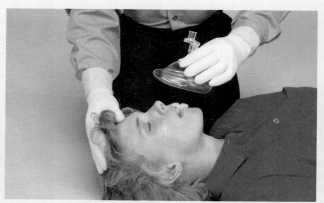

5. When the airway is positioned properly, the flange rests against the patient's lips.

6. The patient is ready for ventilation.

2. Select the largest nasopharyngeal airway that will fit into the patient's nostril without force. The size can be compared to the patient's little finger. Length is not critical but it should be at least as long as the distance between the patient's earlobe and the tip of his nose. It can be longer.

3. Use a water-based lubricant to lubricate the outside of the tube before you insert it. Do *not* use petroleum jelly or any other non-water-based lubricant. These types of substances will damage the nasal cavity and pharynx (throat) and will increase the risk of infection.

4. Keep the patient's head in a neutral position and gently push the tip of the nose upward. Insert the airway through the right nostril straight back, not angled upward toward the eye. If the airway has a beveled (angled) edge, place the angled edge facing toward the septum (divider between the two nostrils). Gently advance the airway until the flange rests firmly against the patient's nostril. Never force the airway. If the airway will not advance into the nostril easily, remove it, relubricate it if necessary, rotate it 180 degrees, and try it in the other nostril. (It does not matter if the natural curve of the airway is arcing in the other direction; it will adjust as you insert it.) If the airway will not advance in the left nostril, make another attempt with an airway that is slightly smaller in diameter.

5. Ventilate via mask.

WARNING:
If you continue to meet resistance while inserting the airway, do not continue your attempts. Do not attempt to insert the airway if there are indications of nasal injury or if you see clear fluid flowing from the nose.

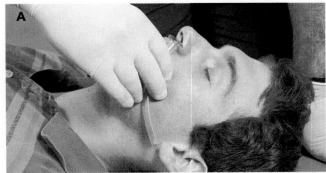

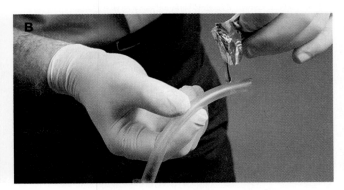

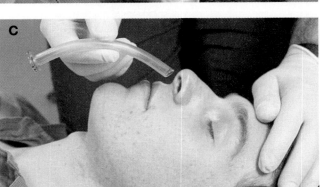

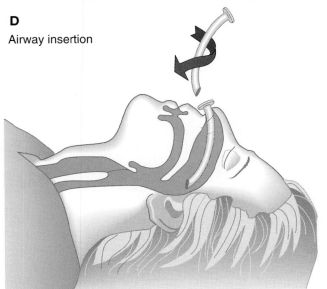

D
Airway insertion

FIGURE 6.26
A Measuring, **B** lubricating, and
C, D inserting a nasopharyngeal airway.

Suction Systems

Typically a First Responder will reposition the patient on his side (recovery position) or use finger sweeps appropriately to clear blood, mucus, and other body fluids from the airway. More and more First Responder units are carrying suction devices, and training programs are including suctioning techniques.

There are several types of portable suction units that range from the hand-operated devices to the mechanically powered ones. They may be manually powered, oxygen- or air-powered, or electrically powered units (Figure 6.27). The vacuum pressure and flow must be adequate for mouth, throat (pharyngeal), and stoma suctioning. All units must have thick-walled, non-kinking, wide-bore tubing; a nonbreakable collection container (bottle); and sterile, disposable semirigid and/or rigid suction tubes or tips. The longer suction tips are usually called *catheters;* the rigid suction tips are sometimes referred to as *tonsil suction tips* (for example, Yankauer suction tip).

FIGURE 6.27
A Oxygen-powered suction unit; **B** Electrically powered suction unit; **C** Portable electrical suction unit, **D** Portable hand-operated suction unit.

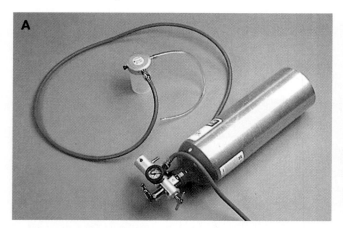

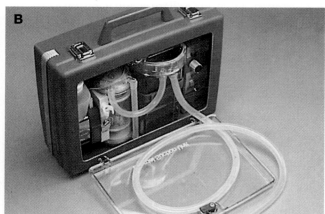

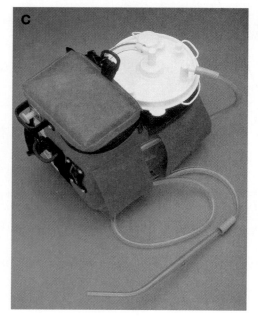

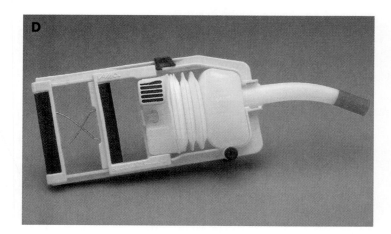

SUCTIONING TECHNIQUES

USE PERSONAL PROTECTIVE EQUIPMENT. Because of droplets in the air, face mask and eye protection are essential. Remember, any patient may be an infection source.

There are many variations to the techniques used to suction the mouth, throat, or stoma. One example of a long-standing procedure is given here. You MUST follow the guidelines established by your local EMS system's Medical Director.

1. Follow all infection control guidelines; use personal protective equipment.

2. Follow standard suctioning rules:

   – NEVER suction for longer than 15 seconds at a time. Some guidelines require a maximum of 10 seconds for the breathing patient; 5 seconds for the nonbreathing patient before attempting to ventilate.

   – Measure the tip of the catheter before inserting it in the patient's mouth. Measure from the patient's earlobe to the corner of the mouth and place your fingers at that point. Insert the tip or catheter no farther than that point where you have your fingers placed.

   – Never suction as you are inserting the catheter; place the suction tip or catheter in the patient's mouth BEFORE starting suction.

   – Suction only as you remove the tip or catheter, and twist and turn the tip or catheter as you are removing it from the mouth, throat, or stoma.

3. If appropriate, turn on the unit. Attach the catheter (tip) and test for suction.

4. Position yourself at the patient's head and turn him to the side. (If practical, turn the entire patient, not just the head; follow guidelines for spinal protection.)

5. Measure the flexible catheter or rigid tip between the earlobe and the corner of the mouth, or from the center of the mouth to the angle of the jaw (just like the oropharyngeal airway). Hold the tip or catheter in your fingers at the point where it reaches the mouth. You will insert the tip or catheter only that far into the patient's mouth.

6. Open the patient's mouth and clear obvious matter and fluid from the oral cavity by turning the patient and draining the mouth or by using finger sweeps.

7. Insert the tip or catheter to your finger position. Usually the tip is inserted to the base of the tongue (Figure 6.28). If you are using a rigid pharyngeal tip, place the convexed (curved-out) side against the roof of the mouth, with the tip at the base of the tongue.

8. Apply suction ONLY when the tip or catheter is in place at the back of the mouth or base of the tongue and as you begin to withdraw it. Twist and turn it from side to side and sweep the mouth. This twisting action prevents the end of the tip or catheter from grabbing mouth tissue. Follow all the rules stated above. REMAIN ALERT FOR THE PATIENT'S GAG REFLEX AND FOR SIGNS OF VOMITING.

> **Note**
>
> If you are using a manually powered unit, it may have a rubber bulb or a hand- or foot-operated device to produce the vacuum. Follow manufacturers' and local EMS system guidelines for generating the vacuum.

FIGURE 6.28
Positioning a rigid pharyngeal (throat) tip. Do not push it down the throat or into the larynx.

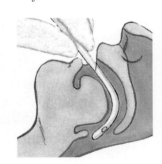

Summary

We breathe to bring in oxygen, remove carbon dioxide, and help regulate the pH level of our blood, a process called **respiration.** The major muscle of breathing, the **diaphragm,** and the muscles between our ribs contract to increase the volume of the chest cavity. Increased volume decreases the pressure in the chest cavity and allows the lungs to expand. As the lungs expand, the pressure inside decreases and allows air to fill the lungs. When we exhale, changes in chest size and pressure cause air in the lungs to flow out. All this is an involuntary, automatic process, which is mainly controlled by the respiratory centers of the brain.

Clinical death occurs when an individual stops breathing and the heart stops beating. **Biological death** occurs when the brain cells start to die. Without oxygen, lethal changes take place in the brain cells within 4 to 6 minutes. Brain death may start within 10 minutes.

In addition to the respiratory centers in the brain and the diaphragm and the muscles between the ribs, the respiratory system includes the nose and mouth, the throat (**pharynx**), the voice box (**larynx**), the **epiglottis,** the windpipe (**trachea**), the bronchial tree, and the lungs.

To assess normal breathing, **look** for chest movements, **listen** and **feel** for air movement, and **observe** skin color for blue, gray, white (pallor), or ashen tints. Suspect problems with changes in breathing rate and depth, skin color, and breathing efforts.

Opening the airway is the first important step in patient care. Simply repositioning the patient's head may solve breathing problems. The **head-tilt, chin-lift maneuver** is used to open the airway of patients without neck or spinal injuries. The **jaw-thrust maneuver** is used when there are possible neck or spinal injuries. Only a **slight head-tilt with chin-lift,** or "sniffing position," is used for children, and the infant's head is kept in the neutral position to maintain the airway.

Mouth-to-mask ventilation is the recommended procedure for performing assisted ventilations. Use a pocket face mask with one-way valve and HEPA filter. Some jurisdictions train First Responders to use the bag-valve mask (see Appendix 2).

Mouth-to-mouth ventilation is another form of pulmonary resuscitation, but it provides no protection from infectious disease. The **mouth-to-nose** method can be used for accident victims or the elderly with no facial support from teeth or dentures, but again it offers no protection from infectious disease. The **mouth-to-stoma** or **mask-to-stoma** method is used for neck breathers. Methods that do not use a mask or some other barrier increase the risk of infectious disease transmission.

Watch for **gastric distention** when you perform assisted ventilations. Reposition the head and adjust your ventilations to correct this. Be on guard for vomiting.

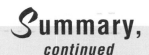

When caring for accident victims, stabilize the head and use the jaw-thrust maneuver to open the airway. If you must reposition an accident victim in order to assist ventilations, open the airway and ventilate the patient while stabilizing the head in the best way you can.

When you begin artificial ventilation, start with two adequate breaths. Assist ventilations for the nonbreathing adult at a rate of one breath every 5 seconds. This rate can also be expressed as 12 breaths per minute. For infants and children, the rate is one breath every 3 seconds or 20 breaths per minute.

A variety of problems can cause **partial or complete airway obstruction.** These include the tongue, the epiglottis, foreign objects, tissue damage, tissue swelling, and disease.

In addition to the signs of inadequate breathing, listen for snoring, crowing, gurgling, and wheezing sounds. For complete obstruction, there will be no chest movements, no sounds of respiration, and no air exchange felt at the nose and mouth.

Encourage patients with partial obstructions to cough. If they cannot cough, if their coughing is very weak, or if there is poor air exchange, provide care as if there is a complete airway obstruction.

To clear an obstructed airway, deliver abdominal thrusts to an adult in rapid succession. Deliver slow, distinct chest thrusts for infants, small children, obese adults, and pregnant patients.

Conscious patients with airway obstructions will look distressed and will often grasp their necks trying to communicate. Ask patients, "Can you speak?" or "Can you cough?" or "Are you choking?" If they can respond, the obstruction is partial.

Relieve airway obstructions with the combined procedures of:

- Attempting to ventilate
- Manual thrusts (back blows for infants only)
- Finger sweeps (Do not perform "blind" finger sweeps.)
- Opening the airway and attempting ventilations again

Airway adjuncts, such as **oropharyngeal** and **nasopharyngeal airways,** help the First Responder maintain the patient's airway while assisting respirations. Measure the oral airway by one of two methods: from the center of the mouth to the angle of the jaw, or from the corner of the mouth to the earlobe. Begin inserting the oropharyngeal airway upside down in adults and turn it to the correct position to seat it properly in the oral cavity. For infants and children, insert the oropharyngeal airway in the right-side-up position. Turning the airway in pediatric patients may damage the oral cavity. The nasal airway should be slightly smaller in diameter than the patient's nostril and at least as long as the distance between the tip of the nose and the earlobe. Lubricate the nasopharyngeal airway with a water-based gel before inserting it. Reassess the patient's airway after inserting any airway adjunct.

Remember and Consider...

Making sure that a patient has an open airway and knowing how to maintain and manage a patient's airway is the most important care you can provide. All other patient care activities are secondary because if people can't breathe, they die. The steps to open an airway are simple and easily performed; the skills required to maintain and manage an airway take practice. Practicing airway maintenance and management skills helps you develop an ability and proficiency that will help you act quickly in a stress-filled emergency.

✔ Do you remember and can you perform the two different ways to open an airway?

✔ Why is it important to recognize and know when to use one technique rather than the other?

You will practice measuring and inserting nasopharyngeal and oropharyngeal airways on manikins in class. You will also practice using pocket face masks and possibly bag-valve masks. Go back to your station and check the response units and aid kits for airways and masks.

✔ What kinds and sizes of airways do you have? Where are they located? Are they kept in several places that are easy to get to?

✔ What kinds of pocket face masks do you have? If you have a variety of manufacturer types, which one is easiest for you to use? Have you tried using one on a person or just a manikin? Ask a member of your family, a friend, or other EMS company member if you can position one on his or her face so you can get used to the placement and grip. Ask the person to breathe in and exhale normally. Check your seal—does air leak out around the cheeks, or does it exit through the one-way valve only? If you feel you have to press hard to get a seal, then you may not have the mask in the correct position. Reposition it until you get a good seal. Be sure to thoroughly wash and dry the mask after practice.

Remember the signs of an obstructed airway and how to manage the patient in all three situations: conscious, becomes unconscious, is unconscious when you arrive.

✔ What do you do if you can't get air into the unconscious patient with your first or second breath? What if you are doing obstructed airway procedures on a conscious patient who is showing signs of obstructed airway and the patient becomes unconscious? Have you ever had to perform obstructed airway procedures on anyone? Ask care providers in your company to tell you their experiences. Ask people you know who are different sizes (tall and short) and various girths (slender and stout) if you can practice your positions on them. Where do you place yourself or the patient when he or she is much taller or shorter than you, when his or her girth is larger than your arms can reach? Is it harder to find the correct position on the abdomen when someone is obese?

Even though obstructed airway procedures do not require extremely forceful thrusts, they can cause discomfort or injury. Therefore, while you can practice positioning on people of different sizes, perform the complete maneuver only on manikins.

Investigate...

✔ How does your company's suctioning unit work?

Is the suction unit a portable battery-operated one, or a hand-operated unit, or do you have both kinds? Do you know how to assemble and disassemble them? Where are the replacement parts and tubing kept? Where do you dispose of the contents? Do you have labels for the collection containers in case the hospital wants the contents? What would you put on a label?

✔ Will you be able to manage a patient with a stoma?

Do you know anyone with a stoma? Where can you get information on stoma patients? Check local directories for the phone numbers of the American Heart Association and the American Lung Association or the health department. They will give you additional information and will probably have speakers willing to give a presentation or show a film at your company on how to manage patients with stomas.

✔ How often do you practice your assisted ventilation skills?

Do you know that motor skills will rapidly deteriorate if you don't use them? Practice makes perfect and in order to be able to assist ventilations quickly and accurately, you must practice them frequently. There are a lot of steps to perform when you assist ventilations, but once you are familiar with them and develop an automatic response, they flow in a very logical sequence. But that automatic response only comes with practice. Check with your company and find out how often they hold drills. Do you have manikins at your station? Find out if you can get them out and practice on them when you are on duty. Even without the actual manikins, you can review the pictures in the text and mentally picture yourself performing each step. Go through the motions even without the manikin—something like playing "air guitar." You can do "air assisted-ventilations."

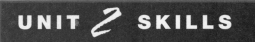
➤ **CHAPTER 6 AIRWAY MANAGEMENT**
➤ **APPENDIX 2 BREATHING AIDS AND OXYGEN THERAPY**

Study the following scenarios. Place check marks in the columns below as appropriate to indicate which skills you would perform for each scenario. You will use skills from the previous unit in these scenarios. Refer to text pages 1–82. Write the skills number of any skills you would use from Unit 1 after each scenario or in the column under "Unit." Discuss answers with other students and your instructor.

SCENARIO 1: Your next door neighbor knows you work with the fire department, and she comes running over with her 2-year-old who doesn't seem to be breathing. She tells you they were eating lunch when the child suddenly started choking, possibly on one of those little hot dogs. You call 911 as you begin to assess the child. You have some basic First Responder equipment in your house and grab your bag to pull out a pocket face mask.

(Skills from Unit 1: _____)

SCENARIO 2: You are riding with the EMTs on their unit when you get a call to respond to a "trouble breathing" call. On the scene, you find a 40-year-old woman with a history of bronchitis. She says she has had this bout of bronchitis for about 4 days and it is getting harder to breathe. While the EMTs take vital signs and get a history, they ask you to set up the oxygen equipment.

(Skills from Unit 1: _____)

Instructors will demonstrate all skills and will give you time to practice them while they coach you.

Skills	Scenarios		Unit
	#1	#2	#1
Opening and clearing the airway (refer to Chapter 6):			
1. Demonstrate look, listen, and feel for air exchange steps to check for breathing (p. 83)			
2. Demonstrate head-tilt, chin-lift (Figure 6.5)			
3. Demonstrate jaw-thrust maneuver (Figure 6.6)			
4. Demonstrate back blows and chest thrusts for infants (Figures 6.17 and 6.21, Scan 6-2)			
5. Demonstrate abdominal thrusts for conscious adults and children (Figure 6.18)			
6. Demonstrate clearing the airway for unconscious adults and children (Scan 6-1)			
7. Demonstrate chest thrusts for conscious and unconscious obese or pregnant adults (Figures 6.19 and 6.20)			
8. Demonstrate the finger sweep (Figure 6.22)			

Skills	Scenarios		Unit
	#1	#2	#1
Ventilation techniques:			
9. Ventilate a manikin with a pocket face mask (Figures 6.8, 6.10, 6.11, 6.12, and 6.14)			
10. Use a bag-valve-mask ventilator with two rescuers (Figure A2-4)			
11. Use a bag-valve-mask ventilator as a single rescuer (Figure A2-3)			
Nasopharyngeal and oropharyngeal airways:			
12. Measure and insert an oropharyngeal airway (Scan 6-3)			
13. Measure and insert a nasopharyngeal airway (Figure 6.26)			
Liter Flow (Appendix 2 and Scans A2-1 and A2-2):			
14. Attach a nasal cannula to supplemental oxygen, adjust to correct liters per minute, apply to patient			
15. Attach a nonrebreather mask to supplemental oxygen, adjust to correct liters per minute, apply to patient			
16. Attach oxygen tubing to a bag-valve-mask ventilator, ventilate a manikin with supplemental oxygen at 15 liters per minute (Figure A2.3)			
Suction (refer to steps on p. 121):			
17. Measure a suction catheter			
18. Suction for the correct amount of time			
19. Ventilate at appropriate time intervals			

Work with a group of classmates to create scenarios that will use listed skills. Exchange the scenarios with other class groups to check your knowledge and to practice your decision-making skills.

CHAPTER 7

ASSESSMENT OF THE PATIENT

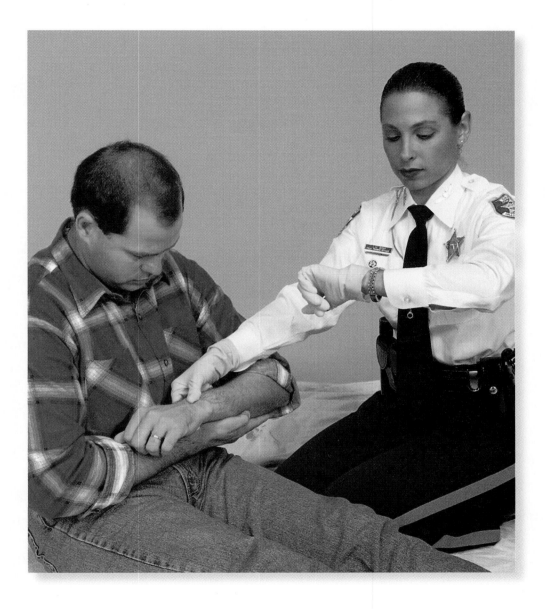

*P*atients cannot receive appropriate care until their medical or traumatic problems have been found and understood by the responders helping them. The First Responder must assess each patient in order to detect the possible illness or injury and to determine the direction of the emergency care needed. Such assessment must be done in a specific and orderly fashion to assure the First Responder that nothing has been missed.

National Standard Objectives

This chapter focuses on the objectives of Module 3, Lesson 3–1 of the U.S. DOT First Responder National Curriculum and serves as an instructional aid to help you meet any specific objectives added to the course by your local EMS system.

By the end of this chapter, you will know how to: (from cognitive or knowledge information) . . .

3–1.1	Discuss the components of scene size-up. (pp. 140–144)
3–1.2	Describe common hazards found at the scene of a trauma and a medical patient. (p. 141)
3–1.3	Determine if the scene is safe to enter. (p. 141)
3–1.4	Discuss common mechanisms of injury/nature of illness. (pp. 141, 143, 154)
3–1.5	Discuss the reason for identifying the total number of patients at the scene. (p. 143)
3–1.6	Explain the reason for identifying the need for additional help or assistance. (p. 143)
3–1.7	Summarize the reasons for forming a general impression of the patient. (p. 145)
3–1.8	Discuss methods of assessing mental status. (p. 145)
3–1.9	Differentiate between assessing mental status in the adult, child, and infant patient. (p. 145)
3–1.10	Describe methods used for assessing if a patient is breathing. (pp. 148, 150, 162–164)
3–1.11	Differentiate between a patient with adequate and inadequate breathing. (p. 150, see also Chapter 6)
3–1.12	Describe the methods used to assess circulation. (pp. 148, 150, 160–162)
3–1.13	Differentiate between obtaining a pulse in an adult, a child, and an infant patient. (pp. 150, 160–162)
3–1.14	Discuss the need for assessing the patient for external bleeding. (pp. 151, 171)
3–1.15	Explain the reason for prioritizing a patient for care and transport. (p. 151)
3–1.16	Discuss the components of the physical exam. (pp. 152–154, 160, 166–171)
3–1.17	State the areas of the body that are evaluated during the physical exam. (pp. 167–171)
3–1.18	Explain what additional questions may be asked during the physical exam. (pp. 156, 158)
3–1.19	Explain the components of the SAMPLE history. (p. 158)
3–1.20	Discuss the components of the ongoing assessment. (pp. 173–176)
3–1.21	Describe the information included in the First Responder "hand-off" report. (p. 176)

Feel comfortable enough to: (by changing attitudes, values, and beliefs) . . .	3–1.22	Explain the rationale for crew members to evaluate scene safety prior to entering. (p. 141)
	3–1.23	Serve as a model for others by explaining how patient situations affect your evaluation of the mechanism of injury or illness. (pp. 140, 141, 143, 153–154)
	3–1.24	Explain the importance of forming a general impression of the patient. (p. 145)
	3–1.25	Explain the value of an initial assessment. (pp. 144–152)
	3–1.26	Explain the value of questioning the patient and family. (pp. 152, 156, 158–159)
	3–1.27	Explain the value of the physical exam. (pp. 152–154, 160, 166–171)
	3–1.28	Explain the value of an ongoing assessment. (pp. 173–176)
	3–1.29	Explain the rationale for the feelings that these patients might be experiencing. (pp. 143, 156, 158)
	3–1.30	Demonstrate a caring attitude when performing patient assessments. (pp. 143, 156, 158)
	3–1.31	Place the interests of the patient as the foremost consideration when making any and all patient-care decisions during patient assessment. (pp. 156, 158–159)
	3–1.32	Communicate with empathy during patient assessment to patients as well as with family members and friends of the patient. (pp. 156, 158–159)

Show how to: (through psychomotor skills) . . .	3–1.33	Demonstrate the ability to differentiate various scenarios and identify potential hazards. (pp. 141, 143–144)
	3–1.34	Demonstrate the techniques for assessing mental status. (pp. 145, 151)
	3–1.35	Demonstrate the techniques for assessing the airway. (pp. 148, 150, 162–164)
	3–1.36	Demonstrate the techniques for assessing if the patient is breathing. (p. 150, see also Chapter 6)
	3–1.37	Demonstrate the techniques for assessing if the patient has a pulse. (pp. 150, 160–162)
	3–1.38	Demonstrate the techniques for assessing the patient for external bleeding. (pp. 151, 171)
	3–1.39	Demonstrate the techniques for assessing the patient's skin color, temperature, condition, and capillary refill (infants and children only). (pp. 151–152, 164–165)
	3–1.40	Demonstrate questioning a patient to obtain a SAMPLE history. (pp. 156, 158)
	3–1.41	Demonstrate the skills involved in performing the physical exam. (pp. 152–155, 160, 166–171)
	3–1.42	Demonstrate the ongoing assessment. (pp. 173, 176)

LEARNING TASKS

In addition to the objectives above, you should also be able to:
- ✔ State the three things you must say to a conscious patient upon your arrival at the scene.
- ✔ Describe the personal protection to be worn by a First Responder during the assessment of the patient.
- ✔ Describe how to ensure an open airway.
- ✔ Differentiate between a sign and a symptom.
- ✔ Define and describe how to take vital signs, and indicate what you are looking for in terms of rate, character, and what is considered normal.
- ✔ List examples of significant mechanisms of injury.
- ✔ List, in correct order, the steps of the focused history and physical exam for the trauma patient with no significant mechanism of injury.
- ✔ List, in correct order, the steps of the rapid trauma assessment for the trauma patient with a significant mechanism of injury.
- ✔ List, in correct order, the steps of the focused history and physical exam for the conscious medical patient.
- ✔ List, in correct order, the steps of the rapid physical exam for the unconscious medical patient.
- ✔ List ten First Responder rules that apply to patient assessment.
- ✔ Define the detailed physical exam and the ongoing assessment.

> ## WARNING:
>
> Patient assessment procedures can bring you into contact with the patient's blood or body fluids. Taking body substance isolation precautions whenever caring for a patient is important. Latex or vinyl gloves should always be worn during the assessment and care of any patient. Eye protection may also be required depending on the type of emergency and patient condition. Wear any other items of personal protection required for your safety and that of your patients. Follow OSHA, CDC, and local guidelines to help prevent the spread of infectious diseases. Review the personal safety and protection information in Chapter 2.

PATIENT ASSESSMENT COMPONENTS

patient assessment the gathering of information to determine the possible nature of the patient's illness or injury. It includes interviews and physical examination.

chief complaint the reason EMS was called, usually in the patient's own words.

Patients cannot receive appropriate care until their problems have been detected and understood by those trying to help them. The **patient assessment** is a procedure that helps to determine the possible illness or injury and provides direction for decisions concerning emergency care.

EMS systems use **assessment-based** prehospital care. In this type of assessment and care, the patient's **chief complaint** is noted, but immediate life-threatening conditions are detected and cared for first. After immediate life-threats have been handled, potential threats are found and cared for. A diagnosis of what may be causing the complaint or problem is not necessary. The patient is cared for based on signs and symptoms, *not* diagnosis. For example, there are many medical reasons a patient may be short of breath. Yet the treatment is the same. We treat the serious problem of breathing difficulty, but do not direct your efforts to trying to determine its cause.

The components of patient assessment and the order in which they are performed may vary from patient to patient based on the nature of the patient's problem. For most patients, the assessment should begin as follows:

1. Ensure your own safety.
2. Ensure the safety of your patient.
3. Determine the level of your patient's responsiveness.
4. Form a general impression of the patient.

The remaining components of patient assessment change slightly, depending on the type of patient. We will discuss each component in detail later in this chapter. Patients will fall into one of four categories and are assessed in a different order for each of the four.

MEDICAL PATIENTS (NO INJURIES)

Responsive Medical Patient (Scan 7-1)

- Begin the interview, which is ongoing throughout the assessment and care of the patient.
- Ask questions to determine what is causing the illness, which is referred to as **nature of illness (NOI).**
- Examine the patient as required based on complaints obtained during the interview.
- Determine vital signs, such as pulse, respirations, skin color, temperature, and condition. Blood pressure and pupil assessment may be included for some First Responders.

nature of illness (NOI) what is medically wrong with a patient.

Unresponsive Medical Patient (Scan 7-2)

- Attempt to interview family or bystanders to determine the chief complaint or the nature of illness (NOI), but simultaneously . . .
- Check to make sure the patient has an open airway, is breathing, and has a pulse. Also check for serious bleeding. Provide care for any problems as you find them.
- Examine the patient for signs of the nature of the illness.
- Take the patient's vital signs.

TRAUMA PATIENTS

No Significant Mechanism of Injury (Scan 7-3)

- Scan the scene to determine what caused the injury, which will be referred to as **mechanism of injury (MOI).**
- Interview the patient while checking for adequate breathing and serious bleeding.
- Conduct a focused history and physical exam of the patient based on the patient's complaint.
- Determine vital signs.
- Perform a detailed physical examination as needed.

trauma physical injury caused by an external force. Common causes other than violence include motor vehicle collisions, falls, burns, and drowning.

mechanism of injury (MOI) a force or forces that may have caused injury.

Significant Mechanism of Injury (Scan 7-4)

- Scan the scene and note the mechanism of injury if possible.
- Begin to question family and bystanders, but simultaneously assess the patient for life-threatening problems. As you stabilize the patient's head

and neck, check for an open airway, adequate breathing, and a pulse. Also, check for serious bleeding. Care for any major problems as you detect them.

- Perform a rapid trauma assessment to look for serious injuries.
- Take vital signs if the patient appears unstable.
- Perform a detailed physical exam of the patient if time allows.
- Reassess the patient's vital signs, looking for any changes.

Note that, at times, the type of patient you are caring for is not so clearly defined. For example, a patient experiencing a medical problem may fall and injure himself. Or a medical problem may have actually caused a motor vehicle collision. Your patient assessment will need to include elements of both medical and traumatic emergencies. What should guide your assessment should be the more serious of the patient's problems.

*S*CAN *7-1*

Patient Assessment—Responsive Medical Patient

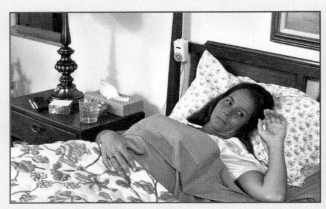

1. Size-up the scene. Is it stable?

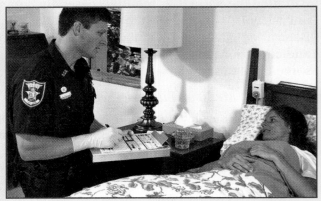

2. Begin the interview, which is ongoing throughout the assessment. Ask questions to determine what is causing the illness.

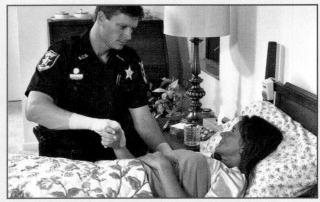

3. Examine the patient as required based on complaints obtained during the interview. Determine vital signs.

Patient Assessment—Unresponsive Medical Patient

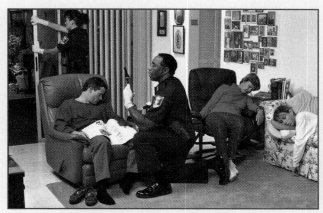

1. Size-up the scene. Attempt to interview family or bystanders to determine the nature of illness, but simultaneously . . .

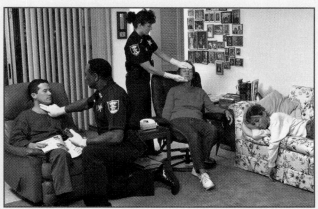

2. Check to make sure patient has an open airway, is breathing, and has a pulse. Also check for serious bleeding. Examine patient for signs of the nature of illness. Take patient's vital signs.

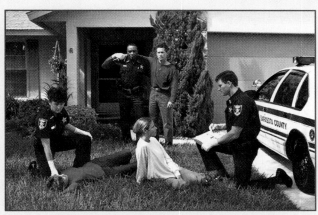

3. Provide care for any problems as you find them.

Patient Assessment—Responsive Trauma Patient
(No Significant Mechanism of Injury)

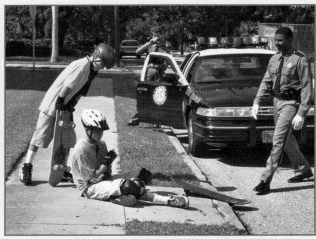

1. Size-up the scene. Scan the scene to determine what caused the injury.

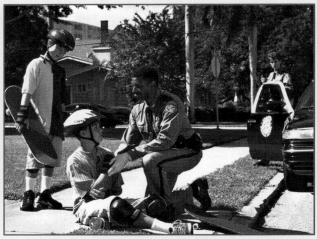

2. Interview the patient while checking for adequate breathing and serious bleeding.

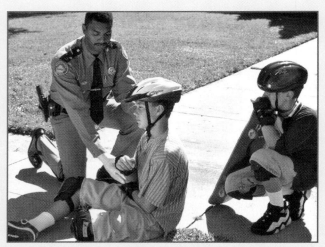

3. Conduct a focused history and physical exam of the patient based on the patient's complaint. Determine vital signs. Perform a detailed physical exam as needed.

Patient Assessment—Unresponsive Trauma Patient

(Significant Mechanism of Injury)

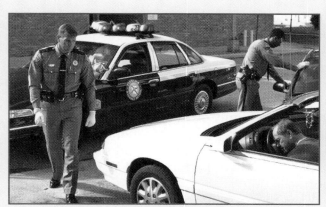

1. Size-up the scene. Scan the scene and note the mechanism of injury if possible.

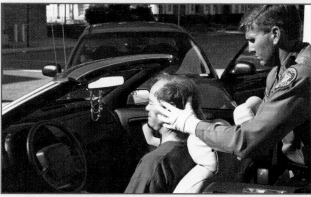

2. Begin to question family and bystanders, but simultaneously assess the patient for life-threatening problems. As you stabilize the patient's head and neck, check for an open airway, adequate breathing, and a pulse. Also, check for serious bleeding. Care for any major problems as you detect them.

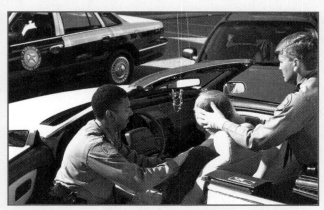

3. Perform a rapid trauma assessment to look for serious injuries. Take vital signs if the patient appears unstable. Perform a detailed physical exam if time permits. Reassess the patient's vital signs, looking for any changes.

FIRST RESPONDER ASSESSMENT-BASED CARE

The First Responder's role in the EMS system may vary. A First Responder may be active in a small part of the initial care of a patient or have responsibilities that may involve all aspects of emergency care. This may include the use of an automated external defibrillator for cardiac arrest patients and continuing care into the emergency department of the hospital.

First | EMS system patient assessment contains seven major components. While only some portions of them apply to the First Responder, you should be familiar with all of them in order to communicate with other EMS responders properly. These components include:

- *Scene size-up*—Note if the scene is safe or has been made safe.
- *Initial assessment*—Detect and correct any life-threatening problems.
- Focused history and physical exam.
  - *Trauma*—Perform a physical exam based on information obtained from the patient, the mechanism of injury, or by completion of an entire body (head-to-toe) exam. Take vital signs, and, if possible, obtain a patient history from the patient or from family or bystanders.
  - *Medical*—Obtain the patient's history, perform any required physical exam, and obtain vital signs. For a significant medical situation, maintain airway, breathing, and circulation; perform CPR if needed; and quickly arrange transport.
- *Detailed physical exam*—When time permits, perform a more detailed head-to-toe physical exam.
- *Ongoing assessment*—Repeat the initial assessment (usually done en route to the hospital), correct any additional life-threatening problems, repeat vital signs, and evaluate and adjust as needed any patient-care interventions that have been performed. The condition of your patient will either improve, stay the same, or get worse. The patient must be monitored to detect any changes.
- *Communications*—Communicate patient information to higher level EMS providers or the hospital ER staff who will be taking over care of the patient on arrival.
- *Documentation*—Accurately and completely fill out all required written reports and forms.

First | The typical First Responder program will stress five major parts of patient assessment. We will discuss these in detail later in this chapter. They include:

- Scene size-up
- Initial assessment
- Focused assessment (trauma and medical)
- Detailed assessment (head-to-toe exam)
- Ongoing assessment

While the responsibilities of the First Responder may differ from one EMS system to another, all use an assessment-based approach to patient assessment and care. After assuring one's own personal safety, a First Responder's first concern is to safely detect and begin to correct life-threatening problems. The second concern is to safely identify those problems that are serious or may become serious and provide care for those problems. The third concern is to safely monitor the patient to quickly detect any changes in his condition.

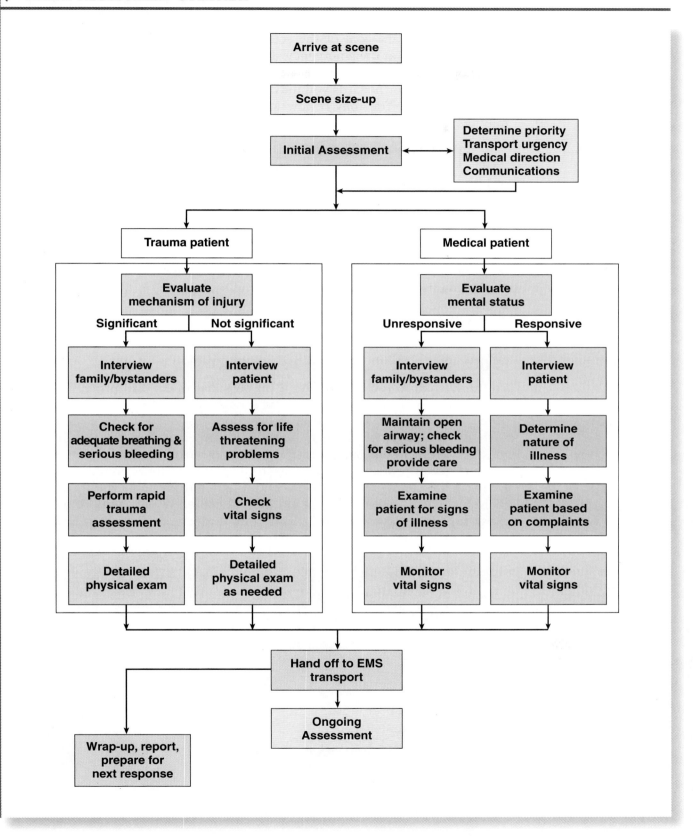

SCENE SIZE-UP

Safety is a primary goal of the scene size-up. Scene size-up actually begins before you arrive at the emergency, often with the information you receive from your dispatcher. While en route to the scene, you may begin thinking about the types of injuries or hazards you may find at a particular scene, such as a motor vehicle collision. You may review in your mind the signs and symptoms you may see in a patient with a particular medical emergency.

First | When you arrive on scene, take appropriate body substance isolation precautions and make sure the scene is safe. Look for the mechanism of injury at calls involving trauma (Figure 7.1), and/or the nature of illness at medical emergencies (Figure 7.2), note the number of patients, and anticipate if any additional resources will be needed. To recap, every patient assessment begins with scene size-up that includes the following (Scan 7-5):

- Body substance isolation precautions
- Scene safety for you, other responders, the patient, and bystanders
- Mechanism of injury or nature of illness
- Number of patients
- Additional resources needed

BODY SUBSTANCE ISOLATION PRECAUTIONS

You may wish to review Chapter 2 on personal safety and protection. *Always* wear latex or vinyl gloves when caring for *any* patient. Wear eye protection and other body substance isolation precautions as needed, depending on the patient's problem. Remember, body substance isolation precautions are as much to protect your *patient* as they are to protect *you*. Apply gloves and any other personal protection as you reach the patient. Gloves applied before or en route to the scene may already be contaminated from items you touch, such as the vehicle door, steering wheel, or other equipment. Contaminated gloves pose a risk for the patient when you touch him or any wounds he may have.

FIGURE 7.1
Clues to the trauma patient's problems may be gathered upon arrival at the scene.

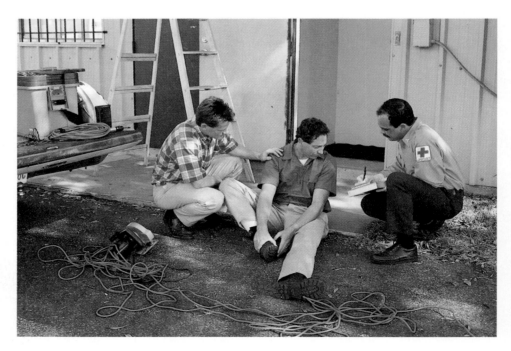

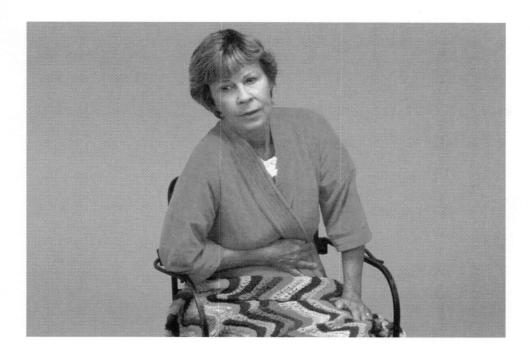

SCENE SAFETY

A dangerous and sometimes fatal mistake that responders make is entering an unsafe or hazardous scene. Never **assume** any scene is safe. If a scene has the potential for violence, and you are not a law enforcement officer, do *not* enter the scene until law enforcement indicates it is safe for you to do so. If there is a potential for a hazardous materials release, remain a safe distance away. You may never actually enter the scene. Often, appropriately trained and equipped hazardous materials team members will bring patients to you after appropriate decontamination.

Other examples of hazardous or unsafe scenes include crash/rescue scenes, the release of toxic substances, violent or crime scenes, scenes involving any weapon, and unstable surfaces. Also look for signs of domestic disturbances, electrical hazards, potential for fire or explosions, and guard dogs or other vicious, wild, or unusual animals. Be especially careful if the emergency is a result of gang activity. Use all your senses to detect unsafe scenes. Establish a "danger zone" to keep yourself and others away from harm. An important rule to remember is, *"Don't take more victims to the scene."* Every year many rescuers are injured and some are killed by being struck by a vehicle while on scene. In some cases, rescuers are not visible or are too close to traffic. In order to ensure scene safety at an accident scene, use adequate emergency lights and properly position emergency vehicles. Also remember that weather conditions, such as icy roads, should be of concern to rescuers.

MECHANISM OF INJURY AND NATURE OF ILLNESS

During the scene size-up, you should note the mechanism of injury for a **trauma patient** and the nature of illness for a **medical patient**. This will often give you clues to what type of injuries or problems to expect. The mechanism of injury, simply defined, is the combined forces that caused the injury. Did this patient fall? Is there a penetrating wound? Was he involved in a motor vehicle collision? A damaged steering wheel of a vehicle, for example, would lead you

trauma patient one who has a physical injury caused by an external force

medical patient one who has or describes symptoms of an illness.

Scene Size-Up

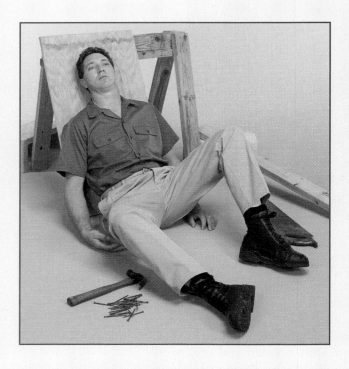

TRAUMA PATIENT (INJURIES). As you approach and perform a scene size-up, put on personal protective equipment.
- Is scene safe?
- Are additional resources needed?
- What is mechanism of injury?
- How many patients are injured?

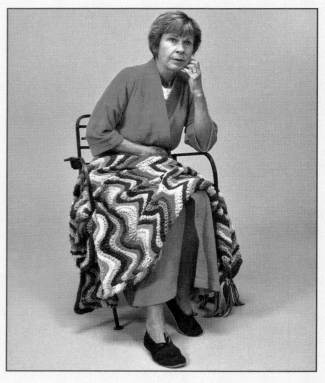

MEDICAL PATIENT (NO INJURIES). As you approach and perform a scene size-up, put on personal protective equipment.
- Is scene safe?
- Are additional resources needed?
- What is the nature of illness?
- How many patients are ill?

to consider the possibility of a chest injury. A cracked windshield could be an indication of a head injury. You would consider spine injuries in a patient who had experienced a fall from a great height. Recalling your reading in anatomy will help you consider what internal structures may be injured under an obvious injury to the body's surface.

The nature of illness for a medical patient is the same as the mechanism of injury for a trauma patient. This may be chest pain, breathing difficulty, abdominal pain, or any number of signs and symptoms. While diagnosing why the patient is having a particular medical problem is not necessary, the nature of illness will guide you in the appropriate direction in providing care. Both the mechanism of injury for trauma patients and the nature of illness for medical patients will allow you to consider what serious complications to watch for that may have not yet developed. For example, if the patient is complaining of chest pain, you should consider the possibility of a heart problem, and potential cardiac arrest, requiring CPR.

To identify the mechanism of injury or nature of illness, begin by scanning the entire scene. Information may be obtained from the patient, if conscious and oriented, from family members or bystanders, and by carefully looking at the scene.

NUMBER OF PATIENTS AND THE NEED FOR ADDITIONAL RESOURCES

The final part of the scene size-up is to determine the number of patients and if you have sufficient resources to handle the call. The number of patients at the scene is important information not only for you, but also for any other responding EMS services. More personnel and transport vehicles may be needed to handle several patients. Your initial call may have been for one patient with "flu-like" symptoms. Yet when you arrive, you find other members of the family with the same symptoms due to a carbon monoxide leak in the furnace. You may require additional resources even on calls with only one patient. You may need additional lifting help if a heavy patient must be carried down stairs. You may require a fire department response to help with extrication or to ensure a motor vehicle collision scene is safe. An important part of scene size-up is recognizing when additional resources are needed, and calling for them early. If you put off calling for assistance, you will become involved in patient care and may forget to call for the additional help. It is also important to account for *all* patients involved. How many people were in the vehicle? Did someone walk away from a crash scene? Did a patient get thrown from the vehicle?

ARRIVAL AT THE SCENE

Upon arrival at the patient's side, you should begin by identifying yourself, even when you believe the patient to be unconscious. A patient who initially appears unconscious may actually be alert. If you wear a uniform, such as a law enforcement officer or firefighter, most bystanders and patients will respond to your uniform and allow you to take charge of the scene without question. If you do not wear a uniform, identifying yourself is critical in allowing you to go about your duties. Simply state your name and then the following: "I am a First Responder, and I've been trained in providing emergency care." While many people may not know what a First Responder is, the statement should allow you access to the patient and the cooperation of bystanders.

Your next statement should be to the patient, "May I help you?" By answering "yes" to this question, the patient is giving you *expressed consent* to care for her. Sometimes a patient's fear may be so great that she is confused, and will answer, "no" or "just leave me alone." Gaining the patient's confidence by simply talking with her is usually easy. If the patient is unconscious or unable to give expressed consent, *implied consent* allows you to care for the patient at the First Responder level. This means that if the patient were able to do so, it is assumed that she would give you expressed consent to care for her. (Review Chapter 3 for a more detailed discussion of consent.)

Remember, upon arrival you must:

1. State your name (and rank or classification).

2. Identify yourself as a trained First Responder, explaining what this means if necessary. Let the patient and bystanders know that you are with the Emergency Medical Services system. (Don't say "EMS" system. The patient may have no idea what that means.)

3. Ask the patient if you may help.

While you are doing this, remember to look for any obvious life threats such as serious bleeding or breathing problems.

If someone is already providing care to the patient when you arrive, identify yourself as a First Responder. If the person's training is equal to or at a higher level than your own, ask if you may assist. You should still identify yourself to the patient and ask if he wishes you to help. Expressed and implied consent laws still apply.

If you have more training than the person who has begun care, respectfully ask to take over responsibility for the patient. Compliment him on what he has done so far and ask him to assist you. Do not criticize or argue with the first provider. Unless you are a law enforcement officer or there are specific emergency care laws in your state, you cannot order the first provider to relinquish care of the patient to you. Check your local laws and protocols.

THE INITIAL ASSESSMENT

initial assessment
the part of a patient assessment that is used to detect and immediately correct life-threatening problems that primarily involve the airway, breathing, and circulation.

The **initial assessment** of a patient is designed to detect and correct life-threatening problems primarily involving the patient's airway, breathing, and circulation. Each problem is corrected as it is found. These problems are serious enough that, if they are not immediately corrected, the patient will die. The initial assessment is begun as soon as you reach the patient. Lifesaving procedures must be done as soon as you discover they are needed.

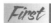 The initial assessment has six components (Scans 7-6 and 7-7).

1. Form a general impression of the patient.

2. Assess the patient's mental status.

3. Assess the patient's airway.

4. Assess the patient's breathing.

5. Assess the patient's circulation (pulse and bleeding).

6. Make a decision on the priority or urgency of the patient for transport.

First | While conducting the initial assessment, you will look for life-threatening problems in three major areas. These are:

- **Airway**—Is the patient's airway open?
- **Breathing**—Is the patient breathing adequately?
- **Circulation**—Does the patient have an adequate pulse to circulate blood? Is there serious bleeding? Did the patient lose a large quantity of blood prior to your arrival? Is the patient developing shock (hypoperfusion)?

These problems and the actions taken to correct them are known as the **ABCs of emergency care** and stand for:

    A = airway (ensure an open airway)
    B = breathing (maintain airway, rescue breathing)
    C = circulation (control of bleeding, chest compressions)

ABCs of emergency care these letters stand for the words *airway*, *breathing*, and *circulation* as they relate to the initial assessment.

FORM A GENERAL IMPRESSION

To begin your initial assessment, form a general impression of the patient and the patient's environment. Note any unusual details such as odors, temperature, or living conditions. EMS providers have always formed a general impression when they first see the patient, even if subconsciously. You notice if the patient looks very ill, pale, or cyanotic (blue coloring to the skin). You may immediately see serious injuries or see a patient who looks very stable. You form an early opinion of how seriously ill or injured the patient is. You may also be given information by the patient or bystanders at this time, such as the reason EMS was called or the chief complaint. Your decision to immediately transport the patient or continue assessment and care on scene may be based solely on your general impression. You may form a general impression on intuition alone, which will be developed with experience.

ASSESS MENTAL STATUS

Your actual assessment of the patient begins with the patient's mental status, or level of responsiveness. If you do not suspect trauma, especially spinal injury, check for responsiveness by gently squeezing the patient's shoulder and shouting, "Are you OK?" Speak loudly enough to wake the patient if he is merely sleeping. You may classify the patient's level of responsiveness by using the letters **AVPU,** which stand for alert, verbal, painful, and unresponsive. The **alert** patient will be awake, talking to you. The patient may appear unconscious at first, but will respond to a loud, **verbal** stimulus. If the patient does not respond to verbal stimuli, he may respond to **painful** stimuli, such as a sternal rub or a gentle pinch to the shoulder. Be careful not to injure the patient if applying painful stimuli. Never stick the patient with a sharp object such as a badge pin or forcefully pinch the skin. If the patient does not respond to either verbal or painful stimuli, he is **unresponsive** (Scan 7-8).

AVPU a system for measuring patient level of responsiveness. The letters stand for <u>a</u>lert, <u>v</u>erbal response, <u>p</u>ainful response, and <u>u</u>nresponsive.

    Try to conduct your assessment without moving the patient. But if the patient is unresponsive, you may need to reposition him to check for breathing, pulse, and serious bleeding, or to perform CPR. Follow the procedures shown in Scan 7-9. You must always assume the presence of neck or spinal injuries in the unconscious trauma patient. Moving this type of patient may cause additional serious injuries, but it may be necessary to check for life-threatening problems. Moving a patient safely was covered in Chapter 5.

Initial Assessment—Responsive Trauma Patient
(No Significant Mechanism of Injury)

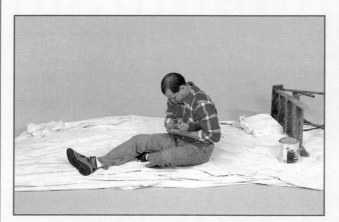

1. General impression.

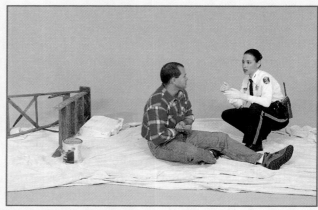

2. Mental status.

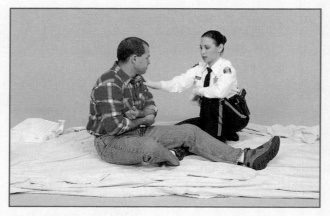

3. Airway/breathing.

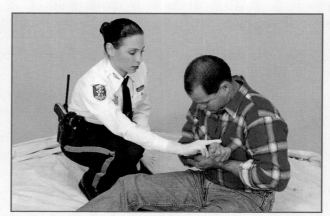

4. Pulse

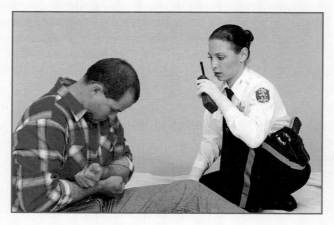

5. Priority

Initial Assessment—Responsive Medical Patient

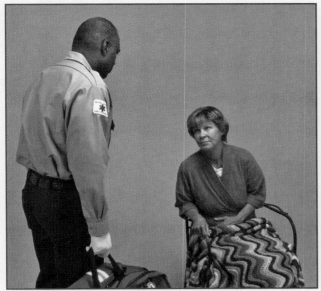

1. General impression.

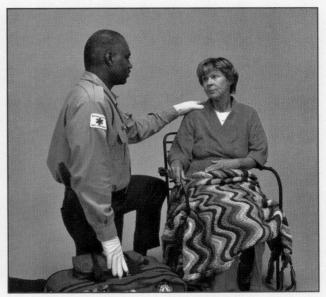

2. Mental status.

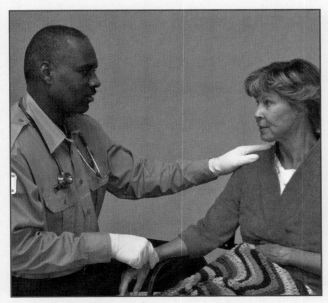

3. Airway/breathing/pulse.

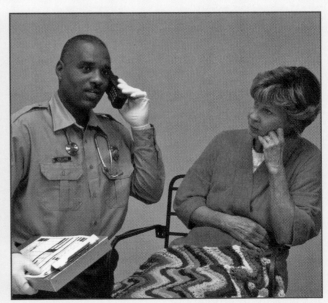

4. Priority.

Initial Assessment—Unresponsive Patient
(Medical or Trauma)

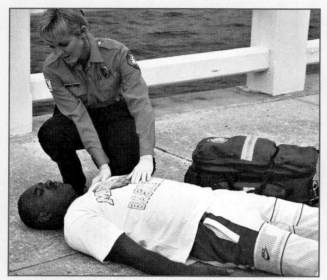

1. Establish unresponsiveness.

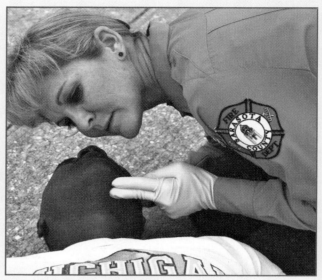

2. LOOK, LISTEN, and FEEL for breathing.

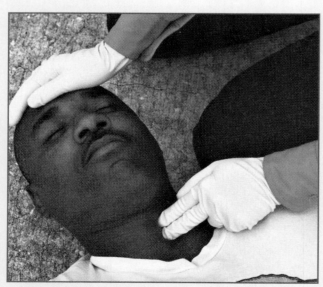

3. Check for a carotid pulse.

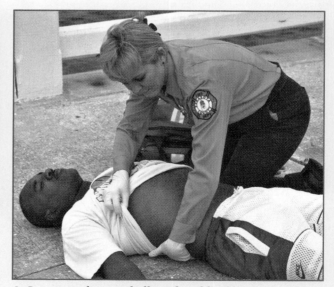

4. Locate and control all profuse bleeding.

Repositioning Patient for Basic Life Support

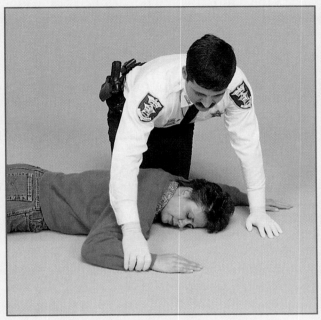

1. Straighten the legs and reposition arms.

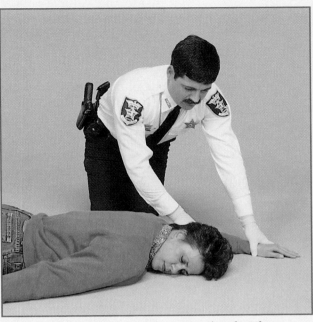

2. Place the arms close to the patient's side. The arms will help splint the torso as you roll the patient.

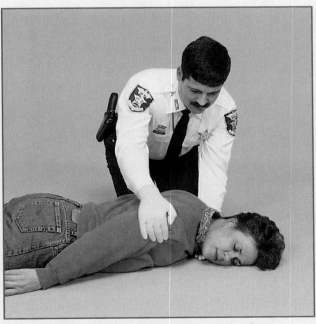

3. Cradle the head and neck and grasp the distant shoulder. Move the patient as a unit onto her side.

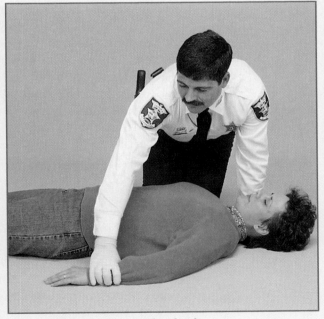

4. Move the patient onto her back.

WARNING: This maneuver is used to initiate basic cardiac life support when you must act alone. For all other repositionings, use a four-rescuer log roll.

ASSESS AIRWAY AND BREATHING

If the patient is unresponsive, stabilize the head and neck and use the jaw-thrust maneuver to ensure an open airway. Check for adequate breathing. If you do not suspect a spinal injury, position the patient lying on his back, and position yourself by his side. (In vehicle collisions, the patient may be seated inside the vehicle.) Use the head-tilt, chin-lift method to open the patient's airway. Remember, the procedure to use for patients with suspected spinal injury is the jaw thrust. See Chapter 6 for step-by-step procedures for both maneuvers.

Check for adequate breathing. With the airway open, place your ear over the patient's nose and mouth, and watch the chest for movement. If the patient is breathing, you will hear and feel the exhaled air on your ear, and you will see the chest rise and fall with each respiration. Listen to the quality of the breaths. Are there any "noises" indicating a possible obstruction? Determining breathing status should take no more than 5 seconds. Even if you hear "noises" coming from the patient's mouth, if there is no chest movement, the patient is not breathing. Sporadic noises from the patient's airway *without* chest movement are called **agonal respirations.** There is no air movement in or out of the lungs. This occurs just prior to death.

If the patient is breathing, there will be a pulse. At this point, you can go on and check for serious bleeding. If the patient is not breathing, or if there is an airway obstruction, you must take immediate action to correct the problem. The procedures to follow were covered in Chapter 6.

ASSESS CIRCULATION

Check for a Pulse

carotid pulse the pulse that can be felt on each side of the neck.

If the patient is not breathing, check for a **carotid pulse** on either side of the neck as shown in Scan 7-8. You do this to determine if blood is circulating. The pulse at the neck is considered more reliable than the pulse at the wrist (radial). A pulse at the wrist may not be present if the patient is in shock, (hypoperfusion). The carotid pulse is taken as follows:

Locate the patient's "Adam's apple." Place the gloved tip of your index and middle fingers directly over the midline (middle) of this structure. Now, slide your fingertips to the side of the patient's neck closest to you. Do *not* slide the fingertips to the opposite side of the patient's neck, as this may apply improper pressure and close the airway. Do *not* attempt to take a carotid pulse on both sides of the neck at the same time. This may interfere with circulation to the brain.

You should detect a pulse in the groove between the trachea (windpipe) and the large muscle on the side of the neck. Very little pressure is needed to feel it. Take the carotid pulse for 5 to 10 seconds. Frequent practice will make this skill easy to master. It is not important during the initial assessment to count the exact rate of the pulse. You only want to determine if there is a pulse at all. If the pulse is very rapid or weak, the patient may be in shock (hypoperfusion). If there is no pulse, alert your dispatcher and begin CPR. If there is a pulse, but no breathing, begin artificial ventilations using a pocket mask or similar device.

If the patient is not breathing but does have a pulse, the patient may have an airway obstruction or be in respiratory arrest. You must take immediate action to ventilate the patient before the heart stops (see Chapter 6). If the chest does not rise during ventilations, the patient may have an airway obstruction.

Check for Serious Bleeding

The next step in the initial assessment is checking for serious bleeding (Scan 7-8). While any uncontrolled bleeding may eventually become life-threatening, you will only be concerned with profuse bleeding during the initial assessment. Blood that is bright red and spurting may be coming from an artery. Because blood in arteries is under a great deal of pressure, large amounts of blood may be lost in a short period of time. Flowing blood, darker in color, is most likely coming from a vein. Even if the bleeding is slow, it may be life-threatening if the patient has been bleeding for a long period of time. Look at the amount of blood that has been lost on the ground, in clothing, and in the hair. Your concern is for the total amount of blood that has been lost, not just how fast or slow the bleeding is. Methods of controlling serious bleeding are covered in Chapter 11. Some EMS systems will have First Responders check skin color, temperature, and condition, as well as a radial pulse at this time. An abnormal finding such as pale, cool, clammy skin could indicate a serious problem with circulation such as shock (hypoperfusion) or heart problems.

One condition in which you may alter this procedure slightly is when you immediately see profuse, spurting, or rapidly flowing bleeding. You may attempt to slow the bleeding at the same time you are evaluating the patient's breathing. Do what you can to control the bleeding, but never neglect the patient's airway and breathing status.

DETERMINE PRIORITY, OR URGENCY, OF PATIENT TRANSPORT

Information you give to the responding EMS dispatcher will help determine the priority of the patient for transport. A high-priority patient should be transported immediately, with little time spent on scene. High priority conditions indicating an immediate transport by EMS include a poor general impression, unconsciousness, conscious but not alert, breathing difficulty, severe bleeding or shock (hypoperfusion), complicated childbirth, chest pain, and any severe pain.

SPECIAL CONSIDERATIONS FOR INFANTS AND CHILDREN

Your assessment of an infant or a child will differ from that of an adult in a few ways. It is important for you to realize that children are not little adults. They react to illness and injury differently. They are often shy and distrustful of strangers. When checking the mental status of an unresponsive infant, talk to the infant and flick the bottom of the feet. An infant or a child who pays no attention to you or what you are doing may be in serious condition. Opening an infant's or a child's airway involves moving the head into a neutral position, not tilting it back as with an adult. Breathing and pulse rates in children are faster than in adults. The pulse of an infant or a small child is taken at the brachial artery in the upper arm, not at the neck or wrist.

An additional part of checking an infant's or a child's circulation is **capillary refill.** When the end of the child's fingernail is gently pressed, it turns white because blood flow is restricted. When the pressure is released, the nail bed turns pink again, usually in less than 2 seconds. This is a good way to evaluate the circulation of blood in an infant or a child. If it takes longer than 2 seconds for the nail bed to become pink again or if it does not return to pink at all, there may be a problem with circulation, such as shock (hypoperfusion), or blood loss. If the infant's nail beds are too small, you may perform the same test on the top of the patient's foot or back of the hand. Count, "one-one thousand, two-one thousand" or simply say "capillary refill."

capillary refill the return (refill) of capillaries after blood has been forced out by fingertip pressure applied by the rescuer to the patient's nail bed. Normal refill time is 2 seconds or less.

Usually, when adult patients have a serious problem, they gradually become worse. The downward trend is often spotted in time to take appropriate action. An infant's or a child's body can compensate so well for a problem such as blood loss that he or she may appear stable for some time, then suddenly become much worse. Children can actually maintain a near-normal blood pressure up to the time when almost half of their total blood volume is gone. That is why blood pressure is not a reliable assessment of a child's circulation. Checking capillary refill time is more reliable. It is vital for the First Responder to recognize the seriousness of a child's illness or injury early, before it is too late. You will learn about other considerations in approaching and assessing infants and children in Chapter 14.

ALERTING DISPATCH

There is a natural tendency for First Responders to contact EMS dispatch as soon as they arrive on the scene of an emergency. If you find an unresponsive adult, you should notify dispatch immediately, even before beginning CPR. Most EMS providers now carry defibrillators. The earlier the defibrillation of a cardiac arrest patient takes place, the greater the chance of survival. In other cases, it is best to gather some information, such as the type of emergency and number of patients, before you call. The information you give EMS dispatch may determine the type and level of response sent. Many EMS dispatch centers are now using an emergency medical dispatch system, or priority dispatching. This system determines if basic life support (BLS) or advanced life support (ALS) is sent, or a combination of both, and what response mode is used, such as "cold" with no lights or siren, or "hot" with lights and siren.

If you have notified EMS dispatch, but then obtain additional information, you may contact them again to update the EMS responders. You should update the responding EMS unit with a brief report by radio including the patient's level of consciousness, age and sex, chief complaint, airway and breathing status, circulation status, and interventions you have done and their results.

FOCUSED HISTORY AND PHYSICAL EXAM

The **focused history and physical exam** comes *after* the initial assessment and assumes that life-threatening problems have been found and corrected. If you have a patient with a life-threatening problem that you must continually care for, such as doing CPR on a cardiac arrest patient, you may not get to this assessment component.

The main purpose of the focused history and physical exam is to discover and care for the patient's specific injuries or medical problems. It is a very systematic approach to patient assessment. It also may assure the patient, family, and bystanders that there is concern for the patient and that something is being done for the patient immediately.

The focused history and physical exam includes a physical exam that may focus on a specific injury or medical complaint, or it may be a rapid exam of the entire body. It also includes obtaining a patient history and taking vital signs. The order in which these steps are accomplished is based on the patient's type of emergency (Table 7-1).

TABLE 7-1: THE FOCUSED HISTORY AND PHYSICAL EXAM

TRAUMA PATIENT	MEDICAL PATIENT (NO INJURIES)
Significant Mechanism of Injury	**Unresponsive Medical Patient**
• Perform a rapid trauma assessment. • Take vital signs. • Gather SAMPLE history.	• Perform a rapid physical exam. • Take vital signs. • Gather SAMPLE history.
No Significant Mechanism of Injury	**Responsive Medical Patient**
• Perform a focused trauma assessment. • Take vital signs. • Gather SAMPLE history.	• Gather SAMPLE history. • Take vital signs. • Perform focused physical exam.

First | Some important terms associated with the focused history and physical exam include:

- *SAMPLE history*—Gathering information by asking questions and listening. Whenever possible, the patient is your primary source for information. Family and bystanders are also sources of information (see p. 158).
- *Rapid or focused physical exam*—Performing a focused physical exam or rapid physical exam (medical patient), or focused trauma assessment or rapid trauma assessment (trauma patient), of the patient that requires you to use your senses in order to find injuries or indications of illness (see p. 160).
- *Vital signs*—Pulse, respirations, pupils, and relative skin color, temperature, and condition (see p. 160).
- **Symptoms**—What the patient tells you is wrong. Symptoms include chest pain, dizziness, and nausea.
- **Signs**—What you see, feel, hear, and smell when examining the patient. Signs include cool, clammy skin or abnormal vital sign measurements.

symptom what the patient tells about his injury or illness.

sign what you see, hear, feel, and smell in relation to the patient's illness or injury.

In some First Responder courses, blood pressure and assessment of the pupils are included among the required vital signs.

Many of the signs and symptoms you will find during the focused physical exam are the result of the body's compensating mechanisms. For example, to compensate for blood loss, the body will increase the pulse and breathing rates and close down, or constrict, the blood vessels in the extremities, resulting in cool, clammy, and pale skin. These actions are attempts to circulate an adequate amount of oxygenated blood to the more important parts of the body. Adequate blood flow to all cells of the body is called **perfusion.** Inadequate blood flow is called hypoperfusion, or shock. *Any abnormal findings during your exam indicate a problem and should not be ignored.*

perfusion the constant flow of blood through the capillaries.

FOCUSED HISTORY AND PHYSICAL EXAM— TRAUMA PATIENT

A *trauma* patient is one who has received a physical injury of some type. Your assessment will consist of a physical exam, vital signs, and patient history. The type of physical exam you perform and the order in which you do the various components of the assessment will be based on your initial assessment, what the patient and bystanders tell you, and the mechanism of injury.

The trauma patient is classified as either having a significant mechanism of injury (probably a serious injury) or having no significant mechanism of injury (probably not a serious injury). The assessment is different for each type of patient.

■ *Significant mechanism of injury*—To detect serious injuries, do a **rapid trauma assessment** of the entire body (a head-to-toe exam, pp. 165–170), and care for injuries. Obtain vital signs and gather a patient history. Then, if time permits, perform a **detailed physical exam.** Provide continued care during the ongoing assessment.

Significant mechanisms of injury include:
- Ejection from a vehicle
- Death in the same passenger compartment
- Falls greater than 15 feet
- Rollover vehicle collision
- High-speed vehicle collision
- Vehicle-pedestrian collision
- Motorcycle crash
- Unresponsive or altered mental status
- Penetrations of the head, chest, or abdomen

Significant mechanisms of injury for a child include:
- Falls of more than 10 feet
- Bicycle collision
- Medium-speed vehicle collision.

■ *No significant mechanism of injury*—Perform a **focused trauma assessment** on the area that the patient tells you is injured (Scan 7-10). Obtain vital signs and gather a patient history. Provide continued care during the **ongoing assessment.** (There is usually no need to perform a detailed physical exam on a patient with no significant mechanism of injury.)

FOCUSED HISTORY AND PHYSICAL EXAM— MEDICAL PATIENT

The focused history and physical exam for the patient with a medical problem has the same components as the exam of the trauma patient, but the *order* and *emphasis* are different. You are more concerned with the medical history of the patient because you are looking for a nature of illness instead of a mechanism of injury.

■ *Unresponsive patient, medical problem*—Perform a **rapid physical exam** to rule out any trauma. Take vital signs. Gather a SAMPLE history (see pp. 156, 158), if possible, from family or bystanders. Provide care as needed. Provide continued care during the **ongoing assessment.**

■ *Responsive patient, medical problem*—(Scan 7-11) Gather a SAMPLE history, observing patient signs and asking about the history of the illness and symptoms. The patient's chief complaint helps direct the questioning. Take vital signs. Perform a **focused physical exam** based on the patient's problem areas. Provide care as needed. Provide continued care during the **ongoing assessment.** Medical patients rarely require a **detailed physical exam.**

Note

The nature of injury is not always related to the mechanism of injury. Older patients and children may have significant injury without a significant MOI.

Focused History and Physical Exam—Responsive Trauma Patient

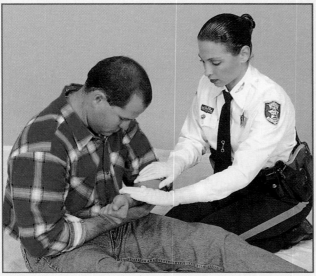

1. Perform a physical exam—focused or head-to-toe. Gather patient history while performing the exam.

TRAUMA PATIENT
- Perform a physical exam—focused or head-to-toe.
- Gather a patient history.
- Take vital signs.
- Render appropriate care.

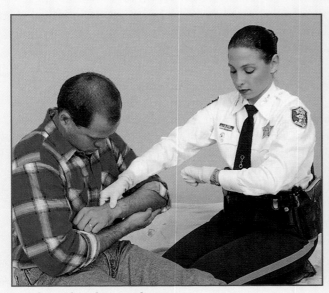

2. Obtain baseline vital signs.

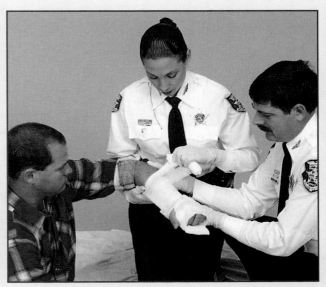

3. Render appropriate care.

REMEMBER: Always assess the patient for chief complaint and signs and symptoms. Continue to gather a patient history throughout the focused assessment, continue to monitor vital signs, and provide appropriate care.

PATIENT INFORMATION AND HISTORY

The Patient Interview

A responsive and alert patient is your best source of information. Direct your questions to him. Ask questions clearly, at a normal rate, and in a normal tone of voice. Avoid leading questions. Do not falsely reassure the patient. Do not say things such as "Everything will be fine" or "Take it easy, everything's OK." The patient knows this is not true and will lose confidence in you if you lie to him. Phrases such as "I'm here to help you" or "I'm doing everything I can to help you" are more appropriate.

 When obtaining information and history from your conscious and alert patient, ask the following questions:

1. *Your patient's name.* Simply ask, "What is your name?" This is an essential piece of information. It shows your patient that you are concerned for him as a person. Remember his name and use it often. Also, if your patient's level of consciousness decreases, you can call him by name to elicit a response.

2. *Children's ages and how to contact their parents.* As a First Responder, you do not need to know more than the general age of your adult patient. But the age of a child is important, as it may determine what type of care is provided. Ask all children their age. Ask adolescents for their age to be certain that you are dealing with a minor. Ask all minors how to contact their parents. Children may already be upset at being hurt or ill without their parents being there to help them. Always reassure them that someone will contact their parents.

3. *What is wrong?* This will usually be the patient's **chief complaint.** No matter what is wrong, ask if there is any pain. When an extremity is involved, ask if there is numbness, tingling, or a burning sensation in the limb. Any of these could indicate possible nerve or spinal injury. As you learn more about various illnesses and injuries, you will also learn additional questions to ask.

4. *How did it happen?* When caring for trauma patients, knowing how the patient was injured will help direct you to problems that may not be noticeable or obvious to you or the patient. If your patient is lying down, determine if she got into that position herself or was knocked down, fell, or was thrown. Do this for patients with medical problems, as well. Remember, the injury to the patient may be the result of a medical problem. This information may indicate the possibility of a spinal injury or internal bleeding.

5. *How long has the patient felt this way?* You want to know if the patient's problem occurred suddenly or if it has been developing for the past few days or over a period of time.

6. *Has this happened before or has the patient felt this way before?* Ask this question if it is appropriate. It is especially important to ask this question of medical patients. Is this the first time this has happened, or is it a recurring, or chronic, problem? This question is not usually asked of trauma patients, unless you suspect a recurring problem. If your patient has been hit by a car, it is not necessary to ask him if this has happened before.

Focused History and Physical Exam—Responsive Medical Patient

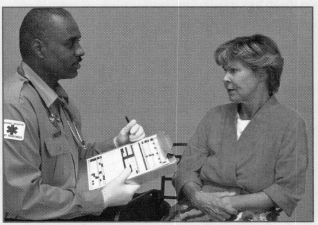

1. Gather patient history.

MEDICAL PATIENT
- Gather a patient history.
- Take vital signs.
- Perform a focused physical exam.
- Render patient care.

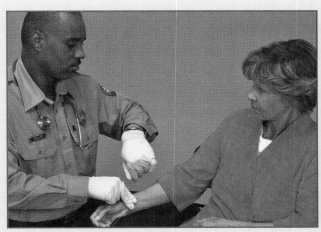

2. Take vital signs.

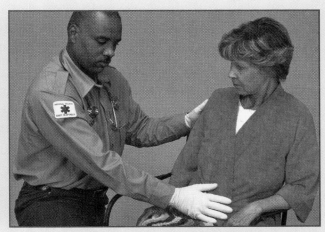

3. Perform a focused physical exam and render patient care.

7. *Are there any current medical problems?* Has the patient been feeling ill lately, seen a doctor, or is he being treated by a doctor for any problems?

8. *Are any medications being taken?* Your patient may not be able to tell you the exact name of a medication she is taking, especially if she is taking several. She may be able to tell you just general medication categories, such as "heart pills" or "water pills." Ask about not only prescription medications but over-the-counter medications as well. Routine use of simple medications such as aspirin may alter the treatment the patient receives at the hospital.

9. *Does the patient have any allergies?* Allergic reactions can vary from simple hives or itching to life-threatening airway problems and shock (hypoperfusion). Knowing what the patient is allergic to will enable you to keep the substance away from him. Be sure to ask specifically about allergies to medications, adhesive tape, and latex (as used in gloves), since the patient may come in contact with any of these during his care.

10. *When did the patient last eat?* This is an important question if your patient is a candidate for surgery. It is also important information when dealing with a patient who is having a diabetic emergency.

When obtaining a patient's history, EMS systems use the word SAMPLE as a memory aid for questions to be asked. Each letter of the word SAMPLE represents a specific question.

SAMPLE history a system of information gathering that allows the rescuer to ask questions about past or present medical or injury problems.

- **S**igns/symptoms?
- **A**llergies?
- **M**edications?
- **P**ertinent past medical history?
- **L**ast oral intake?
- **E**vents leading to the illness or injury?

When taking a history, maintain patient eye contact. This will improve personal communication and build the patient's confidence in you. If you look away while asking questions or listening to answers, it may indicate to your patient that you are not as concerned as you should be or not giving the patient your full attention. A simple touch can also improve communications. You touch the patient's forehead to note skin temperature and condition. But by touching the patient, you are also showing caring and concern. Patients are often fearful and anxious. Your calm, caring, and professional attitude can often do as much for the patient as any medical treatment you provide.

The Bystander Interview

You may encounter a patient who is unresponsive or not alert enough to answer your questions regarding his history. If this is the case, you must depend on family or bystanders for information. Ask specific, directed questions to shorten the time required to obtain the information. Questions to bystanders include:

1. *What is the patient's name?* If the patient is a minor, ask if the parents are there or if they have been contacted.

2. *What happened?* You can receive valuable information when asking this question. If the patient fell from a ladder, did he appear to faint or pass out first? Was he hit on the head by something? Clues from the answers to this question are limitless.

3. *Did they see anything else?* For example, was the patient holding his chest before he fell? This gives the bystander a chance to think again and add anything he remembers.

4. *Did the patient complain of anything before this happened?* You may learn of chest pain, nausea, shortness of breath, a funny odor where the patient was working, and other clues.

5. *Did the patient have any known illness or problems?* Family or friends who know the patient may know her medical history, such as heart problems, diabetes, allergies, or other problems that may cause a change in her condition.

6. *Does the patient take any medication?* Again, family or friends who know the patient may be aware of any medication he takes. When talking with the patient, family, friends, or bystanders, use the word *medication* or *medicine* instead of *drugs*. The public view drugs as illegal substances. Medicines or medications are considered prescriptions for legitimate medical purposes. Remember to ask the patient if he or she is taking over-the-counter medications.

The patient history and physical exams should not be done as isolated parts of the focused history and physical exam. They can be done *simultaneously*. There is no need to wait to take vital signs until the SAMPLE history has been completed. You may obtain the SAMPLE history while performing the physical exam of the patient. You can do them both at the same time. The patient may have moderate bleeding or some other problem that you cannot ignore while you finish conducting the history.

Most of the questions listed above are questions you would normally ask someone who is hurt or ill. You would usually introduce yourself and ask patients their name. If you saw they were sick or injured, you would ask them what was wrong and how it happened. Much of your First Responder training is simply formalized common sense.

When most people see something wrong, they want to take care of it or fix it immediately. Remember, this is correct during the *initial assessment* where you are finding and correcting life-threatening injuries. But you should *not* interrupt a focused history and physical exam to do something about a problem that will not get worse. You can stop bleeding from getting worse, but you cannot stop a broken leg. It is important to complete your focused physical exam or rapid trauma exam before treating injuries that you find. *By stopping to care for an injury, you may delay or forget the remainder of the exam and miss a more important problem.*

Medical Identification Devices

Medical identification devices can provide important information if the patient is unresponsive and a history cannot be obtained from family or bystanders. A common medical ID device is the Medic Alert emblem worn on a necklace or a wrist or ankle bracelet. One side of the device has a Star of Life emblem. Information on the patient's medical problem or allergies is engraved on the reverse side, along with a phone number for additional information. If you must move the patient or any of his extremities, take care to check for a medical ID device. Be sure to alert the EMS responders that the patient is wearing medical identification, and tell them what is on it, such as "diabetes," "heart condition," or "penicillin allergy."

PHYSICAL EXAM

If your trauma patient has no significant mechanism of injury and appears to have an isolated minor injury, supported by the mechanism of injury and what the patient tells you, perform a *focused trauma assessment* on the injury site and the area close to it. If the patient has a significant mechanism of injury or a serious injury or is unresponsive, perform a rapid trauma assessment of the entire body, which is explained later in this chapter.

The physical exam of a medical patient may be brief. If the patient is responsive, perform a *focused physical exam* based on the patient's history. If the patient is unresponsive, conduct a *rapid physical exam* of the entire body, which is explained later in this chapter.

The term **DCAP-BTLS** is used as an aid to remember what to look for during either your focused trauma assessment, rapid trauma assessment, or rapid physical exam. The letters stand for <u>d</u>eformities, <u>c</u>ontusions, <u>a</u>brasions, <u>p</u>unctures and penetrations, <u>b</u>urns, <u>t</u>enderness, <u>l</u>acerations, and <u>s</u>welling. Each part of the body is examined for these injuries and others specific to each body part (see Chapter 12).

DCAP-BTLS a study aid used to remember patient assessment factors. The letters stand for deformities, contusions, abrasions, punctures/penetrations, burns, tenderness, lacerations, and swelling.

VITAL SIGNS

vital signs at the First Responder level, these include pulse, respiration, and relative skin temperature, color, and condition. Vital signs may also include blood pressure and pupil assessment.

First | For most First Responders, the vital signs taken on a patient are pulse, respirations, and relative skin color, temperature, and condition. Some First Responders include determining blood pressure (see Appendix 1) and assessing pupils in the vital signs. Vital signs may alert you to problems that require immediate attention. Vital signs taken at regular intervals can help the First Responder determine if the patient's condition is getting better, worse, or staying the same.

Certain combinations of vital signs point to possible serious medical or traumatic conditions. For example, cool, clammy skin, a rapid, weak pulse, and increased breathing rate can indicate possible shock (hypoperfusion) in the presence of a significant mechanism of injury. Hot, dry skin with a rapid pulse may indicate a serious heat-related emergency. You can determine which patients are a high priority for immediate transport by taking vital signs.

For an adult, a continuous pulse rate of less than 60 beats per minute or above 100 beats per minute is considered abnormal. Likewise, a respiratory rate above 28 breaths per minute or below 8 breaths per minute is considered to be a serious condition. You should be concerned about these conditions because they indicate unstable situations that could become life-threatening; the patient could worsen quickly. Stay alert and monitor the patient closely. Keeping the patient quiet, at rest, caring for shock (hypoperfusion), and reassuring the conscious patient can make a difference in the outcome.

PULSE

radial pulse the wrist pulse. The site is the lateral wrist.

When taking a patient's pulse, you must assess for two factors: *rate* and *character*. Rate is a count of the number of heartbeats per minute and is used to determine if the patient's pulse is normal, rapid, or slow. Character is the rhythm and force of the pulse. The pulse rhythm will be either *regular* or *irregular*, and the pulse force (strength) will be either *full* or *weak* (Figure 7.3).

During the initial assessment, you checked the carotid pulse, in the patient's neck. During the focused history and physical exam, the **radial,** or wrist, **pulse**

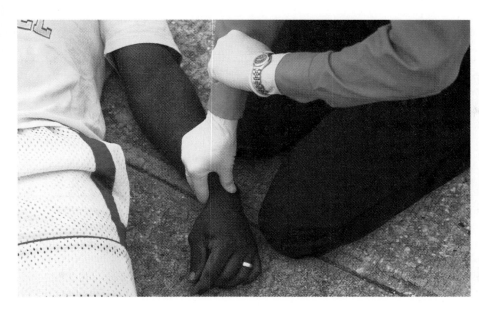

FIGURE 7.3
Pulse rate and character are vital signs.

is measured. The term *radial pulse* refers to the radial artery found in the lateral portion of the forearm, on the thumb side of the wrist. If for any reason you are unable to measure the radial pulse, measure the rate and character of the carotid pulse. The absence of a radial pulse when there is a carotid pulse indicates possible shock (hypoperfusion). A radial pulse may not be detectable if the blood pressure is too low or if there is an extremity injury that is interrupting blood flow to the distal arm. Do *not* start CPR based only on the absence of a radial pulse.

 To measure a radial pulse rate:

1. Use the three middle fingers of your gloved hand. Do *not* use the thumb, as it has its own pulse, and you may be measuring your own pulse rate instead of the patient's.

2. Place the fingertips on the palm side of the patient's wrist, just above the crease between hand and wrist. Slide your fingers from this position toward the thumb side of the wrist (lateral side). Keeping the fingertip of the middle finger on the crease between wrist and hand will ensure you are placing the fingertip over the site of the radial pulse.

3. Apply moderate pressure to feel the pulse beats. If the pulse is weak, you may have to apply more pressure. Too much pressure can cause pain to the patient or slow blood flow. By having all three fingers in contact with the patient's wrist and hand, you should be able to judge how much pressure you are applying.

4. Once you feel the pulse, make a quick judgment as to the rate. Does the pulse feel normal, rapid, or slow?

5. Count the beats for 30 seconds.

6. When counting, judge rhythm and force.

7. Multiply your 30-second count by 2 to determine the number of beats per minute.

> **Note**
>
> If the patient's pulse is irregular, count the pulse rate for a full minute.

While determining the pulse rate, notice if the beats are regular and judge the force of the beats. A rapid, regular pulse means something different than a rapid, irregular pulse. Is the pulse strong and full, or weak and thready? See

TABLE 7-2: ASSESSMENT SIGN: PULSE
[NORMAL ADULT—60–100 BEATS PER MINUTE]

OBSERVATION	POSSIBLE PROBLEM
Rapid, full	Internal bleeding (early stages), fear, heat emergency, overexertion, high blood pressure, fever
Rapid, thready	Shock (hypoperfusion), blood loss, heat emergency, diabetic emergency, failing circulatory system
Slow, full	Stroke, skull fracture, brain injury
No pulse	Cardiac arrest

Table 7-2 for the relationship between pulse and certain emergency problems you may see as a First Responder.

The normal pulse rate for adults at rest is between 60 and 100 beats per minute. Any rate above 100 is considered rapid, and any rate below 60 is considered slow. In emergency situations, because of anxiety or excitement, it is not unusual for the pulse to be about 100 beats per minute. You should consider a pulse rate over 100 or under 60 to be an indication of a serious problem. One exception to this is a well-conditioned athlete whose normal resting pulse may be at or below 50 beats per minute.

Newborn infants can have pulse rates around 120 to 160 beats per minute. Children up to 5 years old will show ranges from 80 to 140 beats per minute, depending on their age. The normal range of the pulse of children from 5 to 12 years of age is 70 to 110 beats per minute. Adolescents typically have a pulse rate ranging from 60 to 105 beats per minute.

Taking pulse rates efficiently takes practice. Practice on both males and females and on adults and children. Take "at rest" pulse rates, and then pulse rates after the person had completed some mild exercise. This practice will help you in judging normal and rapid rates.

Respirations

As with pulse rates, you should determine both *rate* and *character* of the patient's respirations, or breathing. The respiratory rate is a count of the patient's breaths and is classified as *normal*, *rapid*, or *slow*. The character includes *rhythm*, *depth*, *sound*, and *ease* of breathing. A single respiration is the entire cycle of breathing in and out.

While you are counting the respirations, note if the rhythm is regular or irregular. At the same time, decide if the depth of breathing is normal, shallow, or deep. Listen for any abnormal sounds during breathing, such as snoring, gurgling, gasping, wheezing, or "crowing." Notice if the breathing is easy or whether it appears labored, difficult, or painful (Figure 7.4). If the patient is responsive, ask if he is having any problems or pain while he breathes. A patient who has to work at breathing is in serious condition. Table 7-3 shows some of the problems that are associated with variations in respirations.

 To measure respiratory rate and character:

1. After completing the pulse count, leave your hand in the same position at the wrist, as if you were still counting the pulse rate. Many patients will unknowingly alter their respiratory rate if they know someone is watching them breathe.

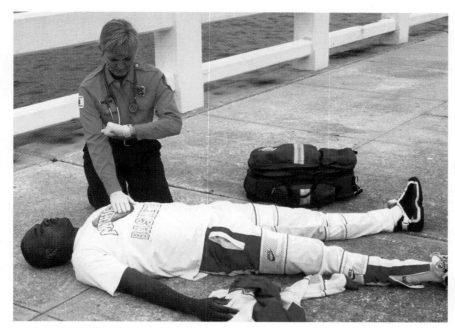

FIGURE 7.4
Breathing rate and character are vital signs.

2. Watch the patient's chest move and listen for sounds.

3. Count the number of breaths the patient takes in 30 seconds. (One breath = one inspiration and one expiration.) Multiply this number by 2 to obtain the number of breaths per minute.

4. While counting respirations, note rhythm, depth, sound, and ease of breathing.

If you have difficulty in visually counting the patient's respiratory rate from watching the chest movement, gently place your hand on the patient's chest near the xiphoid process. Let the patient know you are going to touch his chest and why. This will allow you to feel each inspiration and expiration. However, do *not* do this procedure if there are obvious injuries to the chest or abdomen.

TABLE 7-3: *A*SSESSMENT SIGN: RESPIRATIONS
[NORMAL RESTING ADULT—12–20 PER MINUTE]

OBSERVATION	POSSIBLE PROBLEM
Rapid, shallow	Shock (hypoperfusion), heart problems, heat emergency, diabetic emergency, heart failure, pneumonia
Deep, gasping, labored	Airway obstruction, heart failure, heart attack, lung disease, chest injury, lung damage from heart, diabetic emergency
Slowed breathing	Head injury, stroke, chest injury, certain drugs
Snoring	Stroke, fractured skull, drug or alcohol abuse, partial airway obstruction
Crowing	Airway obstruction, airway injury due to heat
Gurgling	Airway obstruction, lung disease, lung injury due to heat
Wheezing	Asthma, emphysema, airway obstruction, heart failure
Coughing blood	Chest wound, chest infection, fractured rib, punctured lung, internal injuries

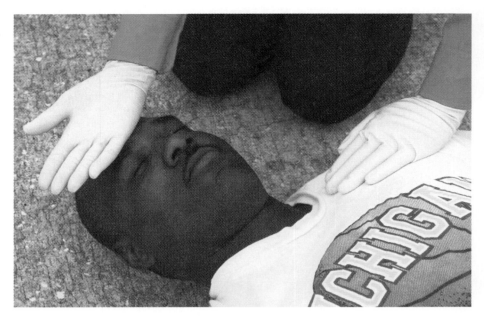

FIGURE 7.5
Relative skin temperature is a vital sign.

Normal respiratory rates for adults at rest are from 12 to 20 breaths per minute. Older adults breathe more slowly than younger adults. For adults, a respiratory rate of over 28 or below 8 breaths per minute is serious. Infants breathe from 25 to 50 times per minute. If the patient is a child between 1 and 5 years of age, a rate over 30 or below 20 breaths per minute is serious. A rate over 30 or below 15 breaths per minute is serious for children 6 to 10 years old.

Skin Temperature, Color, and Condition

First | Skin temperature, color, and condition are measured at the patient's forehead (Figure 7.5), unless this is not possible. The patient's abdomen may also be used as a site for this measurement. Some jurisdictions may have you check the extremities. Use the back of your hand to determine if the skin is normal, hot, cool, or cold. At the same time, notice if the skin is dry, moist, or clammy. Look for goose bumps, which are associated with chills. Table 7-4 shows some of the problems associated with skin temperature and conditions. Check the skin color. Does it appear normal, or is the color changed in any way (see Table 7-5)?

TABLE 7-4: *A*SSESSMENT SIGN: SKIN TEMPERATURE/CONDITION
[NORMAL—98.6°F]

SKIN TEMPERATURE/ CONDITION	SIGNIFICANCE/POSSIBLE CAUSES
Cool, clammy	Shock (hypoperfusion), heart attack, anxiety
Cold, moist	Body is losing heat
Cold, dry	Exposure to cold
Hot, dry	High fever, heat emergency, spinal injury
Hot, moist	High fever, heat emergency
Goose bumps accompanied by shivering, chattering teeth, blue lips, and pale skin	Chills, communicable disease, exposure to cold, pain, or fear

TABLE 7-5: Skin Color

OBSERVATION	SIGNIFICANCE/POSSIBLE CAUSES
Pink	Normal in light-skinned patients; normal in inner eyelids, lips, and nail beds of dark-skinned patients
Pale	Constricted blood vessels possibly resulting from blood loss, shock (hypoperfusion), decreased blood pressure, emotional distress
Blue (cyanotic)	Lack of oxygen in blood cells and tissues resulting from inadequate breathing or heart function
Red (flushed)	Exposure to heat, high blood pressure, emotional excitement; cherry red indicates late stages of carbon monoxide poisoning
Yellow (jaundiced)	Liver abnormalities
Blotchiness (mottling)	Occasionally in patients in shock (hypoperfusion)

Blood Pressure

While patient assessment is more reliable when the patient's blood pressure is taken and monitored, most First Responders do not carry the necessary equipment to measure this vital sign (Figure 7.6). If your EMS system requires that you determine blood pressure, see Appendix 1.

Pupils

Many EMS systems have the First Responder assess the patient's pupils as part of vital sign checks. The technique used and information gathered are given on page 167 as part of the head-to-toe examination. Table 7-6 provides observations

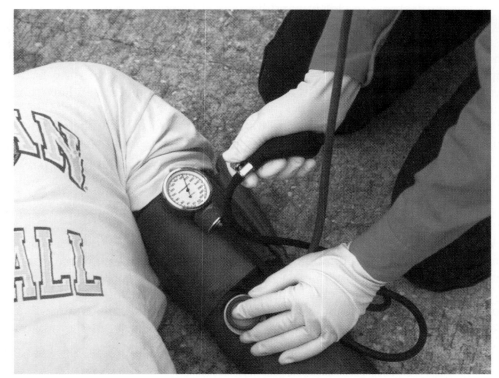

FIGURE 7.6
Blood pressure is a vital sign that some First Responders may be required to determine.

TABLE 7-6: Assessment Sign: Pupils

OBSERVATION	POSSIBLE PROBLEM
Dilated, unresponsive	Unconsciousness, shock, cardiac arrest, bleeding, certain medications, head injury
Constricted, unresponsive	Central nervous system damage, certain medications
Unequal pupils	Stroke, head injury

you may make when assessing a patient's pupils and suggests possible causes. Pupil assessment is usually repeated when vital sign assessment is repeated throughout the assessment and care of the patient.

Types of Physical Exams

The Rapid Trauma Assessment (Trauma Patient with Significant MOI)

The **rapid trauma assessment** is a head-to-toe physical exam of the patient that should take no more than 2 to 3 minutes. The rapid trauma assessment is performed on those patients having a significant mechanism of injury (MOI), as described previously. These patients will most likely have a high priority for transport. Remember, no matter what other injuries a patient has or does not have, a patient who is unresponsive or has an altered mental status has a significant mechanism of injury and is a high priority for immediate transport. Take great care not to move the patient. Neck and spinal injuries may be present. If available, another First Responder can take vital signs while you perform the exam to save time.

Do *not* contaminate wounds or aggravate injuries. Do *not* remove dressings or bandages you have placed to see if the bleeding has been stopped. This may destroy any early stages of clotting and healing. If bleeding continues once the wound has been bandaged, do *not* remove the bandages. Place additional dressings at the site and bandage in place. Most external bleeding can be controlled by direct pressure to the wound. If the wound continues to bleed, you may not be applying enough pressure. Never remove an impaled object in the body unless it is in the cheek and threatens the airway. Leave it in place and attempt to stabilize it as much as possible.

It is usually not necessary for the First Responder to remove the patient's clothing during the head-to-toe exam. You can remove or readjust those articles of clothing that interfere with your ability to examine the patient. Cut away, lift, slide, or unbutton clothing covering a suspected injury site, especially the chest, back, and abdomen, so you can fully inspect the area. If you suspect an injury to the upper leg, you may need to cut away the clothing covering it.

Penetrating wounds may have bleeding that will show or be felt on clothing. You may suspect internal injuries if your responsive patient indicates pain in the area or pain when you touch the area during your exam. If the patient is unresponsive or not alert, you may wish to remove or rearrange clothing covering the chest, abdomen, and back to examine them completely. If you must remove or rearrange the clothing of a responsive patient, tell the patient what you are doing and why. Take great care to protect the modesty of the patient and protect him from harsh weather conditions or temperatures.

Many EMS systems recommend or require having another woman present when a male First Responder examines a female patient. However, do not delay examining any patient. As a trained First Responder in an emergency situation, your intentions should be respected.

When conducting a rapid trauma assessment (head-to-toe physical exam), begin by taking the appropriate body substance isolation precautions. Remember, each area of the body is checked for DCAP-BTLS, plus other problems specific to that area. **If you are dealing with an unresponsive trauma patient, assume the patient has a neck and spinal injury. Immobilize the head and neck before continuing with your assessment.**

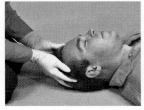

FIGURE 7.7
Examine the scalp.
(Step 1)

 To begin your assessment:

---

1. **Check the scalp for cuts and bruises** (Figure 7.7). Take care not to move the patient's head. Run your fingers through the patient's hair, looking for blood. Gently feel for cuts, swelling, or any other injuries. Do *not* part the hair over a suspected scalp injury. This could restart bleeding. Gently slide your gloved fingers under the back of the patient's neck and upward to the back of the head. Check your gloved fingers for blood.

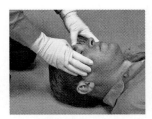

FIGURE 7.8
After examining the scalp, check the skull and face. (Step 2)

---

2. **Check the skull for deformities and depressions and check the face** (Figure 7.8). Note any depressions or bony projections that would indicate an injury to the skull. Check the facial bones for any signs of fracture or crushing, swelling, heavy discoloration, or depressions of the bones.

---

3. **Examine the patient's eyes** (Figure 7.9). Note any cuts, impaled objects, or signs of chemical burns. Have the patient open his eyes, or gently open the eyes of an unconscious patient. Look for cuts, foreign objects, or burns. Check the pupils for size, equality, and reaction to light. A penlight would be helpful for this. If outside in bright sunlight, cover the patient's eye with your hand. Remove your hand quickly and watch for reaction of the pupil to the light. Pupils that are *dilated* or *constricted* may indicate possible drug usage, shock (hypoperfusion), or cardiac arrest. *Unequal pupils* may indicate a brain or spinal injury. *Dull, lackluster* eyes may indicate shock (hypoperfusion).

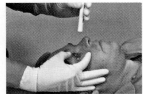

FIGURE 7.9
Examine the eyelids, eyes, and pupils.
(Step 3)

---

4. **Look at the inner surface of the eyelids** (Figure 7.10). A pale color may indicate major blood loss. During the rest of the exam, be alert for external bleeding or signs of internal bleeding. A yellow color (jaundice) may indicate a liver disease or injury.

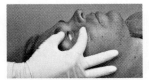

FIGURE 7.10
Are the inner eyelids pale? (Step 4)

---

5. **Inspect the ears and nose for blood, clear fluid, or bloody fluid** (Figure 7.11). Use a penlight or other light source for this. Blood in the nose may be caused by a simple nasal tissue injury. But it could also mean a skull fracture. Blood in the ears or clear or bloody fluids in the ears or nose are strong indications of a skull fracture.

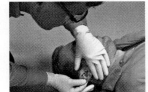

FIGURE 7.11
Check the ears and nose for blood and clear fluids. (Step 5)

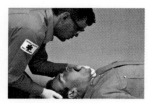

FIGURE 7.12
Examine the mouth for obstructions, bleeding, and tissue damage. (Step 6)

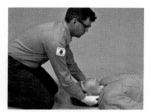

FIGURE 7.13
Check the back of the neck for point tenderness. (Step 7)

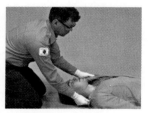

FIGURE 7.14
Check the front of the neck for injuries and openings. (Step 8)

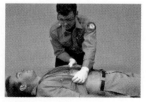

FIGURE 7.15
Inspect the chest for wounds and visible deformities. (Step 9)

6. Inspect the mouth for possible airway obstructions, bleeding, and tissue damage (Figure 7.12). If your patient is unconscious, you will have to open his mouth. Assume that all unconscious trauma patients have neck and spinal injury, so open the mouth gently, without moving the head. Look for broken teeth, bridges, dentures, and crowns. Check for chewing gum, food, vomitus, and foreign objects. In children, take extra care in looking for toys, balls, and other objects in the mouth and the back of the throat. If you find any objects, follow the directions given in Chapter 6. Inspect the mouth for blood and note any odd breath odors.

7. Check the cervical spine for point tenderness and deformity (Figure 7.13). Any point tenderness (pain to gentle finger pressure) or deformity should be considered an indication of possible spinal injury. If you have already immobilized the patient's head and neck, continue with the exam. If not, stop the exam and immobilize the head and neck now, before continuing. Next, gently check the patient's chin for point tenderness and deformity, steadying the patient's chin with one hand. Look for any medical alert identification device. If one is found, do not remove it.

8. Check the front of the neck for injury and deformity (Figure 7.14). The patient may have a surgical opening in the front or side of his neck. See Chapter 6 for details about such patients.

9. Inspect the chest for cuts, bruises, penetrations, and impaled objects (Figure 7.15). If necessary, bare the chest and upper abdomen. Leave impaled objects in place. Do not remove them. Also check for medical alert identification devices.

10. Feel the collarbone (clavicles) for tenderness and look for deformity (Figure 7.16).

11. Examine the chest for possible fractures (Figure 7.17). Gently apply pressure to the sides of the chest with your hands. Warn the patient of possible pain. Pain here indicates possible rib fractures.

12. Check for equal expansion of the chest (Figure 7.18). Feel for equal expansion of both sides of the chest. Look for chest movements and note any portion that appears to be floating or moving in opposite directions to the rest of the chest. This could indicate an injury called a flail chest in which several ribs are fractured in two places, causing them to float in the chest (see Chapter 12). When baring the chest of female patients, provide them with as much privacy as possible.

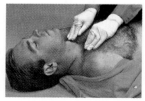

FIGURE 7.16
Check the clavicles for point tenderness and look for deformity. (Step 10)

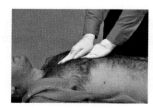

FIGURE 7.17
Gently apply pressure to the sides of the chest to check for fractures. (Step 11)

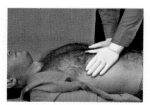

FIGURE 7.18
Check for the equal expansion of the chest. (Step 12)

13. Inspect the abdomen for cuts, bruises, penetrations, distention, and impaled objects (Figure 7.19).

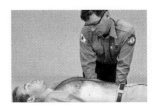

FIGURE 7.19
Inspect the abdomen for wounds and visible deformity. (Step 13)

14. Feel the abdomen for tenderness (Figure 7.20). Prepare the patient for the possibility of pain. If the patient tells you his abdomen already hurts, leave the area alone, but ask where it hurts and what it feels like. Gently press on the abdomen with the palm side of the fingers, noting any areas that are rigid, swollen, or painful. As you press on the area, ask the patient if it hurts. Note if the pain is *local*, just one spot, or *general*, spread over a wide area. Check each abdominal quadrant and note any problems in that specific quadrant.

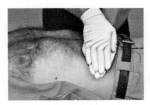

FIGURE 7.20
Check for abdominal tenderness. (Step 14)

15. Feel the lower back for point tenderness and look for deformity (Figure 7.21). Take care not to move the patient. Gently slide your gloved hands into the area of the lower back formed by the curve of the spine. Check your gloves for blood.

16. Feel the pelvis for injuries and possible fractures (Figure 7.22). After checking the lower back, gently slide your hands from the small of the back to the lateral "wings" of the pelvis. Warn the patient of possible pain and gently compress the pelvis. Press in and down at the same time, noting any pain or deformity.

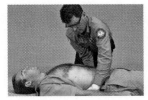

FIGURE 7.21
Check the lower back for point tenderness. (Step 15)

17. Note any obvious injury to the genital (groin) region (Figure 7.23). Look for bleeding and impaled objects. Do *not* expose the area unless you feel there is an injury. In male patients, check for *priapism,* the persistent erection of the penis caused by spinal injury. If there is any reason to suspect spinal injury and clothing prevents you from noting the presence of an erect penis, gently brush the genital region with the back of your hand. Priapism is an important indication of spinal injury and should be noted as a serious consideration during the head-to-toe exam.

18. Examine the legs and feet (Figure 7.24). Examine each leg and foot individually. Compare one limb to the other in terms of length, shape, and any apparent swelling or deformity. Do *not* move or lift the legs. Do *not* change the position of the legs or feet. Note any discoloration, bleeding, bone protrusions, and obvious fractures. If you think there is a fracture, warn the patient about possible pain and apply light fingertip pressure to the site. Note any point tenderness. *Do not touch possible fracture (painful, swollen, or deformed) sites if the skin is broken.*

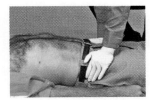

FIGURE 7.22
Gently apply pressure to check for pelvic fractures. (Step 16)

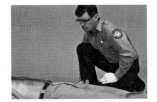

FIGURE 7.23
Look for obvious injuries to the genital region. (Step 17)

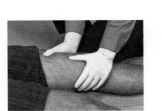

FIGURE 7.24
Examine the legs and feet. DO NOT lift or move the legs or feet. (Step 18)

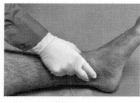

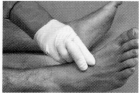

FIGURE 7.25
When possible without risk to the patient, take a distal pulse. (Step 19)

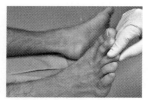

FIGURE 7.26
Check for sensation in the toes of conscious patients. (Step 20)

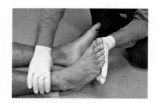

FIGURE 7.27
Can the patient push his foot against the palm of your hand? (Step 20)

19. **Check for distal pulse** (Figures 7.25). Confirm the circulation of blood through the leg and foot by feeling for a distal pulse. The most useful is the *posterior tibial* (TIB-e-al) *pulse*, felt behind the medial ankle, as shown. If the patient is wearing boots, do *not* remove them if the patient has indications of crush injury to the leg or foot, objects impaled in the leg or foot, severe leg or foot fractures, or any indications or possibilities of spinal injury, unless you must to stop obvious bleeding.

Another distal pulse is the *dorsalis pedis* (dor-SAL-is PEED-is) *pulse* located lateral to the large tendon of the big toe. This pulse can be important in assessment because some patients do not have a posterior tibial pulse. Some EMS systems do not have First Responders use the dorsalis pedis pulse in the exam because they would have to unlace or remove the patient's shoe to feel this pulse.

What you can do about the problem of circulation is minimal. Do not cause additional injury to the patient for the sake of taking a distal pulse. When possible, check both legs for a distal pulse. You may also check capillary refill in pediatric patients at this time (see pp. 151–152 and Chapter 14).

20. **Check for sensation and possible paralysis to the legs and feet.** Do *not* perform this on patients with possible fractures or dislocations of the lower limbs. Do *not* aggravate possible injuries by removing shoes. If you cannot rule out paralysis, assume the patient has spinal injury.

Touch each toe and have the patient tell you if he can feel it (Figure 7.26). You may grasp the toes through the patient's shoe if you believe there are no injuries to the toes. Have the patient gently press the sole of each foot against the palm of your hand and, with your hand on the top of his foot, have him pull up, or flex his foot, lifting your hand (Figure 7.27). Then pinch the top of the foot (Figure 7.28). Do these tests on both feet. If the patient does not respond to any one of these tests, consider him to have a spinal injury.

21. **Examine the upper extremities from the shoulders to the fingertips** (Figure 7.29). Examine each limb separately. The procedures are similar to those of the lower extremities.

- Note any cuts, bruises, impaled objects, bleeding, deformities, swelling, discoloration, protruding bones, or obvious fractures. Check for point tenderness at any suspected site of fracture. *Do not touch open fracture sites.*

- Confirm a wrist (radial) pulse in both arms (Figure 7.30). Do not measure pulse rate. Simply confirm circulation. You may also check capillary refill as explained earlier in this chapter.

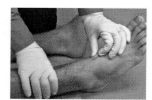

FIGURE 7.28
If the patient is unconscious, pinch the most accessible area of the lower limbs. (Step 20)

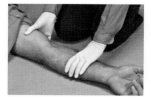

FIGURE 7.29
Check the arms and hands for injuries. (Step 21)

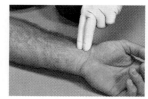

FIGURE 7.30
Take a radial pulse. Remember, you did this for one arm when finding vital signs. (Step 21)

- If alert, have the patient identify the finger you touch (Figure 7.31) and grip your hand (Figure 7.32). When checking grip, test both hands at once to determine equality of strength. Have the patient grip your index finger and middle finger together; having the patient squeeze your whole hand may be painful for you. If the patient is unresponsive, pinch the back of his hand (Figure 7.33).
- Look for a medical alert identification device.

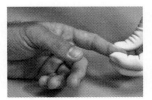

FIGURE 7.31
Can the patient tell you which finger was touched? (Step 21)

WARNING:

You must assume your patient has a spinal injury if he fails to respond properly on any test for leg or arm nerve function. Also, an alert patient who cannot move his hands or arms may suddenly stop breathing due to a spinal injury. Continually monitor the patient.

---

22. **Inspect the back surfaces of the patient for bleeding and obvious injury** (Figure 7.34). Do *not* lift or roll the patient if there is any indication of skull, neck, or spinal injuries. Consider any unresponsive trauma patient as having a neck injury.

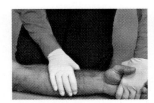

FIGURE 7.32
Can the patient grasp your hand? (Step 21)

Focused Trauma Assessment (Trauma Patient with No Significant MOI)

When your trauma patient has no significant mechanism of injury, the steps of the **focused trauma assessment** are appropriately simplified. Instead of examining the patient from head-to-toe, you *focus* your assessment on just the areas that the patient tells you are painful or that you suspect may be injured because of the mechanism of injury. The assessment includes a physical exam, taking vital signs, and a SAMPLE history.

Your decision on which areas of the patient's body to assess will depend partly on what you see (such as obvious injuries) and the patient's **chief complaint.** The chief complaint is what the patient tells you is the matter. The patient may complain of pain in his leg after falling. You should also consider potential injuries based on the mechanism of injury. For example, if the patient complains of pain in his ankle after falling down several stairs, you may also consider possible back or neck injuries, and treat the patient accordingly. Assess the areas of the body using the memory aid DCAP-BTLS, as previously described.

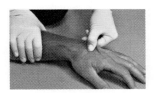

FIGURE 7.33
If the patient is unconscious, pinch the hands. (Step 21)

Rapid Physical Exam (Unresponsive Medical Patient)

The **rapid physical exam** of an unresponsive medical patient is almost the same as the rapid trauma assessment for a trauma patient with a significant mechanism of injury (MOI). You will rapidly assess the patient's head, neck, chest, abdomen, pelvis, extremities, and posterior. As you assess each area of the body, you will look for signs of injury using the memory aid DCAP-BTLS, as with the trauma patient. Other things to look for in the medical patient include:

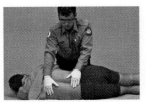

FIGURE 7.34
If there are no injuries to the head, neck, spine, or extremities, inspect the back surface. (Step 22)

NECK	Neck vein distention, and medical identification devices
CHEST	Presence and equality of breath sounds
ABDOMEN	Distention, firmness, or rigidity
PELVIS	Incontinence of urine or feces
EXTREMITIES	Pulse, motor function, sensation, and medical alert devices

Focused Physical Exam (Responsive Medical Patient)

The **focused physical exam** of a responsive medical patient is usually brief. The most important assessment information will be obtained through the SAMPLE history and the taking of vital signs. Focus the exam on the body part that the patient has a complaint about. For example, if the patient complains of abdominal pain, focus your exam on that area of the body. As with the trauma patient, use DCAP-BTLS as a memory aid for what to look for, as well as problems specific to each body part, as in the rapid physical exam.

Completing the Exam

Upon completing the physical exam of the patient, you must consider all the signs found that could indicate an illness or injury. Certain combinations of signs can point to one specific problem. A finding as simple as pain in a certain region of the body may be significant. The lack of certain findings may also lead you to a conclusion. For example, if a patient has an obvious injury but feels no pain at the site, you must consider problems such as spinal injury, brain damage, shock (hypoperfusion), or drug abuse.

During your assessment of the patient, and throughout the time you are caring for him or her, remember the first rule of emergency care: *Do no further harm.* Do only what you have been trained to do. Avoid additional injury and aggravating existing injuries and problems. (See a summary of Rules for Patient Examination in Table 7-7.) Later in your training you will learn what you can do to help the patient based on the findings in your physical exam.

DETAILED PHYSICAL EXAM

Usually, a full detailed physical exam is performed on the patient while en route to the hospital or medical facility. If the response time of EMS is lengthy, the First Responder may perform this exam if time permits (Scan 7-12). Sometimes, the First Responder is a part of the crew or may accompany the ambulance crew to assist in continuing care of the patient. A detailed physical exam

---

TABLE 7-7: RULES FOR PATIENT EXAM

1. Do no further harm.
2. If anything about the patient's awareness or behavior does not seem "right," consider that something is seriously wrong.
3. Patients who appear stable may worsen rapidly. You must be aware of all changes in a patient's condition.
4. Watch the patient's skin for color changes.
5. Look over the entire patient and note anything that appears to be wrong.
6. Unless you are certain that the patient is free of spinal injury, assume every trauma patient has a spinal injury.
7. Tell the patient that you are going to examine him, what you will be doing, and why you are doing it. Stress the importance of the exam.
8. Take vital signs.
9. Conduct a head-to-toe exam. If anything looks, sounds, feels, smells, or "seems" wrong to you or the patient, assume that there is something seriously wrong with the patient.
10. The failure of the patient to respond properly on any test for leg or arm nerve action must be considered to be a sign of spinal injury.

The Head-to-Toe Exam

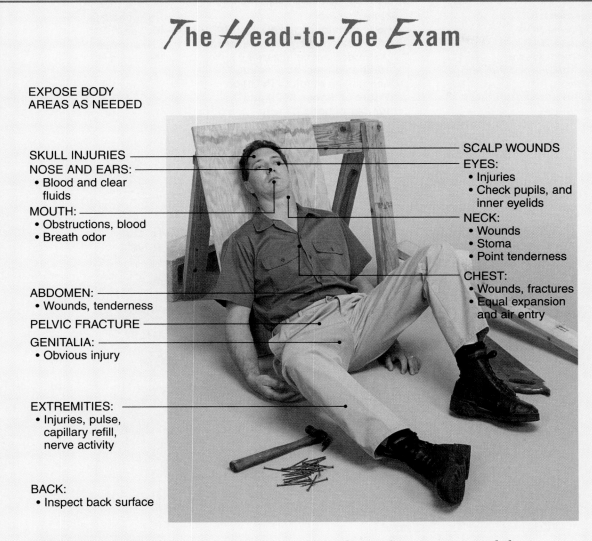

EXPOSE BODY
AREAS AS NEEDED

SKULL INJURIES
NOSE AND EARS:
• Blood and clear
  fluids
MOUTH:
• Obstructions, blood
• Breath odor

ABDOMEN:
• Wounds, tenderness
PELVIC FRACTURE
GENITALIA:
• Obvious injury

EXTREMITIES:
• Injuries, pulse,
  capillary refill,
  nerve activity

BACK:
• Inspect back surface

SCALP WOUNDS
EYES:
• Injuries
• Check pupils, and
  inner eyelids
NECK:
• Wounds
• Stoma
• Point tenderness

CHEST:
• Wounds, fractures
• Equal expansion
  and air entry

NOTE: The head-to-toe exam applies to both the focused assessment and the detailed assessment.

is done by *repeating* the rapid trauma assessment in *much more detail, taking more time.* Detailed physical exams are most often performed on trauma patients with a significant mechanism of injury. First Responders may perform a detailed physical exam on responsive medical patients but may be too involved in necessary patient care to do one on unresponsive medical patients.

ONGOING ASSESSMENT

When performing the *ongoing assessment* either at the scene or en route to the hospital, repeat the initial assessment, reassess vital signs, and check any interventions to assure they are still effective. Reassess the patient, watching closely for any changes in his or her condition. Repeated assessments and the changes

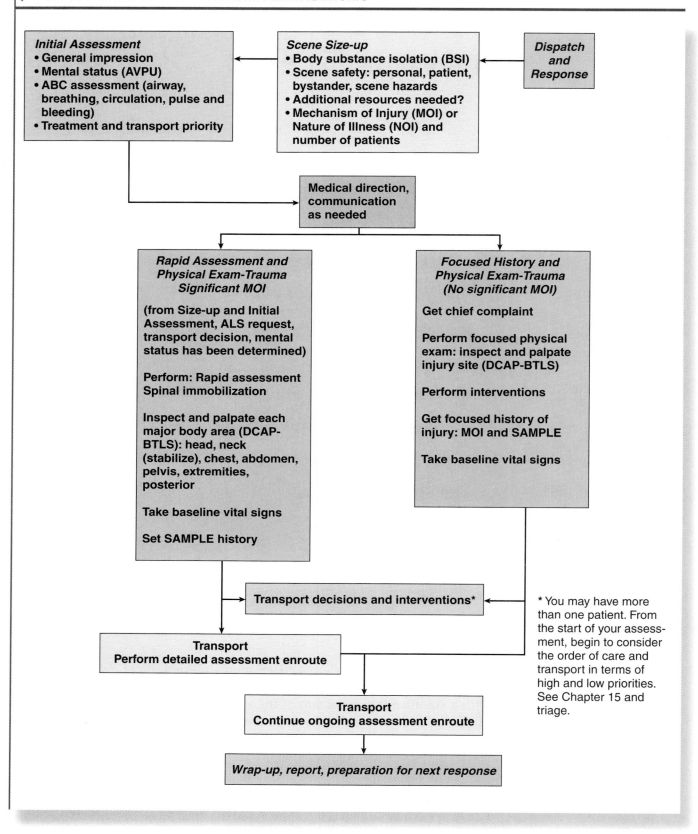

Initial Assessment
- General impression
- Mental status (AVPU)
- ABC assessment (airway, breathing, circulation, pulse and bleeding)
- Treatment and transport priority

Scene Size-up
- Body substance isolation (BSI)
- Scene safety: personal, patient, bystander, scene hazards
- Additional resources needed?
- Mechanism of Injury (MOI) or Nature of Illness (NOI) and number of patients

Dispatch and Response

Medical direction, communication as needed

Rapid Assessment and Physical Exam-Trauma Significant MOI

(from Size-up and Initial Assessment, ALS request, transport decision, mental status has been determined)

Perform: Rapid assessment Spinal immobilization

Inspect and palpate each major body area (DCAP-BTLS): head, neck (stabilize), chest, abdomen, pelvis, extremities, posterior

Take baseline vital signs

Set SAMPLE history

Focused History and Physical Exam-Trauma (No significant MOI)

Get chief complaint

Perform focused physical exam: inspect and palpate injury site (DCAP-BTLS)

Perform interventions

Get focused history of injury: MOI and SAMPLE

Take baseline vital signs

Transport decisions and interventions*

Transport
Perform detailed assessment enroute

* You may have more than one patient. From the start of your assessment, begin to consider the order of care and transport in terms of high and low priorities. See Chapter 15 and triage.

Transport
Continue ongoing assessment enroute

Wrap-up, report, preparation for next response

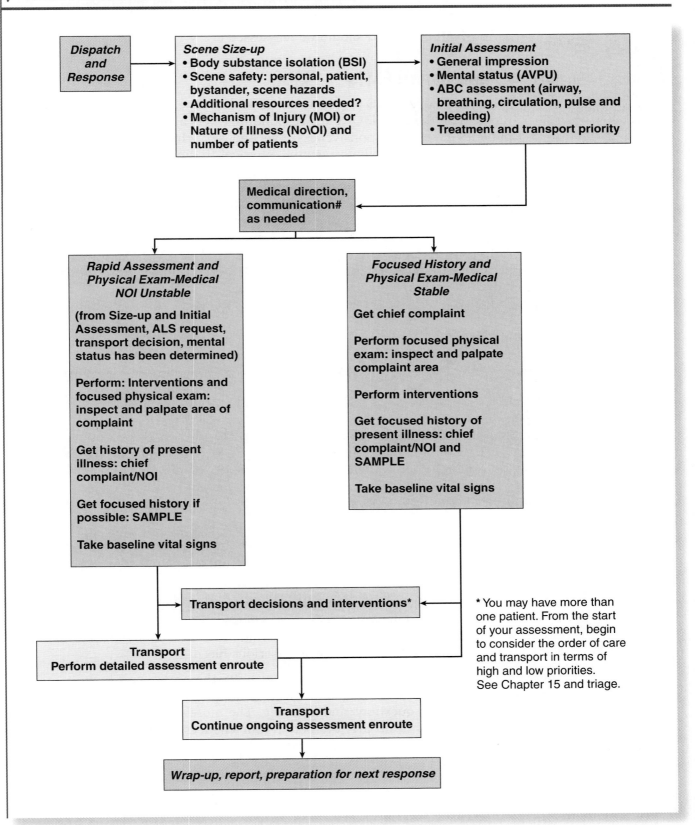

Dispatch and Response

Scene Size-up
- Body substance isolation (BSI)
- Scene safety: personal, patient, bystander, scene hazards
- Additional resources needed?
- Mechanism of Injury (MOI) or Nature of Illness (No\OI) and number of patients

Initial Assessment
- General impression
- Mental status (AVPU)
- ABC assessment (airway, breathing, circulation, pulse and bleeding)
- Treatment and transport priority

Medical direction, communication# as needed

Rapid Assessment and Physical Exam-Medical NOI Unstable

(from Size-up and Initial Assessment, ALS request, transport decision, mental status has been determined)

Perform: Interventions and focused physical exam: inspect and palpate area of complaint

Get history of present illness: chief complaint/NOI

Get focused history if possible: SAMPLE

Take baseline vital signs

Focused History and Physical Exam-Medical Stable

Get chief complaint

Perform focused physical exam: inspect and palpate complaint area

Perform interventions

Get focused history of present illness: chief complaint/NOI and SAMPLE

Take baseline vital signs

Transport decisions and interventions*

* You may have more than one patient. From the start of your assessment, begin to consider the order of care and transport in terms of high and low priorities. See Chapter 15 and triage.

Transport
Perform detailed assessment enroute

Transport
Continue ongoing assessment enroute

Wrap-up, report, preparation for next response

they may find in patient condition are called "trending." Remember that patients will either get better, get worse, or stay the same. Seriously ill or injured patients should be reassessed every 5 minutes. Patients who are not seriously ill or injured should be reassessed every 15 minutes.

Hand-off to EMTs

When additional EMS providers arrive at the scene, it is important to communicate with them well. Give the responding EMTs a verbal report including the patient's level of responsiveness, age and sex, chief complaint, airway and breathing status, circulatory status, physical findings, SAMPLE history, interventions applied, and the patient's response to those interventions.

Some EMS systems include the completion of a written report by the First Responder to be given to the EMS crew. This written form will usually include the same information as the verbal report, previously mentioned. The First Responder's written report and the information in it will become part of the EMS crew's patient care report. Accuracy is vital in any verbal or written report because care given by the responding EMS crew and the hospital ER may be based, in part, on your evaluation of the patient.

Summary

Patient assessment is one of the most important skills you will learn as a First Responder. Even though it may seem time-consuming, it is necessary to properly and completely examine the patient if you are to determine what care the patient requires. You must detect life-threatening problems and correct them as quickly as possible. Then you must detect problems that may become life-threatening if they go untreated. Always keep the following in mind:

Arrival—Perform a scene size-up. Make sure the scene is safe to enter. Gain information quickly from the scene, the patient, bystanders; and determine nature of illness or mechanisms of injury, deformities or injuries, and signs and symptoms.

Initial Assessment—Determine if the patient is responsive. Next, maintain cervical-spine control while you check for an open airway, respirations, circulation, and severe bleeding. Make certain that there is an open airway, adequate breathing, and a pulse. Control all serious bleeding.

Focused History and Physical Exam—Look over the scene, and look over the patient. Look for medical identification devices. Begin gathering information by asking questions and listening. The more organized your interview and physical exam are, the better your chances of gaining the needed information. As part of your examination of the patient, take vital signs. Determine the pulse and respiratory rate and character. Determine relative skin temperature, color, and condition. In some areas, First Responders also measure blood pressure and pupil size.

While EMTs usually complete the detailed physical exam en route to the hospital, in some systems First Responders are part of the team and may assist.

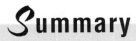

Remember to repeat the initial assessment and the taking of vital signs. If you are assisting with the ongoing assessment, note any changes in patient condition or the need for additional interventions.

The patient assessment varies somewhat depending on whether the patient is a responsive or an unresponsive medical patient or a trauma patient with a significant or with no significant mechanism of injury. Generally, a patient assessment includes a head-to-toe exam:

Head—Check the scalp for cuts, bruises, swellings, and the skull and facial bones for deformities, depressions, and other signs of injury. Inspect the eyelids and the eyes for injury and check pupil size, equality, and reactions to light. Note the color of the inner surface of the eyelids. Look for blood, clear fluids, or bloody fluids in the nose and ears. Examine the mouth for airway obstructions, blood, and any odd odors.

Neck—Examine the cervical spine for injury and tenderness. Recheck to see if the patient is a neck breather. Note obvious injuries and look for medical identification devices.

Chest—Examine the chest for cuts, bruises, penetrations, and impaled objects. Check for possible fractures. Look for equal expansion and note chest movements.

Abdomen—Examine the abdomen for cuts, bruises, penetrations, and impaled objects. Check for local pain and general pain as you examine the abdomen for tenderness.

Lower back—Feel for point tenderness, deformity, and other signs of injury. Check the rest of the back last and only if it is safe to roll the patient (no suspected back injuries).

Pelvis—Use compression to check for possible fractures and note any signs of injuries.

Genital region—Note any obvious injuries. Look for priapism when examining male patients.

Lower extremities—Examine for deformities, swelling, discoloration, bleeding, bone protrusions, and obvious fractures. Check for point tenderness on suspected closed fracture sites. Check for distal pulse in both legs. Do a capillary refill in pediatric patients. Determine motor function.

Upper extremities—Examine for deformities, swelling, bleeding, discoloration, bone protrusions, and obvious fractures. Check for point tenderness on all suspected closed fracture sites. Check for a radial pulse for both arms. Do a capillary refill in pediatric patients. Determine nerve activity. Look for medical identification devices.

Remember and Consider...

It is extremely important that you constantly review and remember the systematic approach to patient assessment.

✔ Take time now to review the rules for patient exam in Table 7-7. You might consider copying each of these rules on a 3″ × 5″ card and keeping these cards as quick reminders of the importance of patient assessment order.

Consider the importance of vital signs and what they can tell you about a patient's condition. Keep in mind:

✔ A pulse rate in an adult of less than 60 beats per minute or above 100 beats per minute is considered serious.

✔ A respiratory rate in an adult above 28 breaths per minute or below 8 breaths per minute is considered serious.

✔ Skin color, temperature, and condition can signal serious conditions such as shock (hypoperfusion), heart attack, decreased blood pressure, and heat and cold emergencies.

✔ Also remember the memory aids DCAP-BTLS and SAMPLE. Work with a partner and practice using these memory aids in various scenarios.

Investigate...

Additional vital signs that some First Responders may be required to take include determining blood pressure and examining the patient's pupils.

✔ Find out if your service requires that you know how to take a patient's blood pressure. If so, review the material on blood pressure determination in Appendix 1. Does your service require examination of the patient's pupils? If so, review Table 7-6.

Study the following scenarios. Place check marks in the columns below as appropriate to indicate which skills you would perform for each scenario. You will use skills from previous units in these scenarios. Refer to text pages 1–81 and 85–123. Write the skill number of any skills you would use from Unit 1 and Unit 2 after each scenario or in the columns under "Units." Discuss answers with other students and your instructor.

SCENARIO 1: Eighteen-year-old Craig has called 911 about his mother. Your First Responder unit is the first on the scene, and you find Craig's mother in bed. The woman is 50 years old and says her chest has been hurting for days, usually when she tries to do some activity, like carry the laundry upstairs. She also tells you that she has trouble catching her breath when she has this pain, but if she sits still for a while and concentrates on breathing deeply and slowly, the chest pain goes away. Her vital signs are within normal range.

(Skills from Unit 1: _____ Skills from Unit 2: _____)

SCENARIO 2: Everyone in the Corbit family has been feeling like they've had the flu all week. Mr. Corbit makes himself go to work on Wednesday, and oddly enough, feels better. When he returns home, he finds his family members unconscious in the family room where they were watching T.V. He calls 911, and while he waits for response units, leaves the door open and tries to rouse his wife and teenage children. The victims are breathing and have a weak pulse when you arrive.

(Skills from Unit 1: _____ Skills from Unit 2: _____)

SCENARIO 3: Your unit and crew are returning to the station after finishing up at another emergency. As you watch a boy skateboarding down the sidewalk, you see him try to jump off the curb. As he tries to land and continue on with his skateboarding acrobatics, he hits a patch of grass and falls. He rolls over, sits up, and grimaces as he cradles his arm against his chest.

(Skills from Unit 1: _____ Skills from Unit 2: _____)

SCENARIO 4: You and your crew are sitting at a traffic light. When it turns green, the car next to you speeds off quickly into the intersection, but a red-light runner crashes into the vehicle on the passenger side and pushes the driver-side front fender into a light pole across the intersection. The driver of the striking vehicle is conscious and alert, but the driver in the other vehicle is unconscious but is breathing and has a pulse.

(Skills from Unit 1: _____ Skills from Unit 2: _____)

Instructors will demonstrate all skills and will give you time to practice them while they coach you. You will learn more about the skills marked with an * and practice them in future lessons. They are listed here to provide an overview and understanding of all skills required for these scenarios.

Skills	Scenarios				Units	
	#1	**#2**	**#3**	**#4**	**#1**	**#2**

Scene size up: Chapter 7, pp. 140–144

1. Use or indicate use of appropriate body substance isolation
2. Check scene safety (self, patient, bystander, hazards)
3. Determine number of patients; perform triage*; state need for additional resources
4. Note and state mechanism of injury or nature of illness

Initial assessment: Chapter 7, pp. 144–152, Scans 7-6, 7-7, 7-8

5. Note and state general impression of patient
6. Determine mental status (AVPU)
7. Assess airway
8. Assess breathing
9. Assess circulation—pulse
10. Assess circulation—bleeding and control as needed*
11. Determine treatment and transport priority

Focused history and physical exam—rapid assessment *(significant MOI—trauma OR unstable—medical)*: **Chapter 7, pp. 167–171, Figures 7.7 through 7.34**

Note: There may not be a figure for each step.

12. Determine chief complaint, take SAMPLE history if possible
13. Stabilize spine; apply collar; perform rapid assessment (DCAP-BTLS)/trauma *OR* focus on and inspect and palpate complaint area/medical
14. Inspect head
15. Inspect neck
16. Inspect chest
17. Inspect abdomen
18. Inspect pelvis
19. Inspect (legs, arms; perform a rapid neurological check (pulse, motor, sensory)
20. Inspect back
21. Take baseline vital signs (pulse, respiration, blood pressure, skin, pupils)

Focused history and physical exam—trauma *(no significant MOI)*: **Chapter 7, p. 171, Scan 7-10**

22. Ask for chief complaint
23. Perform focused physical exam to injury site(s)—DCAP-BTLS
24. Take baseline vital signs (pulse, respiration, blood pressure, skin, pupils)
25. Take a focused SAMPLE history

Skills	Scenarios				Units	
	#1	#2	#3	#4	#1	#2

Focused history and physical exam—medical (stable): Chapter 7, p. 172, Scan 7-11

26. Get history of present illness or chief complaint (NOI)
27. Take a focused SAMPLE history
28. Perform a focused physical exam of complaint area(s)
29. Take baseline vital signs (pulse, respiration, blood pressure, skin, pupils)

Detailed physical exam (usually en route or awaiting EMS arrival): Chapter 7, pp. 172–173

30. Repeat initial assessment; perform focused assessment in more detail
31. Check interventions
32. Reassess vital signs

Ongoing assessment: Chapter 7, pp. 173, 176

33. Repeat initial assessment
34. Reassess and record vital signs
35. Check interventions
36. Repeat focused history and physical exam

Throughout: Communicate, document

Handoff to EMS or hospital: Chapter 7, p. 176

37. Communicate findings to other EMS providers at the scene and/or hospital personnel
38. Give complete verbal report of of patient findings, status
39. Complete written report

Vital signs: Chapter 7, pp. 160–166

40. Pulse, 30 seconds × 2 (Figure 7.3, Table 7-2)
41. Respiration, 30 seconds × 2 (Figure 7.4, Table 7-3)
42. Skin color, temperature, moisture (Figure 7.5, Tables 7-4, 7-5)
43. Blood pressure (Figure 7.6)
44. Pupils (Table 7-6)

SAMPLE history: Chapter 7, p. 158

45. Signs/symptoms and chief complaint
46. Allergies
47. Medications
48. Pertinent past history
49. Last meal or oral intake
50. Events prior to incident

Work with a group of classmates to create scenarios that will use listed skills. Exchange scenarios with other class groups to check your knowledge and to practice your decision-making skills.

CHAPTER 8

CARDIOPULMONARY RESUSCITATION (CPR)

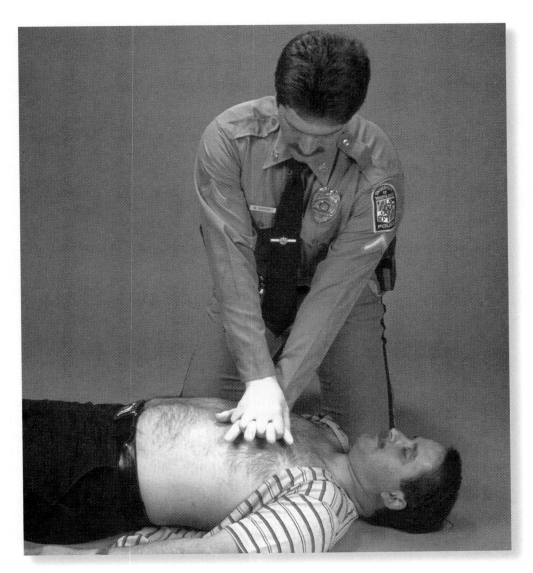

Over 30 years ago, the techniques of cardiopulmonary resuscitation (CPR) were developed. Over those years, researchers have studied and refined CPR so that emergency care providers can easily learn and quickly provide lifesaving techniques to patients in cardiac arrest. This chapter will introduce you to one-rescuer CPR, which includes providing chest compressions and ventilations to adults, children, infants, and neonates.

This chapter focuses on the objectives of Module 4, Lesson 4–1 of the U.S. DOT First Responder National Curriculum and serves as an instructional aid to help you meet any specific objectives added to the course by your local EMS system. **(Note that Objectives 4–1.9 and 4–1.20 are covered in Chapter 9.)**

By the end of this chapter, you will know how to (from cognitive or knowledge information) . . .

4–1.1	List the reasons for the heart to stop beating. (p. 187)
4–1.2	Define the components of cardiopulmonary resuscitation. (pp. 188–190)
4–1.3	Describe each link in the chain of survival and how it relates to the EMS system. (pp. 186–187)
4–1.4	List the steps of one-rescuer adult CPR. (pp. 196–199, 200–201)
4–1.5	Describe the technique of external chest compressions on an adult patient. (p. 193)
4–1.6	Describe the technique of external chest compressions on an infant. (p. 203)
4–1.7	Describe the technique of external chest compressions on a child. (p. 203)
4–1.8	Explain when a First Responder is able to stop CPR. (pp. 210–211)
4–1.10	List the steps of infant CPR. (pp. 199, 202–206)
4–1.11	List the steps of child CPR. (pp. 199, 202–204)

*L*EARNING TASKS

Chapter 8 explains the functions of the heart, lungs, and brain as they work together to circulate life-giving, oxygen-filled blood to your body tissues. You need to understand the relationship of these three vital organs and apply the knowledge you gain from this chapter to performing the ventilation and compression skills of CPR. These simple but special skills have saved many lives. As you work through this chapter, you will need to:

✔ Know and recognize the signs of cardiac arrest.

You will practice ventilation and compression skills, but you will also:

✔ Explain how CPR keeps a patient alive.

It is important that you learn the very specific steps of performing CPR so you may perform them in an emergency without hesitation. One way you can practice to perfection is to work with your classmates and coach one another as you use manikins to:

✔ Locate the CPR compression site on an adult, a child, an infant, and a newborn infant (neonate).

Feel comfortable enough to (by changing attitude, values, beliefs) . . .	4–1.12	Respond to the feelings that the family of a patient may be having during a cardiac event. (pp. 201–211)
	4–1.13	Demonstrate a caring attitude towards patients with cardiac events who request emergency medical services. (pp. 186–190, 208–211)
	4–1.14	Place the interests of the patient with a cardiac event as the foremost consideration when making any and all patient-care decisions. (pp. 186–187, 189–190, 208–211)
	4–1.15	Communicate with empathy with family members and friends of the patient with a cardiac event. (pp. 210–211)
Show how to (through psychomotor skills) . . .	4–1.16	Demonstrate the proper technique of chest compressions on an adult manikin. (p. 193)
	4–1.17	Demonstrate the proper technique of chest compressions on a child manikin. (pp. 203–204)
	4–1.18	Demonstrate the proper technique of chest compressions on an infant manikin. (pp. 203–204, 206)
	4–1.19	Demonstrate the steps of adult one-rescuer CPR on a manikin. (pp. 196–199, 200–201)
	4–1.21	Demonstrate child CPR on a manikin. (pp. 199, 202–204)
	4–1.22	Demonstrate infant CPR on a manikin. (pp. 199, 202–206)

When you gain knowledge, you apply that new knowledge to skills you will perform. You must be able to determine if you are applying new knowledge correctly. Watch one another as you practice and be able to:

✔ Describe how to perform chest compressions and ventilations.

✔ List the rates of compressions and ventilations used during CPR on adults, children, infants, and neonates.

✔ State how you can determine that CPR is being performed correctly.

✔ Describe the complications that can occur during CPR.

Cardiac arrest can result from other situations besides heart attack. Be able to:

✔ Name some other causes of cardiac arrest.

✔ Describe cautions and CPR techniques for accident scenes, electric shock, and drowning.

When you approach any emergency scene, be sure to perform all the patient assessment steps. Remember and be able to:

✔ Demonstrate the steps of the initial assessment to determine if a patient is in cardiac arrest.

You will spend a lot of time practicing the basic techniques of CPR on an adult manikin; but you will use pediatric-sized manikins also. It is important to know how to perform the slightly modified steps for children and to practice on pediatric manikins so you are comfortable and confident if you must perform pediatric CPR. It is unusual for a child to go into cardiac arrest, and if one does, it is usually a result of respiratory failure. Once you have practiced and have begun to feel comfortable with the basic CPR steps, practice these steps on the pediatric manikins. Now you are ready to modify your technique just a little more for the newborn. Be able to:

✔ Perform one-rescuer CPR on an infant manikin to demonstrate neonate CPR techniques.

Your jurisdiction may allow First Responders to use an automated external defibrillator (AED) to defibrillate a patient in cardiac arrest. Your department or organization may have these machines for use on your unit or in your place of work. You *must* complete appropriate training before using an AED, and in your training you will:

✔ Demonstrate how to set up an AED and perform the steps to analyze and safely defibrillate a patient.

THE CHAIN OF SURVIVAL

Chapter 1 described the chain of human resources and services in the EMS system. If each link in the chain works to its full ability, the EMS system can provide effective prehospital emergency care. The chain of survival is another linked system of patient-care events. These events include

- early access
- early CPR
- early defibrillation
- early Advanced Cardiac Life Support (ACLS)

Early access includes the events that start with a patient's illness or collapse, someone recognizing critical signs and symptoms and calling 911, rapid dispatch and information to a response unit, and rapid arrival of EMS personnel who will recognize cardiac arrest and start CPR immediately. *Early CPR* means that bystanders are trained and will begin CPR even before EMS responders arrive. Besides continuing CPR, EMS responders may bring defibrillators. *Early defibrillation* is the link most likely to improve survival rates. Either the first arriving responders or dispatch will contact ALS, which will arrive with a defibrillation unit. If First Responders in your jurisdiction are permitted to use automated external defibrillators (AEDs), your instructor or Medical Director will provide appropriate training. Do not attempt to use an AED without training. Information on using AEDs is provided later in this chapter. Your instructor will have you learn AED protocols and will teach you how to properly use them if your jurisdiction allows First Responders to do so. For patients in cardiac arrest, the highest hospital discharge rate has been for patients who had CPR started within 4 minutes of arrest and had ALS respond and act within 8 minutes. In addition to defibrillators, ALS units bring other *early intervention* equipment such as oxygen to support ventilation and intravenous access for fluids and medications that control heart rate and rhythm, relieve pain, and stabilize the patient.

Each event, or link, is critical in improving patient survival; and each part of the EMS system works to improve its strength or ability through training, responding quickly, and applying well-practiced skills. Over the years, new skills have been added to training programs, and old standard skills have been perfected. In many jurisdictions, EMTs are being trained to use AEDs.

CIRCULATION AND CPR

The circulatory system keeps blood moving in a constant, one-direction flow. At the center of the circulatory system is the heart. When the heart beats, it acts as a pump. Blood from the body flows into the heart and is sent to the lungs. In the lungs, the blood gives up carbon dioxide gathered while circulating through the body and exchanges it for oxygen. This oxygen-rich blood is then sent back to the heart, where it is pumped back out to the body.

As it flows through the body, blood picks up nutrients from the small intestines and secretions from special glands to carry to organs and tissues. Blood gives up wastes to the kidneys and picks up carbon dioxide from the tissues in exchange for oxygen it picked up in the lungs. This constant exchange of nutrients for wastes and oxygen for carbon dioxide is important for life and body function. One vital organ that needs a constant flow of oxygen is the brain.

First | There is a strong relationship among breathing, circulation, and brain activity (Figure 8.1) that works as follows:

■ If breathing stops, blood pumped to the brain will contain too little oxygen.
■ Without enough oxygen, the brain cannot direct the work of all other body functions. If the brain fails because of a lack of oxygen, the heartbeat becomes irregular, then slows, and finally stops beating altogether.
■ When the heart stops beating, breathing stops almost instantly. When the heart suddenly stops beating, no oxygen can be pumped to the brain and the oxygen supply in the brain is used up in about 4 to 6 minutes.

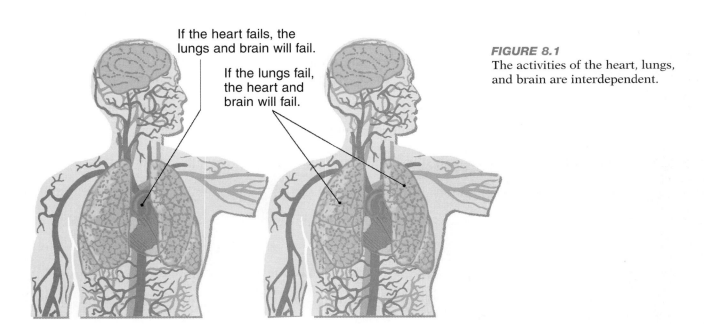

If the heart fails, the lungs and brain will fail.

If the lungs fail, the heart and brain will fail.

FIGURE 8.1
The activities of the heart, lungs, and brain are interdependent.

FIGURE 8.2
Carotid (neck) pulse used for adult and child.

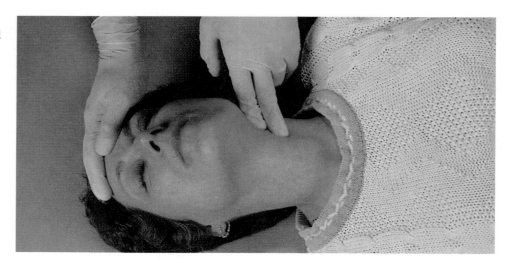

cardiac arrest
when the heart stops beating. Also, the sudden end of effective circulation caused by erratic muscle activity in the lower chambers of the heart (ventricular fibrillation).

brachial (BRAY-key-al) pulse the pulse found on the inside (medial) upper arm of the patient. It is used to evaluate circulation during the initial assessment of an infant.

apical (AP-i-kal) pulse the pulse felt or heard over the apex (lower part where the heart forms a cone at the ventricles) of the heart.

cardiopulmonary resuscitation (KAR-de-o-PUL-mo-ner-e re-SUS-ci-TA-shun; CPR) heart-lung resuscitation. Combined compression and breathing techniques that maintain circulation and breathing.

ℭARDIAC ARREST

First | When the heart stops beating, a person is in **cardiac arrest.** The signs of cardiac arrest are:

■ The patient is unresponsive (to your voice or touch).

■ The patient is not breathing. (Respirations usually stop within 30 seconds of cardiac arrest.)

■ The patient has no pulse. [For an adult or a child, check the carotid pulse in the neck (Figure 8.2); for an infant, check the **brachial pulse** on the inner side of the arm (Figure 8.3A); for a neonate, check the **apical pulse** by listening over the left side of the rib cage just below the nipple with your ear or a stethoscope (Figure 8.3B).]

The above signs are listed in the order in which you check them as you perform the initial assessment.

ℭPR—WHAT IT IS

CPR (cardiopulmonary resuscitation) is an emergency procedure that provides both chest compressions and ventilations when heart and lung actions stop. ("Cardio" refers to the heart, and "pulmonary" refers to the lungs.)

First | Whenever you read about basic life support, you will see references made to the ABCs of emergency care. ABC stands for:

FIGURE 8.3
A Brachial (arm) pulse used for an infant. **B** Apical (over the chest) pulse used for a neonate.

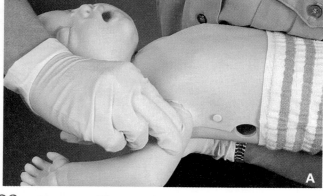

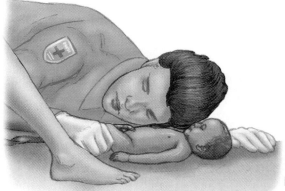

A = Airway

B = Breathing

C = Circulation

In Chapter 7, you were introduced to these terms as part of the initial assessment.

First | In Chapter 6, you learned how to open and maintain an airway and assist breathing on a patient in respiratory arrest. When performing CPR, you will still open and maintain an airway and provide breaths for the patient. In addition to these steps, you will circulate blood to the lungs and the rest of the patient's body with chest compressions. This means that during CPR, you will have to perform a series of steps to:

■ Maintain an open airway.
■ Breathe for the patient.
■ Perform chest compressions to circulate the patient's blood.

CPR—HOW IT WORKS

When you perform the ABC steps on a patient in cardiac arrest, you circulate oxygenated blood to the brain so its tissues continue to live and function. *Clinical death* occurs the instant breathing and heartbeat stop. **Brain tissues use up oxygen and die in 4 to 6 minutes.** This 4-to-6-minute period is the start of *biological death* and when brain damage begins. About 10 minutes after breathing and heartbeat stop, lethal changes take place in the brain and tissues die. By starting early CPR, the breathing and compression techniques you use will circulate oxygenated blood to brain tissues, which help prevent biological death and brain damage.

The time frame for beginning CPR and saving someone in cardiac arrest is not always within 10 minutes. Patients who have been in arrest for more than 20 minutes have been successfully resuscitated in special cases. In cold-water drownings, some people have survived long after 20 minutes. You will not know exactly when a patient's breathing and heartbeat stopped, even though a family member or bystander reported the person unconscious for what seemed to them a long time. Remember that the estimates are generally unreliable.

You will start CPR because you will not be able to pinpoint the exact time that breathing and heartbeat stopped, nor will you be able to predict the outcome of unusual circumstances. The delay between clinical and biological death gives you time to apply CPR. The sooner you begin, the better the patient's chances for survival.

It is possible to provide breaths for a patient who is not breathing, but giving breaths alone will not benefit the patient unless the blood is circulating. In CPR, the rescuer makes the patient's blood circulate by applying **external chest compressions.**

With the patient lying on his back, you will compress the patient's chest straight down along its midline at a point over the lower half of the breastbone (sternum). The patient must be placed on a hard surface so the compressions will cause an increased pressure in the chest (thoracic) cavity. This increased pressure forces blood out of the heart and into the arteries to circulate to all parts of the body (Figure 8.4). When compression is relaxed and pressure is released, blood flows into the veins and back to the heart. One-way valves in the patient's heart and veins keep the blood moving in the proper direction.

external chest compressions measured compressions performed during CPR at a set rate over the CPR compression site. These compressions are applied to help create circulation of the blood.

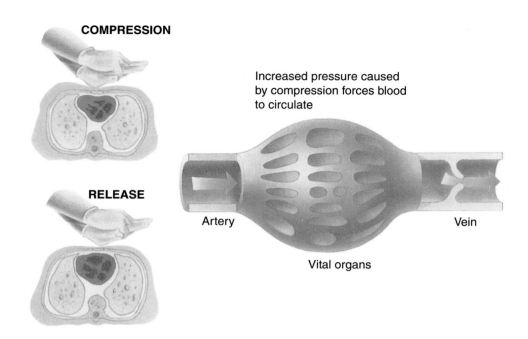

FIGURE 8.4
During CPR, pressure in the chest cavity increases with compression. This forces blood into circulation.

COMPRESSION

Increased pressure caused by compression forces blood to circulate

RELEASE

Artery

Vein

Vital organs

First | When you perform CPR, your breaths provide oxygen to the patient, which is taken up by the blood. Your compressions force this oxygenated blood into circulation to reach the body's tissues.

THE TECHNIQUES OF CPR

CPR techniques include a series of specific steps that must be performed in a certain manner. Although CPR techniques for adults, children, infants, and neonates are similar, there are slight variations. We will begin our discussion of CPR by describing the basic techniques. Next, the complete procedure will be presented, step by step. Finally, we will describe CPR for children, infants, and neonates.

When to Begin CPR

First | As a First Responder, always perform an initial assessment on your patient (see Chapter 7). Your actions leading to CPR should include the following:

1. *Form a general impression of the patient.* As you approach, note what the patient looks like. Form an immediate opinion and react based on that opinion. Does the patient look sick, appear to be having trouble breathing, or seem unresponsive? What is the sex and general age of the patient?

2. *Assess responsiveness.* Remember AVPU (see Chapter 7). Is the patient alert and responsive or unresponsive to your approach and voice? Is the patient responsive to your touch or only to a painful stimulus? Start with a gentle shake or squeeze on the shoulder and shout, "Are you OK?" If there is no response, rub the sternum or pinch the shoulder. If the adult patient is unresponsive, alert the EMS dispatcher. For an infant or a child patient, continue with your assessment and then start the steps of CPR.

3. *Assess airway.* Open the airway by the head-tilt, chin-lift method or by the jaw-thrust method. (Check now to see if the patient is a neck breather [has a stoma].)

4. *Assess breathing.* Look, listen, and feel for breathing for 3 to 5 seconds. If the patient is not breathing, deliver two initial breaths. If the airway is obstructed, perform the steps to clear the airway (Chapter 6) and, when clear, provide two ventilations before assessing pulse.

5. *Assess circulation (pulse, bleeding, skin color, and temperature).* Take 5 to 10 seconds to check a pulse. Check the carotid pulse on the adult and on the child (1 to 8 years); check the brachial pulse on the infant (1 month to 1 year); check the apical pulse over the heart on a neonate (birth to 1 month) by listening for the heartbeat with a stethoscope or your ear placed over the chest. (If the neonate is newly born [just delivered], check for pulsations by placing your fingertips at the base of the umbilical cord.) If there is no pulse . . .

6. *Position the patient and begin CPR.* If the patient is an adult, alert the EMS system dispatcher as soon as you realize the patient is unresponsive. Advanced cardiac life-support personnel with defibrillators and EMTs with oxygen and ventilation devices can be dispatched to the scene while you begin CPR. If the patient is a child or an infant, begin CPR immediately and continue for one minute, then alert the EMS dispatcher. Details of neonatal CPR will be explained later in this chapter.

Locating the CPR Compression Site

External chest compressions are not effective unless they are delivered to a specific site on the patient's chest (Scan 8-1). If you apply compressions to the wrong site, you may injure the patient or provide ineffective CPR.

 After determining that the adult patient needs CPR, you will:

1. Position yourself at the patient's side with your knees next to him and placed between his lower ribs and shoulder.

2. Use your index and middle fingers of the hand closest to the patient's waist to locate the *lower margin* of the rib cage. Do this on the side of the patient's chest closest to your knees.

3. Run your fingers along the patient's rib cage until you find the notch where the ribs meet the breastbone (sternum). The notch is found in the lower center of the patient's chest.

4. Keep your middle finger at the notch. Place your index finger next to your middle finger so it is over the lower end of the sternum.

5. Place the heel of your other hand over the middle of the sternum with the thumb next to and touching the side of the index finger you used to find the notch where the ribs meet the sternum. This is the CPR compression site (Figure 8.5). Do *not* place your hand on top of your index finger.

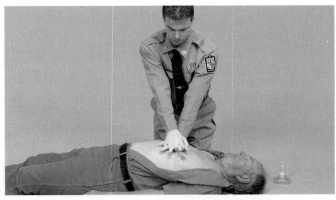

FIGURE 8.5
Positioning the hands at the CPR compression site.

Locating the CPR Compression Site

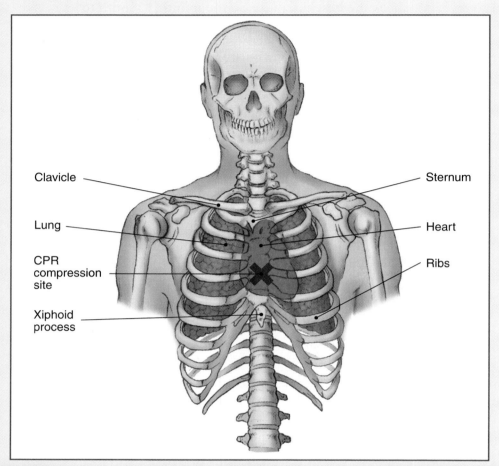

Clavicle

Lung

CPR compression site

Xiphoid process

Sternum

Heart

Ribs

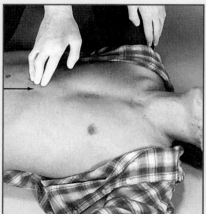

1. Use the index and middle fingers of the hand that is closest to the patient's waist to locate the lower margin of the rib cage.

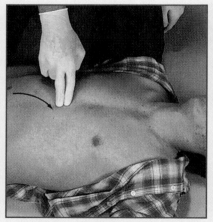

2. Move your fingers along the rib cage until you find the notch where the ribs meet the sternum. Keep your middle finger at the notch.

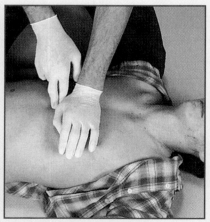

3. With your index finger over the lower end of the sternum, move your other hand to the midline. Place its thumb side against the index finger of the lower hand.

External Chest Compressions

 For external chest compressions to be effective, you must:

■ Place the patient face up on a firm surface such as the ground or floor. If the patient is in bed, move him to the floor or place a board under his back. Do *not* delay CPR to find a board.

■ Carefully find the CPR compression site as described above.

 The correct technique for external chest compressions includes:

1. Place the patient face up on a firm surface and locate the CPR compression site; then reposition the hand you used to locate the notch where the ribs meet the sternum. Place it on top of the hand that is over the CPR compression site.

2. Keep the heels of both hands parallel to each other, with the fingers of both hands pointing away from you.

3. Keep your fingers off the chest, either extended or interlaced (Figure 8.6). For some it may be easier to do compressions by grasping the wrist of the hand placed at the compression site. Practice different positions until you find one that is comfortable for you.

4. Keep your elbows straight and locked. Do *not* bend your elbows when delivering or releasing compression.

5. Position your shoulders over your hands so that you deliver compressions straight down onto the CPR compression site (Figure 8.7). Keep both of your knees on the ground.

6. Deliver compressions straight down (Figure 8.8), and apply enough force to the adult patient to depress the sternum 1½ to 2 inches. CPR will be effective for the patient and less tiring for you if you bend from the hips in a smooth up-and-down motion.

7. Release pressure on the chest to allow the patient's heart to refill. Do not bend your elbows in order to release pressure. Do not lift your hands off the patient's chest. Lift up from your hips to return your shoulders to their original position. The release of pressure should take the same amount of time as compression (50% compression and 50% release).

Providing Breaths During CPR

Along with artificial circulation, you must provide artificial ventilation when performing CPR. Breaths are provided between a set number of compressions. These breaths between compressions are provided to the patient, using the

> **WARNING:**
> Do *not* practice CPR compressions on anyone. This is an emergency care procedure that may cause serious problems when applied to someone with normal lung and heart actions. Practice only on the manikins provided. Finding CPR landmarks (sternal notch and compression site) can be practiced on people as well as on manikins.

FIGURE 8.6
Hand placement showing different ways of keeping your fingers off the ribs during compression.

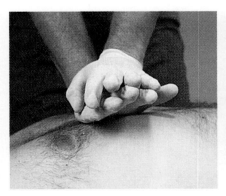 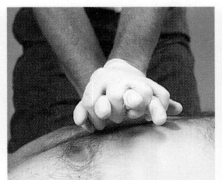 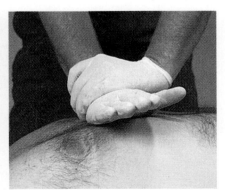

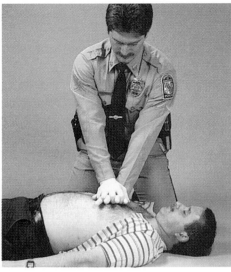

FIGURE 8.7
The shoulders are placed directly over the compression site.

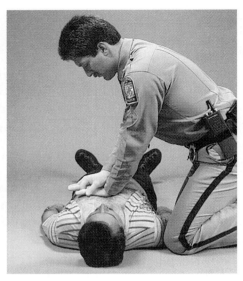

FIGURE 8.8
Compressions are delivered straight down.

same technique as used in mouth-to-mask resuscitation (or mouth-to-mouth, mouth-to-nose, or mouth-to-stoma). Place the patient's head in the correct position by using the head-tilt, chin-lift maneuver or the jaw-thrust maneuver. Breathe into the patient's lungs until you see the chest rise and feel resistance (usually a 1.5 to 2.0 second ventilation).

There are four special factors to consider when providing ventilations during one-rescuer CPR:

- Deliver each breath in 1.5 to 2.0 seconds.
- Provide **two** slow breaths after every **fifteen** compressions.
- Do *not* overventilate the patient. If you force too much air into the patient's lungs, the excess air will begin to fill the stomach and may eventually cause gastric distention. To prevent this, feel for resistance as you ventilate and watch for the patient's chest to rise.
- Establish a regular pattern of breathing for yourself. Do *not* try to breathe or hold your breath with each compression.

The most effective use of mouth-to-mask ventilations requires the rescuer to be at the patient's head (Figure 8.9) to ensure proper mask placement and mask seal. It is difficult to move quickly to the proper position at the head after

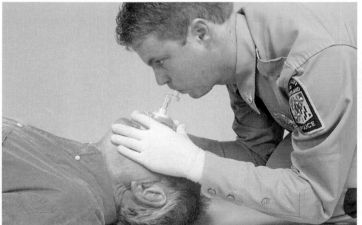

FIGURE 8.9
Position yourself at the patient's head to provide ventilations and deliver each breath in 1.5 to 2.0 seconds.

delivering chest compressions. It is also difficult to move quickly from the head position back to the patient's side in order to deliver compressions directly over the compression site. Practice frequently to develop and perfect your CPR skills so you are able to move quickly from the head to the chest position and back. Remember that your techniques prevent biological death and increase the patient's chance for survival.

Rates of Compressions and Ventilations

First | The rate for delivering compressions and ventilations is critical in CPR. Effective CPR depends on the correct ratio of compressions and ventilations; you must:

- Deliver compressions at a rate of 100 per minute for adults.
- Provide ventilations at a ratio of two breaths every fifteen compressions. Deliver each breath within 1.5 to 2.0 seconds.
- Avoid or minimize CPR interruptions. Interrupt CPR only for pulse and breathing checks and to move the patient for transport or from a dangerous area. If you must move the patient, try to minimize the interruption to 15 to 30 seconds. After the first minute of CPR and every few minutes thereafter, stop CPR to check for a return of the carotid pulse. Take 3 to 5 seconds to check for spontaneous return of pulse and breathing.

In one-rescuer CPR, the chest compression rate should be 80 to 100 per minute. But the time used to provide ventilations between a set of compressions means that only about 60 actual compressions per minute are delivered, which is adequate to prevent biological death. To be sure that you provide compressions at the proper rate of 80 to 100 per minute, count (to yourself) as you deliver compressions: "One-and, two-and, three-and, four-and, . . ." until you reach fifteen. Then, deliver two slow ventilations of 1.5 to 2.0 seconds, quickly relocate the CPR compression site, and continue the next set of compressions.

Effective CPR

First | You can be certain that you are performing CPR correctly if:

- Another trained person feels for the carotid pulse as you compress the patient's sternum. Do *not* try to deliver compressions with one hand while you check for a pulse at the carotid artery with the other.
- You see the chest rise when you provide a ventilation and fall when you allow the patient to passively exhale (see Chapter 6).

If you are performing CPR correctly, you may notice the patient's skin color improve, but this does not always occur. Sometimes the patient may try to swallow, gasp, or move his limbs. These actions do not necessarily mean that the patient is recovering; however, they do mean that you should check for the return of breathing and pulse.

First | Check for a carotid pulse after performing CPR for 1 minute (four cycles of two breaths and fifteen compressions). If the patient has a pulse but is not breathing, stop compressions and continue with ventilations only. If there is no pulse, continue CPR and check for a carotid pulse every few minutes. Most patients will not regain a heartbeat and breathing with CPR alone. Patients will usually require special medical procedures such as defibrillation before they regain heart function. CPR keeps patients biologically alive until special medical procedures can be provided.

ONE-RESCUER CPR

BASIC PROCEDURES

A First Responder must know how to perform both one-rescuer and two-rescuer CPR. In this chapter, we will consider only one-rescuer CPR techniques. The next chapter will cover two-rescuer CPR.

Following is a step-by-step outline for performing one-rescuer CPR (see Table 8-1 for a summary of CPR techniques for the adult, child, infant, and neonate). These procedures follow the American Heart Association (AHA) recommendations. Your instructor will tell you if recent changes were made by the AHA. Otherwise, learn the procedures as they are presented. Do *not* create your own methods or shortcuts. The extensive research done by the AHA has found these procedures to be most efficient in saving lives of patients in cardiac arrest. Remember, the following steps are a part of the initial assessment:

1. **Check for responsiveness.** A responsive patient does not need CPR. Gently shake or squeeze the patient's shoulder and ask, "Are you OK?" If the patient is not responsive, call out for help. If you are alone with an adult patient, call the EMS dispatcher now to get ALS or a defibrillator en route (Figures 8.10 and 8.11).

2. **Position the patient and yourself.** The patient should be placed face up on a hard surface. Kneel beside the patient's chest (Figure 8.12).

3. **Open the airway.** Use the head-tilt, chin-lift maneuver or jaw-thrust maneuver to ensure an open airway (Figure 8.13). Check to see if the patient is a neck breather.

TABLE 8-1: SUMMARY OF ONE-RESCUER CPR TECHNIQUES

PROCEDURE	ADULT	CHILD	INFANT	NEONATE (birth to 28 days)
Compressions				
Method	Heels of two hands	Heel of one hand	2 or 3 fingers	2 thumbs or fingers
Depth	1½" to 2"	1" to 1½"	½" to 1"	½" to ¾"
Rate	80–100/min	100/min	100/min	120/min
Ventilations				
Method	Mouth-to-Mask for all patients Mouth-to-Mouth Mouth-to-Nose	Mouth-to-Mouth Mouth-to-Nose	Mouth-to-Mouth-and-Nose	Mouth-to-Mouth-and-Nose
Ratio of Compressions to Breaths				
	15:2	5:1	5:1	3:1
Counts				
	1 and 2 and 3 and 4 and 5 . . . 15 and breathe, breathe	1, 2, 3, 4, 5, breathe	1, 2, 3, 4, 5, breathe	1, 2, 3, breathe

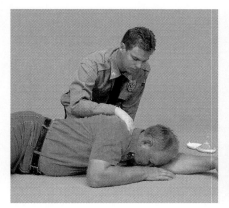

FIGURE 8.10
Determine unresponsiveness.

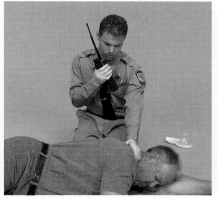

FIGURE 8.11
Alert the EMS dispatcher.

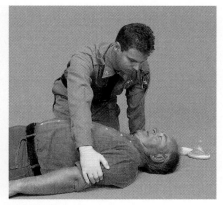

FIGURE 8.12
Properly position the patient and yourself.

4. **Check for breathing.** Look, listen, and feel for air exchange. This should take about 3 to 5 seconds (Figure 8.14).

5. **Provide two breaths** (feel for resistance and watch for chest rise; Figure 8.15). Follow the steps for mouth-to-mask (or mouth-to-mouth, mouth-to-nose, or mouth-to-stoma) ventilation (see Chapter 6 and Appendix 2).

Artificial circulation will not be effective unless oxygen is reaching the air-exchange levels of the patient's lungs.

6. If necessary, **clear the airway.** Use the techniques of manual thrusts, finger sweeps, and ventilations described in Chapter 6.

7. **Check for circulation by feeling for a carotid pulse** (Figure 8.16). This should take **5 to 10 seconds.** If the patient has a carotid pulse, but no respirations, provide one breath every 5 seconds.

8. **Find the CPR compression site.** Slide your index and middle fingers along the lower margin of the ribs until you locate the notch where the ribs meet the sternum (Figure 8.17).

9. **Position your hands on the compression site.** Place your hand closest to the patient's head along the midline of the patient's chest and against (not over) the index finger of the hand used to locate the compression site (Figure 8.18). Next, move the hand used to locate the compression site. Place it on top of the hand on the sternum. The heels of both hands

> **REMEMBER:**
> Oxygen must reach the air-exchange levels of the patient's lungs if artificial circulation is to be effective.

FIGURE 8.13
Open the airway.

FIGURE 8.14
Determine breathlessness (no breathing).

FIGURE 8.15
Provide two breaths.

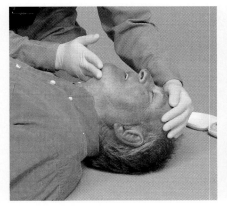

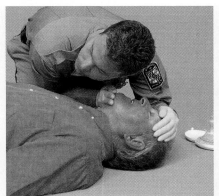

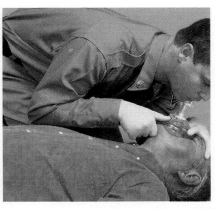

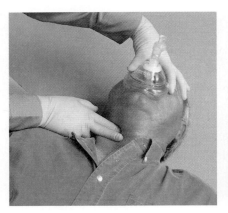

FIGURE 8.16
Determine pulselessness (no pulse).

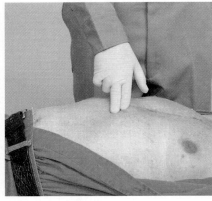

FIGURE 8.17
Locate the CPR compression site.

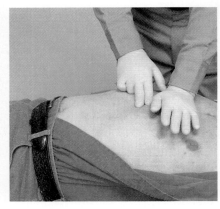

FIGURE 8.18
Properly position your hands.

should be parallel to each other with your fingers pointing away from you. The fingers may be interlocked or extended, or you may grasp the wrist of the hand placed at the compression site. Keep your fingers off the patient's chest (Figure 8.19).

10. **Provide chest compressions.** Keep your arms straight, elbows locked, and shoulders directly over the compression site. Bend at the hips to use your upper body weight when performing compressions (Figure 8.20).

   – Deliver compressions directly over the CPR compression site.

   – Compress the patient's breastbone **1½ to 2 inches.**

   – Deliver compressions at a **rate of 100 per minute,** counting, "One-and, two-and, three-and . . ." etc.

   – Release pressure completely to allow the heart to refill. Each release should take the same amount of time as a compression. *Do not take your hands off the patient's chest while doing chest compressions.*

   – **Deliver 15 compressions, then . . .**

11. **Provide breaths.** Provide ventilations at the **rate of two breaths every 15 compressions** and watch for chest rise (Figure 8.21). Do this at a rate of one ventilation every **1.5 to 2.0 seconds.**

FIGURE 8.19
Keep your fingers off the patient's chest.

FIGURE 8.20
Deliver 15 compressions.

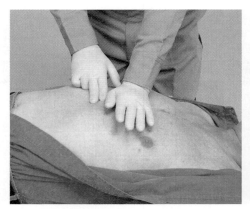

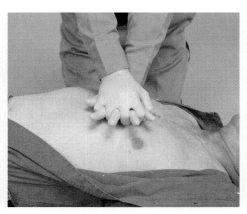

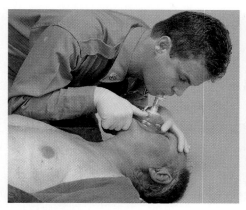

FIGURE 8.21
Provide two breaths.

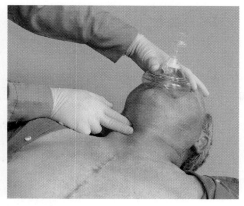

FIGURE 8.22
Reassess the carotid pulse.

12. **Continue CPR.** Deliver **15** compressions at the rate of **100 per minute** followed by **two** ventilations for 1 minute, which is four sets of compressions and ventilations.

13. **Check for a carotid pulse and breathing after the first minute of CPR** (Figure 8.22). Do not interrupt CPR for more than 3 to 5 seconds (but no longer than 7 seconds) to make the check. If there is a pulse and breathing, stop CPR. If there is a pulse but no breathing, continue ventilations at the rate of **one** breath every 5 seconds. If there is no pulse . . .

14. **Continue CPR.** Check for a carotid pulse every few minutes. Provide CPR until another trained person can take over, the patient regains a pulse and breathing, or you are too tired to continue.

For a summary of one-rescuer CPR, see Scan 8-2.

*C*PR TECHNIQUES FOR INFANTS AND CHILDREN

Few children need CPR away from a hospital setting, so many emergency care providers consider performing proper infant and child CPR a major weakness because they have little practical experience. The majority of cases in which CPR has been used for pediatric patients has been for newborns (neonates) in cardiac arrest. Such cases are rare, but anyone who learns CPR needs to continually practice the techniques for children, infants, and neonates.

 The basic principles of adult CPR are generally the same for children, infants, and neonates.

When providing CPR for an infant or a child, it will be necessary to:

1. Determine unresponsiveness.
2. Call for help.
3. Correctly position the patient.
4. Open the airway.
5. Check for breathing.
6. Provide two breaths by pocket face mask or bag-valve-mask (see Appendix 2); clear airway obstructions as necessary.
7. Check for circulation by checking for a carotid pulse on a child, a brachial pulse on an infant, an apical pulse (listening with your ear or a stethoscope over the left side of the rib cage just below the nipple) on a neonate.

REMEMBER:

For the child, infant, and neonate, provide 1 minute of CPR before calling the EMS system dispatcher. For the adult, call after determining unresponsiveness.

One-Rescuer CPR

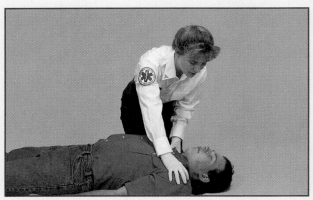

1. Establish unresponsiveness and alert EMS. Position the patient and yourself.

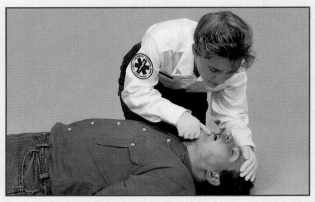

2. Establish an open airway.

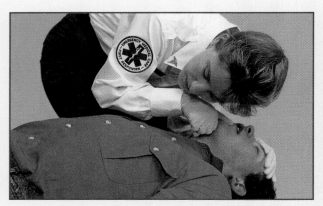

3. Look, listen, and feel for breathing (3–5 seconds).

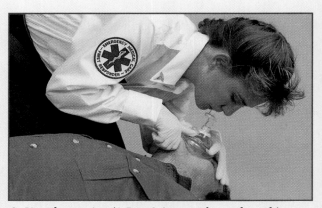

4. Ventilate twice (1.5 to 2.0 seconds per breath).

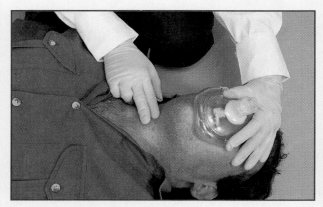

5. Feel for pulse (5–10 seconds).

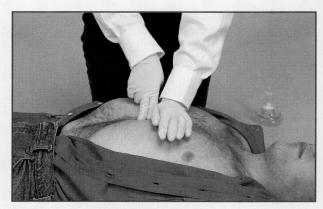

6. Locate compression site.

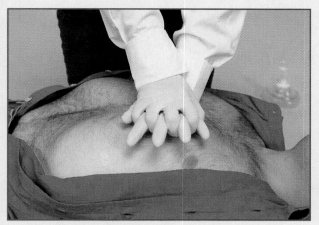

7. Position your hands.

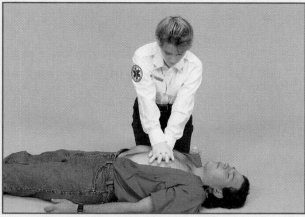

8. Begin compressions.
Compression rate is 100 per minute.

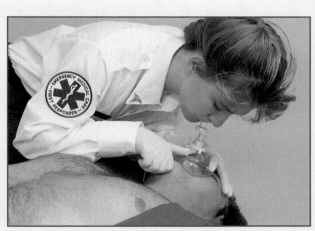

9. Ventilate twice.
Cycle = 2 ventilations every 15 compressions.

WARNING: Mouth-to-mouth and mouth-to-nose ventilation expose rescuers to the dangers of infectious diseases.

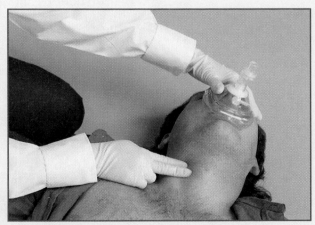

10. Recheck pulse after 4 cycles, then every few minutes.

NOTE: If alone with an unresponsive infant or child, provide 1 minute of CPR before calling EMS dispatch.

8. Provide chest compressions and ventilations (5:1 ratio for children and infants; 3:1 ratio for neonates).

9. Call dispatch.

Determining the Pediatric Patient's Category

First | Since there are large and small infants and children, there is no absolute rule to determine the category of each pediatric patient. Instead, age guidelines have been established for providing CPR. As a First Responder, you need to know the age categories:

- **Neonate**—birth to 1 month
- **Infant**—younger than 1 year of age
- **Child**—1 to 8 years of age

For a child over 8 years old, use adult CPR techniques. Detailed techniques for neonates will be discussed later in this chapter.

The patient's size may cause you to place the patient in a different age category. Many infants and children are large for their age; some adolescents are small enough to be mistaken for children. The above age categories are guidelines, not absolutes. It is more important to begin CPR and check for effective ventilations and compressions than to spend time determining the child's exact age.

Positioning the Patient

As you do for adults, place pediatric patients face up on a flat, hard surface. When the child is on his back, his large head size may cause his head to flex forward and close the airway. To open the airway, place the head in a neutral alignment. However, this maneuver often lifts the child's upper back and prevents contact with the hard surface. To provide support under the back, place a folded blanket or towel under the shoulders to fill the void (Figure 8.23).

Opening the Airway

First | For the infant and child, just as for the adult, use the head-tilt, chin-lift procedure. Tilt the head gently back to a neutral or slightly extended position with one hand. A slight head-tilt is often all that is needed. Place your fingers under the bony part of the chin and lift to finish the technique of opening the airway. Be careful not to compress the soft tissues, causing airway obstruction. Use the jaw-thrust maneuver if you suspect spinal injury. Airway obstructions should be cared for as described in Chapter 6.

Assessing Breathing

To assess for breathing, *look*, *listen*, and *feel* for air exchange. Look for the rise and fall of the chest and abdomen. Listen for exhaled air. Feel for exhaled air from the mouth and nose. If there is breathing, maintain an open airway. If

neonate (AHA standard) newborn to 1 month of age.

infant (AHA standard) younger than 1 year of age.

child (AHA standard) 1 to 8 years of age.

FIGURE 8.23
To provide support under the back, place a folded towel under the shoulders to fill the void.

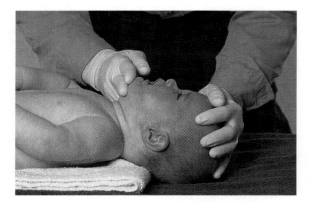

there is no breathing, give two initial breaths through an infection control barrier (pocket face mask) if available; or, if the patient is an infant or a very small child, seal your mouth over the mouth and nose. If the patient is a child or a very large infant, seal your mouth over the mouth and pinch the nostrils closed. Use the steps to clear the airway if no air enters after repositioning the head and attempting to ventilate again (see Chapter 6).

Establishing a Pulse

 Infant—Use the brachial pulse that is found on the medial (inside) upper arm of the patient (Figure 8.24). The brachial pulse is found by:

1. Locating the point halfway between the elbow and shoulder.

2. Placing your thumb on the lateral (outside) side of the upper arm at the midway point.

3. Placing the tips of your index and middle fingers at the midway point on the medial surface of the upper arm.

4. *Gently* pressing your index and middle fingers in toward the bone of the upper arm in order to feel the brachial pulse.

First | **Child**—Determine circulation by checking carotid pulse.

External Chest Compressions

First | **Infant**—The size of the infant's chest and heart places the heart in a slightly different position than in the adult patient. Apply compressions to the breastbone (sternum), one finger-width below an imaginary line drawn directly across the nipples. Deliver compressions with the tips of two or three fingers (Figure 8.25A). Depress the infant's sternum ½ to 1 inch.

First | **Child**—Use the heel of one hand to apply compressions to the sternum (Figure 8.25B), after finding the CPR compression site the same way as you would for an adult. Depress the child's sternum 1 to 1½ inches.

Ventilations

First | **Infant**—After a set of five compressions, provide a breath using the mouth-to-mask (or mouth-to-mouth and nose) technique. Watch carefully for the rise and fall of the infant's chest.

First | **Child**—Provide a breath by mouth-to-mask (or mouth-to-mouth or mouth-to-nose) technique after every set of five compressions. Watch carefully for the rise and fall of the child's chest.

Note

The size of pediatric patients varies, so it is impossible to make precise recommendations about ventilation pressure and volume. The correct volume for each breath is the volume that causes the chest to rise. The pediatric airway may be highly resistant to airflow, and you may have to blow hard to deliver an adequate volume of air and make the chest rise. Compare this airway resistance problem to blowing up balloons: The smaller the balloon, the harder it is to get air in; the larger the balloon, the easier it is to get air in.

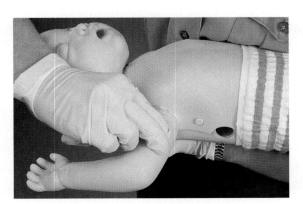

FIGURE 8.24
For infants, determine circulation by feeling for a brachial pulse.

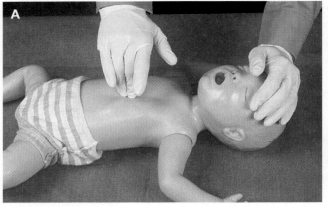
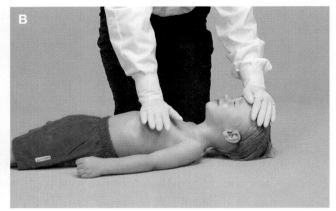

FIGURE 8.25
A For infants, use the tips of fingers for compressions.
B For children, use the heel of one hand.

CPR Rates

REMEMBER:

For infants and children, count "one, two, three, four, five," and provide one breath.

 Infant—Deliver compressions at the rate of at least 100 per minute. Provide a breath after every fifth compression at a ratio of 5:1.

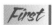 **Child**—Deliver compressions at the rate of 100 per minute. Provide a breath after every fifth compression at a ratio of 5:1.

To assure the correct rate for infants and children, count "One, two, three, four, five," and provide one breath.

Activating the EMS System

After 1 minute of CPR (20 cycles of five compressions and one breath) on the infant or child, call the EMS system dispatcher—911. You may be able to carry the child or infant and continue CPR while calling 911. Note for any patient, if the patient begins breathing and regains a pulse, place her on her side in the recovery position (Figure 8.26). Do not turn the patient if a neck injury is suspected. Monitor the breathing patient or continue CPR on the pulseless, nonbreathing patient until help arrives.

NEONATAL RESUSCITATION

Note

Always keep newborns warm throughout all procedures.

About six percent of all newborns need life support, and for newborns with very low birth weights, the percentage rises. While it may be rare for the First Responder to deliver an infant in the field, it is even rarer for that infant to require basic life support. However, you must have the knowledge and skill to recognize and manage a newborn in distress.

There are five main steps for resuscitating the newborn, but for the majority of cases, the First Responder should only have to perform the first two. The five steps are:

1. Initial stabilization and evaluation (always needed)
2. Blow-by oxygenation if needed.
3. Bag-valve mask ventilation if blow-by oxygenation is inadequate; endotracheal intubation (ALS only) if needed
4. Chest compressions, if necessary, after BVM ventilation is established
5. Administration of medications and fluids if needed (provided only by ALS or hospital personnel)

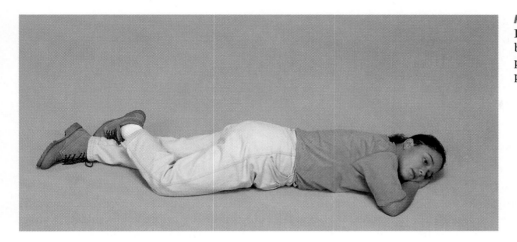

FIGURE 8.26
If the patient begins to breathe and regains a pulse, place her in the recovery position.

Initial Stabilization and Evaluation

Suctioning and Stimulation During delivery, suction the mouth and nose after the head delivers (see Chapter 13). If the newborn needs suctioning because of secretions, use a bulb syringe or neonatal hand suction unit. Suction the mouth first and then the nose. Suctioning will usually stimulate the newborn to breathe if he is not already breathing. If suctioning does not stimulate breathing, first try rubbing the infant's back or flicking the soles of his feet.

Positioning Always keep the newborn warm and dry. Place her on her back or side with the neck in a neutral position. If needed, place a small folded towel under the newborn's shoulders to open the airway and maintain proper head position. If the newborn has a lot of oral secretions, turn her on her side to allow drainage; support her in this position by placing another towel behind her back.

Evaluation Assess and support the ABCs by evaluating respiratory effort, heart rate, and color as described in the following sections. Also assess and support the temperature; the newborn should be warm and dry.

Oxygen, Ventilation and Chest Compressions

Respiratory Effort A newborn who is crying vigorously and is flushed from the effort has good respiratory effort. One who is listless, gasping, and pale or bluish in color has poor respiratory effort and needs oxygen. If you do not have oxygen equipment or have not been trained to use it, call ALS immediately.

If you provide oxygen, deliver it by blow-by through a face mask or makeshift funnel, such as a cup attached to oxygen tubing (see Chapter 14, Figure 14.4) at no less than 5 liters a minute. Hold the oxygen source close to the side of the newborn's face to maximize the inhaled concentration. (Blowing oxygen directly into the face can cause periods of apnea.) If you must assist breathing, use a bag-valve mask attached to 100% oxygen. It is critical to use an appropriate size mask to assure a good seal and proper oxygen delivery to the newborn. (For information on oxygen delivery, see Appendix 2. Follow local protocols *and* medical direction and *only* deliver oxygen if First Responders are allowed to do so in your jurisdiction.)

Deliver 40–60 breaths a minute and watch for the chest to rise as a reliable sign of adequate ventilation. If the chest does not rise, reposition the neonate's head and the mask and try to ventilate again. Suction again if needed. By now, ALS should be on the way. After providing ventilations for 15 to 30 seconds, check heart rate.

Check the heart rate by listening for the apical beat (over the sternum) with your ear or a stethoscope to the chest. In a newborn, you can feel the base of the umbilical cord for a pulse, which will continue to pulsate for several minutes after birth. If the heart rate is at least 100 beats per minute and spontaneous respirations are now present, gradually discontinue assisted ventilations with the bag-valve mask and provide gentle stimulation by rubbing the skin. If respirations are inadequate, continue with assisted ventilations.

Chest Compressions

If the heart rate is less than 60 beats per minute or between 60 and 80 beats per minute and *not* increasing, continue to assist ventilations *and* begin chest compressions. Yes, you will perform chest compressions on a newborn who has a heartbeat. If the heart rate is between 60 and 80 beats per minute and rising, continue to assist ventilations, but compressions are not necessary.

There are two techniques for performing neonate chest compressions. In the preferred technique, place your two thumbs side-by-side on the middle third of the sternum just below the imaginary line drawn across the nipples (Figure 8-27). In very small neonates, you may place one thumb on top of the other (Figure 8-28). Circle the chest and support the back with your fingers. In the second technique, if your hands are too small to encircle the chest, use two fingers. Use the ring and middle fingers of one hand and place them on the sternum just below the nipple line. Use your other hand to support the neonate's back. Depress the sternum 1/2 to 3/4 of an inch, using a smooth compression and relaxation technique. Do not lift your thumbs (or fingers) from the chest during the relaxation phase.

Check the pulse rate periodically and discontinue compressions when the neonate's own heart rate reaches 80 beats per minute or greater. Always provide assisted ventilations with 100% oxygen while you are performing chest compressions. The compression-to-ventilation ratio in neonates is 3:1. Deliver three compressions followed by a pause to allow you to deliver one effective breath. (Check protocols in your jurisdiction to see if the ratio is smaller. Some Medical Directors require a 1:1 ratio.) Compress at a rate of 120 per minute, which actually provides 90 compressions and 30 breaths each minute.

It takes practice to provide effective CPR on neonates. Take every opportunity in class and at your station to practice the procedures on infant manikins. Remember, these cases are rare and you will not get a lot of real-life practice, but you must be ready to provide the skill when needed.

FIGURE 8.27
Place your two thumbs side-by-side on the middle third of the sternum just below an imaginary line drawn across the nipples.

FIGURE 8.28
In very small neonates, place one thumb on top of the other.

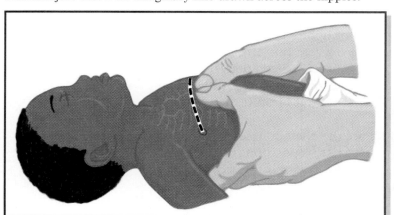

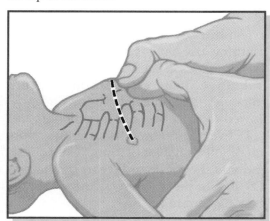

ASSURING EFFECTIVE CPR

CPR is not a simple process. Unless the proper techniques are carried out, CPR will not be effective, and the patient will reach biological death. To assure effective CPR, be sure that:

- The patient is placed face up on a hard surface.
- The airway is opened with the correct technique.
- The mouth and nose are sealed with an infection control barrier (pocket face mask or bag-valve mask; see Appendix 2).
- The nostrils are pinched or sealed, and the patient's mouth is opened wide enough *if you must do mouth-to-mouth ventilation*. First Responders should use a pocket face mask or bag-valve mask (see Appendix 2).
- The hands are placed over the proper compression site.
- The compressions are performed to the proper depth and pressure is relaxed to allow the heart to refill.
- The correct rates and ratios are used.
- The necessary interruptions are limited to 3-to-5 second pulse and breathing checks and to 15-to-30 second patient moves.

Complications can occur during CPR. Some of these complications may be caused by internal injuries from a trauma or from diseased or weakened organs caused by an existing medical condition. First Responders can do nothing about such complications, but regardless of the complication, continue CPR.

First | First Responders are responsible for complications that may be caused by using improper CPR techniques. Certain complications occur because the rescuer places the hands improperly during compressions (Figure 8.29). If you place your hands too high on the patient's chest, you may fracture the collarbones. If your hands are too low, you may cut the liver with the xiphoid process (lower end of the sternum). If you place your hands too far to the right, you may fracture the ribs and possibly cut into the right lung. If you place your hands too far to the left, you might fracture the ribs and cut into the left lung and the heart. You must carefully locate the CPR compression site and properly position your hands to avoid these problems.

In some cases, rib fractures occur even when you are properly performing CPR. In older patients, whose chests are not as pliable and whose bones are more brittle, the ribs may actually break during correct compressions. Children's chests are very pliable; their ribs are not likely to break. On any patient, you may hear a cracking sound while performing compressions, which may be a stretching of the cartilage that connects the ribs to the sternum. This stretching occurs when you compress the sternum to the depth required for appropriate CPR and circulation. If you think you have heard ribs crack, **do not stop CPR.** Check the position of your hands, reposition them properly, and resume CPR. A fractured rib will heal; stopping CPR will result in death.

Another problem occurs if you attempt to force too much air into the patient's lungs. The excess air goes into the stomach. Do not try to force this air out of the stomach. To do so might cause the patient to vomit, which will block the airway. Then, if the patient tries to breathe, vomitus could be aspirated (inhaled) into the lungs; and if you try to provide breaths, you will force the vomitus into the lungs. To avoid or reduce the amount of air forced into the stomach, always look for the patient's chest to rise as you deliver ventilations. Adjust the size of your breaths so that you see the chest rise, then allow the patient to passively exhale. If you see the stomach begin to bulge, reposition the patient's head and adjust your ventilations.

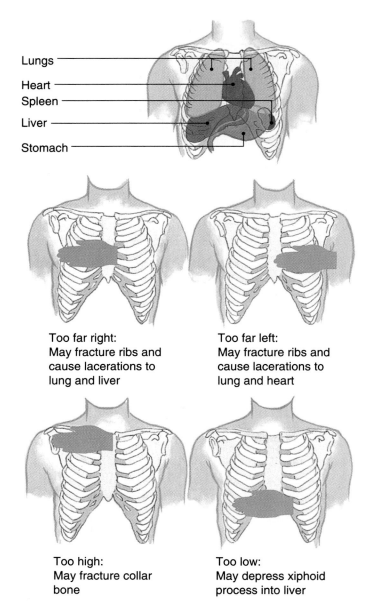

FIGURE 8.29
Improper hand positioning
may cause rib damage and
injury to internal organs.

Lungs

Heart

Spleen

Liver

Stomach

Too far right:
May fracture ribs and
cause lacerations to
lung and liver

Too far left:
May fracture ribs and
cause lacerations to
lung and heart

Too high:
May fracture collar
bone

Too low:
May depress xiphoid
process into liver

If the patient vomits, stop CPR. Take time to clear the patient's airway as best you can by repositioning the patient for drainage and by using your gloved fingers to sweep the mouth. After clearing the airway, resume CPR.

$\mathcal{S}$PECIAL CPR SITUATIONS

Moving the Patient

Usually, there are only two reasons for a First Responder to move a patient who is receiving CPR: transport and immediate danger at the scene. Most of the time, the patient is moved after the EMTs have arrived and assumed responsibility for care. In the majority of moves, you may be asked to help lift and carry the patient. Since EMTs will use special devices and oxygen to assist with ventilations, you probably will not assist in ventilating the patient, but you may be asked to continue compressions. Note that this is a two-rescuer CPR procedure that you will learn about in the next chapter. The two-rescuer procedure is also performed on infants and children as they are moved to the ambulance.

The Accident Scene

Many factors complicate CPR when dealing with an accident victim. Severe injuries to the patient's face may interfere with your attempts to provide ventilations. Crushing injuries to the patient's chest may lessen the effectiveness of chest compressions. Head, neck, and spinal injuries may require that you handle the patient in a special manner.

Your first priority at any accident scene is your own safety. Do not risk your own life. Do not place yourself in a position where someone else will have to rescue you. Be sure you always use the appropriate protective gear and personal protection equipment for patient extrication, assessment, and care. If you are a firefighter or law enforcement officer, you have been taught how to carry out your duties in hazardous situations. You also have been told the limits to the risks that you should take as part of your job. If you have no formal training for the accident scene, proceed with caution. Follow the guidelines or operating procedures of your jurisdiction or agency. More will be said in Chapter 15 about what you may find at the scene of an accident and what will be expected of you as a First Responder.

Many rescuers are unsure about starting CPR on trauma patients. When rescuers find obvious indications of spinal injuries, they may feel it is more important to immobilize the spine before they start CPR. If rescuers find a patient with a crushed chest, they may be afraid of causing internal injuries if they perform chest compressions. **Patient injuries should not prevent you from starting CPR.** If you delay or do not start CPR, the patient will die.

Moving the trauma patient into proper position is a major problem. One concern is spinal injury, but CPR is not effective if the patient is in a seated position. Nor is CPR likely to be effective if the patient is on a soft surface, such as a car seat. Patients must be moved to hard surfaces and placed on their backs. While doing so, take into account the possibility of neck and spinal injury and use your hands and arms to initially control and **stabilize the head and neck** whenever you have to move a patient.

When moving an adult, cradle the head and shoulders in your forearms and attempt to move the patient so that his head stays in line with his body. When moving an infant or a child, always use one hand to support the head and neck of the patient. Again, for CPR to be effective, the patient must be lying face up on a hard surface.

If you must move the patient after starting CPR because of the dangers of the accident scene, then do so. Try not to interrupt CPR for more than 15 to 30 seconds during a move. The total move may have to be done in several stages if conditions allow.

Even if your patient has possible neck and spinal injuries, start CPR as soon as possible. **Do not delay CPR** to fully stabilize the neck and spine with a collar and immobilization devices. Use the jaw-thrust maneuver for ventilations in order to reduce the chances of causing greater injury to the patient.

Drowning Rescuer safety and emergency care procedures at the scene of a drowning or near-drowning incident require special training in water rescue (see Appendix 6). If CPR is needed, begin as soon as possible, but remember your personal safety comes first. You may begin ventilations while the patient is still in the water. Be aware that mouth-to-mask methods may be difficult, if not impossible, to perform under these conditions. In a diving accident, suspect neck injury and use the jaw-thrust maneuver to open the airway. Very little water will be aspirated and any water in the lungs will be absorbed into the circulation as you ventilate the patient. Chest compressions are *not* effective when the patient is in the water. Attempts to begin compressions while the patient is in the water will delay removing the patient from the water and starting effective CPR.

Electric Shock Some of the special problems of accident scenes involving electricity will be covered in Chapter 11. Your first priority is to avoid placing yourself in danger. Assess the patient and start artificial ventilations as soon as possible after you are sure the power is turned off. CPR, when needed, is performed in the same way for a victim of electric shock as it is for any other patient in cardiac arrest.

CPR—RESPONSIBILITIES OF THE FIRST RESPONDER

When dealing with cardiac arrest, your duty is to have someone alert dispatch and to **start CPR immediately.** Only a physician at the scene who has accepted responsibility for the patient may order you not to begin CPR. Bystanders and members of the patient's family may tell you that the patient would not want to be resuscitated. You are not to obey such requests. Even though the patient may have a terminal illness or may be very old, you will still need to **provide CPR** unless there is an official do not resuscitate (DNR) order. Quickly let the family know you understand their feelings, but your duty as a First Responder is to begin CPR. Suggest that they try to contact the patient's doctor to get further directions. If the family does not have advance directives from the patient and doctor, you must begin CPR. Without advance directives confirmed by the patient's doctor or by DNR orders, you have no way of knowing that this is what the patient would have you do. (Be sure you are familiar with prehospital DNR terms in your region; see Chapter 3.) Contact dispatch for assistance, and when EMTs arrive, you or one of them will talk with the family to comfort and reassure them. Offer to call friends or other family members for them, and make sure they know where their family member is being transported.

The longer a patient is in cardiac arrest before CPR is started, the less likely CPR will be effective. However, there are documented cases of adults in cardiac arrest for over 10 minutes who have been resuscitated with no major brain damage. Children and infants usually can survive longer periods of time in cardiac arrest than adults. Do not refuse to begin CPR because someone has been in cardiac arrest for 10 minutes. In most cases, if the patient has been in cardiac arrest for more than 10 minutes, CPR will probably not be effective. However, the moment the patient was seen to collapse and the moment of cardiac arrest are usually not the same. A patient may be unconscious with minimum lung and heart function for quite some time before cardiac arrest occurs. **Always start CPR immediately.**

Cold-water drowning victims can be successfully resuscitated after long periods of cardiac arrest. There are documented cases of arrest that have lasted over 45 minutes before successful resuscitation (see Chapter 10). The same is true of people whose body temperatures are lowered by cold (hypothermia). You must provide resuscitation. The emergency department staff will continue resuscitation while they rewarm the patient's body; they will not declare biological death until the patient is rewarmed and all efforts to revive the patient have failed.

First | Once you have started, continue to provide CPR until:

- Spontaneous circulation begins; then provide ventilations only.
- Spontaneous circulation and breathing begin.

- An equally or more highly trained member of the EMS system or someone certified in CPR can take over for you.
- You turn over responsibility for patient care to a physician.
- You are exhausted and no longer able to continue.

Rescuers are often concerned that they may have to stop CPR when they become exhausted, but you must be realistic. If you reach that point, realize that you have done all you could. CPR has its physical limitations on the rescuer; it also has its physical limitations on the patient. For example, if you performed CPR on a patient for over 30 minutes, then realize that you and the patient may have reached your limits. If you are becoming exhausted and know that you will not be able to continue, look for help from bystanders. Even if they are not trained in CPR, you may be able to tell them what they should do.

If you wish to reduce the chances that you will have to stop CPR because of fatigue, then you should:

1. Keep yourself in good physical condition. Exercise to improve your heart and lung functions.

2. Become a CPR or basic cardiac life-support instructor. Help the American Heart Association (AHA) and American Red Cross in their efforts to train all citizens in basic cardiac life support. This will improve the chances of a bystander being able to assist you in providing CPR.

3. Support your local EMS system so that they may have the personnel and equipment needed to reach all victims in your area.

4. Practice what you have learned about CPR. Your instructor can tell you how to review CPR, keep yourself up-to-date, and have access to manikins for practice.

Almost all jurisdictions have approved and adopted the use of automated external defibrillators (AEDs). Your organization or department may have purchased one or more AEDs and may include AED training in emergency care programs. AEDs assist emergency-care providers in assessing the patient's heart rhythm and in restoring the normal heart beat when certain kinds of abnormal heart beats or arrhythmias are present. The next section will provide information about AEDs and steps on how to use an AED with the steps of CPR. You *must* have the appropriate training and medical direction or protocols before using the AED on a patient in cardiac arrest.

AUTOMATED EXTERNAL DEFIBRILLATION

The fact that most sudden cardiac deaths occur away from hospitals is the reason why there are cardiopulmonary resuscitation (CPR) programs for EMS-level personnel and for laypersons. Two early problems with recognizing and caring for heart attack patients are being resolved. The first problem—delay in starting CPR—has been dramatically reduced through the training of more citizens who can administer CPR before EMS personnel arrive. The second problem stems from the fact that many heart attacks are fatal no matter how soon CPR is started. These deaths are often caused by lethal heart rhythms that must be corrected as soon as possible if the patients are to survive. The special procedure needed to save some of these patients can now be done in the prehospital setting by emergency-care providers such as First Responders and EMTs. This special procedure is called **defibrillation,** which is an electrical shock given to a patient's heart in an attempt to disrupt a lethal (deadly) rhythm and allow the heart to reestablish a normal rhythm.

EMTs and First Responders have been learning how to assess and defibrillate certain lethal cardiac rhythms by using AEDs. Now many non-EMS individuals are being trained to use AEDs because these lifesaving machines are being placed in shopping malls, at golf courses, on airplanes and in airports, and in many other public gathering and recreational places. The United States Senate has passed S.1488, the Cardiac Arrest Survival Act, which does two things. First, it instructs the secretary of Health and Human Services to make recommendations to promote public access to defibrillation programs in federal buildings and other public buildings across the country. This step helps to ensure the health and safety of everyone by encouraging ready access to the tools needed to improve cardiac arrest survival rates. Second, the act extends Good Samaritan protections to AED users and to those who acquire AEDs in those states that do not currently have AED Good Samaritan protections. This Good Samaritan protection will encourage laypersons to respond in a cardiac emergency and use an AED. This legislation will enable and encourage more placement and use of AEDs in public places.

The Cardiac Arrest Survival Act is a critical step toward increasing cardiac arrest survival rates, but just as critical is the training of those who will use AEDs. Training will provide the information needed to understand the heart's electrical system functions and disfunctions and the procedures for assessing and providing initial care for a person complaining of chest pain and going into cardiac arrest. Training will provide information on operation of the AED, and practice time with the AED. Training will also demonstrate the setup and defibrillation steps and emphasize all necessary precautions to take when performing the AED's special procedure. If the defibrillation is successful, the heart can regain or restart its normal rhythm. The next sections will provide information on the heart's electrical conduction system, what causes it to "misfire," and how its rhythm may be restarted by the electrical shock of defibrillation.

THE HEART'S CONDUCTION SYSTEM

The heart is a cone-shaped, hollow muscular organ that is roughly the size of the individual's clinched fist. Its muscular walls are called *myocardium* (mi-o-KAR-de-um). Most of the myocardium is cardiac muscle that maintains the heart's shape and contracts to pump blood. Some of the cells in the cardiac muscle are modified or organized into a system that is known as the **conduction system** (Figure 8.30). These modified cells control the heart's electrical activity.

The normal heartbeat begins at a small region of modified tissue called the *sinoatrial* (si-no-A-tre-al), or SA, node. The SA node is the *natural* pacemaker of the heart, not to be confused with an *artificial* pacemaker that is implanted in some patients with abnormal heart rhythms. An electrical wave is sent out from this site about every 0.8 seconds in the at-rest adult's heart. This wave spreads through the heart's upper chambers (atria) and then is delayed slightly before it is sent on to the lower chambers (ventricles). This delay and transfer take place at a second node called the *atrioventricular* (a-tre-o-ven-TRIK-u-lar), or AV, node.

The impulse that is sent to the lower chambers travels first through the septum, a wall that separates the two lower chambers, and travels through pathways in the septum known as the right and left bundle branches. The wave continues out to the muscular walls by extended pathways called the *Purkinje* (pur-KIN-je) fibers.

SA node

AV node

Bundle of His

Right bundle branch

Left bundle branch

Purkinje fibers

The conduction system initiates the heartbeat, giving time for the upper chambers to prepare for contraction, and then contract with a delay built in before the lower chambers contract. This delay allows for proper chamber filling, contraction, relaxation, and preparation for the next contraction. Any disease of or damage to the heart muscle or arteries may also damage the conduction system. This could lead to an interruption of the heart's rhythm that could stop circulation.

EXTERNAL DEFIBRILLATION

Defibrillators are designed to deliver an electrical shock that will disrupt or stop the heart's dysrhythmic electrical activity. The shock does not start a dead heart, but it will stop certain lethal rhythms and give the heart a chance to spontaneously reestablish an effective rhythm on its own. The entire process is called *defibrillation*.

There are several types of defibrillators. The manual defibrillator requires that the operator look at the patient's heart rhythm on a monitor, interpret the rhythm, decide if it is a shockable rhythm, then lubricate and charge two paddles that will deliver a shock to the patient. The use of manual defibrillators requires special training to determine if a shock should be delivered and to perform the skills to properly deliver the shock. Therefore, they are not usually used by First Responder and EMT-Basic-level providers. Some patients have special implanted automated defibrillators that do not require the help of a rescuer, though the patient will still need rescuer care and transport.

The automated external defibrillators come in two types: semiautomatic and fully automatic, and they are relatively easy to operate (Figure 8.31). AEDs can recognize a heart rhythm that requires a shock, charge itself, and deliver the shock (fully automatic) or advise the rescuer to press an indicated button to deliver the shock (semiautomatic). The limit of usefulness for these devices is related to the nature of the heart problem. The major heart problems that must be considered in a prehospital setting include, but are not limited to:

- *Disorganized rhythm*—A heart rhythm disturbance called **ventricular fibrillation** (ven-TRIK-u-ler fib-ri-LAY-shun), or **VF,** occurs when the heart activity in the lower pumping chambers is disorganized. Instead of

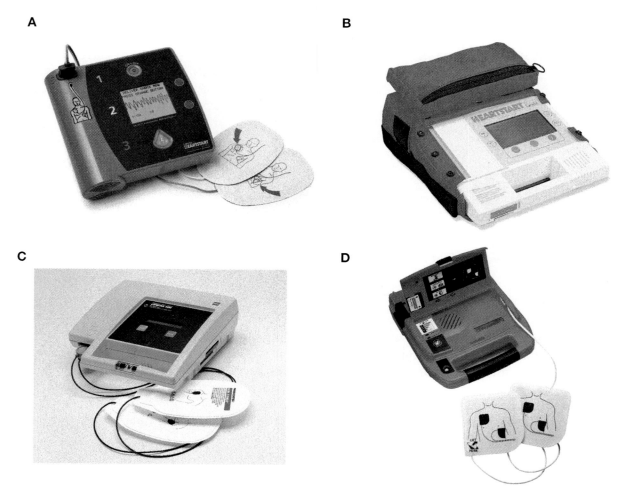

FIGURE 8.31
AEDs from **A** and **B** Laerdal, Medical Corporation; **C** Medtronics/Physiocontrol; **D** Survivalink.

a steady rhythmic pumping action, the muscle "fibrillates" (quivering or spontaneous rapid contraction of the heart's muscle fibers; Figure 8.32). If the rhythm is disorganized in the pumping chambers, the heart cannot pump blood. It is believed that 50 to 60% of all cardiac arrest patients are in ventricular fibrillation (VF) in the first few minutes following cardiac arrest. The sooner the VF dysrhythmia can be defibrillated, the better the patient's chances are for survival.

■ *Organized rhythm, but a very rapid heart rate*—**Ventricular tachycardia** (tak-e-KAR-de-ah) is a very fast heart rate in the heart's lower chambers. Sometimes the rate is so rapid that the heart cannot pump blood. Less than 10% of the prehospital cardiac arrest cases have this problem. Defibrillation may help some of these patients.

■ *Organized rhythm, but a very slow heart rate*—Electromechanical dissociation, also called **pulseless electrical activity (PEA),** is a condition in which the electrical activity of the heart is within normal range, but the heart muscle is too weak and damaged to pump blood efficiently. PEA causes the electrical activity of the heart to separate (dissociate) from the pumping (mechanical) activity. Between 15 and 20% of all cardiac arrest patients have this problem. It cannot be helped by defibrillation.

■ *No electrical impulses*—In **asystole** (ah-SIS-to-le), an absence of electrical impulses, the heart muscle is not stimulated to contract. Defibrillation will not help this problem.

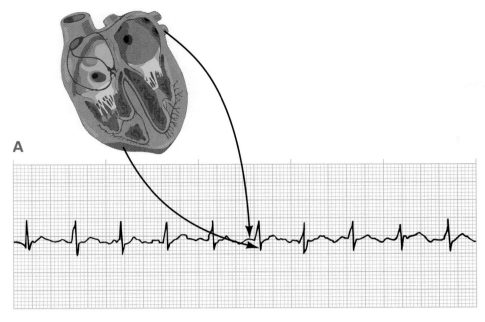

A

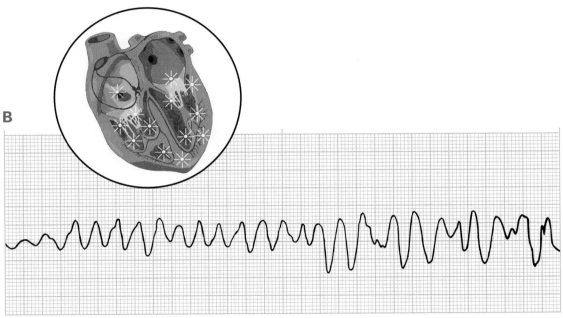

B

FIGURE 8.32
A Normal heart rhythm, or normal sinus rhythm. **B** Ventricular fibrillation.
Many false "pacemaker" sites cause this type of rhythm.

THE ROLE OF THE EMS SYSTEM

The time that passes between the moment a person collapses until the defibrillation shock is delivered is critical. This time can be divided into four segments:

1. *EMS access time*—the time from collapse until the EMS system is alerted.
2. *Dispatch time*—the time from the dispatcher's receipt of the call until the person or crew who will defibrillate the patient is alerted.
3. *Response time*—the time it takes for the alerted person or crew to arrive and reach the patient.

4. *Shock time*—the time it takes from reaching the patient until the defibrillation shock is delivered.

The goal of every EMS system is to reduce the time involved with each stage of the process. In particular, the time from dispatch to the arrival of the defibrillator is being shortened by having rescuers with defibrillators available 24 hours a day. If the patient can receive the first shock within 6 to 8 minutes of collapse, survival is more likely. Table 8-2 shows ideal time components for defibrillation, which if met can improve witnessed cardiac arrest with VF survival rate by 25%.

USING AUTOMATED DEFIBRILLATORS

First Responder defibrillation may be done with either fully automatic or semi-automatic defibrillators. The physician advisory board for your EMS system may have approved one or both of these devices. The operation of both will be covered in this text.

A defibrillator must be ready for use at any given moment. Make certain that you follow your EMS and manufacturer guidelines to ensure that the defibrillators you will use are in working order and prepared for use. Always carry fully charged spare batteries.

BASIC WARNINGS

Certain warnings must be noted when working with automated defibrillators, regardless of type:

- Follow the same precautions that you would for operating any electrical device.
- Do *not* defibrillate a patient who is not in cardiac arrest.

TABLE 8-2: AUTOMATED DEFIBRILLATION

TIME COMPONENT	OBJECTIVE	GOAL	METHOD
EMS Access Time	To minimize the time from collapse until someone places a call for help	1.0 min	An increased community awareness of the need for quickly calling an ambulance; more public CPR programs
Dispatch Time	To minimize the time is takes for an EMS dispatcher to elicit information from a caller and get a defibrillator-equipped unit on the road	0.5 min	Better dispatcher training, improved call-handling procedures
Response Time	To minimize the time it takes to get a trained defibrillator team to the patient	3.0 min	Strategic placement of automated defibrillators with first-response personnel
Shock Time	To minimize the time it takes to deliver the first shock	1.5 min	Use automated defibrillators; continually practice to maintain peak efficiency

Information provided by Kenneth R. Stults, M.S., Director of the University of Iowa Hospitals and Clinics Emergency Medical Services Learning Resource Center. New data suggest that a higher rate of success occurs when patients receive CPR with oxygenation prior to the first shock. Follow your local EMS system guidelines.

- Do *not* defibrillate a patient who is in physical contact with rescuers, bystanders, or other patients.
- Do *not* assess or shock a patient who is moving or when the defibrillator or its leads are being moved.
- Do *not* defibrillate a patient in a moving ambulance or other motor vehicle.
- Do *not* defibrillate a patient who has an obstructed airway. The patient who is in respiratory arrest, but not in cardiac arrest (assess pulse), does not need defibrillation.
- Do *not* defibrillate a patient who is wet, on a wet surface, or in water.
- Do *not* defibrillate a patient who is lying on a metal surface that may transfer the electrical shock to others.
- Do *not* defibrillate a child under 8 years of age. (Note: The American Heart Association has established the age of 8 as the minimum age for AED use. The AHA has found that AED use on 8-year-old children has resulted in successful saves. Prior protocols stated the EMS providers would *not* defibrillate a child under age 12 or weighing less than 30 kilograms (80 pounds) unless directed to do so by a physician. *It is still recommended that you call or radio the emergency department physician or medical direction for all cases involving child patients. Check your local protocols.*)

*N*ote
Make certain that dispatch is informed of the emergency.

The policy of defibrillating trauma patients is established at the state or local level. Follow your EMS system's protocols. Basically, a determination has to be made as to whether the accident was caused by the heart problem, the accident set off a preexisting heart problem, or the heart problem was a direct result of the injury. If you are not certain as to what you are to do, phone or radio the emergency department physician or EMS medical direction.

*F*IRST RESPONDER CARE

The use of a defibrillator must follow other procedures of care and assessment. You must do an initial assessment to confirm that the patient is in cardiac arrest. If an EMT trained in defibrillation is at the scene, you will probably begin CPR. This will allow the EMT to prepare and attach the defibrillator and operate the device. The EMT will alert you before delivering the shock to make certain that you are clear of the patient before a shock is given.

If there is no higher level EMS personnel at the scene and someone else is providing basic life support, your job will be to prepare and attach the defibrillator. Make certain that both of you are clear of the patient before a shock is given.

*A*TTACHING THE DEFIBRILLATOR

The procedure for attaching the defibrillator to a patient is the same for both semiautomatic and fully automatic systems. Electrodes with self-adhesive pads should be properly placed on the patient's bare chest to monitor heart rhythm.

While someone performs CPR, the defibrillator operator should:

1. Bare the patient's chest. If the patient's chest is wet, it should be quickly wiped dry. If the surrounding area is wet, move the patient to a dry surface.
2. Remove two pads from their protective packages.
3. Remove the plastic backing from the first pad and place it adhesive-side down on the patient's upper right chest. (If you are using color-coded pads, this is the white pad.) The top of the pad should touch the skin over

FIGURE 8.33
The correct placement of
defibrillator pads.

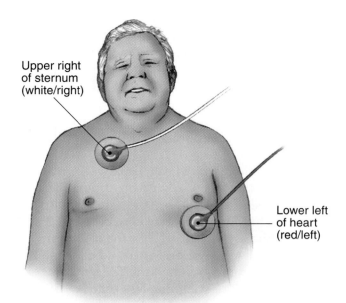

Upper right
of sternum
(white/right)

Lower left
of heart
(red/left)

the top of the clavicle (collarbone), while the medial edge should be on the
skin next to the sternum (Figure 8.33). The pad should *not* be placed over
the top of the patient's sternum.

4. Press the pad so the adhesive makes full contact with the patient's skin.
Do *not* press on the center of the pad, which contains a special gel if it has
a sponge center. Pressing in this region might force the gel onto the adhesive or skin and prevent proper contact.

5. Remove the adhesive backing from the second pad and place it on the
patient's skin below and to the left of the left nipple. (If you are using
color-coded pads, this is the red pad.) Ensure good adhesive contact.

6. Tightly connect the lead cables from the AED to the pads. Follow the
manufacturer's instructions. If the cables are color coded, they should be
placed with the white cable attached to the upper right pad and the red
cable attached to the lower left pad. This placement will allow for the
correct input of the patient's electrocardiogram (ECG) signal into the
AED's circuits.

Automatic external defibrillators will not function unless the pads are fully
adhered to the patient's chest and the cables are tightly secured. If either of
these problems exist, the "no contact" signal or error message will sound or
appear.

*O*PERATING THE FULLY AUTOMATIC DEFIBRILLATOR

*N*ote

Always follow the
manufacturer's
manual and your
EMS system's
guidelines for the
defibrillator you
will be using.

The following is an example of the operational procedures for a fully automatic
defibrillator. Be aware that various defibrillator models are available. Follow
the manufacturer's manual and your EMS system's guidelines for the defibrillator you will be using. Be aware that when three shocks are given, the energy
level of the third shock is usually greater than the first two. You may have to set
the defibrillator for this higher level. This is not necessary with the newer
models.

Once attached to the patient and turned on, the latest models of fully automated defibrillators will automatically assess the patient's heart rhythm, sense
if a shock should be delivered, charge to the preset energy level, and deliver the

shock to the patient. These defibrillators have voice synthesizers to alert the rescuer and give instructions that typically include "Stop CPR," "Stand back," and "Check breathing and pulse." Should this voice system fail, the rescuer is expected to know what to do and how to ensure personal safety.

To operate a fully automatic defibrillator, you should (Scan 8-3):

1. Assess the patient to determine cardiac arrest.

2. Have your partner or someone trained in basic life support begin CPR while you set up the AED.

3. If the rescuer is by himself, he should turn on the AED, attach, analyze, shock up to three times. If no change in rhythm,

    – provide 1 minute of CPR.

    – shock three times (if no change).

    – consider transport.

Each EMS system has its own protocols for First Responders acting alone. You may be required to perform CPR for 1 full minute or perform some other step before you prepare and attach the defibrillator. Follow your local protocols.

4. Make certain that you, your partner, and all other persons at the scene are not in contact with the patient.

5. Press the defibrillator ON button and remain clear of the patient. Note the time this was done. The defibrillator voice synthesizer should state, "Stop CPR." At this time, the defibrillator will perform an analysis of the patient's heart rhythm. If the patient is to be shocked, the voice synthesizer will announce, "Stand back." Make certain that you do not touch or move the patient or the defibrillator. The defibrillator will charge to 200 joules of energy and deliver the shock.

6. Stay clear of the patient and allow the defibrillator to reassess the patient's heart rhythm. If a second shock is required, the voice synthesizer will state, "Stand back," and the defibrillator will again charge (usually to 200 joules) and deliver the second shock.

7. Continue to stay clear of the patient. A third shock may be required. If three shocks have been delivered, the voice synthesizer will announce, "Check breathing and pulse."

8. Assess the patient's breathing and pulse.

    – **If there is a pulse,** leave the defibrillator attached to monitor the patient. Maintain an open airway and continue life-support procedures. The patient would benefit from oxygen therapy and, if necessary, assisted ventilations. Do only what you have been trained to do.

    – If there is **no pulse,** leave the defibrillator attached to the patient and continue CPR.

9. After 60 seconds, the defibrillator will state, "Stop CPR," and do another analysis of the patient's heart rhythm. If a shock is to be delivered, the voice synthesizer will state, "Stand back," and deliver from one to three more electrical shocks.

10. If no more shocks are indicated or if all three additional shocks have been delivered, the voice synthesizer will state, "Check breathing and pulse." You should take the same course of action as stated in step 7.

Automated Defibrillation

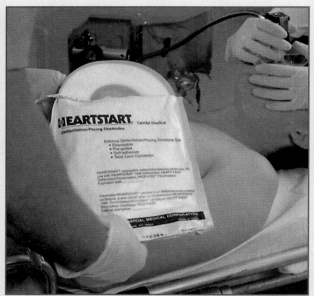

1. The patient's chest is exposed, and the pads are removed from the protective covering.

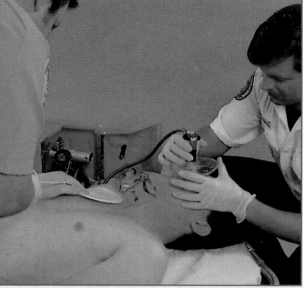

2. The plastic backing is removed from the first pad, and the pad is placed on the chest.

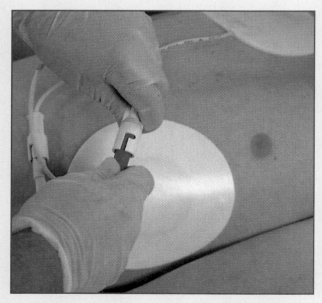

3. The second pad is placed on the patient's chest, and the cables are connected.

4. Turn on the device and follow the defibrillator prompts:

❏ Stop CPR.
❏ Stand back.
❏ Check breathing and pulse.

  Pulse—follow prompts.
  No pulse—begin CPR and follow prompts.

The defibrillator will enter a **perpetual monitoring mode,** allowing it to continue to assess the patient's heart rhythm. It will not be able to deliver additional shocks without rescuer assistance. Instead, it will announce, "Check breathing and pulse." If the patient is still in cardiac arrest, you will have to make certain that you are not touching the patient and then clear everyone away. Press the ON button, note the time that this was done, and continue with steps 4 through 9.

OPERATING THE SEMIAUTOMATIC DEFIBRILLATOR

NOTE: The following is an example of the operational procedures for a semi-automatic defibrillator. Various defibrillator models are available. Follow the instructions given in the manufacturer's manual and your EMS system's guidelines for the defibrillator that you will be using.

Semiautomatic defibrillators are also called *shock advisory defibrillators*. They will automatically monitor and assess the patient's heart rhythm and determine if a shock should be given and, if necessary, charge to a preset level. They will not automatically deliver the shock. The rescuer must push a button to do this (Figure 8.34).

The same basic assessment and safety procedures that apply to the fully automatic defibrillator also apply to the operation of the semiautomatic defibrillator. Some models do not have a voice synthesizer. They all require the rescuer to push a button to deliver the shock. For these reasons, all standard operating procedures for safety must be given extra consideration during semiautomatic defibrillator use.

To operate a semiautomatic defibrillator, you should:

1. Assess the patient to determine cardiac arrest.

2. Have your partner or someone trained in basic life support begin CPR. If you are acting alone, prepare the defibrillator, attach the pads to the

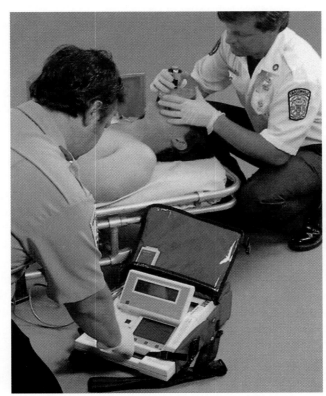

FIGURE 8.34
Operating a semiautomatic defibrillator. Do not apply shock until everyone, including you, is clear of the patient.

patient, and connect the cables. After this is completed, begin CPR and continue for 1 full minute or for the time designated by your EMS medical advisory board.

3. Turn on the defibrillator by lifting open the display model or as directed by the manufacturer. The message screen should show the command PRESS TO ANALYZE with an arrow pointing to the button you need to depress. Do not allow anyone to touch or move the patient or defibrillator. Press the indicated button, and allow the defibrillator to analyze the patient's heart rhythm. If the patient is to be shocked, the defibrillator will automatically charge to 200 joules of energy. A prompt will appear on the message screen telling you to STAND BACK. Your defibrillator may also have a voice synthesizer command that gives the same message.

4. Make certain that you, your partner, and all other persons are clear of the patient.

5. Press the button indicated by the READY PRESS TO SHOCK prompt on the message screen. Note the time that this was done.

6. After the shock is delivered, press the ANALYZE button.
   - **Shock indicated**—Repeat the procedure to deliver a second shock. Press the ANALYZE button to determine if a third shock is necessary. If a third shock is to be delivered, increase the energy level to 360 joules of energy by pressing the indicated button as the defibrillator charges (see the following note). Press the appropriate button when the defibrillator is ready to shock the patient.
   - **No shock indicated**—Assess both respirations and pulse. If they are absent, resume CPR. If they are present, provide appropriate care and ready the patient for transport. Continue to monitor the patient.

NOTE: The number of shocks allowed to be delivered to a patient and the joules of energy delivered for each of these shocks is part of your EMS system's **physician-determined standing orders.** If you are in doubt as to what to do, phone or radio the emergency department physician or medical direction.

PROBLEMS OPERATING A DEFIBRILLATOR

Most of the problems with defibrillator operations that can be corrected by the rescuer involve the attachment of the pads and/or cables. Usually, making certain that the pads are in full contact and the cables are tightly connected will be all that is needed to correct most problems.

There may be times when you cannot secure the pads fully to the patient's chest. The patient's chest should be dry and free of anything in contact with its surface. Make certain that you remove any dressings and nitroglycerin patches that are on the pad placement sites. Wipe off any nitropaste found on the patient's chest. (Your hands should be gloved.) If necessary, you may have to shave the pad placement areas of the patient's chest. Use a disposable safety razor provided for this procedure.

The defibrillators used by First Responders have error message modes. These messages can be audio, visual, or a combination of both. Be sure you know the error messages that apply to your defibrillator and what you should do in response to each message.

ASSESSMENT AND QUALITY ASSURANCE

To be effective, a prehospital defibrillation program requires ongoing evaluation in order to identify and correct any problems. This process of assessment and quality assurance should focus on specific situations that involve standard operating procedures and physician-directed standing orders, care delivered by the rescuers, performance of the equipment, and effectiveness of training programs. Changes in any aspect of the program must be the result of physician evaluation and orders.

All automated defibrillators have a recording device that will provide a record of the resuscitation and defibrillation incident. Since defibrillation incidents are very complex situations and the rescuer must render care without a physician at the scene, certain medical assessments must be made after the fact. The event and how the various aspects of the defibrillation program performed can be evaluated by a physician to help improve patient care. Part of this evaluation will include rescuer performance. You should view this as a helping process, designed to aid you as you improve your skills as a First Responder. This is part of the professional approach needed for patient care.

Be certain to complete your EMS system's records and keep your own notes for each defibrillation incident. Your notes should include when you determined cardiac arrest, how many shocks were delivered, when they were delivered, and the energy level for each shock.

Part of your equipment inspection and assessment should include the operation of your defibrillator recording device. Audiotape devices have caused some field problems. Follow the manufacturer's manual and your EMS system's recommendations to correct any problems before the unit is needed.

Summary

Like the chain of EMS resources, the chain of survival is also a linked system of patient-care events. These events include early access, early CPR, early defibrillation, and early Advanced Cardiac Life Support (ACLS).

There is a strong relationship between breathing, circulation, and brain activity. When the heart stops beating, a patient is in **cardiac arrest** and will be unresponsive. The major signs of cardiac arrest are **no breathing** and **no carotid pulse.**

Determine breathing by the **look, listen,** and **feel** method. Determine circulation by feeling for a carotid pulse on an adult and a child (1 to 8 years). For an infant (under 1 year of age), feel for a **brachial pulse.** For a neonate (birth to 1 month), check the **apical pulse** with your ear or a stethoscope over the chest.

If a patient is unresponsive, check airway, breathing, and circulation (ABCs). After determining that the patient is unresponsive, and after alerting the EMS system dispatcher (for pediatric patients, perform CPR for one minute, then call), you will:

1. Position the patient and open the airway. Do not overextend the head-tilt for infants.

2. Determine that the patient is not breathing.

3. Provide two adequate breaths. (Clear the airway if necessary; see Chapter 6.)

4. Determine that there is no pulse.

5. Find the CPR compression site:
    - **Adult**—next to (not on top of) the index finger of the hand used to locate the notch where the sternum (breastbone) and ribs meet.
    - **Child**—along the midline of the sternum, located in the same way that was done for an adult.
    - **Infant**—along the midline of the sternum, one finger-width below an imaginary line drawn between the nipples.
    - **Neonate**—just below the imaginary line drawn between the nipples.

6. Correctly position your hands for compressions:
    - **Adult**—Place the heel of your hand closest to the patient's head on the CPR compression site. Place your other hand on top of this hand so that the heels of both hands are parallel and your fingers are pointing away from your body. You may extend or interlace the fingers. **Keep your fingers off the patient's chest.**
    - **Child**—Deliver compressions with the **heel of one hand,** positioned over the child's CPR compression site.
    - **Infant**—Deliver compressions with the **tips of two or three fingers,** positioned over the infant's CPR compression site.
    - **Neonate**—Deliver compressions with **two thumbs side-by-side** (or one on top of the other for newborns), positioned over the neonate's CPR compression site.

7. Provide external chest compressions:
    - **Adult**—at a depth of 1½ to 2 inches at a rate of 100 per minute.
    - **Child**—at a depth of 1 to 1½ inches at a rate of 100 per minute.

- **Infant**—at a depth of ½ to 1 inch at a rate of at least 100 per minute.
- **Neonate**—at a depth of ½ to ¾ inch at a rate of 120 per minute.

8. Provide ventilations:
   - **Adult**—2 breaths every 15 compressions.
   - **Child**—1 breath every 5 compressions.
   - **Infant**—1 breath every 5 compressions.
   - **Neonate**—1 breath every 3 compressions.

9. Check for a carotid pulse after 1 minute of CPR. Use the brachial pulse if the patient is an infant, the apical pulse if the patient is a neonate.
   - No pulse, no breathing—continue CPR, checking for a pulse every few minutes.
   - Pulse, but no breathing—stop compressions and provide artificial ventilations. Continue to monitor pulse every few minutes.

NOTE: The patient will not be breathing unless there is heart action.

For neonates, a First Responder may have to perform the first three steps: 1) initial stabilization and evaluation; 2) ventilations; and 3) chest compressions. Make sure the airway is clear and suction if necessary, which may stimulate breathing. Provide ventilations for 15 to 30 seconds at 40 to 60 breaths a minute. Then evaluate heart rate. If the heart rate is 100 beats a minute and the neonate is breathing, discontinue ventilations. If the heart rate is less than 60 or between 60 and 80 but not increasing, assist ventilations and start chest compressions. If the heart rate is 60 to 80 beats per minute and increasing, continue to assist ventilations but discontinue compressions.

Do not stop CPR for more than **5 seconds** other than to move the patient because of danger on the scene (scene safety). If you have to move the patient, do not stop CPR for more than 15 to 30 seconds. Continue CPR until heart or heart and lung functions start, until you are relieved by an equally or more highly trained person, care for the patient is accepted by a physician, or until you can no longer continue because of exhaustion.

Start CPR immediately on a patient in cardiac arrest, even if you may worsen existing injuries. Without CPR, the patient will go from clinical death to biological death within 6 minutes. If the patient has an advance directive (Do Not Resuscitate order), do not start resuscitation. Check with your jurisdiction about advance directives.

First Responders use AEDs in many jurisdictions. These lifesaving units are placed in many public areas, and First Responders will assist the public in using them and performing CPR.

AEDs can convert certain **dysrhythmias** to a normal cardiac rhythm. AEDs are electrical devices and must be used with caution. They are also lifesaving devices and must be used according to protocol. The general steps for use are:

■ Expose the patient's chest and attach the pads
■ Turn on the AED, stop CPR, stand clear, defibrillate, check breathing and pulse
■ Follow AED prompts for a pulse or start CPR if no pulse.

Remember and Consider...

The blood in our body moves in circuits—two of them. One circuit, the pulmonary circuit, is the circulation of unoxygenated blood from the heart to the lungs where it picks up oxygen then returns to the heart. The other circuit, the vascular circuit, is the circulation of oxygenated blood from the heart to the entire body and back to the heart. As long as the heart pumps, the blood circulates. If the heart stops pumping, the blood stops circulating and the First Responder must do CPR to restart and maintain circulation. You will practice CPR in class and may have done so already. Think about what you have read in the text and what you will do during practice.

✔ What equipment do you need to perform CPR?

✔ How many people do you need to perform CPR?

Were the answers easy? Or did you say, "It depends"? Does it depend on the age or size of the patient? On how many people there are to help? On whether you have a pocket face mask, gloves, oxygen? Can you do CPR without these things? Is it safe to do so? What are your obligations for performing CPR on someone in cardiac arrest? Do you think you need to carry your own pocket face mask and gloves with you at all times? What if you don't have a pocket face mask and someone in a restaurant has a heart attack and goes into cardiac arrest before the ambulance gets there? Is there anything handy that you can use as a face shield?

Investigate...

✔ Do public places and stores keep emergency care supplies handy for public use?

When you go to the library, the grocery store, the mall, the theater, or restaurants, do you see signs that tell you they have pocket face masks available? Some places do. If you don't see signs, ask if these items are kept for public use in the event of an emergency. Can they be retrieved quickly? Or are they locked away causing someone to wait while the key is found? Many malls are beginning to keep emergency care supplies at special locations or at a first-aid center. Do the security guards know where these supplies are kept? Do they have access to these supplies? How hard is it to locate and retrieve these supplies? What supplies are kept? Are there pocket face masks, different sizes of airways and bag-valve masks, an AED? What training do mall personnel have for using these items?

Checking public places for these items ahead of the potential incident is called preplanning. Fire department personnel frequently check public places in order to preplan their firefighting strategies. Emergency care personnel carry their own patient care equipment on their units. Off-duty personnel are often in public places where they may need to assist in the care of a patient before the ambulance arrives. Preplanning can help prepare you for such events.

CHAPTER 9

TWO-RESCUER CPR

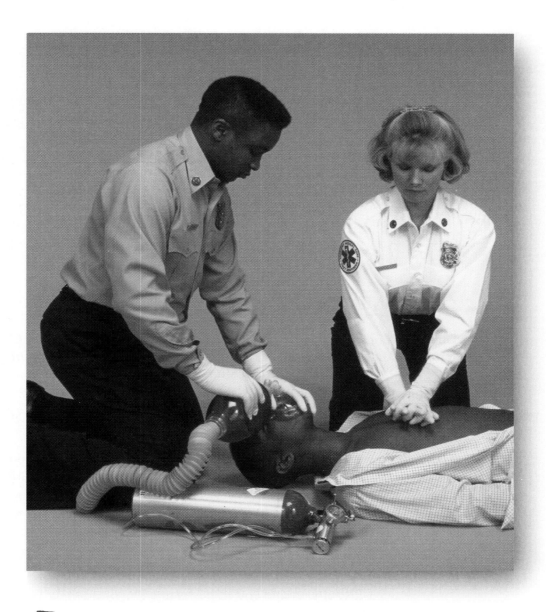

First Responders have or feel a responsibility for the well-being of people in their communities. Too many members of our communities have heart disease. Research and statistics show that there are nearly one million deaths a year from cardiovascular disease; about a quarter of these people die suddenly from heart attacks. First Responders are the closest and quickest source of assistance for those having signs and symptoms of heart attack, but it is often difficult to provide emergency care alone. This chapter introduces you to two-rescuer CPR, which includes the steps of one-rescuer CPR and also addresses the two-rescuer compression-to-breathing ratio and the technique of switching positions.

This chapter focuses on the objectives of Module 4, Lesson 4–1 of the U.S. DOT First Responder National Standard Curriculum and serves as an instructional aid to help you meet any specific objectives added to the course by your local EMS system.

By the end of this chapter, you will know how to (from cognitive or knowledge information) . . .

4–1.9   List the steps of two-rescuer adult CPR. (pp. 229–236)

Show how to (through psychomotor skills) . . .

4–1.20   Demonstrate the steps of adult two-rescuer CPR. (pp. 229–236)

*L*EARNING TASKS

Chapter 8 concluded with the difficulty of maintaining one-rescuer CPR for any length of time. Two-rescuer CPR has some distinct advantages, but it takes a little more training and practice. After this chapter, you will be able to:

✔ State the advantages of two-rescuer CPR over one-rescuer CPR.

✔ State the qualifications needed by those who wish to help a First Responder in performing two-rescuer CPR.

The techniques for two-rescuer CPR are basically the same, but you will need to remember and perform a different ratio of compressions to ventilations. As you practice and coach each other, be able to:

✔ Cite the rate of compressions and the rate of ventilations used when providing two-rescuer CPR.

✔ State how often you should check for a carotid pulse when providing two-rescuer CPR.

Two-rescuer CPR may enable you to perform CPR for a longer period of time, when needed. When you become tired during two-rescuer CPR, you may switch or change positions with your partner. This switch takes practice so that CPR efforts remain effective. Practice the steps, but also be able to:

✔ List, step by step, the sequence of procedures for changing positions during two-rescuer CPR.

At first, you may find it hard to adjust to the switch. With practice, you will get better and will find you can change positions with anyone, and not just with your classmates. While your are practicing and adjusting to two-rescuer CPR, compare the steps to one-rescuer CPR. Do you find that most steps are the same? What steps are different? Be able to:

✔ State how long compressions may be interrupted when checking for breathing and a carotid pulse.

✔ Repeat the skills demonstrated in two-rescuer CPR, but with a different partner.

Your jurisdiction may allow First Responders to use an automated external defibrillator to defibrillate a patient in cardiac arrest. Your department or organization may have these machines for use on your unit or in your place of work. You *must* complete appropriate training before using an AED, and in your training you will:

✔ Demonstrate how to set up an AED and perform the steps to analyze and safely defibrillate a patient.

/NTRODUCTION

Two-rescuer CPR, when performed correctly, is a more efficient procedure than one-rescuer CPR. More oxygen is provided to the patient, chest compressions are not interrupted for as long, the compression rate allows for better filling of the heart, and rescuer fatigue is reduced.

First When you are working with another member of the EMS system, you should find no major problems when the two of you perform CPR because you both will have the same training (Figure 9.1).

Sometimes, bystanders are doing CPR when you arrive, and sometimes First Responders will start CPR before other members of the EMS system arrive. Bystanders will often offer to assist and, if they have been trained by the American Heart Association (AHA) or the American Red Cross, you can begin two-rescuer CPR. Though the bystander may have had two-rescuer CPR training, his skills may not be perfect if he has not had opportunity to practice. You may have to coach the individual during CPR, or even ask that the individual stop so you may resume effective one-rescuer CPR.

Since two-rescuer CPR has not been a part of the AHA citizen training for a number of years, you may find that your helper is not up-to-date on CPR techniques. Also, it is unlikely that bystanders will know how to use a pocket face mask, nor will they be likely to have their own mask with them. Today, most people are very aware of infectious diseases and will be reluctant to perform mouth-to-mouth breathing on a stranger. If a bystander is willing to help, you will perform the ventilations with your pocket face mask, and the bystander will take over chest compressions. You will be able to quickly determine if the bystander is performing proper compressions, and you can direct him to adjust his compressions or to stop if necessary.

With two rescuers, not only is it more efficient to perform CPR, it is also more efficient to use the AED. One rescuer will begin to set up the AED and attach the electrodes to the patient, while the other rescuer begins the ABC steps of CPR. Refer to the information in Chapter 8 on how to use the AED and practice using it until you are proficient in setting it up and feel confident in performing the steps. You may arrive on the scene of a cardiac arrest and find that an AED has been set up and is in use. When you arrive and an AED is being used, assure that the individuals are performing the steps properly and taking the necessary safety precautions. Offer to assist the rescuers and support their

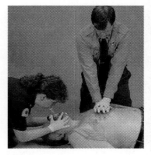

FIGURE 9.1
Positioning in two-rescuer CPR.

actions. You may also need to relieve or guide someone who is unsure of the procedures.

CHANGING TO TWO-RESCUER CPR

NOTE: For an adult who has collapsed, your first action is to find out if the person is unconscious by checking for unresponsiveness. Tap or gently shake the victim and shout "Are you OK?" If there is no response, activate the EMS system (usually by calling 911). If you are alone and there is no telephone, start CPR. If someone arrives where you are performing CPR and dispatch has not been called, have that person call dispatch immediately.

In many cases, one-rescuer CPR is started by a bystander before another rescuer arrives. When a second rescuer arrives, he should activate the EMS system, if it has not yet been done, and should perform one-rescuer CPR when the first rescuer becomes tired. The second rescuer will assess breathing and pulse before he resumes CPR. If you determine that the bystander's CPR techniques are inadequate or incorrect, take over one-rescuer CPR.

First If a First Responder member of the EMS system is performing CPR when you arrive, begin two-rescuer CPR. The following steps will help you make a smooth transition from one-rescuer to two-rescuer CPR:

1. A First Responder is performing one-rescuer CPR. Another First Responder arrives and identifies herself.

2. The first rescuer accepts the help and continues one-rescuer CPR while the second rescuer activates the EMS System if not yet done.

3. While the first rescuer continues the cycle of 15 compressions and two breaths, the second rescuer checks for the pulse in the carotid artery, which is generated each time the first rescuer provides a compression.

4. At the end of the compression and breathing cycle, the first rescuer stops for a 5-second check for return of spontaneous breathing and pulse just after he has provided the two breaths. If there is no pulse, the second rescuer, who has moved to the chest, resumes chest compressions. There is no need to provide another breath since two breaths were just given. The first rescuer, now the ventilator, resumes ventilations, providing *one ventilation after every fifth compression* (AHA *Guidelines 2000:* two ventilations after 15 compressions at a rate of 100 per minute).

5. The second rescuer, now the compressor, provides compressions at the rate of 80 to 100 per minute with a pause after every fifth compression to allow for a ventilation (AHA *Guidelines 2000:* two ventilations after 15 compressions at a rate of 100 per minute).

6. If the compressor becomes tired, she signals, and at the end of a compression cycle, moves to the ventilator position. The ventilator moves to the compressor position and resumes compressions (see the section on Changing Positions).

COMPRESSIONS AND VENTILATIONS

During two-rescuer CPR, five compressions are delivered every 3 to 4 seconds at a rate of 80 to 100 compressions a minute. With the pause for ventilations,

Note

The American Heart Association's *Guidelines 2000* (effective January 2001) recommends that two rescuers provide two ventilations after every 15 compressions at a rate of 100 per minute. Check with your jurisdiction to find out if it has adopted the new guidelines or when it plans to do so.

you will actually deliver at least 60 compressions a minute. One ventilation is delivered after every five compressions to provide a rate of 12 breaths a minute.

 ■ Compressions: 80 to 100 per minute to actually deliver at least 60 per minute
■ Ventilations: 12 per minute

The rescuer providing compressions will count aloud so that both rescuers will be able to establish and maintain the correct rate. By hearing the count, the other rescuer will be prepared to provide a breath after every fifth compression (while the first rescuer pauses to allow for adequate ventilation). While providing compressions, that rescuer will repeat the count 1 through 5 in every cycle as long as two-rescuer CPR is provided for the patient.

CPR PROCEDURE

Scan 9-1 outlines the complete sequence for two-rescuer CPR. Note that one rescuer is called the ventilator, and the other rescuer is called the compressor. Both rescuers are shown on the same side of the patient for teaching purposes. In actual two-rescuer CPR, rescuers normally place themselves on opposite sides of the patient. If the ventilator uses a pocket face mask or a bag-valve mask and supplemental oxygen (see Appendix 2), his position is usually at the top of the patient's head so he can provide the most effective ventilation technique. Your instructor will demonstrate how to ventilate a patient using the masks, supplemental oxygen, and oxygen delivery equipment that your jurisdiction requires First Responders to use.

The ventilator will check frequently for a carotid pulse, which should be generated with each compression. If this pulse cannot be found, the ventilator will have the compressor check hand position, body position (arms straight, shoulders over sternum, bend at hips), and depth of compressions.

The ventilator will check periodically for return of spontaneous breathing and pulse. After the first minute of CPR, and every few minutes thereafter, the rescuers will stop CPR. After delivering a breath, the ventilator will take 5 seconds to determine if there is breathing and a pulse and take appropriate action:

■ Pulse, no breathing—say "There is a pulse." Continue rescue breathing only.
■ No pulse, no breathing—say, "No pulse, continue CPR."
■ Pulse and breathing—say, "Stop CPR." Monitor the patient.

If CPR is continued, the ventilator will check for spontaneous breathing and pulse every few minutes. This interruption should last for no more than 5 seconds.

CHANGING POSITIONS

Either rescuer may request a change in position if he or she becomes tired, but it is usually the compressor who needs the break. Unless the ventilator finds that the compressor cannot generate a pulse during compression, the compressor will decide when to change positions. At the beginning of a cycle, the compressor will give a clear signal to the ventilator to switch places, but will complete a set of five compressions before any moves are made. At the end of the fifth compression, the ventilator will provide one ventilation, then the rescuers will quickly change positions (Scan 9-2). (Your instructor will teach you the preferred switching signals to use.)

Note

Each rescuer should use his or her own pocket face mask with one-way valve and HEPA filter insert.

Two-Rescuer CPR

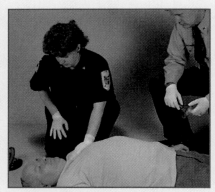

1. Determine unresponsiveness. Alert EMS. Reposition.

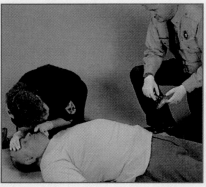

2. Open the airway. Look, listen, feel for 3–5 seconds.

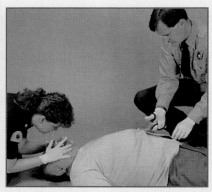

3. Ventilate twice (1.5 to 2.0 seconds per breath).

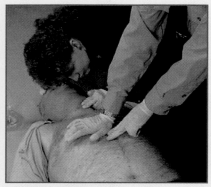

4. Determine pulselessness (no pulse). Locate CPR compression site.

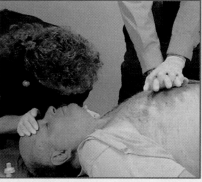

5. Say "No pulse." Begin compressions. Deliver five compressions in 3–4 seconds (80–100 per minute).

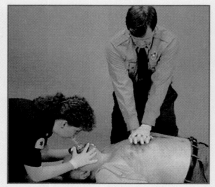

6. Ventilate once (1.5 to 2.0 seconds). Stop compressions for mouth-to-mask ventilation.

7. Continue with one ventilation every five compressions (AHA *Guidelines 2000:* two ventilations after 15 compressions at a rate of 100 per minute).

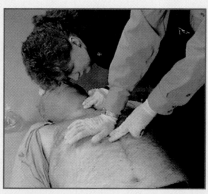

8. Check compression effectiveness. Deliver five compressions in 3–4 seconds (80–100 per minute).

NOTE: Assess for spontaneous breathing and pulse for 5 seconds at the end of the first minute, then every few minutes thereafter.

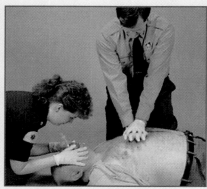

9. After twelve cycles, reassess breathing and pulse. No pulse—say "Continue CPR." Pulse—say "Stop CPR."

Changing Position

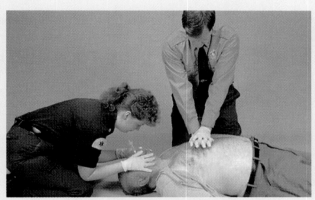

1. When fatigued, the compressor calls for a switch; gives a clear signal to change.

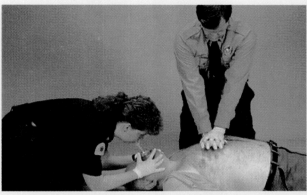

2. Compressor completes fifth compression. Ventilator provides one ventilation.(**NOTE:** AHA *Guidelines 2000* recommends 15 compressions and two ventilations.)

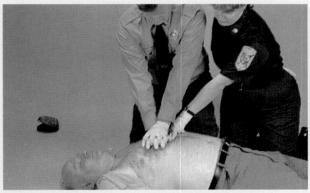

3. Ventilator moves to chest and locates compression site.

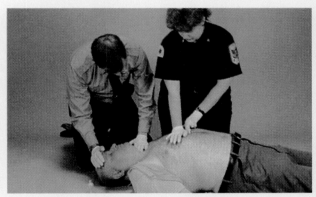

4. New compressor positions hands. New ventilator checks carotid pulse (5 seconds) and says "No pulse, continue CPR." (**NOTE:** Another breath is not given.)

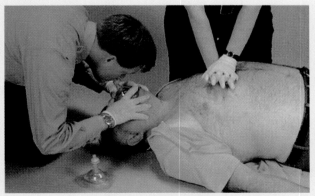

5. New compressor begins compressions and new ventilator breathes after every fifth compression (1.5 to 2.0 seconds for each breath). (**NOTE:** AHA *Guidelines 2000* recommends breathing after every fifteenth compression.)

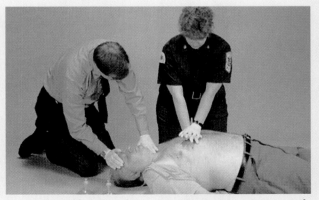

6. New ventilator and new compressor continue until compressor is fatigued and calls for a change.

CHAPTER 9 ■ Two-Rescuer CPR   **233**

The ventilator will check for a generated carotid pulse periodically, but the best time to check for return of respiration and pulse is at the time of the position change. The compressor, when he moves to the ventilator position, can do both of these checks simultaneously for 5 seconds.

PROBLEMS

When two people begin to perform two-rescuer CPR, there are always adjustments to be made as they change positions. Each person performs the change a little differently than the next. For this reason, practice two-rescuer CPR with several different partners.

After the fifth compression, the ventilator must provide a breath within 1.5 to 2.0 seconds. Resistance from the patient's airway, rescuer fatigue, and many other factors can cause the ventilator to miss providing the breath to the patient at the appropriate time. If you should miss a breath, do not wait another five compressions. Provide a ventilation after any compression as soon as possible during the next set of compressions. Resume your normal ventilations after the fifth compression.

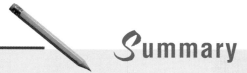

Summary

Scan 9-3 provides a summary of both one-rescuer and two-rescuer CPR for adults. Remember that two-rescuer CPR:

- is a more efficient procedure than one-rescuer CPR
- provides more oxygen to the patient
- reduces interruptions between chest compressions
- allows for better filling of the heart
- reduces rescuer fatigue

In two-rescuer CPR:

- Compressions = 5 within 3 to 4 seconds at a rate of 80–100 per minute to actually deliver at least 60 a minute.
- Provide one ventilation every 5 compressions = 12 per minute.
- The ventilator monitors the carotid pulse to check the effectiveness of the compressions.
- The compressor counts out loud each 1–to–5 cycle.
- The compressor signals the change of position.
- Check for breathing and carotid pulse after the first minute and then every few minutes. The best time to check for return of pulse and breathing is when changing positions. The new ventilator should make this check.
- Do not interrupt CPR for more than 5 seconds.
- If you miss a breath, provide a ventilation after any compression as soon as possible during the next cycle of compressions.

Use the AED in your basic life-support procedures if First Responders are trained to do so in your jurisdiction (review Chapter 8).

CPR Summary—Adult Patient

ONE RESCUER	FUNCTIONS		TWO RESCUERS
	• Establish unresponsiveness • If no response, call 911 • Position patient • Open airway • Look, listen, and feel (for 3–5 seconds)		
	• Deliver two breaths (1½–2 sec each). If unsuccessful, reposition head and try again. Clear airway if necessary.		
	• Check carotid pulse . . . (5–10 seconds) If no pulse . . . • Begin chest compressions		
	DELIVER COMPRESSIONS		
	1½–2 inches 100/min (15/9–11 sec)	1½–2 inches 100/min (5/3–4 sec)	
	DELIVER VENTILATIONS **10–12 breaths/min**		
	15:2	5:1 (AHA *Guidelines 2000*: 15:2)	
	• Pause to allow ventilations		
	• Do four cycles • Ventilator checks pulse for effective CPR		
	CONTINUE PERIODIC ASSESSMENT		

Changing Positions

• Compressor—signal to change; finish compression cycle • Ventilator—one ventilation (AHA *Guidelines 2000:* two ventilations)	New ventilator checks pulse. If no pulse, says "No pulse, continue."	Continue CPR sequence

NOTE: Wear latex or vinyl gloves. Rescuers should have their own pocket face masks with one-way valves and HEPA filter inserts.

Remember and Consider...

✔ If you start CPR on a cardiac arrest patient in a public place, how do you work with someone who wants to help but is doing CPR incorrectly?

Do you feel that you could coach someone or give directions while you are performing CPR? Would you ventilate and tell the person how to do chest compressions, or would you do chest compressions and tell the person how to ventilate? Would it be better to send the person for help or to ask him or her to control the crowd while you perform one-rescuer CPR?

✔ Practice doing chest compressions while you coach a classmate or station member on ventilations. Switch your position and practice giving ventilations while you coach someone on doing chest compressions. Do you think this is effective? Can it work? Or do you think it is easier to just do it yourself? How long can you last? Have someone time you while you do CPR until you get tired. How long were you able to do CPR before you felt you were no longer effective?

Investigate...

Part of the learning experience and an effective quality assurance step is wanting to know if your emergency care delivery was correct.

✔ How do you find out if the CPR that you performed on a patient was effective? Does your department get follow-up information on patients that you cared for in the prehospital setting? If so, check the records for patient outcome information; if not, find out what you must do to get patient outcome information from the hospital.

You may find that your procedures were performed correctly, but the patient could not be resuscitated because of other medical or trauma conditions or circumstances. Knowing that you performed correctly is a positive reinforcement for your efforts. Finding out what you need to do to correct your performance is a learning experience.

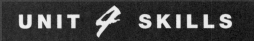
➤ **CHAPTER 8** CARDIOPULMONARY RESUSCITATION (CPR)
➤ **CHAPTER 9** TWO-RESCUER CPR

Study the following scenarios. Place check marks in the columns below as appropriate to indicate which skills you would perform for each scenario. You will use skills from previous units in these scenarios. Refer to text pages 1–81; 85–123; 129–178. Write the skill number of any skills you would use from Units 1, 2, and 3 after each scenario or in the columns under "Units." Discuss answers with other students and your instructor.

SCENARIO 1: You and your neighbor, a retired man of 69, have been shoveling snow for most of the morning. You are about finished when you notice the man leaning on his shovel with one fist to his chest. Suddenly he collapses. You run over, roll him to his back, and find he is not breathing and has no pulse.

(Skills from Unit 1: _____ Skills from Unit 2: _____)

(Skills from Unit 3: _____)

SCENARIO 2: Your rescue unit is first on the scene of an outdoor barbeque. The crowd of people part to let you approach a child who appears to be about five and whose face is bluish. The mother is hovering over him and is in tears, pleading with you to do something. Your initial assessment finds that the child is not breathing, but he still has a faint pulse. The mother tells you all the children were eating at another table when she noticed her boy struggling to get up, clutching his throat, and falling over.

(Skills from Unit 1: _____ Skills from Unit 2: _____)

(Skills from Unit 3: _____)

SCENARIO 3: You and a coworker are performing CPR and setting up the AED. The patient is a 50-year-old executive of the airline where you work as a security guard. His secretary said she found him on the floor when she went into his office to have him sign some papers. He had only been in the office about 10 minutes, and he looked ashen and distraught when he came in.

(Skills from Unit 1: _____ Skills from Unit 2: _____)

(Skills from Unit 3: _____)

Instructors will demonstrate all skills and will give you time to practice them while they coach you.

Skills	Scenarios			Units		
	#1	#2	#3	#1	#2	#3
Adult-single rescuer: Chapter 8, pp. 196–201, Scan 8-2						
1. Check response (Figure 8.10)						
2. Alert the EMS dispatcher (Figure 8.11)						
3. Properly position the patient and yourself (Figure 8.12)						
4. Open airway (Figure 8.13)						

Skills	Scenarios			Units		
	#1	**#2**	**#3**	**#1**	**#2**	**#3**
5. Determine breathlessness (Figure 8.14)						
6. Give two breaths with pocket face mask (Figure 8.15)						
7. Determine pulselessness (Figure 8.16)						
8. Locate compression site (Scan 8-1, Figures 8.5, 8.6, 8.7)						
9. Properly position hands (Figures 8.18, 8.19)						
10. Compress at 15:2 (Figure 8.20)						
11. Provide two breaths (Figure 8.21)						
12. Reassess pulse after one minute of CPR (Figure 8.22)						
Child: Chapter 8, pp. 199, 202–204						
13. Check response						
14. Properly position the patient						
15. Open airway						
16. Determine breathlessness						
17. Give two breaths with pocket face mask						
18. Determine pulselessness (carotid)						
19. Locate compression site (Figure 8.25B)						
20. Properly position heel of one hand (Figure 8.25B)						
21. Compress with the heel of one hand at 5:1						
22. Provide one breath						
23. Reassess pulse after one minute of CPR and alert dispatcher						
24. If no pulse, continue CPR until EMTs/ALS arrive						
Infant: Chapter 8, pp. 199, 202–204						
25. Check response						
26. Properly position the patient (Figure 8.23)						
27. Open airway (Figure 8.23)						
28. Determine breathlessness						
29. Give two breaths with pocket face mask						
30. Determine pulselessness (brachial)						
31. Locate compression site (Figure 8.25A)						
32. Properly position fingertips (Figure 8.25A)						
33. Compress with with two fingers, one finger below nipple line at 5:1						
34. Provide one breath						
35. Reassess pulse after one minute of CPR and alert dispatcher						
36. If no pulse, continue CPR until EMTs/ALS arrive						

Skills	Scenarios			Units		
	#1	**#2**	**#3**	**#1**	**#2**	**#3**
Neonatal: (practiced here for early learning reinforcement; reviewed in Unit 6, Chapter 14) Chapter 8, pp. 204–206						
37. Check response						
38. Properly position the patient (Figure 8.23)						
39. Open airway (Figure 8.23)						
40. Suction airway if necessary with bulb syringe						
41. Assess respiratory effort						
42. Provide blow-by oxygen if respiratory effort is poor/weak and skin is pale/bluish						
43. Assist respiratory effort with neonatal-sized bag-valve mask at 40 to 60 breaths per minute for 15 to 30 seconds						
44. Watch for chest to rise; no chest rise—reposition head and mask						
45. Check heart rate (apical site—over the sternum) or umbilical cord if newborn (at least 100 beats per minute and spontaneous respirations)						
46. Gradually discontinue assisted ventilations						
47. Continue assisted ventilations if breathing is still inadequate						
48. Continue assisted ventilations and chest compressions if heart rate is less than 60 or between 60 to 80 beats per minute						
49. Locate compression site (Figures 8.27, 8.28)						
50. Compress with two thumbs and hands circling chest or two fingers at 3:1 (Figures 8.27, 8.28)						
51. Assist ventilations with bag-valve mask and 100% oxygen						
52. Check pulse rate periodically; discontinue compressions when heart rate reaches 80 beats per minute						
Foreign body airway obstruction: Review Unit 2, Chapter 6, pp. 104–114						
53. Demonstrate obstructed airway adult—conscious						
54. Demonstrate obstructed airway adult—becomes unconscious						
55. Demonstrate obstructed airway adult—initially unconscious						
56. Demonstrate obstructed airway child—conscious to unconscious						
57. Demonstrate obstructed airway child—initially unconscious						

Skills	Scenarios			Units		
	#1	#2	#3	#1	#2	#3
58. Demonstrate obstructed airway infant—conscious to unconscious						
59. Demonstrate obstructed airway infant—initially unconscious						
Adult two-rescuer: Chapter 9, pp. 229–235, Scans 9-1, 9-2, 9-3						
Rescuer 1:						
60. Check response						
61. Alert the EMS dispatcher						
62. Properly position the patient and yourself						
63. Open airway						
64. Determine breathlessness						
65. Give two breaths with pocket face mask						
66. Determine pulselessness; report to partner						
Rescuer 2:						
67. Locate compression site						
68. Properly position hands						
69. Compress with heels of two hands at 5:1 (AHA *Guidelines 2000:* 15:2)						
Rescuer 1:						
70. Provide one breath (AHA *Guidelines 2000:* two breaths)						
71. Reassess pulse after one minute of CPR						
72. Check for breathing, give one breath with pocket face mask						
Both rescuers:						
73. Demonstrate a switch and continue CPR						
AED: Chapter 8, pp. 211–223, Scan 8-3						
74. Assess and determine patient is in cardiac arrest						
75. Partner begins CPR while second rescuer sets up AED						
76. Bares patient's chest, correctly places defibrillator pads						
77. Connects lead cables from AED to defibrillator pads						
78. Turn on AED and analyze patient						
79. Defibrillate patient, if indicated, three times						
80. Provide 1 minute of CPR						
81. Repeat three shocks if indicated						
82. Repeat sequence of CPR and shocks one more time if indicated						
83. Continue CPR and transport						

Work with a group of classmates to create scenarios that will use listed skills. Exchange scenarios with other class groups to check your knowledge and to practice your decision-making skills.

$\mathcal{M}$EDICAL EMERGENCIES

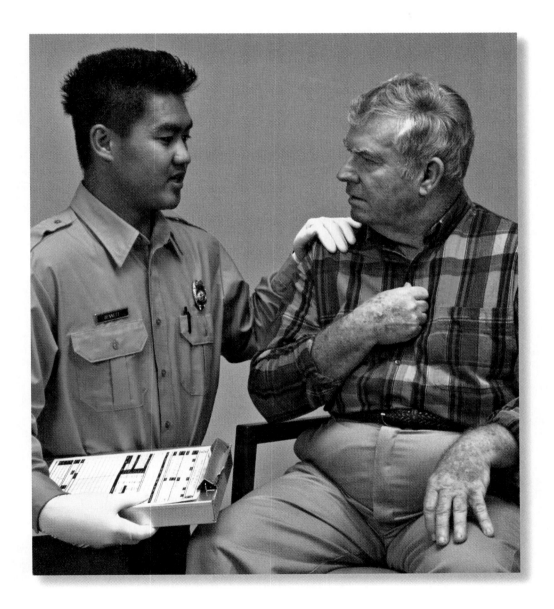

$\mathcal{A}$ wide variety of illnesses and conditions that can affect the body are known as medical emergencies. While some situations may require you to intervene with specific skills, other conditions will be referred to as a common medical complaint. You must be prepared to provide appropriate emergency medical care to the various medical patients that you may encounter.

National Standard Objectives

This chapter focuses on the objectives of Module 5, Lesson 5–1 of the U.S. DOT First Responder National Standard Curriculum and serves as an instructional aid to help you meet any specific objectives added to the course by your local EMS system.

By the end of this chapter, you will know how to (from cognitive or knowledge information) . . .

5–1.1	Identify the patient who presents with a general medical complaint. (pp. 244–245)
5–1.2	Explain the steps in providing emergency medical care to a patient with a general medical complaint. (p. 245)
5–1.3	Identify the patient who presents with a specific medical complaint of altered mental status. (pp. 256–262, 263)
5–1.4	Explain the steps in providing emergency medical care to a patient with an altered mental status. (pp. 257–262)
5–1.5	Identify the patient who presents with a specific medical complaint of seizures. (p. 259)
5–1.6	Explain the steps in providing emergency medical care to a patient with seizures. (pp. 259–260)
5–1.7	Identify the patient who presents with a specific medical complaint of exposure to cold. (pp. 280–283)
5–1.8	Explain the steps in providing emergency medical care to a patient with an exposure to cold. (pp. 280–283)
5–1.9	Identify the patient who presents with a specific medical complaint of exposure to heat. (pp. 276–280)
5–1.10	Explain the steps in providing emergency medical care to a patient with an exposure to heat. (pp. 277–280)
5–1.11	Identify the patient who presents with a specific medical complaint of behavioral change. (pp. 283–284)
5–1.12	Explain the steps in providing emergency medical care to a patient with a behavioral change. (pp. 284–286)
5–1.13	Identify the patient who presents with a specific medical complaint of psychological crisis. (pp. 283–284)
5–1.14	Explain the steps in providing emergency medical care to a patient with a psychological crisis. (pp. 284–286)

Feel comfortable enough to (by changing attitudes, values, and beliefs) . . .

5–1.15	Attend to the feelings of the patient and/or family when dealing with the patient with a general medical complaint. (pp. 244–245)
5–1.16	Attend to the feelings of the patient and/or family when dealing with the patient with a specific medical complaint. (pp. 247, 249, 257, 258, 259, 265, 281)
5–1.17	Explain the rationale for modifying your behavior toward the patient with a behavioral emergency. (pp. 283, 284, 285)

5–1.18	Demonstrate a caring attitude towards patients with a general medical complaint who request emergency medical services. (pp. 244–245)
5–1.19	Place the interests of the patient with a general medical complaint as the foremost consideration when making any and all patient-care decisions. (pp. 244–245)
5–1.20	Communicate with empathy to patients with a general medical complaint, as well as with family members and friends of the patient. (pp. 244–245)
5–1.21	Demonstrate a caring attitude towards patients with a specific medical complaint who request emergency medical services. (pp. 249, 257, 259, 265, 281)
5–1.22	Place the interests of the patient with a specific medical complaint as the foremost consideration when making any and all patient-care decisions. (pp. 249, 257, 259, 265, 281)
5–1.23	Communicate with empathy to patients with a specific medical complaint, as well as with family members and friends of the patient. (pp. 249, 257, 259, 265, 281)
5–1.24	Demonstrate a caring attitude towards patients with a behavior problem who request emergency medical services. (pp. 283, 284, 285)
5–1.25	Place the interests of the patient with a behavioral problem as the foremost consideration when making any and all patient-care decisions. (pp. 283, 284, 285)
5–1.26	Communicate with empathy to patients with a behavioral problem, as well as with family members and friends of the patient. (pp. 283, 284, 285)

Show how to (through psychomotor skills) . . .	5–1.27	Demonstrate the steps in providing emergency medical care to a patient with a general medical complaint. (p. 245)
	5–1.28	Demonstrate the steps in providing emergency medical care to a patient with an altered mental status. (pp. 257, 258, 259–261, 262)
	5–1.29	Demonstrate the steps in providing emergency medical care to a patient with seizures. (pp. 259–260)
	5–1.30	Demonstrate the steps in providing emergency medical care to a patient with an exposure to cold. (pp. 280–283)
	5–1.31	Demonstrate the steps in providing emergency medical care to a patient with an exposure to heat. (pp. 277, 278, 279–280)
	5–1.32	Demonstrate the steps in providing emergency medical care to a patient with a behavioral change. (pp. 284, 286)
	5–1.33	Demonstrate the steps in providing emergency medical care to a patient with a psychological crisis. (pp. 284, 286)

LEARNING TASKS

This chapter gives an overview of medical emergencies and tells how to provide care for specific complaints. In addition to the previously stated objectives, you will need to understand the importance of performing an initial assessment on these patients and identifying any life-threatening conditions. As you work through this chapter, you will also need to know:

✔ The signs and symptoms of a heart attack and the care for patients with chest pain, including those with congestive heart failure.

✔ The signs and symptoms of respiratory difficulty and the care for these patients, including patients who appear to be hyperventilating.

✔ Conditions associated with abdominal pain, including signs and symptoms, causes, and emergency care.

✔ The signs and symptoms of poisonings, bites, and stings, including types and emergency care.

✔ The signs and symptoms of alcohol and drug abuse and the care for patients who appear to be affected by them.

MEDICAL EMERGENCIES

Patients may request emergency services for a variety of medical complaints or emergencies. Medical conditions or illnesses may be caused by infections, poisons, or the failure of one or more of the body's organs and systems.

Medical emergencies may be hidden because of an accident or injury. For example, a diabetic patient may collapse because of very low blood sugar or have a car wreck and be injured by the trauma. As a First Responder, you will have to provide care for the patient's injuries. The medical problem, however, should not go unnoticed. Proper physical assessment and history-taking of the patient should indicate that there is also a medical emergency. The patient might have a medical information emblem (Medic Alert) that could provide information on his condition. The emblem may be worn as a bracelet on the wrist or attached to a watchband; it can be worn on a chain around the patient's neck. Some patients may be taking medications that help their medical problem. In some jurisdictions, First Responders may assist patients in taking certain medications. Check your protocols and always call for medical direction before assisting a patient with medications (see Appendix 3).

Remember, thousands of diseases and conditions have been detected worldwide. There is no way that you, as a First Responder, can be familiar with all or even most of them. In this text, we will discuss the most common medical emergencies and how to deal with a patient with an unknown, general medical complaint. You should assess each patient and determine the chief complaint as well as signs and symptoms present. The patient or bystander may be able to tell you of a known disease or condition. However, in most cases, what you observe and what the patient describes will be your only clues.

> **REMEMBER:**
>
> Part of the patient assessment is to look for medical identification devices.

SIGNS AND SYMPTOMS

Signs are what you observe during an assessment, such as observing that a patient is sweating or pale. **Symptoms** are what the patient tells you about his condition. For example, the patient says, "I am having chest pain." This information is gained during the initial and focused assessments. Review the details of this information in Chapter 7.

To detect a medical emergency, you will have to be aware of the common *signs* of a medical emergency such as unusual:

- Levels of awareness or consciousness
- Pulse rate and character—Pulse rate above 120 or below 50 beats per minute indicates a true emergency for an adult patient.
- Breathing rate and character—Breathing rate less than 8 or greater than 24 breaths per minute may indicate a true emergency for an adult patient.
- Skin temperature, condition, and color; color of the lips
- Pupil size and response
- Breath odors
- Abdominal tenderness or rigidity
- Muscular activities such as spasms and paralysis
- Bleeding or discharges from the body

A patient may complain of some of the following *symptoms*:

- Pain
- A "temperature" or fever, or chills
- An upset stomach and/or vomiting
- Dizziness or feeling faint
- Shortness of breath
- Feelings of pressure or weight on the chest or abdomen
- Unusual bowel or bladder activity
- Thirst, hunger, or odd tastes in the mouth
- Burning sensations

ASSESSMENT

Remember, emergency care for medical emergencies is based on the patient's signs and symptoms. That is why it is so important to complete an appropriate patient assessment. For general medical complaints, you should:

1. Complete a scene size-up before initiating emergency medical care.
2. Complete an initial assessment on all patients.
3. Complete a physical exam as needed.
4. Complete ongoing assessments (as appropriate).
5. Comfort and reassure the patient while awaiting additional EMS resources.

 When assessing the patient, remember:

- If the patient appears or feels unusual in any way, assume that there is a medical emergency.
- If the patient has atypical (unusual) vital signs, assume that there is a medical emergency.

Consider all patient complaints to be valid. If the patient is not feeling normal in any way, assume there is a medical emergency.

Note

If you are a First Responder who determines blood pressure, realize that blood pressure is a vital sign and a diagnostic tool. Remember that a systolic pressure greater than 140 mmHg or a diastolic pressure above 90 mmHg indicates a high blood pressure reading. If you detect a low or a falling blood pressure, assume the patient is developing shock.

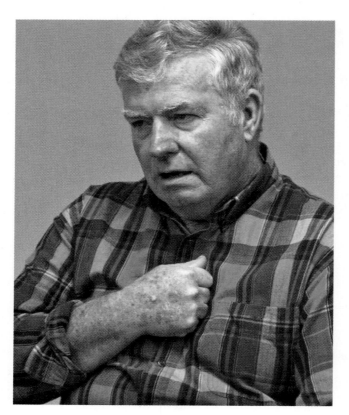

FIGURE 10.1
Chest pain is the primary sign of a heart attack.

SPECIFIC MEDICAL EMERGENCIES

CHEST PAIN AND POSSIBLE HEART ATTACKS

Chest pain is a common medical complaint. There are many conditions that can cause chest pain and give the appearance of being a heart attack. Indigestion, stress, and anxiety can all cause chest pain and other symptoms that may be similar to a heart attack. As a First Responder, you will not be able to tell the difference. Instead, if a patient is having chest pain, you must assume that he or she is having, or is about to have, a heart attack and provide care accordingly (Figure 10.1).

Heart attacks and other problems with the heart are often described using many technical terms, such as *angina pectoris*, *coronary occlusion*, and *acute myocardial infarction* (AMI). You do not need to know these terms. Being able to tell one condition from another requires advanced medical training. Simply realize that the heart is a muscle with its own blood vessels. Any damage to the muscle or to the vessels can prevent the heart muscle from getting enough oxygen and lead to a heart attack. This is a serious condition. You, as a First Responder, must treat all chest pain as a possible heart attack.

First | Whenever you suspect that a patient is having, or is about to have, a heart attack, alert the EMS dispatcher. Report the signs and symptoms gathered. It may be possible for the dispatcher to send an ALS unit.

Signs and Symptoms

First | The following are common signs and symptoms of a heart attack (Scan 10-1):

■ Early symptoms generally include chest or upper abdominal sensations of pressure or burning and are often mistaken for indigestion.

heart attack a general term used to indicate a failure of circulation to the heart muscle that damages or kills a portion of the heart.

Chest Pain and Possible Heart Attack

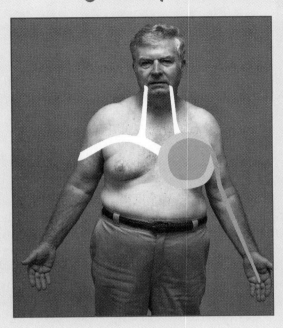

Signs and Symptoms

- Early symptoms generally include chest or upper abdominal sensation of pressure or burning, and are often mistaken for indigestion.
- As an attack worsens, pain may localize behind sternum and radiate to either arm or shoulder (usually the left). Pain may extend to:
  - hand
  - neck, jaws, and teeth
  - upper back
  - upper, middle abdomen
  Some patients have pain only in the jaw, neck, or arm.

Chest pain may be accompanied by other symptoms that suggest a heart attack, including:

- Shortness of breath
- Nausea
- Sweating

Pain may diminish when physical exertion or emotional stress ends or when the patient takes nitroglycerin.

Additional signs may include:

- An increased pulse rate; irregular pulse
- A low (shock-level) blood pressure (usually a result of repeated doses of nitroglycerin, which dilates blood vessels)

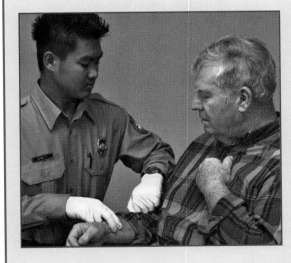

Emergency Care

- Make certain EMS dispatcher has been alerted.
- Provide emotional support; reassure and calm the patient.
- Keep the patient at rest. Do not allow the patient to move himself.
- Place the patient in a comfortable position.
- Assure an open airway and adequate breathing.
- Cover to conserve body heat, but do not overheat.
- Ask if patient took nitroglycerin, when, how much, and over what period of time (see Appendix 3).
- Contact medical facility and let them know:
  - You have a patient with chest pain
  - Patient's history
  - If and when the patient took nitroglycerin
- If local protocols permit, assist patient with prescribed dose of medication. Consult medical direction.
- Do not leave the patient unattended.
- Monitor vital signs.

Note

If you are a First Responder who is trained to administer oxygen (see Appendix 2), follow your EMS system's protocol for chest pain victims. Sometimes the patient's pain will decrease once supplemental oxygen is provided. If this occurs, it does not mean that the patient's problem has grown any less serious.

■ As an attack worsens, pain may localize behind the sternum and may radiate to either of the arms or shoulders (usually the left). In some cases, the pain may extend to:

– The hand
– The neck, jaws, and teeth
– The upper back
– The upper abdomen

The pain may not originate under the sternum. For example, some patients have pain only in the jaw, neck, or arm.

First | Many times, the chest pain is associated with other symptoms, and these are also suggestive of a heart attack in progress. These include:

■ Shortness of breath
■ Nausea
■ Sweating

The pain of a heart attack may diminish when physical exertion or emotional stress ends or when the patient takes nitroglycerin. Additional signs may include an increased pulse rate and an irregular pulse as well (for example, premature ventricular contractions). Patients who have taken repeated doses of nitroglycerin may have low blood pressure as a result of blood vessel dilation.

Sometimes patients who are having a heart attack will deny that they are having one. They will frequently appear frightened and anxious. If there are other signs of a heart attack, or if bystanders report that the patient complained of pain or other discomfort in the areas described above, provide care for a heart attack.

Emergency Care

If the patient is in cardiac arrest (no pulse and not breathing), have someone notify dispatch and perform CPR. Otherwise, complete the assessment as required, carefully noting the patient's vital signs. If the patient is unconscious when you arrive, gain what information you can from bystanders. If no one saw the patient prior to the loss of consciousness, suspect that the patient may have had a heart attack.

First | Upon gathering signs and symptoms indicating a heart attack or the possibility of a heart attack, you should (Scan 10-1):

1. Perform a scene size-up, including scene safety and BSI.

*A*SSESSMENT OF CHEST PAIN

Chest pain → Symptoms progress → YES → Typically pain extending to arm, jaw, sweating → Possible heart attack in progress

Symptoms progress → NO → On-going assessment

Cardiac signs and symptoms begin to develop

Patient becomes unstable

2. Make certain that the EMS system dispatcher has been alerted. Stay with the patient and monitor his condition.

3. Provide emotional support and reassure the patient.

4. Keep the patient at rest. If possible, provide oxygen per local protocols.

5. Place the patient into a comfortable position. You should do all the work for the patient. This position should be one that allows for easiest breathing. Many patients with the signs and symptoms of a heart attack are most comfortable in a semi-sitting position. Assure an open airway and adequate breathing. If the patient is also an accident victim, do not cause additional problems through incorrect or inappropriate repositioning.

6. Loosen any restrictive clothing as needed for taking vital signs.

7. Cover the patient to prevent chill, but do not overheat the patient.

8. Contact medical facility and let them know:
   – You have a patient with chest pain
   – Patient's history
   – If and when nitroglycerin was taken

9. Assist the patient with the prescribed dose of medication (nitroglycerin) if your protocols permit. Consult medical direction.

10. Do not leave the patient unattended.

11. Continue to monitor vital signs.

First Remember, conducting yourself in a calm, professional manner when treating any type of patient is very important. It is of particular importance in treating patients with chest pain who can be very anxious, restless, or in denial. Their chances for survival may be increased if they can be calmed and rested.

A patient may ask if he or she is having a heart attack. It is best to respond by saying, "Your pain could be a lot of things, but let's not take chances." Do all you can to keep the patient calm and still. Do *not* argue with patients and do not try to physically restrain them. The stress caused by such efforts could be very harmful. Remain calm and talk to your patient, keeping eye contact whenever possible. Let the patient know that resting is an important part of his or her care.

Continue to comfort the patient as long as you provide care. Reassure the patient that highly trained help is on the way. Tell the patient that you are a trained First Responder and that you will be there until further help arrives.

CHEST PAIN CARE

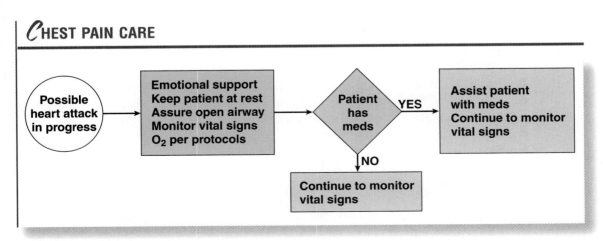

Medications

Normally, First Responders do not administer medications. However, some patients with a history of heart problems have been given medications by their physicians to take when having chest pain. Always ask if a physician has given the patient any medications for the current problem. If medications have been prescribed, then assist the patient in taking them if your local protocols allow (see Appendix 3).

Patients who suffer from **angina pectoris** will usually have nitroglycerin tablets to take when having chest pain. This chest pain indicates that the heart muscle needs more oxygen. Placing a nitroglycerin tablet under the patient's tongue will allow the drug to rapidly enter the bloodstream. Nitroglycerin improves the circulation of blood to the heart muscle. It also reduces the workload of the heart. In doing so, the patient's blood pressure may be lowered. This can cause the patient to become dizzy or lightheaded. Patients receiving nitroglycerin should be sitting or lying down to avoid fainting.

First | Assume a heart attack is in progress and treat as previously described. Help all patients with the signs and symptoms of a heart attack to take their own medications if they have been prescribed by a doctor and you are allowed to do so (unless they have taken the prescribed limit prior to your arrival). Continue to monitor the patient and provide care, even if the pain stops. Do *not* cancel your request for an EMT or more advanced EMS response.

CONGESTIVE HEART FAILURE (CHF)

A medical emergency you might encounter that affects both the lungs and the heart is known as **congestive heart failure.** While often confused with a heart attack or cardiac arrest, it is actually a condition in which the heart cannot pump blood properly. This may be because of problems primarily affecting the lungs or the heart. In either case, fluid builds up in the lungs, leading to respiratory difficulty. In addition to the lungs, fluid can also build up in the feet, ankles, legs, and abdomen. Patients will complain of swelling associated with this fluid buildup.

Signs and Symptoms

First | The signs and symptoms of congestive heart failure include (Figure 10.2):

- Shortness of breath. Breathing will be labored, often rapid and shallow. Unusual breathing sounds may be heard. The rate of breathing can be greater than 30 breaths per minute. This is a true emergency. Patients in this degree of congestive heart failure are frequently very anxious, sweaty, and their blood pressures tend to be very high. These patients may sit upright in a tripod position.
- Rapid pulse rate. The rate can be greater than 120 beats per minute.
- Swelling of the feet, ankles, legs, and/or abdomen. (By themselves, these symptoms are seldom an emergency.)
- Neck veins may appear engorged.
- Skin, lips, and nail beds may turn blue.
- Patients may act confused if they are not getting enough oxygen.

Emergency Care

First | The emergency care for a patient in congestive heart failure is the same as for most patients in respiratory distress (see page 253).

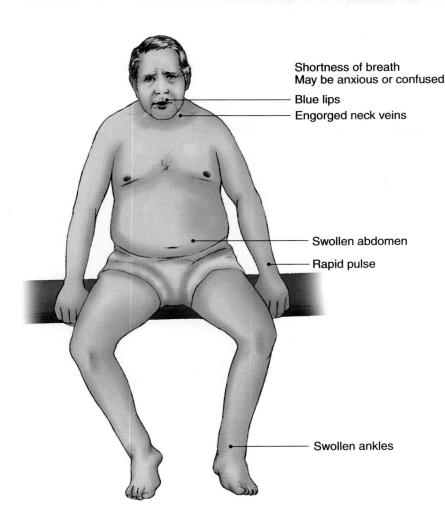

Shortness of breath
May be anxious or confused
Blue lips
Engorged neck veins

Swollen abdomen
Rapid pulse

Swollen ankles

Maintain an open airway. Make certain that someone alerts the EMS dispatcher and requests ALS services if available. Position the patient to provide the greatest ease when breathing. The patient will usually want to remain upright. This should be encouraged. If the patient is alert, he should be assisted to a sitting position with feet off the bed or chair and on the floor. Administer high-flow oxygen by nonrebreather mask if allowed to do so. Keep the patient covered to conserve body heat, but do not overheat. Reassure the patient and calm him or her if possible.

RESPIRATORY EMERGENCIES

Many conditions may cause people to experience difficulty in breathing, or shortness of breath (Scan 10-2). A patient may be unable to stop breathing too rapidly (hyperventilation); muscle spasms may cause narrowing of the airways (asthma), or there may be a disease or condition such as emphysema, bronchitis, or pneumonia. The difficulty in breathing may stem from being exposed to a poison or something to which the patient is allergic. Regardless of the cause or condition, a patient's breathing can be considered *adequate* or *inadequate*.

Adequate breathing is breathing that is sufficient to support life. Breathing should be easy and effortless; patients should not have to work hard to breathe. Patients should be able to speak full sentences without having to catch their breath. Adequate breathing is characterized by a "normal" respiratory *rate*, *rhythm*, and *quality*.

Respiratory Disorders

RESPIRATORY DIFFICULTY

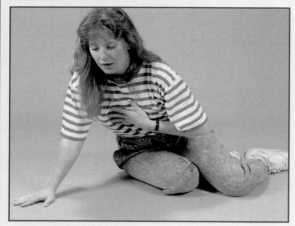

CHRONIC OBSTRUCTIVE PULMONARY DISEASE (COPD)

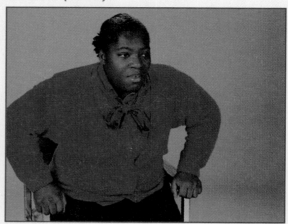

Symptoms and Signs

- Difficult breathing
- Shortness of breath
- Temporary cessation of breathing
- Rapid deep breathing
- Noisy breathing
- Dizziness, faintness, or unconsciousness
- Restlessness, anxiety, or confusion
- Strained muscles: face, neck, chest, abdomen
- Stabbing chest pains
- Numbness or tingling in limbs (hands or feet)
- Pursed lips or mouth open wide to aid breathing
- Blue skin color (cyanosis)

Emergency Care

1. Stay with the patient. Have someone call EMS dispatch.
2. Ensure an open airway. Check for airway obstructions.
3. Check to see if the patient is allergic to anything at scene. (Remove substance or move patient.)
4. Keep patient at rest. Conscious patient may desire to sit upright.
5. Cover to conserve body heat.
6. Monitor patient and provide emotional support.
7. Administer oxygen per local protocols.
8. Assist with inhaler per local protocols and medical direction (see Appendix 3).

Symptoms and Signs

Usually the patient will have emphysema or chronic bronchitis.

- History of respiratory problems or allergies
- Cough
- Shortness of breath
- Tightness in chest
- Swelling in lower extremities (advanced cases)
- Rapid pulse (some cases)
- Barrel chest (some cases)
- Dizziness (some cases)
- Blue discoloration (cyanosis)
- Desire to sit upright at all times. May use hands or elbows to push up on chair arms.

Emergency Care

Provide the same care as you would for respiratory distress. Be certain not to overheat the patient. Do what you can to reduce stress. If appropriate, encourage coughing.

WARNING: If you are allowed to provide oxygen, follow local guidelines for the COPD patient.

NOTE: Refer to local protocols for care. Some EMS systems recommend administration of oxygen. Others recommend only care that consists of calming and reassuring the patient.

Respiratory **rate** is the number of breaths per minute.

- Normal respiratory rate for the adult—12 to 20
- Normal respiratory rate for the child—15 to 30
- Normal respiratory rate for the infant—25 to 50

The **rhythm** of breathing is the pattern of the respirations.

- The respiratory rhythm should be regular. Breaths should be taken at regular intervals and last the same amount of time. Exhaling (breathing out) should take about twice as long as inhaling (breathing in).

The **quality** of breathing is how well the patient is breathing.

- Both sides of the chest should rise and fall equally. The depth of respirations should be adequate, and the breathing should be quiet without added sounds (for example, wheezes or stridor).

Inadequate breathing is breathing that is *not* sufficient to support life. Left untreated, such a condition will eventually result in death. In these patients, you may see the following:

- A rate that is faster or slower than the normal respiratory rate.
- An irregular breathing rhythm, or pattern.
- Decreased quality of respirations, such as diminished volume of air taken in and exhaled with each breath, or abnormal breath sounds, such as wheezes.

Breathing difficulty is a common medical complaint and represents a patient's feeling of difficult or labored breathing. The breathing may be either adequate or inadequate when a patient experiences difficulty breathing. Respiratory difficulty may be caused by a variety of conditions ranging from ongoing medical problems, such as asthma, to sudden illnesses, such as pulmonary embolism. Always listen to what a patient tells you about how he or she perceives the problem before attempting to make a determination of a patient's condition. The patient may have special medication, which is inhaled and helps certain respiratory conditions. A patient who has an inhaler will want to take the medication but may be too upset or frightened to use it properly. Some jurisdictions allow First Responders to help patients use this kind of medication. Check local protocols and always call for medical direction before assisting a patient with medications.

Signs and Symptoms

First | For most cases of respiratory difficulty or **respiratory distress,** any or all of the following signs and symptoms may be noticed (Figure 10.3):

- Labored or difficult breathing; a feeling of suffocation
- Unusual breathing sounds
- Rapid or slowed rate of breathing
- Unusual pulse rate and character
- Changes in the color of the lips, skin, and nail beds—usually, the color will change to blue or gray.
- Confusion, hallucinations, or the patient feels that people want to hurt him. This is sometimes seen in advanced cases.

respiratory distress any difficulty in breathing. Sometimes the problem is severe enough to require emergency care. Once distress begins, it is difficult to predict the short-term course of the problem.

Emergency Care

First | When caring for most cases of respiratory difficulty, you should:

1. Perform scene size-up, including scene safety and BSI.
2. Have someone call the EMS system dispatcher. Arrange for ALS response

FIGURE 10.3

The signs and symptoms of respiratory distress.

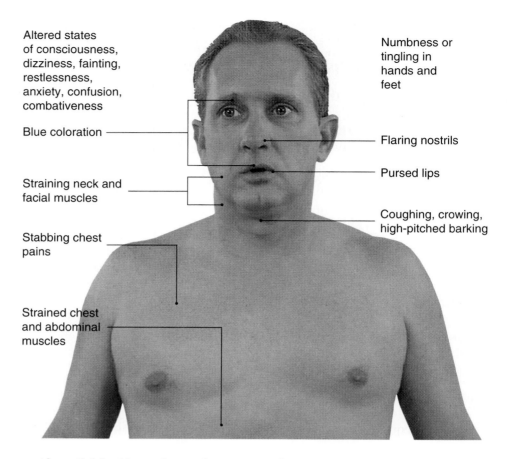

Altered states of consciousness, dizziness, fainting, restlessness, anxiety, confusion, combativeness

Blue coloration

Straining neck and facial muscles

Stabbing chest pains

Strained chest and abdominal muscles

Numbness or tingling in hands and feet

Flaring nostrils

Pursed lips

Coughing, crowing, high-pitched barking

if available. Never leave the patient alone, since respiratory arrest might develop.

3. Maintain an open airway.
4. Make certain that the problem is not caused by an airway obstruction.
5. Make certain that the patient is not allergic to substances at the scene. If this is the case, move the substance or move the patient.
6. Keep the patient at rest.
7. Place the conscious patient in a sitting position, allowing for proper drainage from the mouth. It often helps if the patient can support himself by the forearms when in a sitting position. This eases the patient's efforts in expanding the chest.

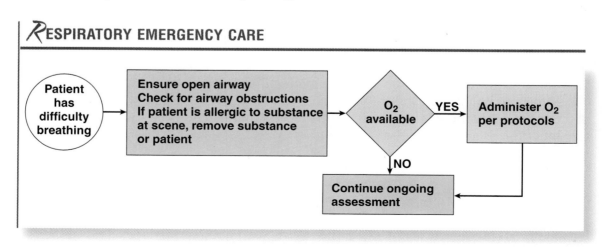

RESPIRATORY EMERGENCY CARE

Patient has difficulty breathing → Ensure open airway / Check for airway obstructions / If patient is allergic to substance at scene, remove substance or patient → O₂ available — YES → Administer O₂ per protocols

O₂ available — NO → Continue ongoing assessment

8. Provide oxygen if allowed to do so; assist with prescribed medication per local protocols and medical direction (see Appendix 3); obtain vital signs.

9. Cover the patient to conserve body heat, but do not allow the patient to overheat.

10. Provide emotional support.

11. Continue to monitor the patient

Hyperventilation

Breathing that is too rapid and too deep is known as **hyperventilation.** Most of the time, it stems from fear or stress, which may cause the patient to appear anxious and frightened. Patients experiencing hyperventilation are receiving an adequate supply of oxygen but not getting rid of enough carbon dioxide. This could lead to numbness and tingling of the lips, arms, and fingers.

First | Since most cases of hyperventilation are related to conditions of anxiety, your priority in treating these patients is to reduce anxiety by reassuring and comforting them. Encourage patients to take slow, deep breaths to slow down their breathing rate. Check with medical direction.

First | **WARNING:** Hyperventilation can be a sign of possible respiratory distress, impending heart attack, or a more serious medical condition. It will be difficult to determine if the condition is related merely to anxiety. Alert the EMS system dispatcher and provide care for respiratory distress. Be alert for cyanosis or other signs and symptoms of inadequate breathing. Monitor vital signs and be prepared in case the patient has a heart attack or respiratory arrest.

Stay alert for the signs of a possible heart attack and changes in vital signs, which may indicate medical problems that are more serious than simple hyperventilation. Do not rule out impending heart attack, poisoning, or other serious medical problems.

Chronic Obstructive Pulmonary Disease (COPD)

A variety of respiratory conditions can be classified as a **chronic obstructive pulmonary disease (COPD).** These include emphysema and chronic bronchitis. Other conditions, such as black lung disease, produce features similar to emphysema and chronic bronchitis. Usually the patient is middle-aged or older, but COPD can occur in children and teenagers.

First | ***Signs and Symptoms*** The signs and symptoms of COPD may include:

■ A history of heavy cigarette smoking, respiratory problems, or allergies
■ A persistent cough
■ Shortness of breath. Sometimes the patient breathes through pursed lips and tries to ease breathing effort by sitting forward and leaning on hands or elbows (tripod position).
■ Weakness or fatigue
■ Tightness in the chest
■ Periods of dizziness (in a few cases)
■ Wheezing

In advanced cases, there may be:
■ Irritability and agitation or lethargy and sleepiness
■ Rapid pulse, sometimes irregular
■ Barrel-chest appearance

hyperventilation uncontrolled rapid, deep breathing that is usually self-correcting. This may occur by itself or as a sign of a more serious problem.

chronic obstructive pulmonary disease (COPD) a variety of lung problems related to disease of the airway passages or exchange levels. The patient will suffer difficulties in breathing.

- Strong desire to remain sitting, even when asleep
- Blue discoloration of the skin, lips, and nail beds

This condition can be very difficult to distinguish from congestive heart failure. For First Responders, this is less important because both conditions are treated similarly by EMS responders at this level.

First **Emergency Care** When caring for COPD patients, you should:

1. Perform scene size-up, including scene safety and BSI.
2. Ensure an open airway, making certain that the problem is not because of obstruction by the tongue or some form of mechanical obstruction.
3. Have someone alert the EMS system dispatcher and report the problem as a possible COPD patient who is in distress.
4. Help the patient into a position to ease respirations.
5. Provide emotional support for the patient.
6. Monitor vital signs.
7. Administer oxygen if permitted and assist with medications if permitted.
8. Loosen any clothing to allow vital sign monitoring.
9. Cover the patient to conserve body heat, but do not overheat the patient.

Note

If you are a First Responder who may administer oxygen, monitor COPD patients carefully. The amount you will administer may have to be adjusted by medical direction.

REMEMBER:

Do not withhold oxygen from a patient with inadequate breathing or respiratory distress, including COPD patients.

ALTERED MENTAL STATUS

Several conditions may cause a patient to experience an altered mental status, or altered level of consciousness. This would be characterized by the patient's alertness and responsiveness to her surroundings. Signs and symptoms such as dizziness or hearing loss may not always indicate altered mental status. An altered mental status may be caused by seizures, strokes, diabetic emergencies, poisonings, breathing problems, and cardiac events.

Regardless of the underlying cause, you will need to look for ways to decide on the appropriate care procedures by observing and questioning to detect altered mental status. To start this process, you will need to know and understand the "normal" mental status. The memory aid AVPU (Alert, Verbal, Painful, Unresponsive) is used to categorize a patient's level of consciousness (Table 10-1).

TABLE 10-1: AVPU

A	Alert	Patient is awake and aware of his surroundings. Often, it is stated that a patient is Alert and Oriented times three (A & O x 3), which means the patient is alert and oriented . . . ×1 to person. He can tell you his name. ×2 to place. He can tell you where he is. ×3 to time. He can tell you what time it is.
V	Verbal	Patient responds only to verbal stimuli (yelling or raised voice).
P	Painful	Patient responds only to painful stimuli (sternal rub).
U	Unresponsive	Patient is not responsive to any stimuli (unresponsive).

Stroke

One potentially serious cause of altered level of consciousness is a **stroke,** or cerebrovascular accident (CVA). Such a condition occurs when blood to the brain is obstructed or if the vessel ruptures. During a stroke, an inadequate supply of oxygen is being supplied to a portion of the brain and damage occurs. In some cases, this damage is so great that it may lead to death (Scan 10-3).

stroke the blocking or bursting of a vessel that supplies blood to the brain. A portion of the brain is damaged or killed by this event. Also known as cerebrovascular (SER-e-bro-VAS-cu-ler) accident (CVA).

 Signs and Symptoms There are many signs and symptoms for stroke, including:

- Headache. This may be the only symptom at first.
- Collapse
- Altered levels of consciousness
- Numbness or paralysis—usually to the extremities and/or to the face
- Difficulty with speech or vision
- Confusion/dizziness
- Seizures
- Altered breathing patterns
- Unequal pupils
- Loss of bowel and bladder control
- May have a history of hypertension

RULE: If a patient has any of the signs or symptoms of a stroke, including nothing more than a headache, assume that the patient may be having, or is about to have, a stroke. Remember, the risk of having a stroke increases with age.

 Emergency Care When caring for a possible stroke patient, you should:

1. Perform scene size-up, including scene safety and BSI.
2. Maintain an open airway. Be prepared to provide rescue breathing or CPR if needed.
3. Make sure someone alerts the EMS dispatcher.
4. Keep the patient at rest.
5. Protect all paralyzed parts.
6. Provide emotional support. Be certain to make an effort to understand everything that the patient says. Remember, the speech centers of the brain may be affected.
7. Position the patient to allow for drainage from the patient's mouth by placing the patient into the recovery position. *Do not* place a possible stroke patient in a head down position (Scan 10-3, bottom).
8. Do not allow the patient to become overheated.
9. Do not administer anything by mouth.
10. Continue to monitor the patient. Shock, respiratory arrest, or cardiac arrest is possible.
11. Administer oxygen per local protocols.

Seizures

Irregular electrical activity in the brain that can cause a sudden change in behavior or movement is called a **seizure.** The most common form of seizure seen by the First Responder involves uncontrolled muscular movements known as *convulsions*. These are known as *grand mal*, or generalized, seizures. Other seizures characterized by a temporary loss of concentration without dramatic body movements are known as *petit mal*, or partial complex, seizures.

seizure in general, any event in the brain that causes uncontrolled muscle contractions (convulsions).

Altered Mental Status—Stroke: Cerebrovascular Accident

CAUSES OF CEREBROVASCULAR ACCIDENTS: STROKE

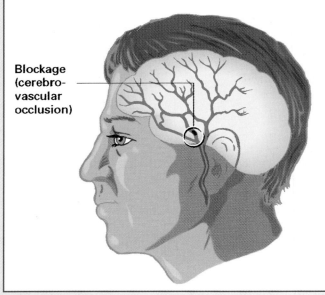

Blockage (cerebro-vascular occlusion)

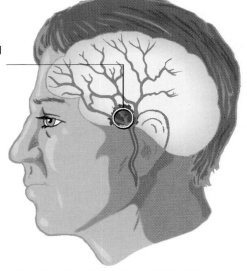

Diseased artery ruptures

Cerebral Thrombosis (Clot): Blockage in arteries supplying oxygenated blood will result in damage to affected parts of the brain.

Signs and Symptoms of Stroke
- Headache
- Confusion and/or dizziness
- Loss of function or paralysis of extremities (usually on one side of the body)
- Numbness (usually limited to one side of the body)
- Collapse
- Facial flaccidity and loss of expression (often to one side of the face)
- Impaired speech
- Unequal pupil size
- Impaired vision
- Rapid, full pulse
- Irregular respiration, snoring
- Nausea
- Convulsions
- Coma
- Loss of bladder and bowel control
- May have history of hypertension

Cerebral Hemorrhage (Rupture): An aneurysm or other weakened area of an artery ruptures. This has two effects:
- An area of the brain is deprived of oxygenated blood.
- Pooling blood puts increased pressure on the brain, displacing tissue and interfering with function. Cerebral hemorrhage is often associated with arteriosclerosis and hypertension.

Emergency Care of Stroke Patients
- Ensure an open airway.
- Keep the patient calm.
- Monitor vital signs.
- Give nothing by mouth.
- Provide care for shock.
- Place the patient into the recovery position.
- Administer oxygen per local protocols.

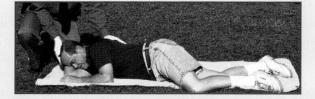

Seizures can be very frightening for a patient's family, friends, and others to witness. Even though most seizures do not last longer than a minute, it can seem like a much longer period to bystanders. Talk to witnesses to determine what the patient was doing prior to the seizure and if this has happened in the past. While some people have seizures on a regular basis, the patient should still be evaluated by someone with advanced medical training.

A seizure is not a disease, but a sign of an underlying condition. Some of the causes of seizures are:

- Drugs, alcohol, or poisons
- Brain tumors
- Infections, high fever
- Diabetic problems
- Trauma
- Stroke
- Heat stroke
- Epilepsy
- Unknown

Note

Tonic-clonic, or grand mal, seizures *usually* only last a *few minutes* and consist of dramatic body movements.

Absence (petit mal) seizures *usually* only last *10–30 seconds*, and there are no dramatic body movements.

First | **Signs and Symptoms** In cases of severe seizures, such as the grand mal seizure, any or all of the following may be present:

- Sudden loss of consciousness with the patient falling to the ground.
- The patient may report a bright light, bright colors, or the sensation of a strong odor prior to losing consciousness.
- The patient's body will stiffen.
- Sometimes the patient will temporarily stop breathing and lose bladder and bowel control.
- The patient will go into convulsions, jerking all parts of the body. Breathing will be labored, and there may be frothing at the mouth.
- After convulsions, the patient's body completely relaxes.
- The patient becomes conscious, but is very tired and confused.
- The patient may complain of a headache.

First | **Emergency Care** The basic emergency care for seizures producing convulsions is to:

1. Perform scene size-up, including scene safety and BSI.

2. Place the patient on the floor or the ground. Do *not* force anything into the patient's mouth.

3. Loosen restrictive clothing.

4. Do not try to hold the patient still during the convulsions. Your primary job as a First Responder is to protect the patient from injury (Figure 10.4). Keep the patient from striking any nearby objects.

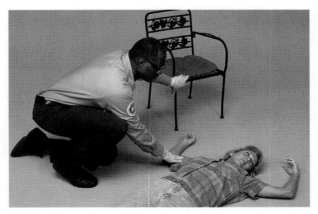

FIGURE 10.4
During a seizure, protect the patient from injury.

glucose (GLU-kohs) a simple sugar that is the primary source of energy for the body's tissues.

insulin (IN-su-lin) a hormone produced in the pancreas that is needed to move sugar (glucose) from the blood into the cells.

diabetes usually refers to **diabetes mellitus.** This is the condition in which there is a decrease or absence of insulin produced by the pancreas or the body does not respond appropriately to insulin. The glucose level of the blood will increase and the movement of this sugar into the cells will decrease as the insulin level falls.

hyperglycemia the sugar (glucose) level increases in the blood and decreases in the tissue cells. The problem can be serious enough to produce a coma.

5. After convulsions have passed, keep the patient at rest, with the head positioned to allow for drainage in case of vomiting.

6. Protect the patient from embarrassment by asking onlookers to give the patient some privacy.

If the patient says that this is the first attack, alert the EMS system dispatcher. If the patient is aware of the problem and has had other attacks, ask if you may phone the patient's doctor. It is possible that the doctor may wish to see the patient, change medications, or have the patient transported to a medical facility. Remember, the patient has the option to refuse additional care.

After a seizure, the patient will generally feel tired and weak and may not be fully alert. Do *not* let the patient wander away. It is best to keep the patient at rest and to provide emotional support for the patient and family members until additional medical help arrives.

Diabetes

Glucose, a form of sugar, is the main source of energy for the body's cells. This sugar is carried to the cells by way of the bloodstream. To enter the cells, however, **insulin,** a hormone secreted by the pancreas, must be present. Insulin allows the sugar to enter the blood cells so it may be utilized effectively. In normal, healthy adults this process works well to balance the glucose levels within the body.

Diabetes is a disease that prevents individuals from producing enough insulin or utilizing insulin effectively. While some cases of diabetes can be managed by diet, others require the patient to take doses of insulin or oral hypoglycemic agents. These patients are susceptible to fluctuations in their glucose levels.

Hyperglycemia (High Blood Sugar)
Hyperglycemia is usually a gradual event, taking several days to develop. Should the individual not take enough insulin, or eat too much sugar (carbohydrates) for the amount of insulin being taken, or if the diabetes has not been diagnosed, hyperglycemia may occur.

First | The **signs and symptoms** of hyperglycemia are (Figure 10.5):

- Difficult breathing—Typically the patient will take deep, rapid breaths, often heaving or sighing. This may appear to be hyperventilation.
- Dry, warm skin—Sometimes the skin may become reddened.
- Rapid, weak pulse
- In some cases, the eyes will appear sunken.
- A sweet or fruity odor on the patient's breath, called "acetone breath"
- Dry mouth
- Restless and in a stupor
- Becomes unresponsive and goes into a coma

First | The **emergency care** for hyperglycemia consists of the following:

1. Perform scene size-up, including scene safety and BSI.
2. Have someone alert the EMS system dispatcher. This patient will have to be transferred to a medical facility.
3. Keep the patient at rest. If the patient is alert, try to gain additional information through a focused history and physical examination. Ask if the patient is diabetic. Find out if the patient has taken insulin and has eaten recently.

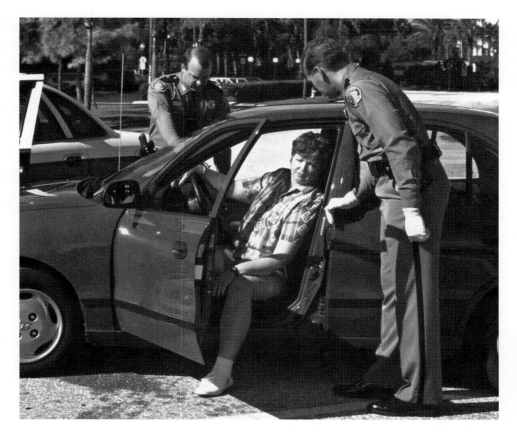

4. If you are not certain if you are dealing with a patient with too much sugar (hyperglycemia) or too low (hypoglycemia), give the patient sugar, candy, orange juice, or a soft drink (make certain that the substance contains real sugar, not an artificial sweetener). Some jurisdictions may allow First Responders to give oral glucose. Check local protocols and always call for medical direction before assisting a patient with medications (see Appendix 3). Do not give any liquids to patients unless they are fully alert. Granulated sugar can be placed under the tongue of an unconscious patient; however, you must sprinkle a few granules at a time from your fingers and constantly monitor the patient to ensure an open airway. **Follow your local EMS system guidelines.**

5. Care for shock and provide oxygen per local protocols.

Hypoglycemia (Low Blood Sugar) The diabetic who has taken too much insulin, has eaten too little sugar, or is overexerted may develop hypoglycemia, which usually comes on suddenly.

 The **signs and symptoms** for <u>hypo</u>glycemia and developing **insulin shock** include:

- Pale, moist skin, often cold and clammy
- A full and rapid pulse
- Dizziness. The patient may become disoriented, faint, and go into convulsions or a coma.
- Headache
- Normal or shallow breathing with no unusual odors
- Being very hungry
- Some patients will develop convulsions if they do not receive early care.
- Some patients develop stroke-like symptoms, including weakness or numbness.

> **WARNING:**
> Some patients who are hyperglycemic may appear to be drunk at first. Do not assume someone is drunk unless there is obvious alcohol abuse and you have ruled out hyperglycemia. Keep in mind that an alcoholic may also be diabetic.

hypoglycemia too little sugar in the blood.

insulin shock severe hypoglycemia. A form of shock usually caused by too high a level of insulin in the blood, producing a sudden drop in blood sugar. The causes are too much insulin injected by the diabetic or too little food taken in for the amount of insulin injected or produced by medication.

First **Emergency care** for hypoglycemia and developing insulin shock consists of the following:

1. Perform a scene size-up, including scene safety and BSI.

2. Keep the patient at rest.

3. Provide sugar for the patient in the form of granulated sugar, sugar cubes, candy, orange juice, a soft drink, syrup, or honey. Make certain that the substance contains sugar and not an artificial sweetener. Do not give liquids or foods to the patient who is not fully alert.

4. Have someone alert the EMS system dispatcher. If you are not sure that you are dealing with severe hypoglycemia or insulin shock, if the patient does not respond to sugar, if this is the patient's first case of insulin shock, or if the patient went into convulsions or a coma, be sure that the dispatcher has this information.

5. Care for shock, including oxygen per local protocols.

ABDOMINAL PAIN

First The sudden onset of severe abdominal pain is sometimes called an **acute abdomen** or **acute abdominal distress.** The presence of pain alone is enough to indicate that the patient must be seen as soon as possible by someone with more advanced training.

The cause of the pain may be anything from simple indigestion to a very serious medical problem. Your role is to assess the patient and provide the needed care, making certain that the EMS dispatcher has been alerted. Do *not* attempt to diagnose the patient's problem. If the pain is severe enough for the patient to seek emergency care, then his problem must be considered to be serious.

Many medical problems are associated with severe abdominal pain. Some examples include appendicitis, ulcers, inflamed abdominal cavity membranes, pancreatitis, obstruction of the intestine, serious liver disease, gallstones, and kidney stones. Female patients may have severe abdominal pain related to problems with pregnancy. Detecting the exact nature of the pain is not possible at the First Responder level of care.

Do not assume that pain over the top of a specific organ means that this organ is the location of the patient's problem. Abdominal pain is usually *referred*, or spread out over one or more areas. The pain may not be over the top of or near the sick or damaged organ (Figure 10.6).

Signs and Symptoms

First The signs and symptoms associated with acute abdomen may include:

- Abdominal pain
- Back pain
- Nausea and vomiting
- Fear
- Rapid pulse
- Rapid and shallow breathing
- Fever
- Signs of developing shock
- Guarding the abdomen—The patient may also fold his arms across his abdomen and draw up his knees. Usually, the patient tries not to move.
- Bulging (distention) and/or rigid abdominal wall

acute abdomen the sudden onset of severe abdominal pain. Abdominal distress related to one of many medical conditions or specific injury to the abdomen.

Note

The location of abdominal pain may not be the actual site of the patient's problem.

*D*iabetic *E*mergencies

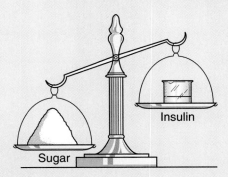

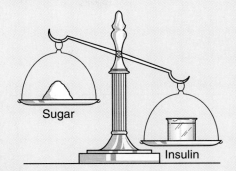

Hyperglycemia

Causes
- ■ The diabetic's condition has not been diagnosed and/or treated.
- ■ The diabetic has not taken his insulin.
- ■ The diabetic has overeaten, flooding the body with a sudden excess of carbohydrates.
- ■ The diabetic suffers an infection or other stress that disrupts his glucose/insulin balance.

Emergency Care
- ■ Immediately transport to a medical facility.

Signs and Symptoms
- ■ Gradual onset of signs and symptoms over days
- ■ Patient complains of dry mouth and intense thirst
- ■ Abdominal pain and vomiting common
- ■ Gradually increasing restlessness, confusion, followed by stupor
- ■ Coma, with these signs:
  - – Signs of air hunger—deep, sighing respirations
  - – Weak, rapid pulse
  - – Dry, red, warm skin
  - – Eyes that appear sunken
  - – Breath smells of acetone—sickly sweet, like nail polish remover

Hypoglycemia

Causes
- ■ The diabetic has taken too much insulin.
- ■ The diabetic has not eaten enough to provide her normal sugar intake.
- ■ The diabetic has overexercised or overexerted herself, thus reducing her blood glucose level.
- ■ The diabetic has vomited a meal.

Emergency Care
- ■ Conscious patient: Administer sugar, granular sugar, honey, a Lifesaver, or other candy placed under the tongue, or orange juice.
- ■ Unconscious patients: Avoid giving liquids. Sprinkle granulated sugar under the tongue or give oral glucose per local protocols and medical direction (see Appendix 3).
- ■ Turn head to side or place on side.
- ■ Transport to the medical facility.

Signs and Symptoms
- ■ Rapid onset of signs and symptoms in minutes
- ■ Dizziness and headache
- ■ Abnormal, hostile, or aggressive behavior, which may appear to be alcohol intoxication
- ■ Fainting, convulsions, and occasionally coma
- ■ Full rapid pulse
- ■ Patient intensely hungry; drooling
- ■ Skin pale, cold, clammy; profuse perspiration

When faced with a patient who may be suffering from one of these conditions:
- ■ Determine if the patient is diabetic. Look for medical alert devices or information cards; interview patient and family members.
- ■ If the patient is a known or suspected diabetic, and hypoglycemia (insulin shock) cannot be ruled out, assume that it is hypoglycemia and administer sugar.

Often a patient suffering from these conditions may appear drunk. Always check for underlying conditions—such as diabetic complications—when treating someone who appears intoxicated.

FIGURE 10.6
Patterns of abdominal pain.

**REFERRED AND ACTUAL
PAIN AREAS**

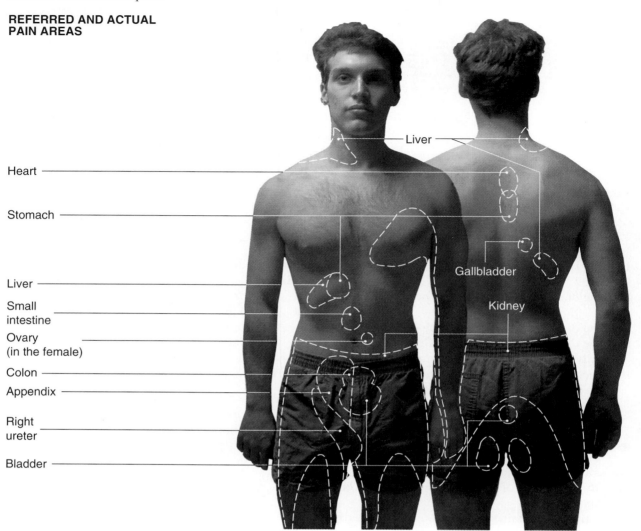

- Abdominal tenderness
- A protrusion, lump, or mass is seen or felt
- Rectal bleeding; dark, tarry stools or changes in stools; blood in the urine; or nonmenstrual vaginal bleeding

As you gather signs and symptoms, be sure to carefully watch the patient. Does the person appear ill? Does he or she continue to guard the abdomen? Is the person reluctant to move?

Emergency Care

First The basic care for patients with abdominal complaints requires you to:

1. Perform scene size-up, including scene safety and BSI.
2. Maintain an open airway. Stay alert for vomiting.
3. Provide care for shock, including oxygen per local protocols.
4. Make certain that EMS dispatch is alerted.
5. Keep the patient at rest. Sometimes the patient's pain may be reduced

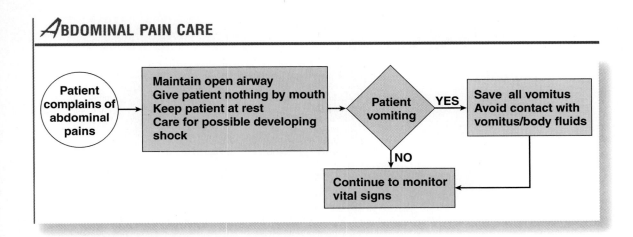

if he or she is positioned on the back with the knees flexed. Do not force the patient to assume this position.

6. Save all vomitus. Avoid contact with the vomitus, discharges, mucous membranes, and body fluids.

7. Reassure the patient and continue to gather information. Ask if the pain came on suddenly, the nature of the pain (sharp, dull, stabbing), if there were any fevers or chills, any unusual bowel movements (dark, light, tarry, bloody, loose, or hard), or any problems with urination (inability to urinate, frequent urination, or blood in the urine). Ask the patient when he last ate and what was consumed. Make sure you document the patient's answers. Ask the female patient about her menstrual history.

First | **WARNING:** Do not give the patient anything by mouth. To do so may cause the patient to vomit or may set off organ or gland activity that could prove harmful.

POISONINGS, BITES, STINGS

Any substance that can be harmful to the body is known as a **poison.** There are more than one million incidents of poisoning reported annually in the United States. While some cases might be related to murder or suicide attempts, most are accidental and often involve children.

ROUTES OF POISONS

We usually think of a poison as a liquid or solid chemical that has been ingested, but there are actually several types of poisons that can be classified into four categories. These categories are arranged according to how a substance may enter the body:

■ **Ingestion**—*Poisons taken into the body by way of the mouth.* Ingested poisons can include various household and industrial chemicals, certain foods and improperly prepared foods, plant materials, petroleum products, medications (particularly if taken in improper doses), and poisons made specifically to control rodents, insects, and crop diseases (Figure 10.7). Severe abdominal pain, nausea, and vomiting may occur.

FIGURE 10.7
Household poisons.

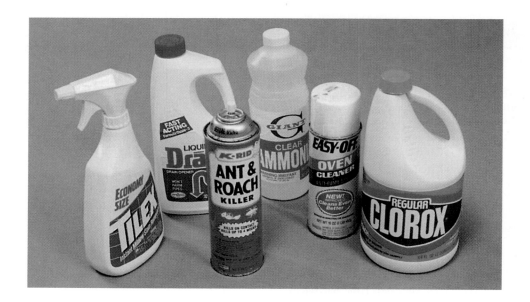

- **Inhalation**—*Poisons taken in by breathing.* Inhaled poisons take the form of gases, vapors, and sprays, including carbon monoxide (from car exhaust, kerosene heaters, and wood-burning stoves), ammonia, chlorine, volatile liquid chemicals (including many industrial solvents), and insect sprays. Allergic reactions may occur, including respiratory difficulties.
- **Absorption**—*Poisons absorbed through the skin and through body tissues.* Poisons absorbed through the skin may or may not damage the skin. Many contact poisons will do harsh damage to the skin and then be slowly absorbed into the bloodstream. Some insecticides and agricultural chemicals can be absorbed through the skin. Corrosive chemicals may damage the skin and then be absorbed by the body. Contact with a wide variety of plant materials and certain forms of marine life can cause allergic reactions and/or damage to the skin, with the poison (toxin) being absorbed into tissues under the skin.
- **Injection**—*Poisons entered directly into the bloodstream.* Insects, spiders, snakes, and certain marine life are able to inject poisons into the body. Injection might be self-induced by way of a hypodermic needle. Unusual industrial accidents producing cuts or puncture wounds also can be a source of poisons being injected into the body.

In this section, we will consider general signs and symptoms and some basic courses of action to take for various poisonings. Table 10-2 lists some of the types of poisons you may see that require emergency care. This information is provided so that you may learn more about various poisons as part of your continued training. The table is not meant to be memorized as part of your basic course.

POISON CONTROL CENTERS

First In most areas, a poison control center can be reached 24 hours a day. The staff at the center can tell you what should be done for most cases of poisoning. Your instructor will tell you which center serves your area and give you the phone number for this center. Place this number on your home and work phones and on the gear you take on calls (Figure 10.8).

TABLE 10-2: *Common Poisons*

POISON	SIGNS AND SYMPTOMS
Acetaminophen (Tylenol, Comtrex, Bancap, Datril, Excedrin P.M.)	Nausea, vomiting. The victim is usually a child.
Acids	Burns on or around the lips. Burning in the mouth, throat, and stomach, often followed by heavy vomiting.
Alkalis (ammonia, bleaches, detergents, lye, washing soda, certain fertilizers)	Check mouth to see if the membranes appear white and swollen. There may be a soapy appearance in the mouth. Abdominal pain is usually present. Vomiting may occur, often full of blood and mucus.
Arsenic (most rat poisons and now warfarin)	"Garlic breath," with burning in the mouth, throat, and stomach. Abdominal pain can be severe. Vomiting is common.
Aspirin	Delayed reactions, including ringing in the ears, rapid and deep breathing, dry skin, and restlessness.
Chloroform	Slow, shallow breathing with chloroform odor on breath. Pupils are dilated and fixed.
Corrosive agents (disinfectants, drain cleaners, household acids, iodine, pine oil, turpentine, toilet bowl cleaners, styptic pencil, water softeners, strong acids)	(See Acids.)
Food poisoning	Difficult to detect since signs and symptoms vary greatly. Usually, you will note abdominal pain, nausea and vomiting, gas and bowel sounds, and diarrhea.
Iodine	Upset stomach and vomiting. If a starchy meal has been eaten, the vomitus may appear blue.
Metals (copper, lead, mercury, and zinc)	Metallic taste in mouth, with nausea and abdominal pains. Vomiting may occur. Stools may be bloody and dark.
Petroleum Products (some deodorizers, heating fuel, diesel fuels, gasoline, kerosene, lighter fluid, lubricating oil, naphtha, rust remover, transmission fluid)	Note characteristic odors on patient's breath and clothing or in vomitus.
Phosphorus	Abdominal pain and vomiting
Plants: Contact (poison ivy, poison oak, poison sumac)	Swollen, itchy areas on the skin, with quickly forming blisterlike structures
Plants: Ingested (azalea, castor bean, poison elder, foxglove, lily of the valley, mountain laurel, mushrooms, nightshade, oleander, mistletoe and holly berries, rhododendron, rhubarb leaves, rubber plant, some wild cherries)	Difficult to detect, ranging from nausea to coma. Always question in cases of apparent child poisoning.
Strychnine	The face, jaw, and neck will stiffen. Strong convulsions occur quickly after ingesting.

FIGURE 10.8
Poison control phone sticker.

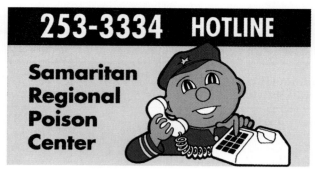

In some EMS systems, rescuers must receive directions for the care of poisoning patients from a physician. This is not always the case for every poison control center. If directions must come from a physician, the First Responder should phone or radio the emergency department or EMS dispatch. This is termed "seeking help from medical direction." You are to follow the method used by your EMS system. Remember, a nurse or the dispatcher may relay the physician's directions. You may not have a chance to speak directly to a physician. In your jurisdiction, First Responder care for ingested poison may include giving the patient syrup of ipecac or activated charcoal. Check local protocols and always call for medical direction before assisting a patient with medications (see Appendix 3).

To aid the poison control center or medical direction, note and report any containers at the scene of the poisoning. Let them know if the patient has vomited and describe the vomitus (check for pill fragments). When possible, and if it can be done quickly, gather information from the patient or from bystanders before you call the center.

TYPES OF POISONS

Ingested Poisons

In cases of possible ingested poisoning, you must gather information quickly. If at all possible, do so while you are doing the focused history and physical exam. Note any containers that may hold poisonous substances. See if there is any vomitus. Check if there are any substances on the patient's clothes or if the patient is wearing clothing that may indicate the nature of work (farmer, miner, and so on). Can the scene be associated with certain types of poisonings? Question the patient and any bystanders.

First | **Signs and Symptoms** The signs and symptoms for ingested poisons can be gathered during the initial and focused assessments. They can include any or all of the following:

- Burns or stains around the patient's mouth
- Unusual breath odors, body odors, or odors on the patient's clothing or at the scene
- Abnormal breathing
- Abnormal pulse rate and character
- Sweating
- Dilated or constricted pupils
- Excessive saliva formation or foaming at the mouth
- Pains in the mouth or throat, or painful swallowing
- Stomach or abdominal pain
- Upset stomach or nausea, vomiting, diarrhea
- Convulsions
- Altered mental status, including unconsciousness

You should contact your local poison control center to obtain advice on appropriate treatment for specific poisons. But do *not* provide any treatment until you have contacted medical direction.

Emergency care directions from a poison control center may consist of diluting the poison in the patient's stomach or using activated charcoal to absorb the poison. Never attempt to dilute the poison or give activated charcoal (see Appendix 3) if the patient is not fully alert and conscious. Follow your local guidelines and the instructions given by the poison control center.

 Providing liquids by mouth to ingested poisoning patients may be dangerous for some victims. This is especially true if the patient has been convulsing, or if the source of the poison is a strong acid, alkali, or petroleum product. Included in these groups of substances are oven cleaners, drain cleaners, toilet bowl cleaners, lye, ammonia, bleaches, kerosene, and gasoline. Always check for burns around the patient's mouth and the odor of petroleum products on the patient's breath. Follow the poison control center's instructions.

 Emergency Care For conscious patients, the typical procedures include:

1. Perform scene size-up, including scene safety and BSI.

2. Maintain an open airway.

3. *Call the poison control center or medical direction.*

4. You may be directed to dilute the poison by having the patient drink one or two glasses of water or milk, or you may be directed to give syrup of ipecac or activated charcoal. Check local protocols, and always call for medical direction before assisting a patient with medications. The poison control center or medical direction may tell you to have the patient consume the fluids in sips to prevent vomiting. Do *not* give anything by mouth if the patient is having convulsions, unless otherwise directed by a physician or the poison control center.

5. If supplies are available and you are directed to do so, give activated charcoal. For an adult, give 25 to 50 grams. For a child, give 12.5 to 25 grams (see Appendix 3).

6. In case of vomiting, position the patient so that no vomitus will be aspirated (inhaled). Put him on one side or in a semi-sitting position with the head turned to the side.

7. Save all vomitus.

8. Provide care for shock, keeping the patient positioned to drain the mouth should vomiting occur.

9. Provide oxygen according to local protocols. Assisted ventilations may be required.

In cases of ingested poisons, be realistic about the limits of emergency care. Some poisons kill instantly. Some patients can be helped only by very special antidotes, and there are no antidotes at all for some poisons. Understand that you may do your best as a First Responder and the patient may still die from ingested poison.

In addition to the usual risks, if the patient has ingested a highly concentrated dose of certain poisons, such as arsenic or cyanide, and if deposits remain on the patient's lips, there is a chance the rescuer may be harmed. The current recommendation is to use a pocket mask with HEPA filter, a bag-valve

> **WARNING:**
> Always follow the poison control center's instructions before giving liquids by mouth to ingested poisoning patients.

mask, or your EMS system's approved protective barrier (see Chapter 2) on all patients who need rescue breathing. Keep in mind that patients receiving a high dose of these poisons usually die within seconds.

Inhaled Poisons

Gather information from the patient and bystanders as quickly as possible. Look for indications of inhaled poisons. Possible sources can be automobile exhaust systems, stoves, charcoal grills, industrial solvents, and spray cans.

First | **Signs and Symptoms** The signs and symptoms of inhaled poisons vary depending on the source of the poison. Shortness of breath and coughing are common indicators. Pulse rate is usually too fast or too slow. Often, the patient's eyes will appear irritated.

First | **Emergency Care** Emergency care consists of safely removing the patient from the source of the inhaled poison, maintaining an open airway, giving oxygen (see Appendix 2) providing needed life-support measures, contacting the poison control center or medical direction, and making certain that the EMS system dispatcher has been notified. Remember to gather information from the patient and bystanders (substance inhaled, length of time exposed, early care measures, patient's initial reactions and appearance).

It may be necessary to remove contaminated clothing from the patient. Avoid touching this clothing since it may cause skin burns. Wear latex or vinyl gloves to protect yourself.

Fire presents problems other than thermal burns. One such problem is smoke inhalation. The smoke from any fire source contains poisonous substances. Modern building materials and furnishings often contain plastics and other synthetics that release toxic fumes when they burn or are overheated. It is possible for the substances found in smoke to burn the skin, irritate the eyes, injure the airway, cause respiratory arrest, and, in some cases, cause cardiac arrest. Do *not* attempt a rescue unless you have been trained to do so and have all the required personnel and equipment.

As a First Responder, you will probably see irritation to the eyes and injury to the airway associated with smoke. Irritations to the skin and eyes may be treated by simple flooding with water. Your first priority will be the patient's airway. In cases of smoke inhalation, you should:

1. Move the patient to a safe, smoke-free area.
2. Perform an initial assessment and supply life-support measures as needed.
3. If the patient is conscious and without signs of neck or spinal injury, place him in a sitting or semisitting position. The patient may find it easier to breathe in a different position. Let the patient assume the position that proves best. Always provide support for the back and be prepared if the patient loses consciousness.
4. Provide care for shock.
5. Provide oxygen if you have been trained and your jurisdiction permits First Responders to do so.

Carbon monoxide poisoning is often seen at fire scenes. This gas enters the patient's bloodstream, where it is picked up by red blood cells that should be carrying oxygen. The patient's nervous system is affected. She will complain of headache and dizziness. Other signs and symptoms include confusion,

Note

The body's reaction to toxic gases and foreign matter in the airway often can be delayed. It is good First Responder practice to alert 911 for all cases of smoke inhalation.

seizures, and coma. Other inhaled gases from combustion can cause injuries to the respiratory system.

Proper care requires moving the patient away from the source and the same basic procedures as would be provided for any smoke inhalation or inhaled poison victim. EMT-level care and transport are required in all cases of carbon monoxide poisoning.

Absorbed Poisons

As mentioned earlier in this chapter, absorbed poisons usually irritate or damage the skin or eyes. However, there are cases in which a poison can be absorbed through the skin with little or no damage to the skin. The patient, bystanders, and the scene will help you determine if you are dealing with such rare cases. In First Responder care, most cases of absorbed poisoning will be detected because of skin reactions related to chemicals or plants at the scene.

First | ***Signs and Symptoms*** The signs and symptoms of absorbed poisoning include any or all of the following:
- Skin reactions—ranging from mild irritations to chemical burns
- Itching
- Eye irritation
- Headache
- Increased skin temperature
- Anaphylactic (allergy) shock

First | ***Emergency Care*** Emergency care for absorbed poisons includes moving the patient from the source of the poison (when safe to do so) and immediately flooding with water all the areas of the patient's body (including the eyes) that have been exposed to the poison. After flooding with water, remove all contaminated clothing (including shoes and jewelry), and wash the affected areas of the patient's skin with soap and water. If no soap is available, continue to flood the exposed areas of the patient's skin. Be certain to have someone contact the poison control center and the EMS system dispatcher or medical direction. More specific directions for chemical burns appear in Chapter 11.

Injected Poisons

Insect stings, spider bites, marine life stings, and snakebites can all be sources of injected poisons. Some of these poisons cause true emergencies for all patients. Others are only problems for those patients sensitive to the poison. In all cases of injected poisons, be alert for anaphylactic (allergy) shock (see pages 237–238).

Poisons can also be injected into the body by a hypodermic needle. Drug overdose and drug contamination can produce serious medical emergencies. This topic will be covered later in this chapter.

First | ***Signs and Symptoms*** Gather information from the patient, bystanders, and the scene. The signs and symptoms of injected poisoning may include:
- Noticeable stings or bites to the skin
- Puncture marks to the skin—Pay careful attention to the fingers and hands, forearms, toes and feet, and lower legs.
- Pain at or around the wound site
- Itching
- Weakness, dizziness, or collapse
- Difficult breathing and unusual pulse rate
- Headache

Note
Carbon monoxide poisoning may also occur under circumstances other than a fire. Malfunctioning furnaces and other heating devices are common sources.

Note
You are responsible for all clothing, jewelry, documents, and monies removed from the patient. Obtain a receipt for these items when you turn them over to the proper authorities. The receipt must be one that your EMS system accepts as a legal document, and it must be proper for inclusion in the patient's medical records at the medical facility as well as in your system. Your instructor will inform you of such forms in your state.

- Nausea
- Allergy shock

 Emergency Care Since a patient may go into anaphylactic (allergy) shock, alert the poison control center and the EMS system dispatcher or medical direction as soon as possible for all cases of injected poisoning. Emergency care for injected poisons (except snakebite) includes:

1. Perform scene size-up, including scene safety and BSI.

2. Provide care for shock. This is done even if the patient does not show any of the signs of anaphylactic (allergy) shock.

3. Scrape away bee and wasp stingers and venom sacs. Do not pull out stingers. Always scrape them from the patient's skin. A plastic credit card works well as a scraper.

4. Place an ice bag or cold pack over the bitten or stung area.

Some patients sensitive to stings or bites carry medication to help prevent anaphylactic (allergy) shock. Help all such patients to take their medications (see Appendix 3). (Your First Responder course may include training in how to administer injectable medications for cases when the patient cannot do so. *Do only what you have been trained to do.*) Remember to look for medical identification devices.

Snakebites

Thousands of people in the United States are bitten by poisonous snakes each year, with fewer than ten deaths being reported annually. (In the United States, more people die each year from bee and wasp stings than from snakebites.) The signs and symptoms of poisoning may take several hours to develop. Death from snakebite is usually not a rapidly occurring event unless anaphylactic (allergy) shock also occurs. Staying calm and keeping the patient calm is critical. There is time to alert the EMS system dispatcher and to provide care for the patient.

Consider all snakebites to be from poisonous snakes. The patient or bystanders may indicate that the snake was not poisonous. They could be mistaken. If you see the live snake, do not approach it to gather information for determining its species. If safe to do so, note its size and coloration. Unless you are an expert in capturing snakes, do not try to catch the snake. However, if possible, do contact animal control authorities.

 Signs and Symptoms The signs and symptoms of snakebite may include:

- A noticeable bite to the skin—This may appear as nothing more than a discoloration.
- Pain and swelling in the area of the bite—This may be slow to develop, taking 30 minutes to several hours.
- Rapid pulse and labored breathing
- Weakness
- Vision problems
- Nausea and vomiting

 Emergency Care The emergency care for snakebite includes:

1. Perform a scene size-up, including BSI.

2. Keep the patient calm and lying down.

3. Have someone alert the EMS system dispatcher.

4. Locate the fang marks and clean this site with soap and water.

5. Remove from the bitten extremity any rings, bracelets, and other constricting items.

6. Keep any bitten extremities immobilized. The application of a soft splint will help. A rigid splint may cause problems if there is swelling at the site of injury. Try to keep the bitten area at the level of the heart, or when possible, below the level of the heart.

7. Provide care for shock, conserve body heat, and monitor vital signs.

Note
The coral snake has a small mouth. Usually, its bites are limited to the patient's finger or toe. When the bite is known to be from a coral snake, apply one constricting band above the wound site.

If you know that the patient will not reach a medical facility within 5 hours after having been bitten, or if the signs and symptoms of the patient begin to worsen, apply a constricting band above and below the fang marks (Figure 10.9). Each band should be about 1½ to 2 inches wide, placed about 2 inches from the wound, or above and below the swelling. (*Never* place one band on each side of a joint, such as above and below the knee.) The constricting bands should be from a snakebite kit or made of wide, soft rubber. If only one band is available, place it above the wound (between the wound and the heart). If no bands are available, use a handkerchief.

The constricting bands should be placed so that you can slide your finger underneath them. Do *not* place them so that they cut off arterial flow. Monitor for a pulse at the wrist or ankle, depending on the extremity involved.

Many EMS systems recommend constricting bands for all cases of snakebite. Check with your instructor.

Do *not* place an ice bag or cold pack on the bite unless you are directed to do so by a physician or the poison control center. Do not cut into the bite and/or apply suction unless you are directed to do so by a physician. Never suck the venom from the wound, using your mouth.

ANAPHYLACTIC SHOCK

Anaphylactic (allergy) shock occurs when people come into contact with a substance to which they are allergic. The body considers the substance an invader and reacts to counteract it. This is a true life-threatening emergency. There is no way of knowing if patients will stabilize, grow worse slowly or rapidly, or overcome the reaction on their own. Many patients decline rapidly. For some, death is a certain outcome unless special treatment is given quickly.

anaphylactic (AN-ah-fi-LAK-tik) shock a severe allergic reaction in which a person goes into shock. Also called *allergy shock*.

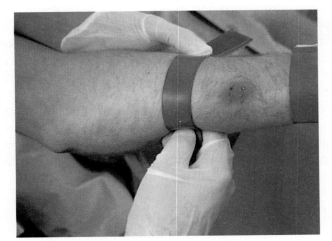

FIGURE 10.9
Constricting bands must not be too tight.

Many different things can cause anaphylactic (allergy) shock, such as:

- Insect bites and stings, including bee stings
- Foods (nuts, spices, shellfish, and so on)
- Inhaled substances, including dust and pollens
- Chemicals, inhaled or when in contact with the skin
- Medications, injected or taken by mouth, including penicillin

Signs

First | The signs of anaphylactic (allergy) shock are:

- **Skin**—burning, itching, or "breaking out" (such as hives or some type of rash)
- **Breathing**—difficult and rapid, with possible chest pains and wheezing
- **Pulse**—rapid, very weak or not detected
- **Face**—the lips often turn blue (cyanosis); the face and tongue may swell.
- **Level of consciousness**—restlessness, often followed by fainting or unconsciousness

REMEMBER:

When you interview patients, ask if they are allergic to anything and if they have been in contact with that substance. Look for a medical identification device, which may indicate that there is an allergy problem. If you are in the patient's residence, look for a "Vial of Life" or similar type sticker on the main entrance, the closest window to the main door, or the refrigerator door. This sticker indicates the presence of patient information and medications in a vial kept in the refrigerator.

Emergency Care

First | To care for patients in anaphylactic (allergy) shock, follow the same procedures used for shock (see pages 326–330). Even though the danger to the patient may be immediate, do not attempt to transport the patient unless you are allowed to do so. It is usually better to wait for the EMTs to respond. In many cases, EMTs or paramedics can respond to the scene and administer the medications required to stabilize the patient before transport. Some jurisdictions may allow First Responders to give medications to counteract the effects of allergic reaction or anaphylactic (allergy) shock. Check local protocols, and always call for medical direction before assisting a patient with medications.

Patients in anaphylactic (allergy) shock need medications as soon as possible. In some states, certain First Responders are allowed to transport anaphylactic (allergy) shock patients immediately to a hospital. The EMS system dispatcher in those areas may decide that the EMT response time is too long and recommend that the First Responder provide transport. The First Responder may be allowed to transport anaphylactic (allergy) shock patients to a medical facility only if they have no injuries. Your instructor can tell you the policy for your own state or certain areas within your state. If you do transport anaphylactic (allergy) shock patients, be prepared for them to grow worse and be ready to provide pulmonary resuscitation or CPR.

Some people who are sensitive to bee stings or have other allergy problems carry medications to take in case of an emergency. These medications, usually

REMEMBER:

Anaphylactic (allergy) shock is a true emergency.

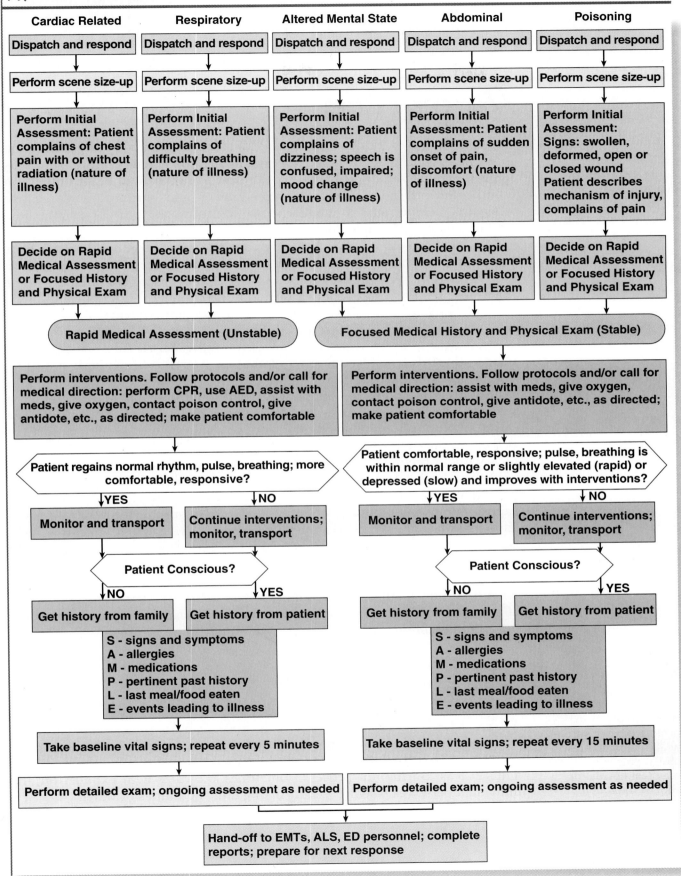

Cardiac Related	Respiratory	Altered Mental State	Abdominal	Poisoning
Dispatch and respond	Dispatch and respond	Dispatch and respond	Dispatch and respond	Dispatch and respond
Perform scene size-up	Perform scene size-up	Perform scene size-up	Perform scene size-up	Perform scene size-up
Perform Initial Assessment: Patient complains of chest pain with or without radiation (nature of illness)	Perform Initial Assessment: Patient complains of difficulty breathing (nature of illness)	Perform Initial Assessment: Patient complains of dizziness; speech is confused, impaired; mood change (nature of illness)	Perform Initial Assessment: Patient complains of sudden onset of pain, discomfort (nature of illness)	Perform Initial Assessment: Signs: swollen, deformed, open or closed wound Patient describes mechanism of injury, complains of pain
Decide on Rapid Medical Assessment or Focused History and Physical Exam	Decide on Rapid Medical Assessment or Focused History and Physical Exam	Decide on Rapid Medical Assessment or Focused History and Physical Exam	Decide on Rapid Medical Assessment or Focused History and Physical Exam	Decide on Rapid Medical Assessment or Focused History and Physical Exam

Rapid Medical Assessment (Unstable)

Focused Medical History and Physical Exam (Stable)

Perform interventions. Follow protocols and/or call for medical direction: perform CPR, use AED, assist with meds, give oxygen, contact poison control, give antidote, etc., as directed; make patient comfortable

Perform interventions. Follow protocols and/or call for medical direction: assist with meds, give oxygen, contact poison control, give antidote, etc., as directed; make patient comfortable

Patient regains normal rhythm, pulse, breathing; more comfortable, responsive?

Patient comfortable, responsive; pulse, breathing is within normal range or slightly elevated (rapid) or depressed (slow) and improves with interventions?

YES → Monitor and transport

NO → Continue interventions; monitor, transport

YES → Monitor and transport

NO → Continue interventions; monitor, transport

Patient Conscious?

NO → Get history from family

YES → Get history from patient

Patient Conscious?

NO → Get history from family

YES → Get history from patient

S - signs and symptoms
A - allergies
M - medications
P - pertinent past history
L - last meal/food eaten
E - events leading to illness

S - signs and symptoms
A - allergies
M - medications
P - pertinent past history
L - last meal/food eaten
E - events leading to illness

Take baseline vital signs; repeat every 5 minutes

Take baseline vital signs; repeat every 15 minutes

Perform detailed exam; ongoing assessment as needed

Perform detailed exam; ongoing assessment as needed

Hand-off to EMTs, ALS, ED personnel; complete reports; prepare for next response

epinephrine and/or antihistamines, can be administered by the patient (see Appendix 3). Your jurisdiction may allow First Responders to help the patient take medications. State laws and protocols will govern if you can administer the medication. Your instructor will inform you of local policies for the care of these patients.

*H*EAT EMERGENCIES

hyperthermia an increase in body core temperature above its normal temperature.

Exposure to hot and humid environments can cause the body to generate too much heat, which can create an abnormally high body temperature, known as **hyperthermia.** Such a condition could result from a patient being outside on a hot, humid afternoon for a prolonged period of time, or exposure to excessive heat while indoors, such as a boiler room. Left unchecked, this condition could lead to death.

Dry heat can often fool individuals, causing them to continue to work in or be exposed to heat far beyond the point that can be accepted by their bodies. For this reason, the problems caused by dry heat exposure are often far worse than those seen in moist heat exposure.

The body regulates body heat by creating energy during digestion and metabolism. Heat is lost through the lungs and skin. The entire process is controlled by a structure in the brain (hypothalamus) that acts as the body's thermostat. It is responsible for regulating all processes to maintain a normal body temperature (98.6°F).

Sweating is one of the body's ways of ridding itself of excess heat. On a really hot day, you can lose up to 1 liter (about 2 pints) of sweat per hour. The sweat, in turn, is evaporated from the motion of the wind or gentle breeze. Heat is then evaporated at the same time. The problem develops on humid days or days without breezes, which inhibit the evaporative process.

When dealing with problems created by exposure to excessive heat, keep in mind that you must do patient assessments and interviews. Collapse due to heat exposure may break bones. A history of blood pressure or heart or lung problems may have quickened the effects of heat exposure. What appears to be a problem related to heat exposure could be a heart attack. Also remember that certain types of patients are at risk for heat emergencies. Children, the elderly, the chronically ill, and alcoholics are more susceptible to temperature extremes. Individuals who are taking certain heart or other medications may also be more prone to such conditions along with anyone with a preexisting illness or condition (Scan 10-5).

*H*EAT EXHAUSTION

heat exhaustion prolonged exposure to heat, which creates moist, pale skin that may feel normal or cool to the touch.

A typical heat emergency patient with *moist, pale, normal-to-cool skin* is a healthy individual who has been exposed to excessive heat while working or exercising. The circulatory system of the patient begins to fail because of fluid and salt loss. During this process, sometimes known as **heat exhaustion,** the individual perspires heavily, often drinking large quantities of water.

Heat-Related Emergencies

NOTE: All heat-related emergencies require alerting EMS dispatch.

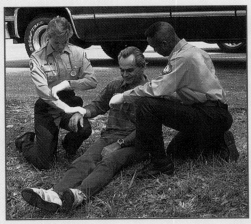

Heat exhaustion

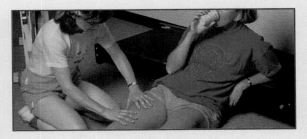

Heat cramps

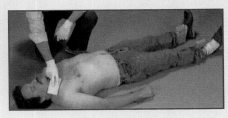

Heat stroke

Heat emergency patient with moist, pale, normal-to-cool skin (heat cramps, heat exhaustion)

Signs and Symptoms
- Severe muscle cramps in legs and abdomen
- Exhaustion, possible dizziness, faintness, and loss of consciousness
- Weak pulse and rapid, shallow breathing
- Heavy perspiration

Emergency Care
- Move patient to nearby cool place, and loosen or remove clothing; do not chill—watch for shivering.
- Provide oxygen at 15 liters per minute (LPM) by nonrebreather mask if allowed.
- Give water to the responsive patient.
- Position the patient; responsive patient on his back with legs elevated; unresponsive patient on the left side, monitoring airway and breathing.
- Help ease cramps by applying moist towels over cramped muscles or, if the patient has no history of circulatory problems, apply gentle but firm pressure on the cramped muscle.

Heat emergency patient with hot, dry or moist skin (heat stroke)

Signs and Symptoms
- Rapid, shallow breathing
- Rapid pulse
- Weakness, loss of consciousness
- Scant or no perspiration
- Large (dilated) pupils
- Seizures or muscular twitching
- Coma

Emergency Care
- Rapidly cool the patient in any manner. Move to a cool place, remove clothing; keep skin wet by applying wet towels. Fan the patient.
- Wrap cold packs or ice bags, if available, and place them at the neck, armpits, wrists, ankles, and groin. Fan the patient to increase heat loss.
- If transport is delayed, find tub or container and immerse patient up to face in cool water. Monitor to prevent drowning.
- Continue to monitor the patient's vital signs.
- Provide oxygen at 15 liters per minute (LPM) via nonrebreather mask if allowed.

Signs and Symptoms

> **First** | Signs and symptoms of heat exhaustion (moist, pale, normal-to-cool skin) include:

- Heavy perspiration
- Moist, pale skin that may feel normal or cool
- Weakness, exhaustion, or dizziness
- Muscle cramps (usually in legs or abdomen)
- Rapid, shallow breathing
- Weak pulse
- Possible loss of consciousness

Emergency Care

> **First** | Emergency care for heat exhaustion includes:

1. Complete a scene-size up, including scene safety and BSI.
2. Make sure EMS dispatch has been alerted.
3. Perform an initial assessment.
4. Remove the patient from the hot environment and place into a cool area (ambulance with air-conditioning running on high).
5. Loosen or remove clothing.
6. Cool patient by fanning—be sure not to chill the patient.
7. Place patient in the recovery position.
8. Provide emotional support and reassure patient.

*H*EAT CRAMPS

heat cramps typical layperson's term for muscle cramps in the lower limbs and abdomen associated with the loss of fluids and possibly salts while active in a hot environment.

Heat cramps are painful muscle spasms following strenuous activity in a hot environment, usually caused by an electrolyte (such as salt) imbalance. Sometimes, these cramps are accompanied by signs and symptoms of heat exhaustion. In most cases, however, the patient will be mentally alert and sweaty with a normal body temperature. The care for these victims is to simply remove them from heat and replenish fluids by having them drink water. If symptoms persist, contact the EMS dispatcher for an EMT or more advanced response.

*H*EAT EMERGENCY ASSESSMENT

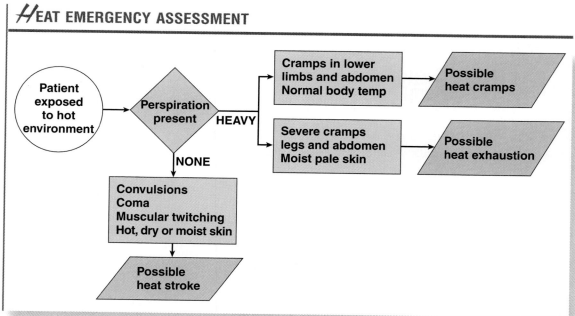

Heat Stroke

Sometimes, the body's temperature-regulating mechanism fails and is unable to rid the body of excess heat. The temperature then rises significantly, causing the patient to become very hot. This condition is known as **heat stroke** and should be considered a life-threatening condition. A patient's body temperature may increase to 105°F or higher and the patient begins to have signs and symptoms of a decreased level of consciousness. The skin will be hot and dry or moist.

heat stroke
prolonged exposure to heat, which creates dry or moist skin that may feel warm or hot to the touch.

Signs and Symptoms

 Patients suffering from this condition may also present with the following signs and symptoms:

- Rapid, shallow breathing
- Full and rapid pulse
- Generalized weakness
- Hot, dry, or possibly moist skin
- Altered mental status
- Little or no perspiration

Emergency Care

 Emergency care for heat stroke (hot, dry or moist skin) includes the following:

1. Complete a scene-size up, including scene safety and BSI.
2. Make sure EMS dispatch has been alerted.
3. Perform an initial assessment.
4. Remove the patient from the hot environment and place into a cool area (ambulance with air-conditioning running on high).
5. Loosen or remove clothing. Pour cool water over wet wrappings.
6. Cool patient by fanning—be sure not to chill the patient.
7. Wrap cold packs or ice bags, if available, and place one under each of the patient's armpits, one on each wrist and ankle, one on the groin, and one on each side of the neck.

Heat Emergency Care

```
Patient exposed to hot environment → Perspiration present?
    HEAVY → Possible heat cramps → Fluids/H₂O to responsive patient
    HEAVY → Possible heat exhaustion → Move patient to cool place / H₂O to responsive patient / Moist towels ease cramps
    NONE → Possible heat stroke → Rapidly cool patient / Cool H₂O wrappings / Armpit icebags
```

8. Place patient in the recovery position.

9. Provide oxygen at 15 liters per minute via nonrebreather mask and monitor vital signs.

10. Provide emotional support and reassure patient.

COLD EMERGENCIES

HYPOTHERMIA (GENERALIZED COLD EMERGENCY)

hypothermia (HI-po-THURM-e-ah) a general cooling of the body. Severe forms can lead to death.

In cold environments, body heat can be lost faster than it can be generated. This creates a state of low body temperature known as **hypothermia,** or a **generalized cold emergency.** To prevent this condition from occurring, the body will attempt to compensate by increasing muscle activity by shivering to increase metabolism and maintain body heat. But as core body temperature continues to drop, shivering stops and the body can no longer attempt to warm itself.

As with heat exposure, young children and the elderly are more susceptible to cold emergencies. Those with previous medical problems might also be more prone to such problems. Many cold exposures are more obvious than others, such as a victim who is often working or playing outside in a cold environment during the winter months. Sometimes, however, the exposure can be more subtle. Elderly patients who do not maintain the thermostat at a proper level during the winter are often affected by cold exposure. Refrigeration accidents and incidents in mild climates also occur.

The patient experiencing a generalized cold emergency will present with cool or cold abdominal skin temperature. Place the back of your hand against the patient's abdomen to assess the general temperature of the patient. In healthy adults, the abdomen should be warm, dry, and pink.

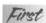 Remember the temperature does not have to be below freezing for hypothermia to occur.

Signs and Symptoms

 Signs and symptoms of a generalized cold emergency may include the following:

- Cool/cold skin temperature
- Shivering
- Decreased mental status such as drowsiness
- Lack of coordination
- Stiff or rigid posture
- Muscle rigidity
- Poor judgment
- Complaints of joint/muscle stiffness

Emergency Care

 Emergency care for generalized cold emergencies includes:

1. Perform a scene size-up, including scene safety and BSI.
2. Make sure that someone alerts the EMS dispatcher.
3. Perform an initial assessment.
4. Remove the patient from the cold environment.
5. Protect the patient from further heat loss.
6. Remove any wet clothing and place a blanket over the patient.

7. Handle the patient gently.

8. Do *not* allow the patient to walk or exert himself in any way.

9. Do *not* give the patient anything to eat or drink (including hot coffee or tea).

10. Comfort the patient and reassure him while awaiting additional EMS resources.

11. Monitor vital signs.

Some cases of generalized cold emergency are extreme. The patient might be unconscious and show no vital signs, with skin cold to the touch. You cannot assume that this patient is dead. Assess the pulse for 30–45 seconds. If there is no pulse, begin CPR immediately. Arrange for transportation to an emergency room. The doctors at the hospital will pronounce a patient biologically dead.

LOCALIZED COLD INJURY

Another environmental emergency that is characterized by the freezing or near freezing of a body part is known as a **localized cold injury,** or **frostbite.** It is caused by a significant exposure to cold temperature and mainly occurs in the extremities and in areas of the fingers, toes, ears, face, and nose (Scan 10-6).

A classic example of a victim of a cold emergency is someone who is outdoors during the winter for a prolonged period of time. Perhaps she is unprotected by scarves, gloves, or boots. The core of the body continues to be warmed by metabolism, but the exposed areas are susceptible to the impact of cold and wind. Most patients will describe a localized cold injury as starting with a cold sensation to the extremities that leads to pain, followed by numbness. This is the classic progression of symptoms.

frostbite localized cold injury. The skin is frozen, but the layers below it are still soft and have their normal bounce.

Signs and Symptoms

First | Signs and symptoms of a localized cold injury may include the following:

Early

■ Blanching of the skin (palpation of the skin in which color does not return)
■ Feeling of cold, pain, or loss of feeling and sensation to the injured area
■ Skin remains soft.
■ If thawed, tingling sensation present

Late

■ White, waxy skin
■ Firm to frozen feeling upon palpation
■ Swelling may be present.
■ Blisters may be present.
■ If thawed, may appear flushed with areas of purple and blanching

Emergency Care

First | Emergency care for a localized cold injury is as follows:

1. Perform a scene size-up, including scene safety and BSI.

2. Perform an initial assessment.

3. Make sure that someone alerts the EMS dispatcher.

4. Remove the patient from the cold environment.

Note

As a First Responder, never listen to bystanders' myths and folktales about the care of frostbite. *Never* rub a frostbitten or frozen area. Do not allow the patient to smoke or drink alcohol or caffeine. These substances may constrict blood vessels and worsen the condition.

Cold-Related Emergencies

CONDITION	SKIN SURFACE	TISSUE UNDER SKIN	SKIN COLOR
Early, Superficial	Soft	Soft	White
Late, Deep	Hard	Initially soft, progressing to hard	White and waxy progressing to blotchy white, then to yellow-gray to blue-gray

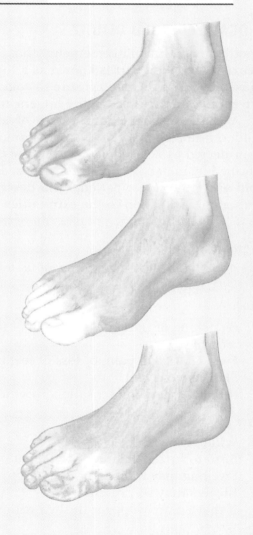

EARLY, SUPERFICIAL

Slow onset with numbing of affected part. Have the patient rewarm the part with his own body heat. Tingling and burning sensations are common during rewarming.

LATE, DEEP

Tissues below the surface initially will have their normal bounce. Protect the entire limb. Handle gently. Keep the patient at rest and provide external warmth to injury site. Untreated, this will progress to where the tissue below the surface will feel hard. Provide the same care you would for early superficial cooling. Immediate EMS transport is recommended.

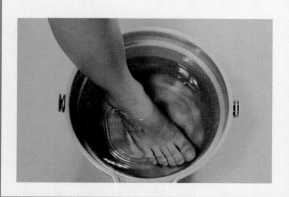

Rewarming: Only if transport is delayed in case of late or deep local cooling and if medical direction allows, rewarm the affected part by immersing it in warm water (100°F to 105°F). Do not allow the body part to touch the container bottom or side. After rewarming, gently dry the part and pad between fingers or toes. Dress the affected area, cover and elevate the limb, and keep the patient warm.

5. Protect the patient from further cold exposure.
6. Remove any wet or constrictive clothing.
7. If it is an *early* injury,
   – Manually stabilize the extremity.
   – Cover the extremity.
   – Do *not* rub or massage.
   – Do *not* re-expose to cold.
8. If it is a *late* injury
   – Remove jewelry.
   – Cover with dry, sterile dressings.
   – Do *not:*
      . . . Break blisters.
      . . . Rub or massage area.
      . . . Apply heat.
      . . . Rewarm. (Some jurisdictions allow rewarming. Check with medical direction.)
      . . . Allow the patient to walk on the affected extremity.
9. Comfort and reassure the patient.

BEHAVIORAL EMERGENCIES

Behavior is a manner in which a person acts or performs. This includes any or all activities of a person including physical and mental activity. The behavior of most people is considered **normal** because it is accepted by our families and society. It does not interfere with our daily activities of life.

As a First Responder, you might encounter patients whose behavior is unacceptable or intolerable to others. This is known as **abnormal behavior.** While caring for this type of patient might be challenging, it is crucial that you remain professional and provide appropriate care.

CAUSES

A **behavioral emergency** exists in situations where the patient exhibits abnormal behavior that is unacceptable or intolerable to the patient, family, or community. Such behavior may be because of extremes of emotion or a psychological or medical condition. Refer back to earlier portions of this chapter that discuss conditions such as heat exhaustion, hypothermia, or low blood sugar in diabetes. Other causes of behavioral change include:

1. Situational stress
2. Mind-altering substances
3. Psychiatric problems
4. Psychological crises
   a. Panic
   b. Agitation
   c. Bizarre thinking
   d. Danger to self
   e. Danger to others

FIGURE 10.10
Evaluate the scene and maintain a comfortable distance from the patient as you begin to ask questions and reassure the patient

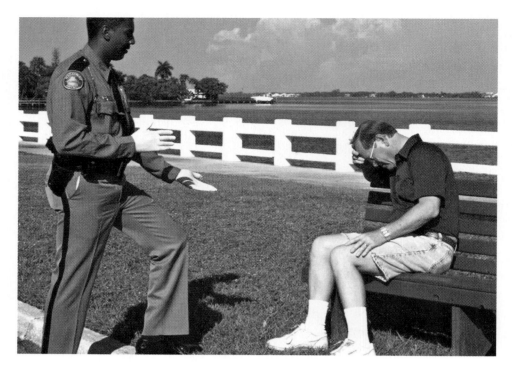

ASSESSMENT

 Remember, when performing an assessment on behavioral emergency patients (Figure 10.10):

- Identify yourself and let the person know you are there to help.
- Inform the person of what you are doing.
- Ask questions in a calm, reassuring voice.
- Without being judgmental, allow the patient to tell what happened.
- Show you are listening by rephrasing or repeating part of what is said.
- Assess the patient's mental status
  - Appearance
  - Activity
  - Speech
  - Orientation to person, place, time

EMERGENCY CARE

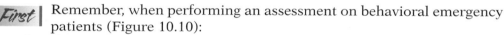 Emergency care methods to calm behavioral emergency patients include:

1. Perform a scene size-up, including scene safety and BSI.
2. Consider the need for law enforcement.
3. Make sure that someone has alerted the EMS dispatcher.
4. Perform an initial assessment.
5. Acknowledge that the person seems upset and restate that you are there to help.
6. Inform the person of what you are doing.
7. Ask questions in a calm, reassuring voice.
8. Maintain a comfortable distance.
9. Encourage the patient to state what is troubling him or her (Figure 10.11).

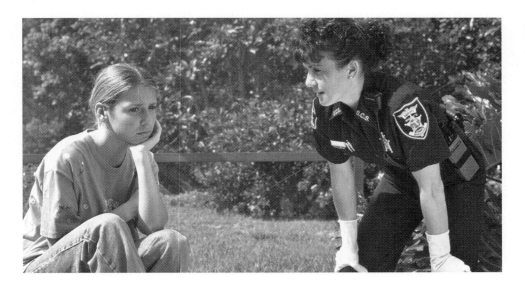

10. Do not make quick moves.

11. Answer questions honestly.

12. Do *not* threaten, challenge, or argue with disturbed patients.

13. Do *not* "play along" with hallucinations or auditory disturbances.

14. Involve trusted family members or friends.

15. Be prepared for an extended scene time.

16. Avoid unnecessary physical contact.

17. Maintain eye contact.

18. Leave yourself a way out. Never let the potentially violent patient come between you and your exit.

> **CAUTION:**
> If the patient creates an unsafe scene and you are not a trained law enforcement officer, *get out* and find a safe place until the police arrive.

*P*OTENTIAL VIOLENCE

Assessment

Sometimes patients experience such conditions that cause them to become violent and uncooperative. As a First Responder, your priority is to prevent the patient from harming himself or others while protecting yourself. Consider contacting law enforcement (Figure 10.12). You should also utilize the following when assessing the potential violence of patients:

■ **Scene size-up.** Use caution when approaching a scene. Observe the patient and the surroundings for any indication that he might be a danger

FIGURE 10.12
Law enforcement officers may be needed to approach and control a behavioral patient who may become violent.

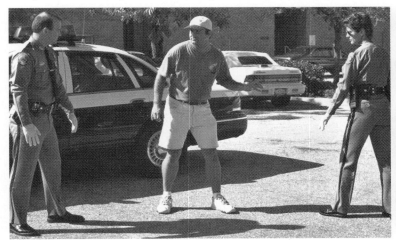
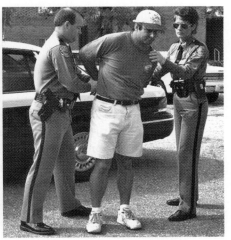

to himself or others. Assure that he has no weapons or anything that may be used as a weapon.

- **History.** Often, patients who have exhibited violent behavior in the past will repeat it again. Take such past history into consideration during your assessment.
- **Posture.** How is the patient standing? Is he in an offensive stance? What does his body language tell you? Are you positioned at a safe distance?
- **Verbal activity.** Often, verbal abuse is a precursor to violence. If a patient continues to use foul language or raise his voice, consider such action as a possible warning sign for violent behavior.
- **Physical activity.** Patients may begin to pace or wave their arms in the air with increased activity. Such movements may escalate into more violent behavior.

Restraining Patients

In some cases, behavioral emergency patients might become violent to the point that it is necessary to physically restrain them. While this task should be avoided, it is often necessary to protect the patient, yourself, and/or others. If you make the decision that it is necessary to restrain a patient, it is typically because the patient is a danger to self or others. In these situations, follow your local guidelines for contacting police and consulting medical direction. Remember that there may be a medical condition causing the emotional disturbance that the patient is not aware of, does not understand, or cannot control. Because of this, emotionally disturbed patients may threaten those who are trying to help and will often resist treatment.

You cannot treat a patient without consent, so in order to provide care, you must have a reasonable belief that the patient will harm himself or others and would want help if he were able to understand and consent to help. Contact medical direction for guidance and before attempting to treat or transport a patient without consent. In these cases, local protocols may direct you to contact law enforcement for assistance. You do not want to approach a violent patient alone. While waiting for assistance, try the following:

- Talk and listen to the patient to divert his focus and keep him from harming himself and others.
- Sit or stand passively but remain alert to the patient's actions and responses.
- Avoid any action that may alarm the patient and cause him to react violently.
- Wait for law enforcement assistance to arrive if restraining the patient is necessary and let the police officers take the lead in restraining the patient.
- Use reasonable force only to defend yourself against attack.

ALCOHOL AND OTHER DRUGS

For all situations involving patients with alcohol or other drug emergencies, perform your scene size-up. Your safety is especially important. Once you can approach the patient, let him know who you are and what you are going to do before you start the initial assessment and focused history and physical exam. You may have to modify your approach and communication techniques as you try to determine whether the situation also involves a medical or a trauma problem. It may be difficult to perform the detailed physical exam, the ongoing assessment, or any care procedures until you can calm the patient and gain his confidence.

ALCOHOL ABUSE

Alcohol is a drug, socially acceptable in moderation, but still a drug. Abuse of alcohol, as with any other drug, can lead to illness, poisoning of the body, antisocial behavior, and even death. A patient under the influence of alcohol is not funny. He or she may have a medical problem or an injury requiring your care. The patient may be injured or could hurt others while under the influence of alcohol.

As a First Responder, try to provide care for the patient suffering from alcohol abuse as you would any other patient. Quickly determine that the problem has been caused by alcohol and that alcohol abuse is the only problem. Remember, diabetes, epilepsy, head injuries, high fevers, and other medical problems may make the patient appear drunk. If the patient allows you to do so, conduct a patient assessment that includes an interview. In some cases, you will have to depend on bystanders for meaningful information.

Signs

 The signs of alcohol abuse in an intoxicated patient may include:

- The odor of alcohol on the patient's breath or clothing. This is not enough by itself unless you are sure that this is not "acetone breath," a sign of the diabetic patient.
- Swaying and unsteady, uncoordinated movement
- Slurred speech and the inability to carry on a conversation. Do not be fooled into thinking that the situation may not be serious because the patient jokes or clowns around.
- A flushed appearance, often with the patient sweating and complaining of being warm
- Nausea and vomiting or feeling the need to vomit

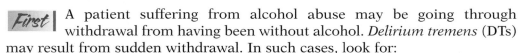 A patient suffering from alcohol abuse may be going through withdrawal from having been without alcohol. *Delirium tremens* (DTs) may result from sudden withdrawal. In such cases, look for:

- Confusion and restlessness
- Atypical behavior, to the point of being "mad" or demonstrating "insane" behavior
- Some DT patients will hallucinate.
- Gross tremor (obvious shaking) of the hands

As you see, some of the signs displayed in alcohol abuse are similar to those found in medical emergencies. **Be certain that the only problem is alcohol abuse.** Remember, persons who abuse alcohol may also be injured or ill. The effects of the alcohol may mask the typical signs and symptoms used in assessment. Also, be on the alert for other signs, such as depressed vital signs because of the patient mixing alcohol and drugs. Never ask if the patient has taken any "drugs." The patient may think that you are gathering evidence of a crime. Ask if any "medications" have been taken while drinking. Most patients, however, will not report recreational drugs or even over-the-counter medications when questioned in this way.

Emergency Care

 The basic care for the alcohol abuse patient consists of the following:

- Perform a proper history and physical exam to detect any medical emergencies or injuries. Remember, alcohol may mask pain. Look carefully for mechanisms of injury and the signs of illness.

- Monitor vital signs, staying alert for respiratory problems.
- Talk in an effort to keep the patient alert.
- Help the patient when vomiting so the vomitus will not be aspirated (inhaled).
- Protect the patient from further injury without the illegal use of restraint.
- Alert dispatch and let them decide if the police must be alerted or if EMTs are to respond on their own.

DRUG ABUSE

First | Drugs may be simply classified as uppers, downers, narcotics, hallucinogens (mind-affecting drugs), or volatile chemicals. **Uppers** are stimulants affecting the nervous system to excite the user. **Downers** are depressants meant to affect the central nervous system to relax the user. **Narcotics** affect the nervous system and change many of the normal activities of the body. Often they produce an intense state of relaxation and feelings of well-being. **Hallucinogens,** or mind-altering drugs, act on the nervous system to produce an intense state of excitement or distortion of the user's surroundings. **Volatile chemicals** give an initial rush, but then depress the central nervous system.

Some courses that train rescuers, EMTs, and others in the EMS system have spent considerable time in the past teaching specific drug names and reactions. As a First Responder, you will not need such knowledge. For you, it is important to be able to detect possible drug abuse at the overdose level and to relate certain signs to certain types of drugs. Your care for the drug abuse patient will be basically the same for all drugs and will not change unless you are ordered to do something by a poison control or drug abuse center. Figure 10.13 and Table 10-3 provide some of the names and illustrations of common drugs being abused. You do not need to memorize the chart.

Signs and Symptoms

The signs and symptoms of drug abuse and drug overdose can vary from patient to patient, even for the same drug. The scene, bystanders, and the patient may be your only sources for finding out if you are dealing with drug abuse and the substance involved. When questioning the patient and bystanders, you will get better results if you ask if the patient has been taking any medications, rather than using the word "drugs." If you have any doubts, then ask if the patient has taken drugs or is "using anything." Patients may not give information about their drug use.

First | Some significant signs and symptoms related to specific drugs include:
- *Uppers*—excitement, increased pulse and breathing rates, rapid speech, dry mouth, dilated pupils, sweating, and the complaint of having gone without sleep for long periods.
- *Downers*—sluggish, sleepy patient lacking normal coordination of body movements and speaking with slurred speech. Pulse and breathing rates are low, often to the point of a true emergency.
- *Hallucinogens*—fast pulse rate, dilated pupils, and a flushed face. The patient often "sees" things, hears voices or sounds that do not exist, has little concept of real time, and may not be aware of the true environment. Often, the patient makes no sense when speaking. Many show signs of anxiety and fearfulness. They have been described as "paranoid." Some patients become very aggressive, while others tend to withdraw.

upper a stimulant that will affect the central nervous system to excite the user.

downer a depressant that will depress the central nervous system to relax the user.

narcotic a class of drugs for the relief of pain that affects the central nervous system. Illicit use is to provide an intense state of relaxation.

hallucinogen a mind-altering drug that acts on the central nervous system to excite the user or to distort his or her surroundings.

volatile chemicals vaporizing chemicals that will cause excitement or produce a "high" when they are inhaled by the abuser.

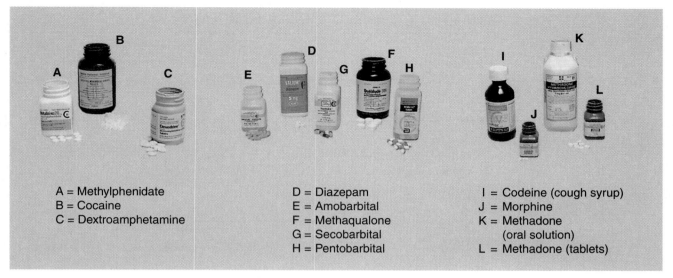

FIGURE 10.13
Abused substances.

A = Methylphenidate
B = Cocaine
C = Dextroamphetamine

D = Diazepam
E = Amobarbital
F = Methaqualone
G = Secobarbital
H = Pentobarbital

I = Codeine (cough syrup)
J = Morphine
K = Methadone
      (oral solution)
L = Methadone (tablets)

- *Narcotics*—reduced rate of pulse and breathing, often seen with a lowered skin temperature. The pupils are constricted, muscles are relaxed, and sweating is heavy. The patient is very sleepy and does not wish to do anything. In overdoses, coma is a common event. Respiratory arrest may occur.
- *Volatile chemicals*—dazed or showing temporary loss of contact with reality. The patient may go into a coma. The inside of the nose and mouth may show swollen membranes. The patient may complain of a "funny numb feeling" or "tingling" inside the head or a headache. The face may be flushed and the pulse rate accelerated. There may be a chemical odor to the patient's breath, skin, or clothing.

These signs and symptoms have a lot in common with many medical emergencies. *Never* assume drug abuse or drug abuse occurring by itself.

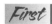 Withdrawal varies from patient to patient and from drug to drug. In most cases of drug withdrawal, you will see shaking, anxiety, nausea, confusion, irritability, sweating, and increased pulse and breathing rates.

Emergency Care

First When providing care for drug abuse patients, you should:

1. Provide life-support measures if required.
2. Alert dispatch as soon as possible. They should be informed that the problem may be caused by drugs.
3. Monitor vital signs and be alert for respiratory arrest.
4. Talk to the patient to gain his confidence and to maintain his level of consciousness.
5. Protect the patient from further harm.
6. Provide care for shock.
7. Continue to reassure the patient throughout all phases of care.

Your area may wish to have First Responders induce vomiting if an overdose was taken within 30 minutes of your arrival at the scene. Your instructor will give you the rules and exceptions for your area. In most cases, vomiting is

Note
Many drug abusers will abuse more than one drug, often mixing several at one time. It may be impossible through simple physical examination to tell what drugs are causing the patient's problem.

Note
For all cases of possible drug overdose, first contact medical direction. Then contact your local poison control center if directed to do so.

TABLE 10-3: *C*OMMONLY ABUSED SUBSTANCES

UPPERS

Amphetamine (Benzedrine, bennies, pep pills, ups, uppers, cartwheels)
Biphetamine (bam)
Cocaine (coke, snow, crack)
Desoxyn (black beauties)
Dextroamphetamine (dexies, Dexedrine)
Methamphetamine (speed, meth, crystal, diet pills, Methedrine)
Methylphenidate (Ritalin)
Preludin

DOWNERS

Amobarbital (blue devils, downers, barbs, Amytal)
Barbiturates (downers, dolls, barbs, rainbows)
Chloral hydrate (knockout drops, Noctec)
Ethchlorvynol (Placidyl)
Glutethimide (doriden, goofers)
Methaqualone (Quaalude, ludes, Sopor, sopors)
Nonbarbiturate sedatives (various tranquilizers and sleeping pills; Valium or Diazepam, Miltown, Equanil, meprobamate, Thorazine, Compazine, Librium or chlordiazepoxide, reserpine, Tranxene or chlorazepate, and other benzodiazepines)

NARCOTICS

Codeine (often in cough syrup)	Morphine
Demerol	Opium (op, poppy)
Dilaudid	Meperidine
Heroin (H, horse, junk, smack, stuff)	Paregoric (contains opium)
Methadone (dolly)	

HALLUCINOGENS AND MIND-ALTERING DRUGS

Hallucinogenic	Psilocybin (magic mushrooms)
DMT	STP (serenity, tranquility, peace)
LSD (acid, sunshine)	*Nonhallucinogenic*
Mescaline (peyote, mesc)	Marijuana (grass, pot, weed, dope)
Morning glory seeds	Hash
PCP (angel dust, hog, peace pills)	THC

VOLATILE CHEMICALS

Cleaning fluid (carbon tetrachloride)	Nail polish remover
Furniture polish	Paint thinner
Gasoline	Amyl nitrate (snappers, poppers)
Glue	Butyl nitrate (locker room, rush)
Hair spray	

REMEMBER: The most commonly abused substance in the United States is alcohol (ethanol). In addition to its direct effects, alcohol is often mixed with other abused substances, worsening both short- and long-term effects on the body.

induced the same as in cases of ingested poisons. For all cases of possible drug overdose, it is good practice to contact medical direction and your local poison control center.

CAUTION: Many drug abusers may appear calm at first and then become violent as time passes. Always be on the alert and be ready to protect yourself. If the patient creates an unsafe scene and you are not a trained law enforcement officer, *get out* and find a safe place to wait until the police arrive.

CAUTION: PCP is a dangerous drug that is being abused more and more each year. Patients on PCP can be very dangerous, even though they may appear calm when you arrive. If PCP is the cause of the problem, wait for police to arrive, unless the patient is unconscious or in need of life-support measures. PCP usage leads to aggressive behavior. The drug can build up in the body and cause a violent reaction without warning. Many patients on PCP no longer display the qualities considered "human." Always consider a PCP user to be dangerous.

Summary

Various illnesses and conditions can bring about a **medical emergency.** The signs and symptoms gained from patient assessment and history-taking will help you recognize a medical emergency. Abnormal pulse, breathing, temperature, and skin color are some of the important signs in determining a medical emergency. Note lip color, any odors of the breath, abdominal tenderness, nausea, vomiting, bleeding, and altered mental status, which are also important signs. Listen to the patient and bystanders for reports of other symptoms, including pain, fever, nausea, dizziness, shortness of breath, problems with bowel and bladder activities, burning sensations, thirst, hunger, and odd tastes in the mouth. Look for medical identification devices and question the patient. There may be medication that should be taken during medical emergencies.

If the patient appears or "feels" unusual or has unusual vital signs and there is no injury present as a result of an accident, assume that there is a medical emergency. An accident may mask a medical emergency or problem that caused the accident. Always check for medical emergencies.

Consider chest pain in any patient as a possible **heart attack.** Ask if the patient has chest, arm, neck, and jaw pains. Nausea, shortness of breath, sweating, weakness, and restlessness also may indicate a heart attack. Alert the EMS dispatcher. Keep the patient at rest and in a position to ease difficult breathing. Loosen restrictive clothing and prevent chill. Monitor vital signs and provide emotional support.

Respiratory difficulties, including those seen in **congestive heart failure,** may produce the same signs and symptoms regardless of the cause of the distress. Check for labored breathing, unusual breath sounds, rate, and quality. Make sure there is no airway obstruction. Skin color change is an important sign in serious cases. Check for altered mental status. Look for swelling at the ankles and engorged neck veins, which indicate congestive heart failure.

In all cases of respiratory difficulty, have someone call dispatch. Breathing can either be *adequate* or *inadequate,* so care for all respiratory difficulty cases: maintain an open airway and check that nothing is causing an allergic reaction. Place the patient in a sitting position and conserve body heat. Keep the patient at rest and provide emotional support.

Numerous conditions may cause a patient to experience an **altered mental status:** seizures, strokes, diabetic emergencies, poisonings, breathing problems, and cardiac

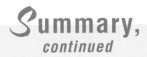

events. Signs and symptoms may include dizziness, impaired speech, hearing loss, confusion, or rapid mood changes. To check patient status, use the AVPU process to categorize a patient's level of consciousness: Alert, Verbal, Painful, Unresponsive.

A **stroke** patient may complain of nothing more than a headache. Consider all headaches to be a serious complaint. In case of possible stroke, you may notice altered mental status, numbness or paralysis, speech or vision difficulty, confusion, convulsions, breathing difficulty, and unequal pupils. Maintain an open airway, keep the patient at rest, and place in the recovery position. Protect all paralyzed limbs. Provide emotional support and monitor vital signs.

A **seizure** patient may have a sudden loss of consciousness and collapse. The body will stiffen and there may be a loss of bowel and bladder control. Convulsions may occur, followed by body limpness. On regaining consciousness, the patient is usually confused and tired. Protect the patient from physical harm during the seizure and from embarrassment after the seizure. Keep the patient at rest.

Diabetics may have trouble with **hyperglycemia** or **hypoglycemia.** In both cases, the patient may become unresponsive and go into a coma. In severe hyperglycemia, expect to find labored breathing with a fruity or sweet odor on the breath, rapid and weak pulse, and dry and warm skin. In severe hypoglycemia, there is no labored breathing and no fruity odor, but the pulse is full and rapid, and skin is cold and moist. The only indication of a diabetes-related problem may be an altered mental status. Alert the EMS dispatcher and keep the patient at rest. When in doubt as to whether the condition is hyperglycemia or hypoglycemia, give the patient sugar.

In cases of **acute abdomen,** keep the patient at rest and as comfortable as possible. Monitor for vomiting, give nothing by mouth, and alert the EMS dispatcher.

Anaphylactic (allergy) shock is a life-threatening emergency. It is brought about when people come into contact with a substance to which they are allergic (bee stings, insect bites, chemicals, foods, dusts, pollens, drugs). Signs may include burning or itching skin, breaking out (hives), rapid and difficult breathing, very weak pulse, swelling of the face and tongue, blue lips, and sudden loss of consciousness. Care for anaphylactic shock is the same as for other cases of shock. Transport the patient to a hospital as soon as possible and care for the patient according to local protocol. Ask the patient about allergies during the interview. Be certain to look for a medical identification device.

When dealing with a possible **poisoning,** look for evidence of the nature of the poison. Signs and symptoms associated with **ingested poisons** include burns or stains around the patient's mouth, unusual breathing and pulse rate, and sweating. Abdominal pain, nausea, and vomiting are common. (Save all vomitus.) **Inhaled poisons** can cause shortness of breath or coughing, irritated eyes, rapid or slow pulse rate, and changes in skin color. **Absorbed poisons** can be severe, irritating or damaging the skin and eyes. **Injected poisons** usually cause pain and swelling at the site, difficulty breathing, and unusual pulse rate.

In cases of poisoning, contact the poison control center and medical direction. (Follow your EMS guidelines.) Emergency care of ingested poisons may include diluting with water or milk, or using activated charcoal to absorb the poison. Be prepared for vomiting. If an unconscious patient vomits or convulses, assure an open airway and alert EMTs.

In cases of inhaled poisons, remove the patient from the source (when safe to do so), provide life-support measures as needed, and remove contaminated clothing. For absorbed poisons, remove the patient from the source, flood with water all areas of the

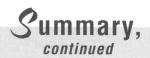

body that came into contact with the poison, and remove contaminated clothing and jewelry. When providing care for injected poisons other than snakebite, care for shock, scrape away stingers and venom sacs, and place an ice bag or cold pack over the area. For snakebite, keep the patient calm and lying down, clean the site, keep bitten extremities immobilized, alert the dispatcher, and provide care for shock.

A hot and humid environment can cause the body to generate too much heat, which can create an abnormally high body temperature, known as **hyperthermia.** **Heat exhaustion** results from prolonged exposure to heat, which creates moist, pale skin that may feel normal or cool to the touch. Signs and symptoms include excessive sweating, rapid weak pulse, weakness, and possible altered level of consciousness. **Heat stroke** results from prolonged exposure to heat and causes hot, dry or moist skin, altered mental status, and rapid breathing. This is a life-threatening emergency. Emergency care for heat emergencies includes removing patients from the hot environment, cooling them with water, and fanning them. Alert the dispatcher.

In cold environments, body heat can be lost faster than it can be generated. Rapid heat loss creates a state of low body temperature known as **hypothermia,** or a **generalized cold emergency.** Patients will have cool skin temperature, shivering, decreased mental status, stiff or rigid posture, and poor judgment. The temperature does not have to be below freezing for hypothermia to occur. Another environmental emergency that is characterized by the freezing or near freezing of a body part is known as a **localized cold injury,** or **frostbite.** Frostbite patients will experience a feeling of cold followed by pain and finally numbness or tingling. Emergency care includes removing the patient from the cold environment, removing any wet clothes, keeping the patient calm and warm, and stabilizing any cold extremity.

First Responders might encounter patients whose behavior is unacceptable or intolerable to others. This is known as **abnormal behavior.** There are many causes for a patient to act in this manner, such as stress, mind-altering substances, psychiatric problems, psychological crises, and medical causes. When assessing a patient with abnormal behavior, it is important to:

- Identify yourself and let the person know you are there to help.
- Inform the person of what you are doing.
- Ask questions in a calm, reassuring voice.
- Without being judgmental, allow the patient to tell what happened.
- Show you are listening by rephrasing or repeating what is said.
- Assess the patient's mental status.

Patients may experience conditions that cause them to become violent and uncooperative. Exercise caution in approaching these patients during the scene size-up. Consider any past history of behavioral difficulties or violence. Remember that a patient's posture and verbal activity may be warning signs of potential violent behavior. Notify law enforcement to assist you in dealing with these patients.

In some cases, behavioral emergency patients might become violent to the point that it is necessary to physically restrain them, but the patient must be endangering himself or others in order for First Responders to have the legal right to restrain him.

Patients suffering from **alcohol abuse** should receive the same professional level of care as any other patient. The problem may be because of alcohol or alcohol withdrawal, but there may be a medical problem or injuries. Try to detect the odor of alcohol, slurred speech, swaying, and unsteadiness of movement. Find out if the patient is nauseated. Be alert for vomiting. In cases of alcohol withdrawal, look for tremors that

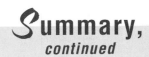

may indicate the DTs. In all cases of alcohol abuse, monitor vital signs and be alert for respiratory arrest.

Drug abuse can show itself in many ways, depending on the drug, the patient, and whether it is withdrawal or overdose. Withdrawal from most drugs will produce shaking, anxiety, nausea, confusion, irritability, sweating, and increased pulse and breathing rates.

Uppers usually speed up activity, speech, pulse, and breathing, and tend to excite the user. **Downers** do just the opposite. **Hallucinogens** increase pulse rate, dilate pupils, and cause the patient to see things and lose touch with reality. **Narcotics** reduce pulse and breathing rates. The pupils are usually constricted. The patient may appear sleepy and may not wish to do anything. **Volatile chemicals** act as depressants, causing the patient to be dazed.

In cases of drug overdose or drug withdrawal, provide life support as needed and alert the dispatcher. Monitor vital signs and talk to the patient. Protect the patient and provide care for shock. Reassure the patient through the entire process.

Remember and Consider...

Medical emergencies are very common. As a First Responder, you will more than likely encounter many patients with medical complaints. In this chapter and in your classes, you will discuss how to assess these patients and manage certain specific conditions. Remember the overview of medical emergencies and how to approach a victim with a generalized medical complaint or a specific illness.

✔ What will you do for a victim of a seizure in a public place?

✔ What are the various causes of an altered mental status?

✔ Are your CPR skills up-to-date?

✔ How do you feel about treating a patient with a behavioral emergency?

You should feel comfortable answering these questions. Review what you have learned in this chapter and in class and try applying it to your life. How will these things be useful to you, your coworkers, family, friends, and others?

Investigate...

Regardless of where you live or what type of job you have, you should be prepared to handle any medical emergency. Remember, by definition, an emergency happens when and where you least expect it. There are several things you may be able to predict and prepare for ahead of time, based on the area in which you live. For example, many areas in the United States are exposed to extreme heat and humidity conditions.

✔ What are the major types of medical emergencies you might encounter in your area?

✔ What can you do to prepare for an emergency in your area or organization?

CHAPTER 11

BLEEDING AND SOFT-TISSUE INJURIES

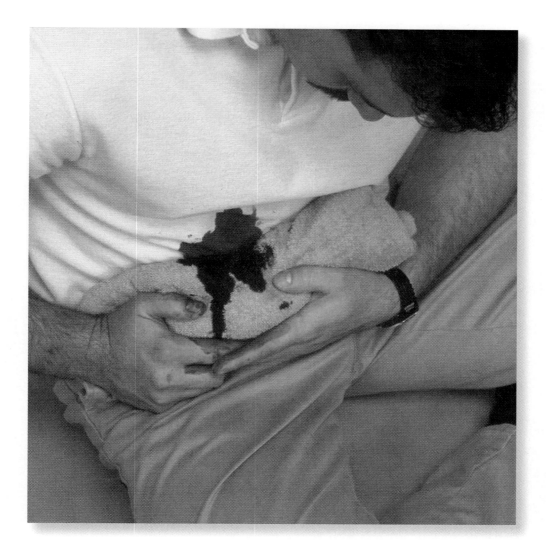

*A*ccidents are responsible for thousands of cases of bleeding and soft-tissue injuries every year. Early assessment and intervention is crucial in order to properly care for these patients. As a First Responder, you must know how the body responds to bleeding and how to provide care for bleeding victims. This chapter covers bleeding, shock, and various soft-tissue injuries and provides the knowledge and skills you will need to care for such emergencies.

National Standard Objectives

This chapter focuses on the objectives of Module 5, Lesson 5–2 of the U.S. DOT First Responder National Curriculum and serves as an instructional aid to help you meet any specific objectives added to the course by your local EMS system.

By the end of this chapter, you will know how to (from cognitive or knowledge information) . . .

5–2.1	Differentiate between arterial, venous, and capillary bleeding. (pp. 302–303)
5–2.2	State the emergency medical care for external bleeding. (pp. 304–317)
5–2.3	Establish the relationship between body substance isolation (BSI) and bleeding. (pp. 301–302, 304)
5–2.4	List the signs of internal bleeding. (pp. 316, 318–320)
5–2.5	List the steps in the emergency medical care of the patient with signs and symptoms of internal bleeding. (p. 321)
5–2.6	Establish the relationship between body substance isolation (BSI) and soft-tissue injuries. (p. 335)
5–2.7	State the types of open soft-tissue injuries. (pp. 331–333)
5–2.8	Describe the emergency medical care of the patient with a soft-tissue injury. (pp. 333–349)
5–2.9	Discuss the emergency medical care considerations for a patient with a penetrating chest injury. (pp. 349–352)
5–2.10	State the emergency medical care considerations for a patient with an open wound to the abdomen. (pp. 352–353)
5–2.11	Describe the emergency medical care for an impaled object. (pp. 336, 340–341, 342, 352)
5–2.12	State the emergency medical care for an amputation. (p. 338)
5–2.13	Describe the emergency medical care for burns. (pp. 357–362)
5–2.14	List the functions of dressing and bandaging. (pp. 306, 312–316)

Feel comfortable enough to (by changing attitude, values, beliefs) . . .

5–2.15	Explain the rationale for body substance isolation when dealing with bleeding and soft-tissue injuries. (pp. 302, 304, 335)

	5–2.16	Attend to the feelings of the patient with a soft-tissue injury or bleeding. (pp. 329, 337, 338, 342, 354, 362)
	5–2.17	Demonstrate a caring attitude towards patients with a soft-tissue injury or bleeding who requests emergency medical services. (pp. 329, 337, 338, 342, 354, 362)
	5–2.18	Place the interests of the patient with a soft-tissue injury or bleeding as the foremost consideration when making any and all patient-care decisions. (pp. 302, 310, 312, 316, 318, 321–322, 333–334, 361)
	5–2.19	Communicate with empathy to patients with a soft-tissue injury or bleeding, as well as with family members and friends of the patient. (pp. 329, 337, 338, 342, 354, 362)
Show how to (through psychomotor skills) . . .	5–2.20	Demonstrate direct pressure as a method of emergency medical care for external bleeding. (pp. 304–305, 306–307)
	5–2.21	Demonstrate the use of diffuse pressure as a method of emergency medical care for external bleeding. (pp. 304–305, 306–307)
	5–2.22	Demonstrate the use of pressure points as a method of emergency medical care for external bleeding. (pp. 304, 305, 307–310)
	5–2.23	Demonstrate the care of the patient exhibiting signs and symptoms of internal bleeding. (pp. 321, 326, 328–329)
	5–2.24	Demonstrate the steps in the emergency medical care of open soft-tissue injuries. (pp. 333–349)
	5–2.25	Demonstrate the steps in the emergency medical care of a patient with an open chest wound. (pp. 349–352)
	5–2.26	Demonstrate the steps in the emergency medical care of a patient with open abdominal wounds. (p. 353)
	5–2.27	Demonstrate the steps in the emergency medical care of a patient with an impaled object. (pp. 336–337, 340–341, 342, 352)
	5–2.28	Demonstrate the steps in the emergency medical care of a patient with an amputation. (p. 338)
	5–2.29	Demonstrate the steps in the emergency medical care of an amputated part. (p. 338)

LEARNING TASKS

This chapter explains the functions of blood and the blood vessels, and describes the effects bleeding has on the body. You will need to understand the relationship between profuse bleeding and shock. As you work through this chapter, you will also need to know and recognize:

✔ The difference between internal and external bleeding and what actions should be taken for each during the initial assessment.

✔ The methods used to control **profuse** bleeding versus the methods used to control **mild** bleeding.

You will learn how to perform the steps of controlling bleeding, including:

✔ How to apply a pressure dressing.

✔ The use of elevation in controlling external bleeding, including the situations when elevation should *not* be used.

✔ The use of the two major pressure point sites used by First Responders.

✔ Why tourniquets are used as a last resort, only after other methods to control bleeding have failed.

✔ The step-by-step procedure for applying a tourniquet, including all precautions for the procedure.

✔ The procedures used to care for:

- cuts, burns, and foreign objects in the eye

- impaled objects

- injuries to the ear

- nosebleeds and other nonfracture injuries to the nose

- injuries to the mouth

- venous bleeding from the neck

- injuries to the genitalia

It will be important for you to learn about internal bleeding, what causes it, and how it can affect the body. As you gain knowledge, you will also be able to:

✔ List various conditions associated with internal bleeding.

✔ Define shock.

✔ List the signs and symptoms of shock.

✔ Describe the step-by-step procedures used in treating shock.

✔ Describe how to reduce a patient's chances of fainting.

As you work through this chapter, you will learn about the assessment and treatment for burns and will be able to:

✔ Distinguish among superficial, partial-thickness, and full-thickness burns.

✔ Use the rule of nines.

✔ Demonstrate the appropriate dressings for burn injuries.

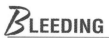

BLEEDING

THE HEART

The heart is the center of the circulatory system. It pumps blood with its nutrients and oxygen as fuel through the many miles and types of vessels to all the body's tissues, organs, and systems. If the heart stops functioning, as in cardiac arrest, blood does not circulate, or carry the blood and its fuel to the body's parts, and they die. The heart has four separate chambers (Figure 11.1A). The top two chambers are called *atria* (plural), or the right and left *atrium* (singular). The right atrium receives unoxygenated blood from the body; the left atrium receives oxygenated blood from the lungs. Each atrium pumps blood to the ventricle below it. The bottom two chambers are called *ventricles* (plural), or the right and left ventricle (singular). The right ventricle receives the unoxygenated blood from the right atrium and pumps it to the lungs through the *pulmonary artery* (the only artery that carries unoxygenated blood and is named so because *arteries* carry blood away from the heart). The left ventricle receives oxygenated blood from the left atrium, which received it from the lungs through the *pulmonary vein* (the only vein that carries oxygenated blood and so named because *veins* carry blood to the heart). The ventricles are larger than the atria because they do the harder (and unending) task of pumping blood to the lungs and body. The atria only have to pump blood to the ventricles below them.

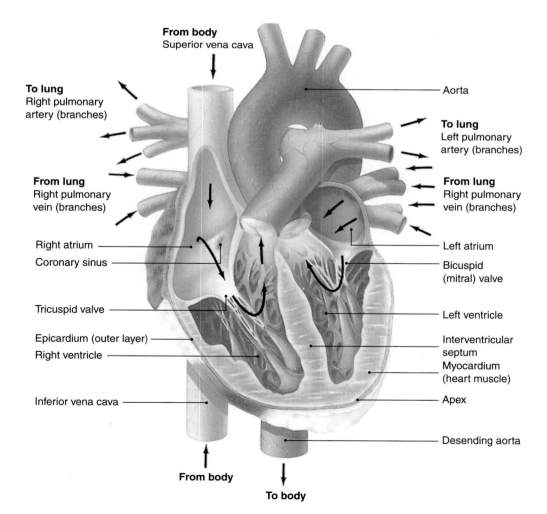

From body
Superior vena cava

To lung
Right pulmonary
artery (branches)

From lung
Right pulmonary
vein (branches)

Right atrium

Coronary sinus

Tricuspid valve

Epicardium (outer layer)

Right ventricle

Inferior vena cava

From body

To body

Aorta

To lung
Left pulmonary
artery (branches)

From lung
Right pulmonary
vein (branches)

Left atrium

Bicuspid
(mitral) valve

Left ventricle

Interventricular
septum
Myocardium
(heart muscle)

Apex

Desending aorta

FIGURE 11.1A
The heart.

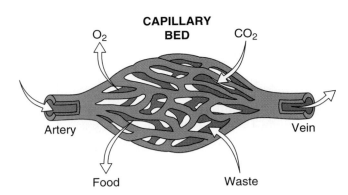

FIGURE 11.1B
The blood vessels.

CAPILLARY BED

O_2 CO_2

Artery   Vein

Food   Waste

THE BLOOD

Blood performs many invaluable functions necessary to sustain life. Blood carries oxygen to the body's cells and carries away carbon dioxide (Figure 11.1B). It transports nutrients to the cells and carries away certain waste products. The blood contains cells that destroy bacteria and cells that produce substances to help you resist infection (immunity). There are elements in the blood that act with chemical factors and calcium to enmesh blood cells and form a sticky clot around cuts to help control bleeding. Compounds carried in the blood called *hormones,* such as insulin, regulate most body activities. Without blood circulating through your body, you would quickly die.

First | The functions of blood are to:

■ carry oxygen and carbon dioxide (Respiration)
■ carry food to the tissues (Nutrition)
■ carry wastes from the tissues to the organs of excretion—kidneys, lungs, and skin (Excretion)
■ carry hormones, water, salts, and other compounds needed to keep the body's functions in balance (Body Regulation)
■ protect against disease-causing organisms (Defense)

Blood contains red blood cells, white blood cells, and elements involved in forming blood clots. All of these are carried by a watery, salty fluid called **plasma,** which comprises over half of the blood volume. The volume of blood in the typical adult's body is approximately 6 liters (about 12 pints). When bleeding occurs, the body not only loses blood cells and clotting elements, it also loses plasma and total blood volume. This loss can be very significant since the volume of blood must be maintained at a certain level in order to have proper heart action, blood flow, and exchange between the blood and the body's cells. The body has more blood than is needed to produce minimum circulation. During bleeding, once this reserve is gone, the patient experiences circulatory system collapse, followed very quickly by death. See Table 11-1 for blood volumes and lethal blood loss volumes for adults, children, and infants.

BLOOD VESSELS

Arteries carry blood away from the heart and to the tissues, organs, and systems of the body. The largest artery is the **aorta** (Figure 11.1A). The smallest artery is called an *arteriole.* All other sizes are just referred to as *arteries.* At certain points on the body, where arteries are close to the skin surface, you

REMEMBER:

The typical adult has 6 liters (about 12 pints) of blood. This volume must be maintained for proper circulatory function.

plasma (PLAZ-mah)
the fluid portion of the blood; the blood minus the blood cells and other structures.

artery any blood vessel that carries blood away from the heart.

TABLE 11-1: Blood Volumes and Serious Blood Loss

PATIENT	TOTAL BLOOD VOLUME	LETHAL BLOOD LOSS (RAPID)
Adult male (154 pounds)	6.6 liters	2.2 liters
Adolescent (105 pounds)	3.3 liters	1.3 liters
Child (early to late child-hood: depends on size)	1.5 to 2.0 liters	0.5 to 0.7 liters
Infant (newborn, normal weight range)	300+ milliliters	30 to 50 milliliters

Note: One liter equals about 2 pints. One milliliter is about the same as 20 drops from a medicine dropper.

can feel the blood pumping through the artery. These points are called *pulse points*, places where you can feel the heart as a pump at work and where you take a pulse rate (see Chapter 7).

Veins carry blood from the tissues, organs, and systems of the body back to the heart. The largest veins are the **superior** and **inferior** vena cava (Figure 11.1A). The smallest vein is called a *venule*. All other sizes are just referred to as *veins*. On some parts of the arms (inside wrist and elbow) and legs (lower leg and ankle), and sometimes the face (temple), you can see the blue of veins showing through skin where they are close to the surface. Veins appear blue because they are carrying unoxygenated blood.

vein any blood vessel that returns blood to the heart.

The oxygen and nutrients carried by arteries are passed off to body cells when the blood reaches a small system of vessels called **capillaries.** Capillaries act as an exchange for nutrients and wastes. Some of our organs act as disposal and maintenance organs, such as the kidneys and liver, but the heart is the organ that works with the lungs to replenish the oxygen. Since the blood has dropped off all its supply of oxygen for the body's cells to use, unoxygenated blood travels from the capillary system into the veins and back to the heart, through the lungs to pick up oxygen, and back to the heart again to be pumped through vessels to the body. By the time blood reaches the capillaries, pressure and speed are greatly reduced and the beating action of the heart no longer causes pulsations. Blood moving through the capillaries in a constant flow is called **perfusion.** (A reduction in blood volume can seriously affect perfusion.)

capillary the microscopic blood vessels that connect arteries to veins; where exchange takes place between the bloodstream and the body tissues.

First | For now, you should know:

- *Arteries*—carry blood away from the heart
- *Veins*—return blood to the heart
- *Capillaries*—where oxygen, nutrient, and waste exchange takes place

perfusion the constant flow of blood through the capillaries.

General Considerations

Having an idea of how blood and blood vessels work within the body will assist you in assessing patients with bleeding problems. Keep these general considerations in mind while learning how to treat these patients:

- *Body substance isolation (BSI)*—The risk of infectious disease should be kept at the forefront when treating bleeding patients. BSI precautions must be taken routinely to avoid skin and mucous contact with bodily fluids. Gloves should be used on every patient encounter and additional equipment (goggles, gown, mask) used in situations in which there is an increased risk of contact with blood or other body fluids (for example, childbirth).
- *Severity of blood loss*—The severity of blood loss should be based on the patient's signs and symptoms and an estimation of blood loss. If signs and symptoms of shock are present, bleeding should be considered serious.
- *Body's normal response to bleeding*—The body's natural response to bleeding is blood vessel constriction and clotting. In cases of major bleeding, however, clotting might not occur. The factors affecting the body's response will be discussed throughout this chapter.

First Uncontrolled bleeding should be taken seriously. If not stopped, it will lead to shock and subsequent death.

TYPES OF BLEEDING

Bleeding can be classified as **external** or **internal.** Both kinds are based on the type of blood vessel involved. Since a discussion of the vessels involved in internal bleeding is not very practical for First Responders, only external bleeding will be considered in relation to blood vessel type. Both kinds of bleeding will be presented in terms of assessment and care.

EXTERNAL BLEEDING

First External bleeding may be classified by the First Responder as (Figure 11.2):
- *Arterial bleeding*—Blood is *spurting* from an artery, often pulsating as the heart beats. The color of the blood is bright red since it contains oxygen. A great deal of blood can be lost in a short amount of time (profuse bleeding).
- *Venous bleeding*—Blood is *flowing steadily* from a vein. The color of the blood is dark red, often appearing deep maroon (since it contains little oxygen) however, it may look or become a brighter red when exposed to oxygen. Venous bleeding can also be profuse.

Note

Large veins may produce profuse bleeding, but there is not the pulsation typically seen with arterial bleeding. Look at the rate of flow and pulsation as more significant factors in determining if the bleeding is arterial or venous than the color. Venous blood saturated with oxygen in the air may quickly turn to a brighter red than when it is inside the veins or bleeding has just begun.

FIGURE 11.2
Three types of bleeding.

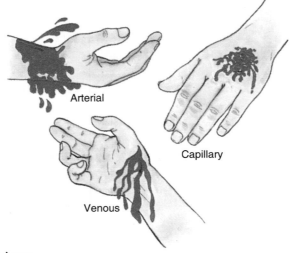

Arterial

Capillary

Venous

- *Capillary bleeding*—Blood is oozing from a bed of capillaries. The color of the blood is red, usually less bright than arterial blood. The flow is slow, as seen in minor scrapes and shallow cuts to the skin.

Evaluating External Bleeding

Arterial Bleeding Of the three types of external bleeding, arterial bleeding is usually the most serious. The action of the heart and the pressure in the arteries prevent blood clot formation because of the rapid, pressurized flow. The muscular nature of walls creates problems in stopping the flow of blood. Sometimes the end of a completely severed artery will collapse and seal off the flow. In small arteries, the pulsation of the muscular wall may slow bleeding. In larger arteries, the thickness of the vessel walls prevents this collapse from being complete and the flow remains profuse. Since arteries are located deep within body structures, capillary and venous bleeding are seen more often than arterial bleeding.

Venous Bleeding Venous bleeding can range from very minor to very severe, leading to death within minutes. Some veins are located near the body surface. Many of these are large enough to be seen through the skin. Other veins are deep in the body and can be as large as arteries. Bleeding from a deep vein will produce rapid blood loss. Surface vein bleeding can be profuse, but the blood loss is not as rapid as that seen from arteries and deep veins because of the smaller vessel diameter. Veins have a tendency to collapse as soon as they are cut. This often reduces the severity of venous bleeding.

Capillary Bleeding Most individuals experience little difficulty with capillary bleeding. The blood flow slowly oozes and clotting is very likely to occur within 6 to 8 minutes. The larger the area of the wound, however, the more likely is the chance of infection. Capillary bleeding requires care to stop blood flow and reduce contamination.

Arterial and large vein bleeding are given priority over small vein and capillary bleeding. If bleeding is severe and considered an immediate threat to life, control of the bleeding will have to begin while you are noting signs of breathing during the initial assessment. Even though it may prove awkward, a First Responder may be faced with the task of stopping severe bleeding while, at the same time, evaluating airway and pulse.

Determining blood loss because of external bleeding requires some experience (Figure 11.3). The ability to make such a determination is of value to the First Responder in cases where slow bleeding has been occurring for a long time or in cases where both internal and external bleeding are present. A bleeding rate that normally could wait until after patient assessment may be life-threatening because the patient has already lost a large quantity of blood.

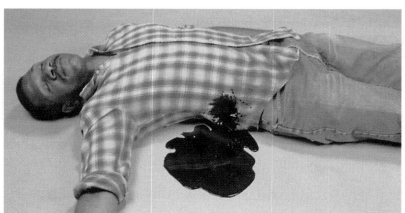

FIGURE 11.3
Estimating external blood loss; ½ liter (approximately 1 pint).

To get a better idea of how to estimate blood volume loss, pour a pint of water on the floor next to a fellow student or a manikin. Also, try soaking an article of clothing with a pint of water and then note how much of the article is wet and how wet it feels.

Controlling External Bleeding

In the following section, a **dressing** is defined as the material placed over a wound, and a **bandage** is the material that holds a dressing in place.

Regardless of the method used to control bleeding, you must wear latex or vinyl gloves to avoid direct contact with the patient's blood.

Prior to initiating emergency medical care for bleeding, you should first . . .

- Complete a scene size-up. (Assure that you include BSI.)
- Complete an initial assessment. (Assure that you maintain ABCs.)

First | Four major procedures can be used by First Responders to control external bleeding (Scan 11-1):

- Direct pressure (including use of pressure dressing)
- Elevation (used with direct pressure)
- Pressure points (arm/leg)
- Tourniquet (used only as a last resort when other bleeding control steps fail to control bleeding)

First | **Direct Pressure** Most cases of external bleeding can be controlled by applying **direct pressure** to the site of the wound. Ideally, a sterile dressing should be used. However, hunting in your pocket for a sterile dressing, going back to your car, going to a kit found in the next room, or other such activities are a waste of precious time.

If *profuse* bleeding is found during the initial assessment, you should:

1. Use your gloved hand if necessary; do *not* waste time hunting for a dressing (Figure 11.4).
2. Place your gloved hand directly over the wound and apply pressure.
3. Keep applying steady, firm pressure.

If bleeding is *mild* or well-controlled (Figure 11.5):

1. Apply firm pressure using a sterile dressing or clean cloth. (You may have to use a clean handkerchief or towel.)
2. Apply pressure until bleeding is controlled. In some cases, this may take 10 minutes, 30 minutes, or longer.
3. Hold the dressing in place with bandages only after you are certain that the bleeding is controlled.

dressing any material used to cover a wound that will help control bleeding and reduce contamination.

bandage any material that is used to hold a dressing in place.

REMEMBER:

Finding and stopping profuse bleeding is a component of the initial assessment.

direct pressure the quickest, most effective way to control most forms of external bleeding. Pressure is applied directly over the wound site.

FIGURE 11.4
In cases of profuse bleeding, use your gloved hand; do not waste time hunting for a dressing.

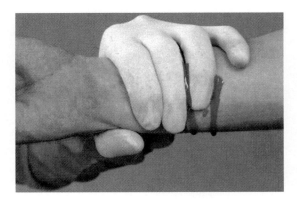

Methods of Controlling External Bleeding

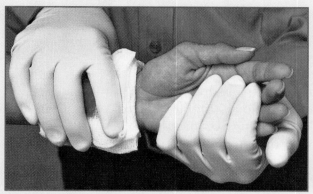

1. Direct pressure.

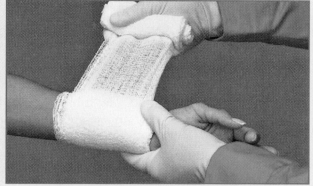

2. Pressure dressing.

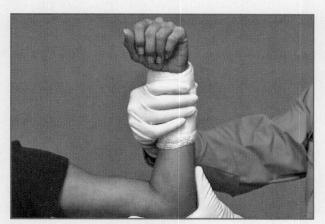

3. Direct pressure and elevation.

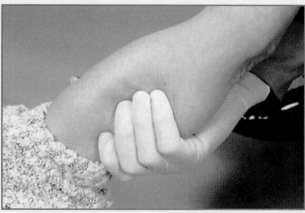

4. Pressure point: arm.

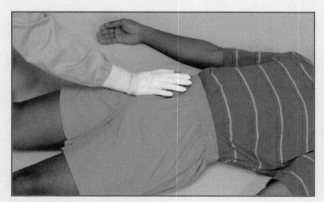

5. Pressure point: leg.

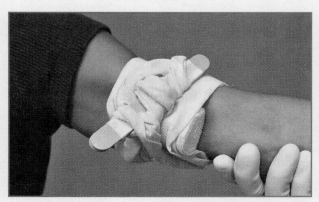

6. Tourniquet.

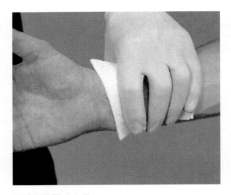
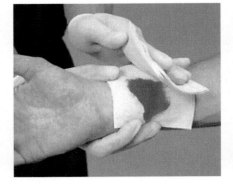
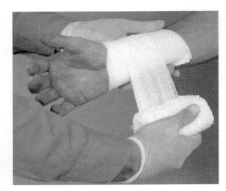

FIGURE 11.5
Apply direct pressure with a dressing.

4. *Never* remove or attempt to replace any dressing once it is in place. To do so may interrupt clot formation and restart bleeding or cause additional injury to the wound site. If a dressing becomes soaked with blood, place another dressing directly over the blood-soaked one and hold both in place with firm pressure.

Most bleeding can be controlled by a special form of direct pressure, the *pressure dressing* (Figure 11.6). To apply a pressure dressing:

1. Place several sterile gauze dressing pads directly on the wound and maintain pressure with your gloved hand.
2. Set a bulky dressing pad (multitrauma or universal dressing, sanitary pad, or several handkerchiefs) over the gauze dressing pads. Continue to apply hand pressure.
3. Use a self-adherent roller bandage to hold the entire dressing in place. It should be wrapped over the dressing and above and below the wound.
4. Wrap the bandage to produce enough pressure to control the bleeding.
5. Check for a distal pulse to be certain that the pressure has not restricted blood flow.

A pressure dressing should not be removed once it is in place. If bleeding continues, you can add more pressure by using the palm of your gloved hand, applying more dressing pads, and continuing the process of bandaging (do not remove the bandage to add more pads), or apply more bandages to increase the

FIGURE 11.6
The pressure dressing.

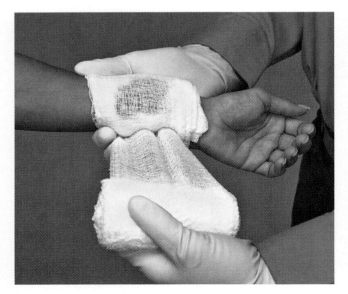
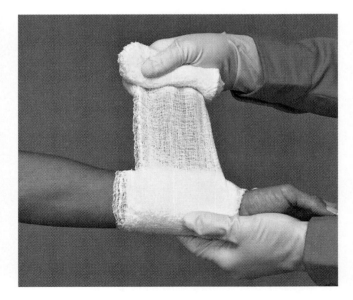

pressure. In very few cases (amputations and severe tearing injuries), you will have to create more bulk by using additional dressings.

If you use your gloved hand or a dressing to apply direct pressure, you can apply a pressure dressing once the bleeding is controlled. If you are dealing with bleeding from an armpit, the abdominal wall, a large artery, or a deep vein, attempting to apply a pressure dressing may not be of any real use. Your best approach to such situations is to maintain pressure using your gloved hand and a dressing.

First | ***Elevation*** Elevation may be used in combination with direct pressure when dealing with bleeding from the arm or leg (Figure 11.7). The effects of gravity will help reduce blood pressure and slow the bleeding. This method should not be used, however, with possible fractures to the extremities, objects impaled in the extremities, or possible spinal injury. To use elevation:

- Elevate the injured extremity. When practical, raise the extremity so that the wound is above the level of the heart. If the forearm is bleeding, you do not have to elevate the entire arm. Simply elevate the forearm.
- Continue to apply direct pressure to the site of bleeding as explained earlier in this chapter.

First | ***Pressure Points*** Pressure points are sites where an artery that is close to the skin surface lies directly over a bone (Figure 11.8). The flow of blood through such an artery can be interrupted if pressure is applied to the artery. This procedure should be employed only after direct pressure or direct pressure with elevation has failed to control the bleeding.

Twenty-two major pressure point sites are used to control bleeding. They occur at 11 sites on each side of the body. Only the upper arm and thigh are commonly part of First Responder training. These sites are:

- **Brachial artery pressure point** in the upper arm for controlling bleeding from the arm
- **Femoral artery pressure point** in the thigh for controlling bleeding from the leg

REMEMBER:

Direct pressure is the quickest, most effective way to control bleeding.

brachial (BRAY-ke-al) artery pressure point the pressure point in the upper arm that can be used to help control serious external bleeding from the upper limb.

femoral (FEM-o-ral) artery pressure point the pressure point in the thigh that can be used to help control serious external bleeding from the lower limb.

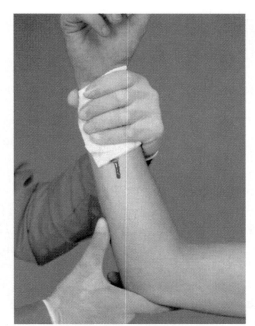

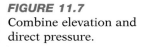

FIGURE 11.7
Combine elevation and direct pressure.

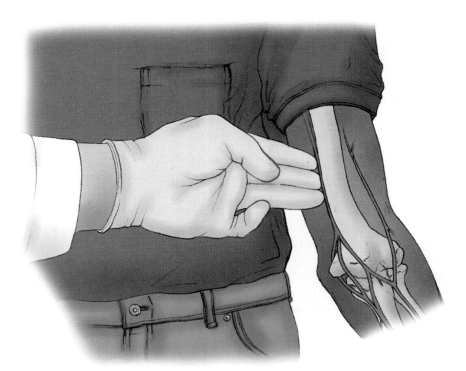

FIGURE 11.8
Pressure points are sites where an artery that is close to the skin surface lies directly over a bone.

REMEMBER:

Use pressure point techniques only after direct pressure and elevation have failed.

WARNING:

Exercise care when practicing pressure point techniques.

First | Pressure point techniques are to be used only after direct pressure and elevation have failed to control bleeding.

First | Care must be exercised in the practice of pressure point techniques. As with most emergency care procedures, the application of pressure to an artery must be viewed as a drastic measure. A single compression of short duration will not harm a healthy adult. However, repeated practice on someone, applying pressure for more than a few seconds, and too much pressure applied to children can all cause problems. Do not attempt to practice or demonstrate this technique on children, infants, or adults with a history of heart problems, blood clot problems, or inflamed blood vessels.

First | For bleeding from the arm:

1. Make sure someone alerts EMS dispatcher.
2. Perform scene size-up.
3. Assure body substance isolation (BSI).
4. Perform initial assessment (assure ABCs).
5. Apply direct pressure.
6. If this fails, apply direct pressure with elevation.
7. Should this fail, extend the patient's arm, placing it at a right angle, lateral to the body. This angle will provide the best results, but may be reduced if a 90-degree extension is not possible. Place the palm of the patient's hand in the anatomical position.
8. Cradle the patient's upper arm in the palm of your gloved hand and position your fingers in the groove found below the biceps muscle (Figure 11.9).
9. Apply pressure to the brachial artery by pressing your fingers into this groove. Bleeding should stop and you should no longer be able to feel a radial (wrist) pulse.
10. Reassure the patient and keep patient calm.
11. Treat for shock (hypoperfusion).

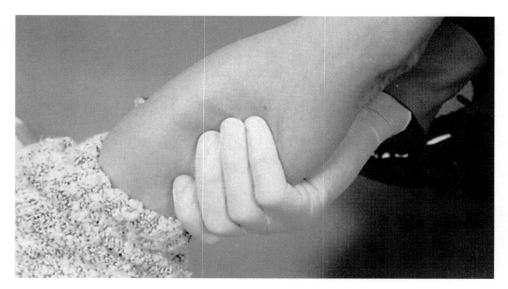

FIGURE 11.9
Apply pressure to the brachial artery pressure point to control bleeding from the arm.

 For bleeding from the leg:

1. Make sure someone alerts EMS dispatcher.
2. Perform scene size-up.
3. Assure body substance isolation (BSI).
4. Perform initial assessment (assure ABCs).
5. Apply direct pressure.
6. If this fails, apply direct pressure with elevation.
7. Should this fail, locate the anterior, medial side of the leg where the thigh joins the lower trunk (Figure 11.10). The femoral artery has a pulse that can be felt at this location.
8. Use the heel of your gloved hand to apply pressure to this site. Keep your arm straight, using your body weight to help apply the pressure. The number of leg muscles, their size, and the fat content of the thigh require that you exert much more pressure than you would use to compress the brachial artery in the arm.
9. Apply the necessary pressure to stop the bleeding.
10. Reassure the patient and keep patient calm.
11. Treat for shock (hypoperfusion).

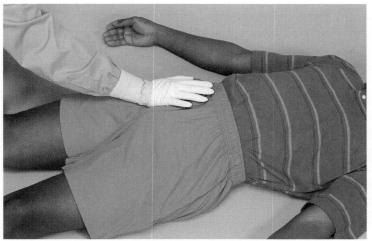

FIGURE 11.10
Apply pressure to the femoral artery pressure point to control bleeding from the leg.

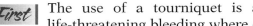 Keep in mind that the upper arm and thigh pressure points are not to be used if there are possible fractures to the bone under the pressure point site. To do so could produce severe pain and could cause serious damage to the bone, soft tissues, nerves, and blood vessels in the area. You could cause more bleeding to take place rather than reduce the bleeding. If there are no indications of possible fractures of the extremity or spinal injury (remember to consider the mechanism of injury), elevation and pressure point techniques can be combined to control bleeding.

First *Tourniquet* Consider the use of a tourniquet as one of the most extreme measures that can be applied by First Responders when providing emergency care. **A tourniquet is a last resort,** used only when the other methods of controlling life-threatening bleeding have failed. In most cases when you think you should use a tourniquet, a pressure dressing would be the better choice.

A partial amputation of the arm or leg may leave you with no other choice than to use a tourniquet. However, many total amputations do not have uncontrollable, profuse bleeding since the ends of the blood vessels tend to collapse. In cases in which there is profuse bleeding from an arm or leg wound, a tourniquet should be applied to stop life-threatening bleeding after direct pressure, elevation, and pressure point techniques have failed. Be aware that the procedure could lead to the eventual loss of the arm or leg to which the tourniquet has been applied. If there is not another way to stop the bleeding and save the patient's life, then this is acceptable action.

First The use of a tourniquet is a last resort, used only to control life-threatening bleeding where other methods have failed.

First The application of a tourniquet is an extreme method of emergency care. Do *not* practice tightening a tourniquet on anyone. Once a tourniquet has been applied, it should not be loosened.

First If all other methods have failed and you must apply a tourniquet, carefully follow these steps (Figure 11.11):

1. Locate the site for the tourniquet. This should be between the wound and the patient's heart, as close to the wound as possible without being on its edge. The most effective and safest location is about 2 inches from the wound.

2. Place a tourniquet pad on the site you have selected, over the artery. This pad can be a roll of dressing, a folded handkerchief, or a piece of cloth folded to about the same thickness as a folded handkerchief.

3. If you are using a manufactured tourniquet, carefully place it around the limb at the site. Pull the free end of the band through the friction catch or buckle and draw it tightly over the pad. You should tighten the tourniquet to the point where bleeding is stopped. Do *not* tighten it beyond this point. If you do not have a commercially manufactured tourniquet or you would have to leave the patient to retrieve one, use a flat belt, necktie, stocking, or long dressing material. Flat materials are best. The band should be at least ½ inch wide. Do *not* use any material that could cut into the patient's limb. Carefully slip the tourniquet around the patient's limb and tie a knot with the ends of the tourniquet. The knot should be over the pad. A device such as a long stick, wooden dowel, or metal rod should then be inserted into the knot. (Pens and pencils tend to break.) Turn the device until bleeding has been stopped. Do *not* tighten the tourniquet beyond this point.

tourniquet the last resort used to control bleeding from an extremity. A wide, flat band or belt is used to constrict blood vessels to help stop the flow of blood.

REMEMBER:

Use a tourniquet only as a last resort.

WARNING:

Never practice tightening a tourniquet on anyone.

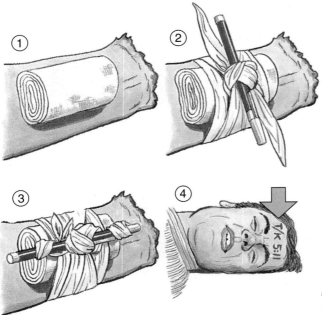

FIGURE 11.11
Application of a tourniquet.

4. Once it is in place, **do not loosen the tourniquet.** To do so may cause great harm to the patient. Tie it or tape it in place.

5. Attach a note to the patient stating that a tourniquet has been applied and the time at which it was applied (for example: T/K—5:11 P.M.). If you do not have a tag, write the information, in ink, on the patient's forehead. If you do not have a pen, write the note in lipstick, crayon, or whatever is available at the scene. This note must be written so that the tourniquet does not go unnoticed and so that the hospital staff will know how long it has been in place.

6. Deliver care for shock (hypoperfusion) (pages 326–330), but do *not* cover the tourniquet. This is an additional safeguard to prevent it from being missed by others who provide care for the patient.

Splinting Splinting is usually not considered a First Responder-level method of controlling bleeding; however, some First Responders are trained to use air-inflatable splints. For long wounds on an arm or leg, the application of an air splint can help to control bleeding. This is actually a form of direct pressure. Using an inflatable splint requires special training in its application and knowledge of its limitations (see Chapter 12). The air splint can be used even when there is no fracture to the bones of the limb.

Combining the use of an air splint and elevation can work well on long, bleeding wounds. The splint also serves to immobilize the limb, helping to reduce the chance of patient movement restarting the bleeding. Since time is consumed by obtaining and applying air splints, this procedure is best done in cases of minor bleeding. The skilled rescuer can use air splints to control more serious bleeding if the splint is immediately at hand.

Any patient who has suffered moderate to severe blood loss will benefit form receiving oxygen. If you are a First Responder who carries oxygen, administer 50% to 100% oxygen by mask as needed. (Follow local protocols.)

Note

As a First Responder, you have the responsibility to advise the EMTs or other more highly trained personnel about the application of a tourniquet and the time it was applied.

EXTERNAL BLEEDING—CONTROL AND ASSESSMENT

```
┌─────────┐                                    ┌─────────────────────────┐
│ Profuse │         ╱ Direct  ╲    SUCCESS     │  Bleeding is controlled │
│ external │───────▶╲ pressure ╱───────────────▶│                         │
│ bleeding│         ╲         ╱                 └─────────────────────────┘
│ present │              │
└─────────┘           FAILURE
                         │
                         ▼
              ┌──────────────────┐
              │ Elevation with   │
              │ direct pressure  │
              └──────────────────┘
                         │
                      FAILURE          ┌──────────────────────────────────────┐
                         │             │          Use of Tourniquet           │
              ┌──────────────────┐     ├──────────────────────────────────────┤
              │ Pressure points  │  FAILURE │ The use of a tourniquet is a last resort │
              │ are applied      │─────────▶│ Use only when all other bleeding     │
              └──────────────────┘     │ control measures have failed          │
                                       └──────────────────────────────────────┘
```

Special Cases of External Bleeding

Bleeding from the eye, ear, nose, mouth, and around impaled objects presents special cases that will be considered elsewhere in this text. For now, do not consider these sites while you are learning how to control bleeding.

There are situations where a deep cut will open a major artery or vein and then the cut will partially close. Such cuts do not always appear to be major, and the bleeding from these cuts is often mild. Be alert for blood flow from wounds to change quickly from mild to profuse. If there is a wound to the arm and you cannot detect a wrist pulse, or if there is a wound to the leg and you cannot detect a distal pulse, be prepared for profuse bleeding.

Do not let cuts to the chest and abdomen fool you. Some may appear minor, but they could be very deep and have produced internal injuries that are causing a great deal of internal bleeding. When you find an external wound, you must consider the possibility of internal injuries. **Do not open the wound to determine its depth.**

First | You must have someone alert the EMS dispatcher for all patients with external bleeding except for the mildest cases (small areas of capillary bleeding) in which there are no other signs of injury.

Dressing and Bandaging

Bandaging is not a difficult skill to learn. In First Responder care, there are few "special" techniques and most bandages are simple and easy to apply. However, there are some patients who will benefit from a special bandaging procedure that will be presented. Otherwise, if you follow the basic principles of dressing and bandaging wounds, you will provide effective care for the patient.

First | To begin, review the following definitions (Figure 11.12):

- Dressing—any material placed over a wound that will help control bleeding and help prevent additional contamination
- Bandage—any material used to hold a dressing in place

Types of Dressings Dressings, whenever possible, should be *sterile*. This means that they have been processed so that all germs and the spores that can grow

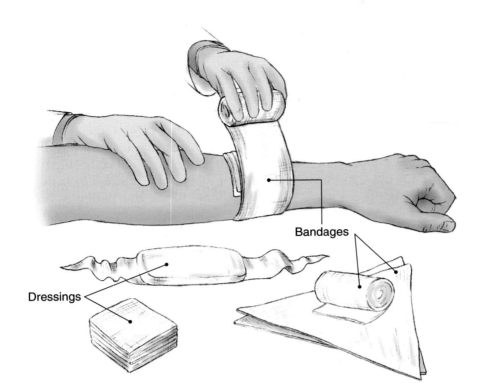

FIGURE 11.12
Dressings cover wounds. Bandages hold dressings in place.

into active germs are killed. Dressings are also *aseptic*, meaning that all dirt and foreign debris have been removed. Commercially prepared dressings are aseptic and are usually sterile. They come in a variety of sizes, with the most common size being 4 inches square. They are referred to according to size, such as 2 × 2s and 4 × 4s.

Throughout this text, you will find reference to **bulky dressings** and multitrauma dressings. These are thick dressings, often large enough to allow for the complete covering of large wounds. They are used to help control very serious bleeding and to stabilize impaled objects. Sanitary pads can be used in place of these dressings. They are available individually wrapped. While sanitary pads are not sterile, they are very clean on their surfaces. (Avoid applying any adhesive surface directly to the wound.) Bulky dressings can be formed by applying many layers of simple gauze dressings.

Another type of special dressing is the **occlusive dressing**, which is a dressing used to create an airtight seal to a wound or body cavity. It is used when it

bulky dressing a thick single dressing or a buildup of thin dressings used to help control profuse bleeding, stabilize impaled objects, or cover large open wounds.

occlusive dressing a dressing used to create an airtight seal or to close an open wound of a body cavity. Usually, it is made of plastic.

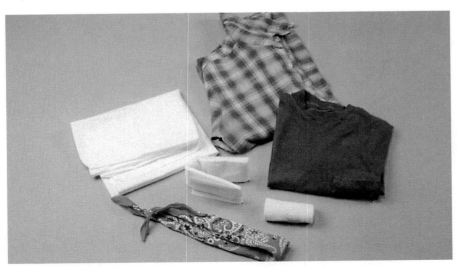

FIGURE 11.13
Dressings for use in emergencies.

is necessary to close an open wound that penetrates a body cavity. Commercially prepared occlusive dressing pads are available. If these are not on hand, you can use folded plastic wrap or a plastic bag to help seal off a penetrating wound to the chest or abdomen. (Some EMS systems have allowed aluminum foil to be used instead of plastic, but there are reports that this foil can cut internal organs. Follow local protocols.)

Often, a First Responder will not have any dressing materials at the scene of an emergency. In such cases, you might have to use clean handkerchiefs, towels, sheets, a piece of clothing, or other similar materials (Figure 11.13). When you improvise to make a dressing, it will not be sterile, but it can be used to help provide proper care for the patient. Since the patient's wound has already been contaminated, your task is to avoid further contamination by using the cleanest material available. The hospital has special wound-cleansing procedures and antibiotics to care for wound contamination and infection. In the field, you must be concerned with controlling bleeding and reducing contamination.

Bandaging Materials Dressings are more effective if they are held in place. Usually, this is done by taping or tying. The adhesive bandage has a sticky backing that will adhere to the patient's skin. If no such bandaging material is on hand, tie a dressing in place by using a gauze roller bandage, a **cravat,** a handkerchief, strips of cloth, or any other material that will not cut into the patient's skin. *Do not use elastic bandages* that are often used for strains and sprains to the joints. This type of bandage may restrict circulation and will apply undesired pressure to the injured tissues.

The use of the self-adherent, form-fitting, gauze roller bandage eliminates the need for highly specialized bandaging techniques (Figure 11.14). Most of these techniques were developed for use with the ordinary gauze roller bandage. The self-adherent roller bandage does not have an adhesive backing, yet clings to itself, making the task of wrapping the bandage around the dressing easier, quicker, and more efficient.

First | *Rules for Dressing and Bandaging* The following rules apply to dressing wounds:

1. **Control bleeding.** A dressing and bandage are of little value if they do not help to control bleeding. Continue to apply dressing material and pressure as needed to control bleeding.

2. **Use sterile or clean materials.** Avoid touching the dressing in the area that will come into contact with the wound.

cravat a piece of cloth material that can be used to secure a dressing or splint.

FIGURE 11.14
Application of self-adherent roller bandage.

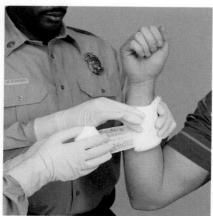 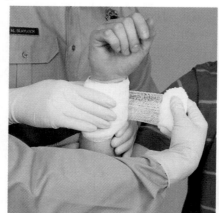 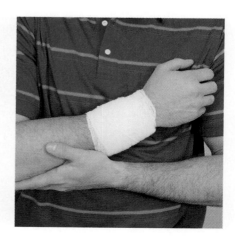

3. **Cover the entire wound.** The dressing should cover the entire surface of the wound and, if possible, the immediate area surrounding the wound.

4. **Do not remove dressings.** Once a dressing is applied to a wound, it must remain in place. Add new dressings on top of blood-soaked dressings. When a dressing is removed from a wound, there may be a restart of bleeding or an increase in the rate of bleeding. Because of this, a dressing should remain in place once it is applied to a wound. Removal should be done in the emergency department. There is an exception to this rule in some EMS systems. (Do only what you have been trained to do.) If a bulky dressing becomes blood-soaked, you may have to remove it so that direct pressure can be reestablished or a new bulky pad or dressing can be applied.

It is best to apply simple gauze pads to wound sites before applying a bulky dressing. This will allow removal of the bulky dressing if necessary without directly disturbing the wound.

 The following rules apply to bandaging (Figure 11.15):

1. **Do not bandage too tightly.** Hold the dressing snugly in place, but do not restrict blood supply to the affected area.

2. **Do not bandage too loosely.** The dressing must *not* be allowed to move on top of the wound or slip from the wound.

3. **Do not leave loose ends.** Keep in mind that the patient will have to be moved. Loose ends of tape, dressing, or cloth might get caught on objects when the patient is being moved.

4. **Do not cover fingers and toes.** Dressing materials and bandages should not cover the tips of the patient's fingers or toes unless they are injured. These areas must be exposed so that you can watch for color changes indicating a change in circulation or that the bandage is too tight. Blue skin, pale skin, and complaints of numbness, pain, and tingling sensations all indicate that the bandage may be too tight.

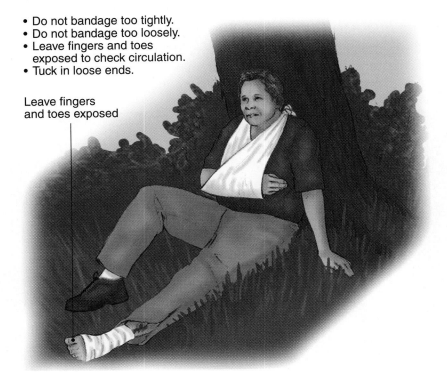

- Do not bandage too tightly.
- Do not bandage too loosely.
- Leave fingers and toes exposed to check circulation.
- Tuck in loose ends.

Leave fingers and toes exposed

FIGURE 11.15
The rules of bandaging.

5. **Bandage from the bottom of a limb to the top** (distal to proximal). The bandage should be wrapped around the limb starting at its far (distal) end and working toward its origin or near (proximal) end. Taking such action will reduce the chances of restricting circulation and wrapping too tightly.

Two additional rules for bandaging must be considered when the wound is on a limb:

1. Avoid applying the bandage to a narrow area. This can produce enough pressure to restrict circulation. Instead, wrap a large area of the limb, making certain to maintain uniform pressure as you wrap the bandage.

2. Do not bend a joint if it is bandaged. Once the bandage is in place, movement of the joint may restrict circulation or cause the bandage and dressing to loosen.

See Scan 11-2 for examples of general dressing and bandaging.

INTERNAL BLEEDING

Significance of Internal Bleeding

Internal bleeding can range from minor importance to a major life-threatening problem. Most small, simple bruises are examples of minor internal bleeding. Such small blood loss is not of great significance. Of primary concern to First Responders are those cases of internal bleeding that produce a blood loss that could bring about shock (hypoperfusion), heart and lung failure, and eventual death. Some cases of internal bleeding are so severe that the patient dies in a matter of seconds. Other severe cases of internal bleeding take minutes to hours before death. First Responder-level care might keep these patients alive until the EMTs arrive.

Even when internal bleeding is not profuse, it does not take very long for serious reactions to occur in the body. The most important of these, shock, will be covered later in this chapter. The care you provide for internal bleeding and shock, even when the bleeding is not profuse, may save the patient's life.

Detecting Internal Bleeding

Internal bleeding can occur in many ways (Figure 11.16). It can be caused by wounds that are deep enough to sever major blood vessels or the vessels in organs, such as a deep wound to the chest or abdomen. Open wounds that have

FIGURE 11.16
Certain types of injuries may indicate serious internal bleeding.

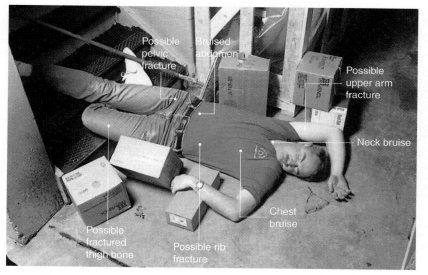

Possible pelvic fracture

Bruised abdomen

Possible upper arm fracture

Neck bruise

Chest bruise

Possible fractured thigh bone

Possible rib fracture

Examples of General Dressing and Bandaging

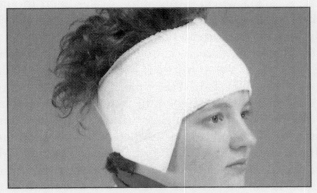

FOREHEAD (NO SKULL INJURY) OR EAR. Place dressing and secure with self-adherent roller bandage.

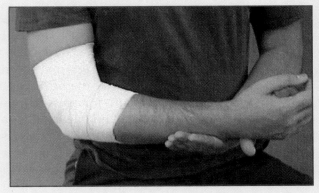

ELBOW OR KNEE. Place dressing and secure with cravat or roller bandage. Apply roller bandage in figure-eight pattern.

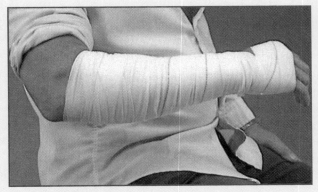

FOREARM OR LEG. Place dressing and secure with roller bandage, distal to proximal. Better protection is provided if palm or sole is wrapped.

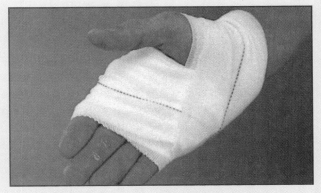

HAND. Place dressing, wrap with cravat, and secure at wrist. Use the same pattern for roller bandage.

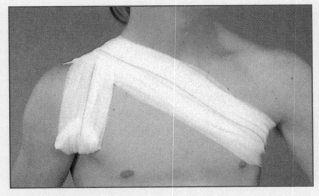

SHOULDER. Place dressing and secure with figure-eight of cravat or roller dressing. Pad under knot if cravat is used.

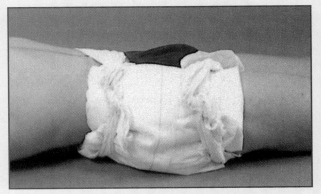

HIP. Place bandage and large dressing to cover hip. Secure with first cravat around waist and second cravat around thigh on injured side.

cut through major vessels to produce profuse internal bleeding may show only minor external bleeding. Many cases of internal bleeding occur even when there are no cuts in the skin or cavity walls. Internal organs and blood vessels may have been ruptured or crushed by a severe blow to the body that did not produce any external wounds. This is an example of **blunt trauma,** or injury caused by an object that was not sharp enough to penetrate the skin. The blunt instrument can be fairly large, such as the steering wheel of an automobile. Even though they do not tend to cause penetrating wounds, blunt instruments can deliver a great deal of force to the body, causing life-threatening internal bleeding.

Pay special attention to bruises on the neck, chest, and abdomen. Severe injury with internal bleeding may show no more than a bruise at first, to be followed by the rapid decline of the patient. Bruise detection can be particularly important in assessing possible internal bleeding when the patient is unconscious and thus unable to tell you of symptoms that would clearly indicate the problem.

To complicate your assessment of the patient, in some cases a blow to one side of the body may cause internal bleeding on the opposite side of the body cavity. In automobile accidents, blunt trauma to the lower right side of the rib cage can cause the spleen, which is on the left side of the body, to rupture and bleed freely, releasing about 1 liter (2 pints) or more of blood.

First | **REMEMBER:** Internal bleeding can be life-threatening. This may be hard to detect since it can occur in cases where bleeding from external wounds is minor, away from the site of noticeable injury, or where there is no obvious external injury. Considering the mechanism of injury (falls, steering wheel injuries, and the like) and conducting a proper patient assessment are of major importance in detecting internal bleeding.

First | Assume there is internal bleeding whenever you detect any of the signs listed below (Figure 11.17). Notice how the signs follow the order of the head-to-toe physical exam:

■ Wounds that have penetrated the skull
■ Blood or bloody fluids in the ears and/or nose
■ The patient vomits or coughs up blood (coffee-grounds or frothy red in appearance).
■ Bruises on the neck
■ Bruises on the chest, possible fractured ribs (possible cuts to the lungs and liver), and wounds that have penetrated the chest
■ Bruises or penetrating wounds to the abdomen
■ Hardness or spasms of the abdominal muscles
■ Abdominal tenderness
■ Bleeding from the rectum or vagina
■ Fractures (with special emphasis on the pelvis, the long bones of the upper arm and thigh, and the ribs)

Always assume there is internal bleeding if the patient has been injured and the signs and symptoms of shock are present (Figure 11.18). We will say more about shock later in this chapter, but for now you should know the basic signs and symptoms of shock used to detect possible internal bleeding.

First | The **symptoms** of shock associated with internal bleeding are:

■ Patient feels weak.
■ Patient is thirsty.
■ Patient may feel cold.
■ Patient feels anxious or restless.

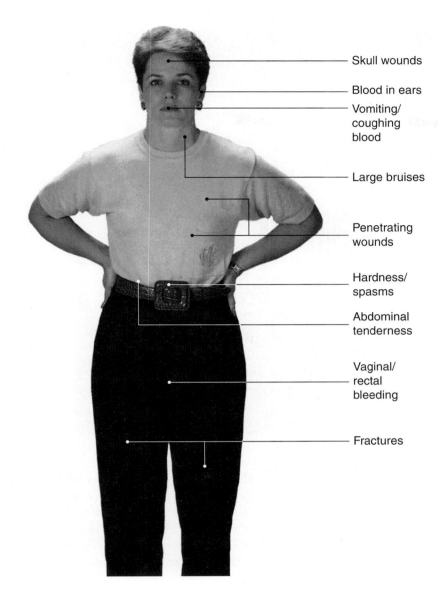

FIGURE 11.17
Signs and symptoms of possible internal bleeding.

Skull wounds

Blood in ears

Vomiting/
coughing
blood

Large bruises

Penetrating
wounds

Hardness/
spasms

Abdominal
tenderness

Vaginal/
rectal
bleeding

Fractures

First | The **signs** of shock associated with internal bleeding include:

■ Awareness—altered levels of consciousness
■ Behavior—restlessness or combativeness
■ Body—may be shaking and trembling (rare)
■ Breathing—shallow and rapid
■ Pulse—rapid and weak
■ Skin—pale, cool, and clammy (There may be profuse sweating.)
■ Eyes—Pupils are dilated.

Stop now and note how these signs fit into your assessment of the patient during the physical exam. Remember, none of these signs and symptoms may be present in the early stages of internal bleeding. If the mechanism of injury is severe enough to make you think that there may be internal bleeding, assume that there is such bleeding and provide the necessary care.

First | You can detect internal bleeding by looking for injuries and mechanisms of injury that may cause internal bleeding, wounds, and the signs and symptoms of shock.

Some severe medical emergencies that can produce internal bleeding were discussed in Chapter 10.

FIGURE 11.18
Signs and symptoms of
shock associated with
internal bleeding.

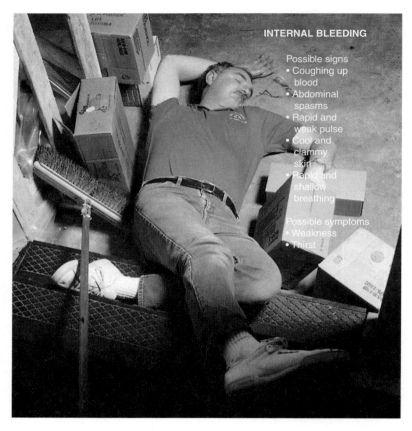

INTERNAL BLEEDING

Possible signs
• Coughing up
  blood
• Abdominal
  spasms
• Rapid and
  weak pulse
• Cool and
  clammy
  skin
• Rapid and
  shallow
  breathing

Possible symptoms
• Weakness
• Thirst

Evaluating Internal Bleeding

It is very difficult to determine the amount of blood lost in cases of internal
bleeding. Special hospital procedures and tests are required. However, estimates
can be made. Consider blood loss to be severe if there is penetration of the chest
cavity over or immediately above the heart, if the spleen or liver may have been
injured, or if the pelvis is fractured. Blood loss of at least 1 liter (2 pints) must
be suspected if there is a major fracture in the upper arm or thigh bone. Where
you find badly bruised skin, assume there is a 10% loss of total blood volume for
each bruise the size of the patient's fist (Figure 11.19). For an adult, this is about
a 1-pint loss. Such estimates will help you evaluate the chance of the patient
going into shock, lung or heart failure, or cardiac arrest.

FIGURE 11.19
Estimating internal
blood loss.

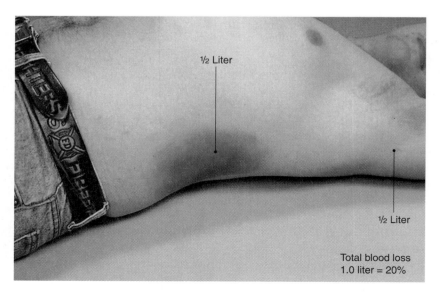

½ Liter

½ Liter

Total blood loss
1.0 liter = 20%

Management of Internal Bleeding

First | The techniques for preventing or reducing the severity of shock will be covered later in this chapter. These techniques will help control internal bleeding. In general, the steps in the care for patients with suspected internal bleeding include:

1. Make certain that someone alerts the EMS dispatcher.
2. Perform scene size-up, including BSI.
3. Perform initial assessment. (Maintain the airway and monitor breathing and pulse.)
4. Keep the patient in the proper position and lying still.
5. Loosen restrictive clothing and provide care for shock.
6. Be alert in case the patient starts to vomit.
7. Do *not* give the patient anything by mouth.
8. Apply pressure dressings if internal bleeding is in an extremity.
9. Reassure patient and keep patient calm.
10. Report the possibility of internal bleeding as soon as more highly trained EMS personnel arrive at the scene.

If you are a First Responder who carries oxygen, remember that any patient with possible internal bleeding will benefit from receiving 50% to 100% oxygen delivered by mask.

Internal bleeding in the abdominal cavity or the chest cavity is a life-threatening situation requiring quick, safe transport to a hospital. Most areas in the country do not consider transport to be a First Responder's duty. Most EMS directors believe it is better if First Responders keep patients at the scene. You must recognize that a patient unattended in the back seat of your car could go into cardiac arrest and die while you are trying to rush to the hospital. Improper transport could also aggravate spinal injuries, leading to the death of the patient.

Patients with internal bleeding need oxygen as part of their care. By transporting such patients to the hospital without oxygen, you may place them in greater risk than if you waited for EMS personnel to arrive with oxygen (and IV fluids).

Some localities may have special rules for First Responders in terms of patient transport (isolated areas with long EMT response time, and others). Follow the guidelines set for your local or regional system.

Internal bleeding is very serious, often leading to death, even in cases in which the bleeding begins once the patient is at the hospital. You may provide excellent First Responder care for a patient with internal bleeding, only to have him die on the scene. To be a good First Responder, accept the fact that there are limits to emergency care at all levels. Some patients will die no matter what you do. The patient has a better chance to survive, however, if you do as you have been trained to do.

SHOCK

DEVELOPMENT OF SHOCK

When providing patients with emergency care, there is the concept of the "golden hour." This is the first hour after serious injury or the sudden onset of certain illnesses occurs. Providers must make every effort to provide care and assist in delivering seriously injured patients to the hospital as quickly as possible. The first 60 minutes are critical. If shock can be prevented or if its severity can be reduced during this period, the patient's chances for survival are greatly improved.

First | Any injury or illness must be considered more severe once the patient enters a state of shock. **Keeping patients from going into shock and helping to stabilize patients who are in shock are two of the most important responsibilities of First Responders.** If nothing is done for the patient who is in shock, death will almost always result.

Whenever the body is hurt, either by injury or illness, it reacts by trying to correct the effects of the damage. If the damage is severe, one reaction is shock, which indicates a problem with the circulatory system. The problem can be related to the:

- *Heart*—The heart may be compared to a pump and should be pumping blood and doing so efficiently. If the heart fails to pump an adequate volume of blood or if it stops pumping altogether, shock will develop. If
- *Vessels*—Blood circulates throughout the body through a closed system. If there is any opening in this system, such as a cut or rupture, with enough blood loss, shock will develop. Shock can also develop when blood vessels dilate and there is not enough blood to fill the now larger system.
- *Volume*—An adequate amount of blood must be present to fill the vessels. If there is loss of blood volume or if the vessels enlarge (dilate) to a size that no longer allows the system to be properly filled, shock will develop.

shock the reaction of the body to the failure of the circulatory system to provide enough blood to all the vital organs of the body. The failure of perfusion, or the state of *hypoperfusion*.

Basically, **shock** is the failure of the body's circulatory system to provide enough blood to all vital organs. There must be enough blood being pumped efficiently to allow for a steady flow through the capillaries so that exchange can occur (perfusion). Oxygen and carbon dioxide are exchanged, food and waste are exchanged, and fluid and salt balance must be maintained between the blood and the tissues. When this cannot take place, shock, or hypoperfusion (lack of adequate perfusion), develops.

The term "develops" means that shock occurs in a step-by-step process. This development can be rapid, or it can come about slowly. For most cases, you will have warning that the patient is going into shock. There is a saying used by EMS personnel: "Be alert for shock."

Caring for patients with shock cannot be delayed. The problem worsens with time, and early intervention is crucial. Think of shock as a reaction to a problem such as blood loss. This reaction causes more problems that, in turn, cause more problems. For example, if there is bleeding, the heart rate increases, attempting to circulate blood to all the vital parts of the body. By doing this, more blood is lost. The body's immediate response to this problem is to try to circulate more blood by increasing the heart rate even further. This process will continue until death occurs (Figure 11.20). This cycle of decline must be stopped. The initial problem, such as bleeding, must be corrected, and shock must be treated. First Responder-level care should begin to correct problems and stop the decline.

REMEMBER:

Shock will be fatal if action is not taken.

First | Shock occurs when there is a failure of the circulatory system to provide enough blood to all the vital parts of the body. Unless action is taken, shock will lead to death.

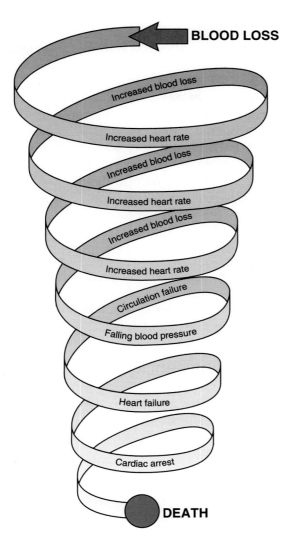

BLOOD LOSS

Increased blood loss

Increased heart rate

Increased blood loss

Increased heart rate

Increased blood loss

Increased heart rate

Circulation failure

Falling blood pressure

Heart failure

Cardiac arrest

DEATH

FIGURE 11.20
The body's attempt to solve the circulatory problem may worsen the situation.

TYPES OF SHOCK

Shock can be classified into several categories since there is more than one cause of shock. It is not necessary to memorize the following list. It is provided so that you can see the many ways shock develops. A patient in shock may have any of the following:

- **Hypovolemic** (HI-po-vo-LE-mic) **shock** is bleeding shock, caused by blood loss or by the loss of plasma (a component of blood) in cases of burns. This term includes all shock caused by fluid loss, such as bleeding, vomiting and diarrhea, burns, and severe dehydration.
- **Cardiogenic** (KAR-di-o-JEN-ic) **shock** is heart shock, caused by the heart failing to pump enough blood to all parts of the body, and may be due to the damage of the heart itself.
- **Neurogenic** (NU-ro-JEN-ic) **shock** is nerve shock, caused when something goes wrong with the nervous system (such as from an injury produced in an accident) and there is a failure to control the diameter of blood vessels. The vessels become dilated. There is not enough blood in the body to fill this new space, causing improper circulation.
- **Anaphylactic** (AN-ah-fi-LAK-tik) **shock** is allergy shock, a life-threatening reaction of the body caused by something to which the patient is

extremely allergic. This is such a serious problem that it is covered as a special topic in Chapter 10.

- **Psychogenic** (SI-ko-JEN-ic) **shock** is fainting. It usually occurs when some factor, such as fear, causes the nervous system to react and rapidly dilate the blood vessels. The proper flow of blood to the brain is interrupted. In most cases, fainting is a self-correcting form of shock, with the interruption of proper blood flow being a temporary condition. Fainting is not the same as neurogenic shock.
- **Metabolic** (MET-ah-BOL-ic) **shock** is body fluid shock, caused by the loss of body fluids as seen after severe diarrhea and/or vomiting. This type of fluid loss is covered under hypovolemic shock.
- **Septic shock** is bloodstream shock, caused by infection. Poisons are released that cause the blood vessels to dilate. As in other cases of shock, the blood volume is too low to fill the circulatory system. This type of shock is seldom seen by First Responders.

As a First Responder, you do not have to classify shock, with the exception of anaphylactic, or allergy, shock. For all other cases, report that the patient has the signs and symptoms of shock and any factors you notice usually associated with shock (bleeding, loss of body fluids).

SIGNS AND SYMPTOMS OF SHOCK

First The **symptoms** of shock are (Figure 11.21):

- Weakness (This may be the most significant symptom.)
- Nausea with possible vomiting
- Thirst
- Dizziness
- The patient indicates restlessness and fear. You may observe both of these conditions, thus considering them to be signs of shock. With some patients, such behavior may be the first indication of shock.

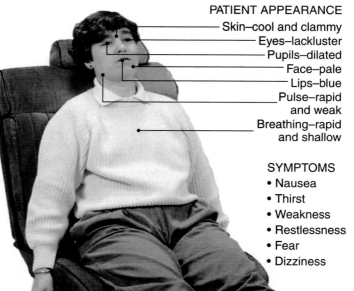

SIGNS
- Restlessness or combativeness
- Becomes unresponsive
- Profuse bleeding
- Vomiting
- Shaking and trembling

PATIENT APPEARANCE
- Skin–cool and clammy
- Eyes–lackluster
- Pupils–dilated
- Face–pale
- Lips–blue
- Pulse–rapid and weak
- Breathing–rapid and shallow

SYMPTOMS
- Nausea
- Thirst
- Weakness
- Restlessness
- Fear
- Dizziness

FIGURE 11.21
Signs and symptoms of shock.

First | The **signs** of shock are:

- **Entire body assessment:**
  - Restlessness or combativeness
  - Profuse external bleeding
  - Vomiting or loss of body fluids (diarrhea)
  - Shaking and trembling (rare)
- **Altered mental status**—The patient may become disoriented, confused, unresponsive, faint, or suddenly unconscious.
- **Breathing**—shallow and rapid
- **Pulse**—rapid and weak
- **Skin**—pale, cool, and clammy (may be profuse sweating)
- **Face**—pale, often with blue color (cyanosis) seen at the lips, tongue, and earlobes
- **Eyes**—lackluster, pupils are dilated

The above list of signs and symptoms follows the order in which they may be detected during the initial assessment of the patient. However, all the signs and symptoms of shock are not present at once, and they do not necessarily occur in the order listed above. Since shock is a changing process, becoming worse with time, you should look for the following patterns (Scan 11-3 and Figure 11.22):

- *Increased pulse rate*—The body is trying to adjust to the loss of blood or inefficient circulation. Unlike the rapid pulse rate associated with the stress of an accident or the fear of needing help during an emergency, this increased rate will not slow down.
- *Increased breathing rate*—When the body is not receiving enough oxygen and the level of carbon dioxide increases, the body tries to compensate by increasing the breathing rate. This increased rate will not slow down as it usually does after experiencing stress.
- *Restlessness or combativeness*—The patient is reacting to the body's attempt to adjust to the loss of proper circulatory function. The patient "feels" that something is wrong and may often look afraid. In some cases, this behavioral change may be the first sign of developing shock.
- *Skin changes indicating possible shock*—Skin, nail bed, and other color changes occur. The skin feels cool to the touch. Sweating will be profuse. Thirst, weakness, and nausea are noted.
- *Rapid, weak pulse and labored, weakened respirations*—The body is failing in its attempt to adjust to the circulatory system failure.
- *Changes in mental status*—As adequate circulation to the brain continues to fail, the patient will become confused, disoriented, sleepy, or unconscious.
- *Respiratory arrest*, then *cardiac arrest*, can develop.

First | Provide care for all injured patients as if shock will develop. Do the same for all patients with problems involving the heart, breathing, abdominal distress, diabetes, drug abuse, poisoning, and abnormal childbirth. Carefully monitor all medical emergency patients for the early warnings of shock. If any are noticed, provide care as if the patient is developing shock.

Note

Children and young adults may compensate for a loss of blood volume better than adults over age 35. This will delay the early indications of developing shock. However, once children and young adults begin to show the first signs of shock, its development may be rapid.

FIGURE 11.22
The development of shock.

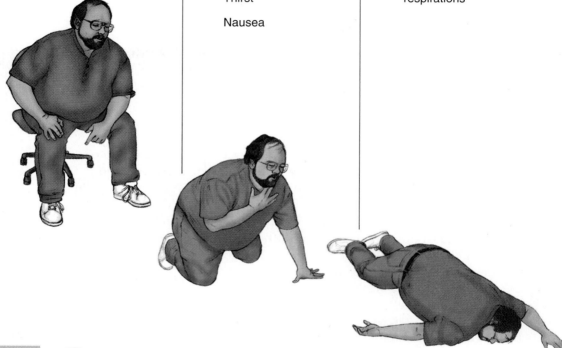

EARLY DEVELOPMENT

Increased pulse rate

Increased respirations

Combativeness

Fearfulness

LOSS OF COMPENSATION

Changes in skin color

Rapid, weak pulse

Labored breathing

Weakness

Thirst

Nausea

LATE DEVELOPMENT

Changes in levels of consciousness

Marked drop in blood pressure

Weak pulse

Weakened respirations

REMEMBER:

It takes prevention of energy loss to conserve body heat. Use a suitable covering to improve the conservation of body heat. Do not overheat. Under certain conditions, you will have to control exposure to harsh environmental conditions.

PREVENTING AND CARING FOR SHOCK

First | As a First Responder, you may help keep a patient from going into shock by doing the following:

1. Make sure someone alerts the EMS dispatcher.

2. Perform scene size-up.

3. Perform initial assessment. (Keep the patient's airway open and prevent the forward tilting of the head.)

4. Assist the patient in lying down. Remember to explain that it is very important for the patient to remain at rest.

5. Control external bleeding and splint major fractures.

6. Maintain the patient's normal body temperature with suitable covers. Prevent loss of body heat, but take care not to overheat the patient. This will worsen the condition. You simply want to conserve body heat. Place at least one blanket under and one blanket over the patient, covering all body parts except the head. Do not try to place a blanket under a patient with possible spinal injuries.

Developing Shock

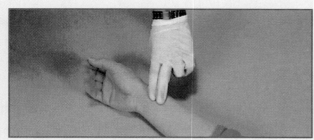

1. Increased pulse: 100+.

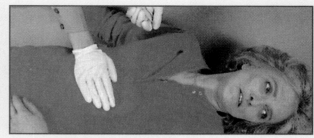

2. Increased breathing rate.

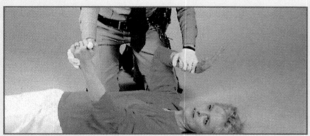

3. Restlessness or combativeness.

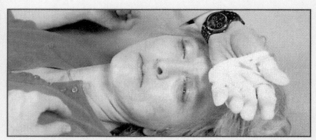

4. Skin changes and sweating.

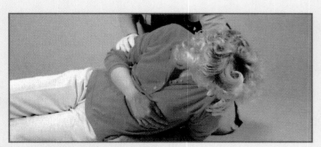

5. Thirst, weakness, and nausea.

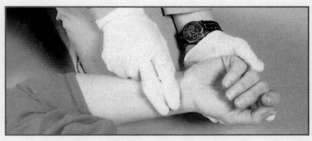

6. Rapid, weak pulse; labored, weak respirations.

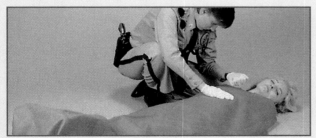

7. Loss of consciousness.

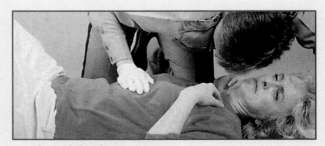

8. Clinical death may occur.

7. Properly position the patient (Figure 11.23). Regardless of the position used, make certain that the patient has an open airway and be alert for vomiting. If there is no indication of spinal injuries, use one of the following positions:

- *Elevate the lower extremities*—This procedure is performed in most cases. Place the patient flat, face up, and elevate the legs 8 to 12 inches. Do *not* tilt the patient's body. Do *not* elevate any fractured limbs unless they have been properly splinted. Do *not* elevate the legs if there are suspected fractures to the pelvis. Remember to consider the mechanism of injury involved with every patient.

- *Lay the patient flat, face up*—This is the supine position, used for patients with serious injuries to the extremities. If the patient is placed in this position, you must constantly be prepared for vomiting.

- *Slightly raise the head and shoulders*—This position should be used only for conscious patients with no possible neck, spinal, chest, or abdominal injuries *and* only for patients having difficulty breathing, but who have an open airway. A semi-seated position can also be used for patients with a history of heart problems. It is *not* recommended for moderate to severe cases of bleeding shock. Be certain to keep the patient's head from tilting forward.

> ### WARNING:
> Do not follow this procedure if there is a possibility of neck injury, if head injuries are severe, or if the patient is having any difficulty in maintaining an adequate airway.

FIGURE 11.23
Properly position the patient in shock. Administer oxygen as soon as possible. Remember, do not move the patient if you suspect spinal injuries.

- Ensure airway.
- Ensure breathing.
- Elevate lower extremities.
- Prevent loss of body heat.
- Do not give anything by mouth.

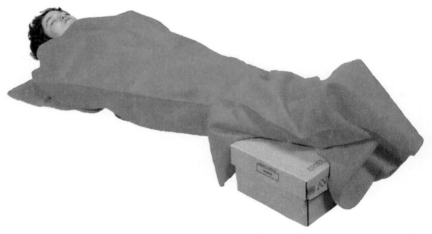

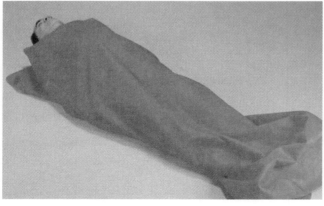

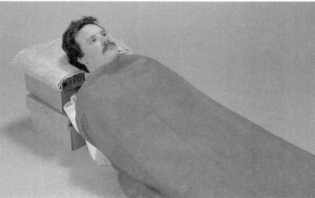

CARE FOR THE PATIENT DEVELOPING SHOCK

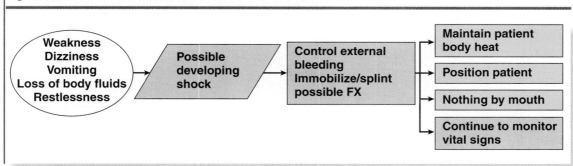

8. Do *not* give the patient anything by mouth. Even if the patient expresses serious thirst, do *not* give any fluids or food.

9. Monitor the patient's vital signs. This must be done no less than every 5 minutes. Stay alert for vomiting, give nothing to the patient by mouth, and provide emotional support to the conscious patient.

Restlessness may be a sign of someone going into shock. The patient may want to assume a sitting position even when there are no problems with breathing. A patient has less chance of going into shock if kept lying down and at rest.

You will not be able to bring a patient out of shock, but you may be able to prevent shock or keep it from worsening by following the previous procedures. The care you provide may reverse the severity of certain aspects of shock and may help the patient avoid immediate danger.

If you are trained to do so and if your state laws allow you to do so, oxygen can be very significant in helping shock patients. Provide the patient with 100% oxygen by mask. (Follow local protocols.)

> **REMEMBER:**
>
> Keeping the patient lying down and at rest reduces the risk of shock.

Fainting

Fainting is usually a self-correcting form of mild shock. However, the patient may have been injured in a fall due to fainting. Be certain to examine the patient for injury. Even if there appear to be no other problems, keep the patient lying down and at rest for several minutes.

In some cases, fainting is caused by a sudden drop or elevation of blood pressure. If you are trained to do so and have the needed equipment, check the patient's blood pressure. Otherwise, have the patient's blood pressure checked by an EMT, a Paramedic, or a nurse.

Fainting can also be a warning of some serious condition, including brain tumors, heart disease, undetected diabetes, and inner ear problems. (Do not cause the patient to faint again by telling him all these possibilities.) Always recommend that the person see a physician as soon as possible. In a polite but firm manner, tell anyone who has fainted not to drive or operate any machinery until after having been seen by a physician. Make certain that you have witnesses to this warning.

Your patient may have fainted because of fear, stress from problems, bad news, the sight of blood, or being in an accident. Be ready to provide emotional support when the patient is alert.

First You can often prevent a person from fainting by lowering the patient's head (Figure 11.24). Have the patient sit down and then lower the head between the knees. You *must* keep the patient from falling from this position. This procedure is *not* recommended for patients with fractures or

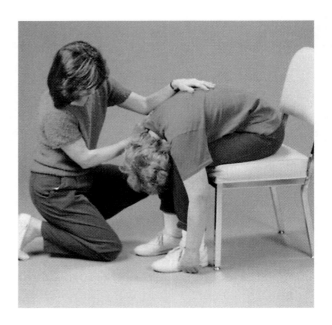

FIGURE 11.24
To help prevent fainting, lower the patient's head.

possible spinal injuries. Do *not* carry out this procedure on anyone who is having difficulty breathing or on anyone with a known heart problem. For this type of patient, lying down with the feet slightly elevated and receiving emotional support will often prevent fainting.

RECOGNIZING INJURIES

Since childhood, we have learned about injuries such as bruises, scratches, and cuts. The idea of amputations and crush injuries are at least known, if not witnessed, before we enter our teens. Our own experiences and those of the people around us lead to our general understanding of injuries.

This prior knowledge will be useful to you. To be a First Responder, you will have to refine this knowledge, learning how to recognize and provide care for various injuries. However, you should not forget your basic understanding of injuries. Most of your patients will, at best, have the same level of understanding that you had when you started this course. Remembering this will help you with patient interviews and in providing explanations and reassurance. Also, recalling what you knew about injuries as you went through childhood will help when dealing with children who have suffered injuries.

Except for cases of spinal injury and certain types of internal injury, most adults can look at someone and often tell if there is an injury. Your training will build upon this ability so that you will not miss detectable injuries. This is why there has been so much emphasis on patient assessment. As you progress through this course, you will be trained to determine the extent of injury and what specific emergency care procedures to use for given injuries.

TYPES OF INJURIES

soft tissues the tissues of the body that make up the skin, muscles, nerves, blood vessels, fatty tissues, and the cells that line and cover organs and glands. Bones, cartilage, and teeth are *hard* tissues.

This section will describe injuries to the **soft tissues** of the body that include skin, muscles, nerves, blood vessels, fatty tissues, and cells (Figure 11.25).

When considering soft-tissue injuries, two general classifications—closed wounds and open wounds—can be used.

Closed Wounds

First A **closed wound** is an internal injury in which the skin is not broken. As noted earlier in the chapter, internal injuries are usually caused by the impact of a blunt object. Bleeding can range from minor to major, while the extent of injury can range from a simple bruise to the rupturing of internal organs.

■ **Bruises.** The vast majority of closed wounds detected during First Responder care are **bruises** (contusions) (Figure 11.26). There is always some internal bleeding associated with a bruise. Since the skin is not broken, the blood flows between tissues, causing discoloration over time ranging from a brownish-yellow to black and blue. Keep in mind that large bruises can mean serious blood loss and that there may be fractures or extensive tissue damage under the site of the bruise.

Open Wounds

First In cases of **open wounds,** the skin is opened. The extent of injury can range from a single scrape to a tearing or cutting open of the skin. A simple scraping of the skin may produce no bleeding, while more severe open wounds may be associated with minor to life-threatening bleeding.

Open wounds may be classified as:

■ **Scratches and scrapes.** Wounds such as skinned elbows and knees, "road rash," "rug burns," and thorn scratches are minor open wounds known as *abrasions* (Figure 11.27). Although scratches and scrapes may be painful, tissue injury is usually not serious since the skin is not fully penetrated and the force causing the injury does not crush or rupture underlying structures. There may be no detectable bleeding or only minor capillary bleeding. Wound contamination tends to be the most serious problem faced when caring for abrasions to the skin.

■ **Cuts.** In cases of cuts, the skin is fully penetrated, with injury also occurring to tissues lying under the skin. Cuts may be classified as **smooth** or **jagged:**

closed wound an internal soft-tissue injury in which the skin is not broken.

bruise simple closed wound in which blood flows between soft tissues, causing a discoloration; a *contusion* (kun-TU-zhun).

open wound an injury to the body in which the skin or its outer layers are opened.

scratches and scrapes the simplest forms of open wounds that damage the skin surface but do not break all the layers of skin. Collectively, these injuries are called *abrasions* (ab-RAY-zhuns).

cut soft-tissue injury in which all the layers of skin are opened and the tissues immediately below the skin are damaged. Smooth cuts are incisions and jagged cuts are lacerations.

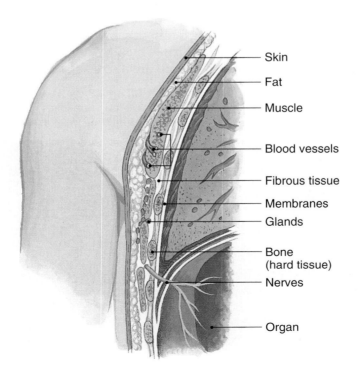

- Skin
- Fat
- Muscle
- Blood vessels
- Fibrous tissue
- Membranes
- Glands
- Bone (hard tissue)
- Nerves
- Organ

FIGURE 11.25
Soft tissues.

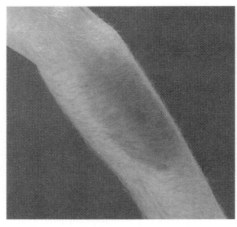

FIGURE 11.26
Bruises are the most common form of closed wounds.

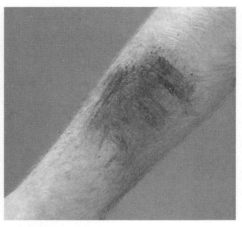

FIGURE 11.27
Scratches and scrapes (abrasions) are the least serious form of all open wounds.

– *Smooth cuts* are called **incisions** (Figure 11.28). They are produced by very sharp objects, such as razor blades, knives, and broken glass. The edges of a smooth cut appear straight, with no apparent tears or jagged areas. Deep incisions can cause severe tissue damage and life-threatening bleeding.

– *Jagged cuts* are called **lacerations.** Tissue along the edge of the wound will be torn and a rough edge is produced (Figure 11.29). Sometimes jagged cuts can be produced from the impact of a blunt object. Usually, they occur when the skin is cut by an object that does not have a very sharp edge.

■ **Punctures.** Objects such as knives, nails, and ice picks can produce puncture wounds. An object puncturing the body will tear through the skin and usually proceed in a straight line, damaging all the tissues in its path. A puncture wound may be a **penetrating wound,** ranging from shallow to deep (Figure 11.30). Another type of puncture wound is a **perforating wound.** This injury, often seen with gunshot wounds, has an entrance and an exit wound, as the object passes through the body (Figure 11.31).

■ **Avulsions.** These wounds most frequently involve the tearing loose or the tearing off of large flaps of skin (Figure 11.32). A torn ear, an eyeball removed from its socket, and the loss of a tooth are also examples of avulsions.

puncture an open wound that tears through the skin and damages tissues in a straight line. If there is only an entrance wound, the puncture is called a *penetrating wound*. If there is an entrance and an exit wound, the puncture is called a *perforating wound*.

avulsion (ah-VUL-shun) a soft-tissue injury in which flaps of skin are torn loose or torn off.

FIGURE 11.28
The edges of a smooth cut (incision) are straight.

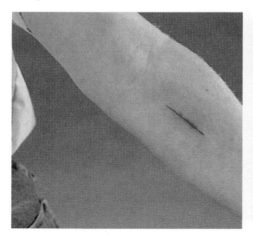

FIGURE 11.29
Tissues along the edges of a jagged cut (laceration) will be torn and rough.

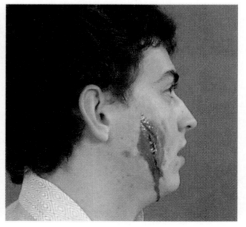

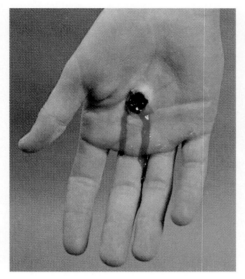

FIGURE 11.30
A penetrating puncture wound.

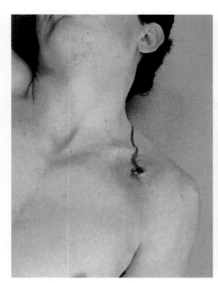

FIGURE 11.31
A penetrating wound can be perforating, having both an entrance wound and an exit wound. Often the exit wound is the more serious of the two.

- **Amputations.** These wounds involve the cutting or tearing off of the fingers, toes, hands, feet, arms, or legs (Figure 11.33). Since amputation can be done as a surgical procedure, the *injury* is often called a *traumatic amputation*.
- **Crush injuries.** Most of the time, when people see an accident in which a body part has been crushed, their first thoughts are of fractures. Soft tissues and internal organs are also crushed, often rupturing (Figure 11.34). Both external and internal bleeding can be profuse.

amputation soft-tissue injury that involves the cutting or tearing off of a limb or one of its parts. Often, hard tissues are also injured.

crush injury soft-tissue injury produced by crushing forces. Soft tissues and internal organs are crushed, and hard tissues are usually damaged.

BASIC EMERGENCY CARE

ONGOING CARE

Bystanders at emergency scenes may begin care before First Responders or other members of the EMS system arrive to begin professional-level assessment and care. Untrained individuals often focus on soft-tissue injuries. Your EMS system may require that you do not attempt to "undo" what has been done

FIGURE 11.32
Avulsions are open wounds.

FIGURE 11.33
Amputation.

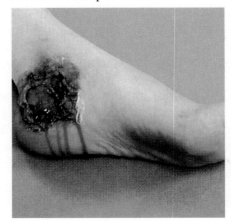

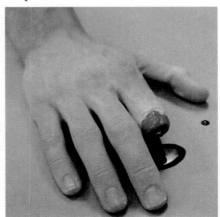

FIGURE 11.34
Both soft tissues and internal organs are damaged in crush injuries.

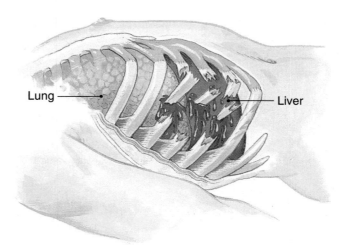

Lung ——— ——— Liver

before your arrival until EMTs or other more highly trained personnel arrive. Usually, EMS system protocols do state that obvious harmful care must be stopped and corrected. For example, persons at the scene may have applied a very tight bandage and stopped circulation in an extremity. In such a situation, you may be required to reestablish distal circulation. Your instructor will alert you to specific protocols for your EMS system.

A special problem associated with soft-tissue injuries and sporting events involves the application of ice or ice and pressure to injury sites before EMS system assessment. Even though the *RICE method* (rest, ice, compression, and elevation) is a time-honored procedure used by many coaches and trainers, it is usually *not* part of EMS system protocols. Improperly done, the RICE method may contaminate wounds, expose the patient to excessive cold, injure tissue, or reduce circulation. The RICE method typically employs elastic bandages to hold a bag of ice to the injury site. Removal of this bandage may cause additional problems, especially if the RICE method was used over a fractured bone or dislocated and/or fractured joint.

In situations where care has been rendered by individuals having less training than a First Responder, follow your EMS system protocols for assessment and care. If there is any doubt, call or have someone call 911.

CARE DURING ASSESSMENT

A limited amount of care may be initiated during the patient assessment (see Chapter 7). In your assessment of some patients, you may quickly detect some injuries that will require the start of simple care procedures (Figure 11.35). Immediately treat injuries involving airway, breathing, and circulation (major bleeding and arrest). As a First Responder, you may begin certain types of soft-tissue injury care during assessment, but take care to avoid a "tunnel vision" approach.

Remember, each patient care case is different. You should follow local protocols and begin care when safe to do so. You should treat any life-threatening injuries as you encounter them, but always remember to continue to monitor the ABCs as they generally take precedence. Do not be in such a hurry to start patient care that you miss detecting serious injuries.

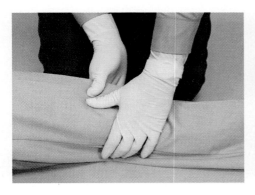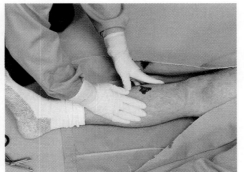

CARE OF CLOSED WOUNDS

As mentioned earlier in this chapter, the most frequently seen closed wound is the bruise. Generally, bruises do not require emergency care in the field. However, bruises can be a warning sign of possible internal injuries and related bleeding. Look for large bruises or large areas of the body covered with bruises. Remember that a deep bruise the size of the patient's fist equals a serious blood loss of about 10%. Be certain to look for swellings and deformities that may indicate fractures. Note if the patient's abdomen is rigid, if the patient is coughing up blood, or if there is blood in the mouth, nose, or ears.

CARE OF OPEN WOUNDS

First | In general, to care for open wounds, you should (Figure 11.36):

1. **Expose the wound.** Clothing over and around an open wound must be cut away. Avoid aggravating the patient's injuries. Do *not* try to remove clothing by pulling the items over the patient's head or limbs. Simply lift aside or cut the clothing away from the site of injury.

2. **Clear the wound surface.** Remove superficial foreign matter from the surface of the wound with a sterile gauze pad. This method will reduce the chances of contamination from your gloved fingers and will protect your fingertips. Do *not* try to clean the wound or pick out any particles or debris. If bleeding from the wound is controlled, take care not to restart or increase the flow of blood.

3. **Control bleeding.** Start with direct pressure or direct pressure and elevation. If the bleeding continues, try pressure point control. A tourniquet should be used as a last resort for life-threatening bleeding from a limb.

4. **Prevent further contamination.** Use a sterile dressing, clean cloth, or clean handkerchief to cover the wound. After the bleeding has been controlled, bandage the dressing in place.

5. **Keep the patient lying still.** Any patient activity increases circulation. Keep the patient lying down, using a blanket or other form of covering to provide protection from the elements.

6. **Reassure the patient.** This will reduce patient movement and may help to lower the patient's blood pressure toward a normal level.

7. **Care for shock.** This applies to all but the simplest of wounds. Do *not* elevate a limb if there is the possibility of a fracture.

Note

Remember, providing care for soft-tissue injuries may place you in contact with blood and body fluids. Take body substance isolation precautions (latex or vinyl gloves). Also, remember to wash your hands after each patient contact.

FIGURE 11.36
Care for open wounds.

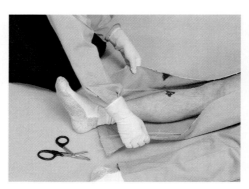

A. Expose the wound.

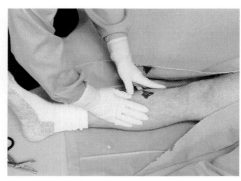

B. Clear the wound surface.

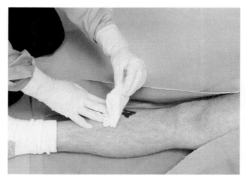

C. Control bleeding with direct pressure.

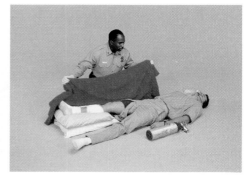

D. Keep the patient lying still, and provide care for shock.

REMEMBER:

Do *not* remove a dressing once it is in place.

If you have to control bleeding from an extremity or if the wound on the limb is a long cut, dress the wound and immobilize the limb with a splint (see Chapter 12). If an air-inflated splint is part of your First Responder equipment, use it to help control the bleeding.

CARE OF SPECIFIC INJURIES

Thus far, we have discussed the treatment of wounds and how to control bleeding. Now we will build on those concepts and discuss how to manage specific injuries.

Puncture Wounds

First | When dealing with any puncture wound, assume that there is extensive internal injury and internal bleeding. Always check for an exit wound, realizing that exit wounds can be more serious than entrance wounds (in the case of gunshot wounds). Care for entrance and exit wounds as you would any open wound in soft tissue.

If the puncture wound contains an impaled object (such as glass, a knife, wood, metal, or plastic), do the following (Figure 11.37):

1. **Do *not* remove an impaled object.**

2. Expose the wound, without disturbing the impaled object. Do *not* lift clothing over the object.

3. Control bleeding by direct hand pressure. (Wear gloves.) **CAUTION:** Take special care not to cut your gloves or hand on the impaled object. Spread your fingers around the object and apply pressure to the wound site. Do *not* put any pressure on the object or the tissues that are up against the edge of a sharp impaled object.

*N*ote

Remember, providing care for soft-tissue injuries may place you in contact with blood and body fluids. Take body substance isolation precautions (latex or vinyl gloves). Also, remember to wash your hands after each patient contact.

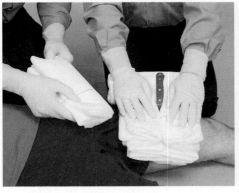

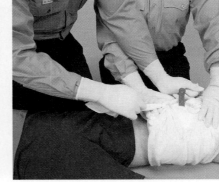

FIGURE 11.37
Impaled objects.

A. Control bleeding.   **B.** Stabilize the object in place.

4. Attempt to stabilize the impaled object by using bulky dressings. Several layers of dressings, cloths, or handkerchiefs placed on the sides of the object will help stabilize it. An alternative approach is to cut a hole in the center of a bulky dressing, making the cut slightly larger than the impaled object. *Gently* pass the dressing over the object. Bandaging these dressings in place will improve stability.

5. Keep the patient at rest and reassured.

6. Care for shock. Do *not* elevate a limb if the object is impaled in it. Do *not* elevate or bend the legs if an object is impaled in the abdomen.

The above procedures do *not* apply to objects impaled in the eye or in the cheeks. The correct procedures for these two cases will be covered later in this chapter.

Adhesive tape often does not stick to the skin around an impaled object wound site. Blood and sweat on the skin, even when the surface is cleared, may cause the tape to slip. Cravats (cloth ties) can be used to tie the dressings in place. These cravats should be made from folded cloth. Once folded, the cravats should be at least four inches wide. If the object is impaled in the chest or abdomen, a thin splint or coat hanger can be used to push the cravats under the natural void in the patient's back so that the cravat can be tied around the patient's trunk (Figure 11.38).

Avulsions

 If flaps of skin have been torn loose, but not off, you should:

1. Clear the surface of the wound.

2. Gently fold the skin back to its normal position. Follow local protocols for procedures.

3. Control bleeding and care as you would for any open wound, using bulky pressure dressings.

 If skin or another body part is torn from the body, you should:

1. Care for the wound with bulky pressure dressings.

2. Save and preserve the avulsed part. This is best done by placing the avulsed part into a plastic bag or wrapping the part in plastic wrap or sterile dressing. If possible, keep the part cool (not cold; avoid freezing). Do *not* place the avulsed part in water or in direct contact with ice.

FIGURE 11.38
A flat splint or coat
hanger can be used to
position the cravat.

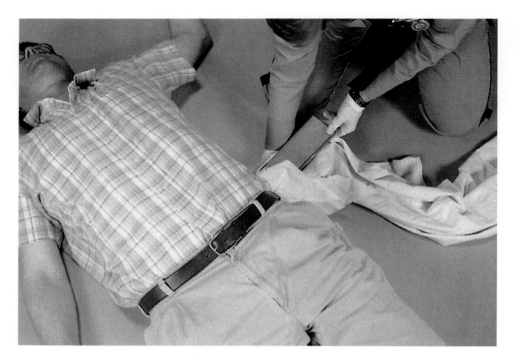

Amputations

| First | In most cases, bleeding can be controlled by direct pressure applied with a dressing held firmly over the stump. Pressure point techniques should be tried along with direct pressure if the bleeding continues. Should this fail, then apply a tourniquet. If possible, wrap or bag the amputated part in plastic and keep it cool.

Protruding Organs

| First | A deep open wound to the abdomen may cause organs to protrude through the wound opening. In such cases:

■ Do *not* try to replace the organ(s).
■ Place a plastic covering over the exposed organs. If possible, apply a thick pad dressing over the top of this covering to help conserve heat.
■ Provide care for shock. Do *not* give the patient anything by mouth.

The Scalp and Face

Injuries to the scalp and face can be difficult to treat because of the numerous blood vessels found in both regions. Many of these vessels are close to the surface of the skin, producing profuse bleeding even from minor wounds. Additional problems arise if the bones of the skull are involved, the airway is obstructed, and neck injuries occur.

Injuries to the scalp and face require an extra effort on the part of the First Responder to provide emotional support for patients. These injuries tend to be very painful, produce bleeding that frightens many patients, and are in a body region where people have concern for their appearance. Talk to patients in a calm, professional manner. Always let them know what you are going to do before you do it. Make certain that they know additional help is on the way.

| First | The procedures for the care of soft-tissue injuries covered earlier in this chapter apply to the care you should provide for injuries to the soft tissues of the scalp and face. However, there are three exceptions:

- **Exception 1:** *Do not* attempt to clear the surface of a scalp wound. This will often cause additional bleeding and may cause great harm if there are fractures to the skull.
- **Exception 2:** *Do not* apply finger pressure to the wound if there is any chance of skull fracture.
- **Exception 3:** *Do* remove impaled objects from the cheek if the object has penetrated the cheek wall and may become an airway obstruction.

 Care of scalp wounds (Figure 11.39):

1. Do *not* clear foreign matter or dirt from the wound. It will cause more bleeding.
2. Control bleeding with a dressing held in place with controlled pressure. Avoid exerting any finger pressure if there are signs of a fractured skull or the injury site feels "spongy."
3. Adhesive bandages will not work well. A roller bandage or gauze can be wrapped around the patient's head to hold dressings in place once bleeding has been controlled. If there is any indication of neck or spinal injuries, do *not* attempt to wrap the patient's head. Do *not* wrap the bandage around the patient's lower jaw or neck.
4. If there are no signs of skull fracture or injuries to the spine, neck, or chest, you may position the patient so that the head and shoulders are elevated.

An optional approach to holding a dressing in place over a scalp wound is to use a commercially prepared triangular bandage or one made from gauze or some other cloth. The steps for this procedure are shown in Figure 11.40.

Facial Wounds

The first concern when caring for facial injuries is to make certain that the patient's airway is open and breathing is adequate. Even though bleeding appears to be the only problem, check the airway and establish the presence of a carotid pulse. Continue to watch the patient to be sure that the airway remains open and clear of fluids and obstructions (tongue, teeth, blood clots).

 When caring for patients with facial injuries, you should (Figure 11.41):

1. Correct breathing problems, taking care to note and properly care for neck and spinal injuries.

FIGURE 11.39
Providing care for scalp wounds.

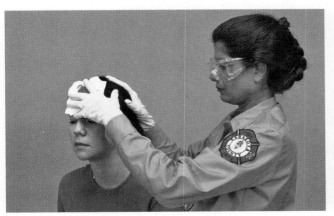
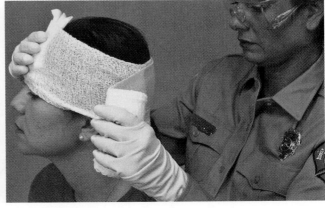

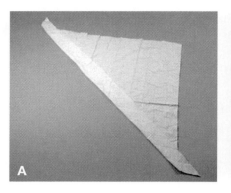

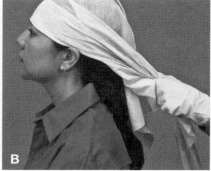

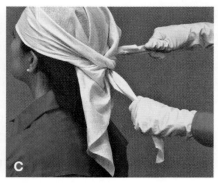

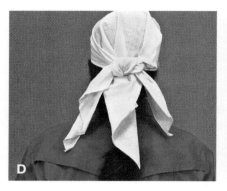

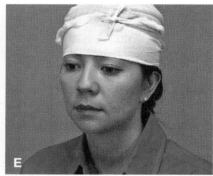

FIGURE 11.40
A Fold the bandage to make a 2-inch hem along its base. **B** Have the folded edge face out when you position the bandage on the patient's forehead, just above the eyes. Make certain that the point of the bandage hangs down behind the patient's head. **C** Draw the ends of the bandage behind the patient's head and **D** tie them over the point of the bandage. **E** Next, pull the ends to the front of the patient's head and tie them together. Finally, bring the point of the bandage down and tuck it into the crossed folds.

2. Control bleeding by direct pressure, taking care not to press too hard since many facial fractures are not obvious.

3. Apply a dressing and bandage.

First If you find the patient has an object that has passed through the cheek wall and is sticking into the mouth, you may have to remove it. This should be done if the object blocks the airway or is loose and may fall into the airway. To remove an impaled object from the cheek (Figure 11.42):

1. Look into the mouth and probe to see if the object has passed through the cheek wall.

FIGURE 11.41
Care of soft-tissue injuries to the face.

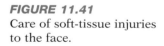

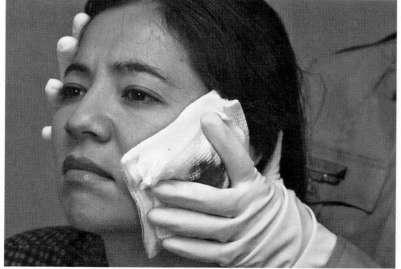

2. If you find penetration, *pull* or safely and carefully *push* the object out of the cheek wall, back in the direction from which the object entered the cheek. Avoid cutting your gloves and yourself. If the object has not penetrated the cheek wall, or if you cannot easily remove the object, stabilize it with dressings applied to the outer surface of the cheek.

3. In all cases, except for neck and spinal injuries, turn the patient so that blood will drain from the mouth. If there are neck or spinal injuries, do *not* turn the patient. Use dressing material packed against the inside wound to control the flow of blood.

4. If you remove an impaled object, pack the inside of the patient's mouth with dressing material. Place the material between the wound and the patient's teeth, leaving some of the dressing outside the mouth so that it can be held to prevent swallowing it. Watch closely to be sure this material does not work its way loose and into the airway. Do *not* assume that the patient's swallow reflex will prevent this material from becoming a major obstruction.

5. Dress and bandage the outside of the wound.

Eye Injuries

Two rules of soft-tissue injury care apply when caring for an eye injury. Do *not* remove any impaled objects and do *not* try to put the eye back into its socket. When caring for a cut eyeball, there is one major exception to the procedures listed for soft-tissue injury care:

First | **EXCEPTION:** Do *not* apply direct pressure on a cut eyeball. There are jelly-like fluids inside the eyeball that cannot be replaced. A loose bulky dressing will help the formation of blood clots to control the bleeding.

Problems resulting from foreign objects in the eyes are common. These problems can range from minor irritations to permanent injury caused by sharp objects. If the patient's own tears do not wash away the foreign object(s), use running water to remove them (Figure 11.43). **Do not apply the wash if there are impaled objects or cuts in the eye.**

Apply the flow at the corner of the eye socket closest to the patient's nose. You may have to help the patient hold open the eyelids. As you pour the water into the eyes, direct the patient to look from side to side and up and down. Before completing the wash, have the patient blink several times. When possible, continue the wash for *at least 20 minutes* or for the time recommended by your EMS system's Medical Director.

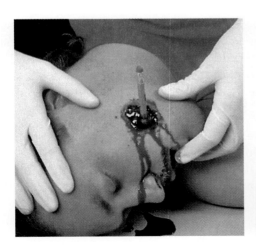 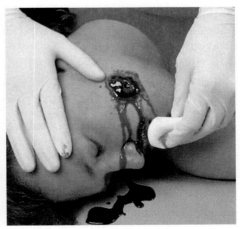

FIGURE 11.42
Removing an impaled object from the cheek.

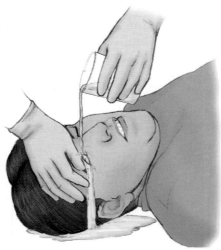

FIGURE 11.43
Foreign objects can be washed from the eye.

Note

After debris is washed from the eye, the patient must be examined by someone with more advanced training. A physician or qualified eye care specialist should see the patient.

First It is critical that you:

- Do *not* remove impaled objects (including what may appear to be small pieces of glass impaled in the globe of the eye).
- Do *not* probe into the eye socket.
- Reduce the patient's eye movements. If there are sharp objects in the patient's eye, do *not* direct the patient to move the eyes during the wash. After the wash, keep the patient's eyes shut. Cover *both* eyes, bandaging the materials in place.

Whenever you are caring for a patient with eye injuries, you will have to cover both of the patient's eyes. In most cases, only one eye will actually be injured. However, when one eye moves, the other eye will also move (sympathetic movement). If you cover the injured eye and leave the uninjured eye uncovered, the uninjured eye will continue to react to activities and movement. Each time the uninjured eye moves, so will the injured eye. Having both of the patient's eyes covered reduces eye movements.

Obviously, a patient with both eyes covered will not be able to see, causing fear and anxiety. Tell the patient why you are covering the uninjured eye. Keep close to the patient or have someone else stay close. Try to maintain contact with the patient through conversation and touch. If a friend or loved one of the patient also has been injured, reassure the patient that care is being provided for others.

If the patient is unconscious, it is best to keep someone with him at all times. This person can reassure the patient if consciousness returns and can help prevent the patient from reaching for his covered eyes. Should the unconscious patient have to be left unattended, you may tie the hands at the waist to prevent the grabbing of the eyes should consciousness be regained. Even though this may produce a fearful moment for the patient, it is better than the additional injury that could take place. Any procedure that requires the tying of the patient's hands must be approved by your EMS system.

First Always remember to close the eyelids of unconscious patients. Since unconscious people do not blink, moisture is quickly lost from the eye surface, damaging the eye. If you notice that the patient is wearing contact lenses, be sure to point this out to the EMTs who take over the care of the patient.

First | Burns to the eye must always be considered serious, requiring special in-hospital care. The actions taken by a First Responder can often make the difference as to whether or not the patient's sight can be saved. As a First Responder, you may have to care for burns to the eyes caused by heat, light, or chemicals (Figure 11.44).

- **Heat burns**—Do *not* try to inspect the eyes if there are signs of heat burn to the eyelids. With the patient's eyelids closed, cover the eyes with loose, moist dressings. If you have no means to moisten the dressings, then apply loose, dry dressings. Do *not* apply any burn ointment to the eyelids.
- **Light burns**—"Snow blindness" and "welder's blindness" are two examples of light burns. Close the patient's eyelids and apply dark patches over both eyes. If you do not have dark patches, then use thick dressings or dressings followed with a layer of an opaque material such as dark plastic.
- **Chemical burns**—Many chemicals cause rapid, severe damage to the eyes. Flush the eyes with water. Do *not* delay care by trying to locate sterile water. Use any source of clean drinking water. If possible, continue the washing flow for **at least 20 minutes.** After washing the patient's eyes, close the eyelids and apply loose, moist dressings.

First | If you find an object impaled in the globe of a patient's eye, you should (Figure 11.45):

1. Use several layers of dressing or small rolls of gauze to make thick pads. Place them on the sides of the object. If you have only enough material for one thick pad, cut a hole, equal to the size of the eye opening, in the

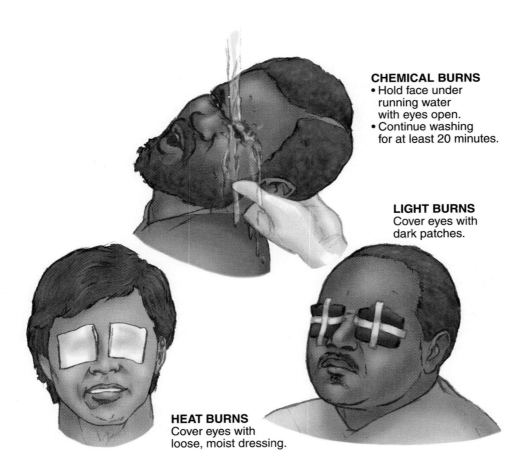

FIGURE 11.44
Basic care for burns to the eye.

CHEMICAL BURNS
• Hold face under running water with eyes open.
• Continue washing for at least 20 minutes.

LIGHT BURNS
Cover eyes with dark patches.

HEAT BURNS
Cover eyes with loose, moist dressing.

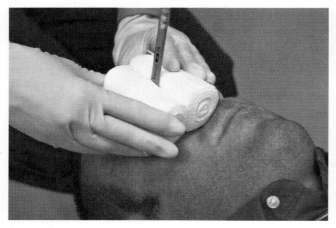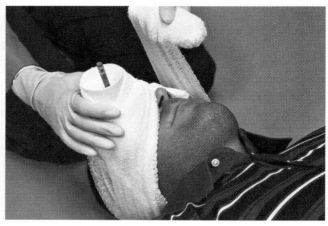

FIGURE 11.45
Care for a patient with an object impaled in the globe of the eye.

center of this pad. Set the pad over the patient's eye, allowing the impaled object to stick out through the opening cut into the pad.

2. Fit a disposable cardboard drinking cup or paper cone over the impaled object. (Do *not* use foam cups since they can break and send flakes into the eye.) This will serve as a protective shield. Rest the cup or cone onto the thick dressing pad, but do not allow this protective shield to come into contact with the impaled object.

3. Hold the pad and protective shield in place with a self-adherent roller bandage or with a wrapping of gauze or other cloth material.

4. Use dressing material to cover the uninjured eye, and bandage this dressing in place. This will reduce eye movements.

5. Provide care for shock.

6. Provide emotional support to the patient.

 Note

Consider any bleeding from the ear as a sign of serious head injury.

Wrapping a paper cup or cone with gauze is very tricky and cannot be done easily unless you practice. Ideally, you should wrap around the cup and then continue around the patient's head and wrap around the cup again. This procedure is repeated until the cup is stable. Do *not* wrap the gauze over the top of the cup. *Take great care* not to push the cup down onto the impaled object or pull the cup out of place.

 If the eye is pulled out of the socket (avulsed eye), the care provided is the same as for an object impaled in the eye.

External Ear Injuries

- *Cuts*—Apply dressing and bandage in place (Figure 11.46).
- *Tears*—Apply bulky dressings, beginning with several layers behind the torn tissue.
- *Avulsions*—Use bulky dressings, bandaged into place. Save the avulsed part in a plastic bag or plastic wrap. Keep the part dry and cool. If no plastic is available, then wrap in dressing material. Be certain to label the bag, wrap, or dressing.

Internal Ear Injuries

Any bleeding from the ear must be considered a sign of serious head injury. Bloody or clear fluids draining from the ear may indicate the presence of cerebrospinal fluid (see Chapter 12) associated with severe head injury. For such

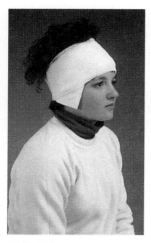

FIGURE 11.46
When caring for injuries to the external ear, apply a dressing and bandage.

cases, assume there is serious injury and provide the necessary care. More will be said about head injuries in Chapter 12.

- *Bleeding from the ears*—Do *not* pack the external ear canal. To do so may cause increased internal injury. Apply external dressings and hold these in place with bandages. Report this bleeding to the EMTs.
- *Foreign objects in the ear*—Do *not* attempt to remove the objects. Apply external dressings if necessary and provide emotional support to the patient.
- *Bloody or clear fluids draining from the ears*—Do *not* pack the external ear canal. Apply a loose, external dressing. This dressing should be sterile, but any clean dressing will do if a sterile dressing is not available.
- *"Clogged" or "stopped up" ear*—Damage to the eardrum, fluids in the middle ear, and objects in the ear canal all can cause the patient to complain of "clogged" or "stopped up" ears. Do not probe into the ears. Many of these problems will go away without care or quickly after hospital care. As a First Responder, your main duty in such cases is to prevent the patient from hitting the side of the head in an effort to clear the ears. These blows may cause severe internal ear damage.

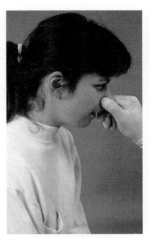

FIGURE 11.47
Caring for nosebleeds. Remember to position the patient for proper drainage.

Nose Injuries

First For now, we will assume that there are no skull fractures or spinal injuries. When dealing with any nasal injuries, you will have two duties: maintain an open airway and stop bleeding. You may be called upon to care for nosebleeds.

Nosebleeds (conscious patients)—Maintain an open airway. Have the patient assume a seated position, leaning slightly forward. This position will help prevent blood and mucus from obstructing the airway or draining down the throat and causing nausea and vomiting. Next, have the patient pinch the nostrils. Bleeding is usually controlled when the nostrils are pinched shut. If the patient cannot pinch them shut, you will have to do so (Figure 11.47). However, if other patients are in need of your help, do not delay their care while you sit pinching someone's nose. Have a bystander put on gloves, pinch the patient's nose, and inform you of any problems as you continue to care for the other patients. Do *not* pack the patient's nostrils.

Nosebleeds (unconscious patients)—If patients are unresponsive or injured in such a way that they cannot be placed into a seated position, lay them back with the head slightly elevated or place them on one side with the head turned to provide drainage from the nose and mouth. Attempt to control bleeding by pinching the nostrils shut.

- *Fluids draining from the nose*—Do *not* pack the nose. Bloody or clear fluids may indicate skull fractures (see Chapter 12).
- *Foreign objects in the nose*—Do *not* remove objects or probe into the nose. Do not allow the patient to blow her nose if she is bleeding from the nostrils or has recently controlled a nosebleed.
- *Avulsions*—Apply a pressure dressing to the site. Save the avulsed part in plastic or a sterile or clean dressing. Keep the part cool.

Nasal fractures will be covered in Chapter 12. Also, see Scan 11-4 for a summary of care for soft-tissue injuries to the head.

Injury to the Mouth

First As with all injuries that occur along the pathway of respiration, your first concern will be to ensure an open airway. If there are no

> **REMEMBER:**
> A First Responder must apply knowledge to make decisions. You must judge the severity of bleeding in cases of nosebleeds. Most are minor, requiring very little attention. However, nosebleeds can be serious, with profuse bleeding. You will have to care for them accordingly.

Care for Soft-Tissue Injury: The Head

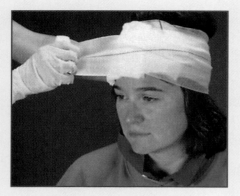

SCALP. Control bleeding, dress, and wrap with roller bandage.

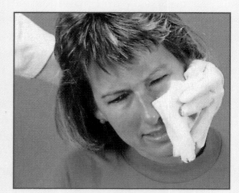

FACIAL. Ensure airway, control bleeding, dress, and wrap with roller bandage.

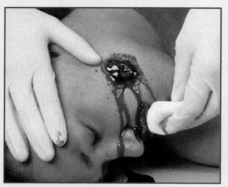

CHEEK. Ensure airway, remove impaled object, and control bleeding. Dress and bandage the external wound.

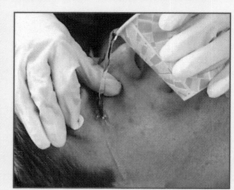

DEBRIS IN EYE. If eye is not cut, wash objects from surface.

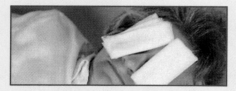

EYE BURNS. Wash chemical burns (20 minutes). Loosely dress heat burns. Apply dark patches for light burns.

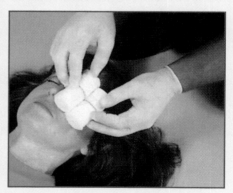

IMPALED OBJECT IN THE EYE. Stabilize the object and apply rigid protection.

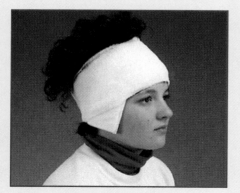

EAR WOUND. Do not pack canal. Dress and bandage.

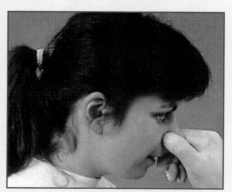

NOSEBLEED. Pinch nostrils shut.

suspected skull, neck, or spinal injuries, position the patient in a seated position with the head tilted slightly forward to allow for drainage. If the patient cannot be placed in a seated position, position him on one side with the head turned slightly downward to provide some drainage for blood and other fluids.

- *Cut lips*—Use a rolled or folded dressing. Place this dressing between the patient's lip and gum. Take great care that the patient does not swallow this dressing.
- *Avulsed lips*—Apply a pressure bandage to the site of injury and save the avulsed part in plastic or a sterile or clean dressing. Keep the avulsed part cool.
- *Cuts to the internal cheek*—Do *not* pack the mouth with dressings. Any dressing positioned between the patient's cheek and gum will have to be held in place by a gloved hand. Always leave 3 to 4 inches of dressing material outside the patient's mouth. This will allow for quick removal. This is necessary to prevent the patient from swallowing the dressing. If possible, position the patient's head to allow drainage.

(Injuries to the bones of the skull and face and avulsed teeth will be covered in Chapter 12.)

Neck Wounds

First Blunt and sharp injuries can occur to the neck. (Fractures will be covered in Chapter 12.) As a First Responder, be aware of the following signs that indicate neck wounds:

- Difficulty with speaking, loss of voice
- Airway obstruction when the mouth and nose are clear and no object can be dislodged from the airway. This is often due to swollen tissues.
- Obvious swelling or bruising of the neck
- Windpipe pushed off to one side (tracheal deviation)
- Depressions in the neck
- Obvious cuts or puncture wounds

First For all profuse bleeding from blood vessels in the neck, make certain that someone alerts dispatch, informing them of the problem and the need for immediate EMS transport. Cut or severed arteries in the neck require the following procedure:

1. *Immediately* apply direct pressure over the wound, using the palm of your gloved hand.
2. Try controlling the bleeding with a pressure dressing, taking care not to close the airway and not to apply pressure to both sides of the neck.
3. Once the bleeding is controlled, place the patient on the left side (Figure 11.48). If possible, lay the patient on a surface that can be slanted (spineboard, table, long bench, plywood) so that the entire body can be tilted into a head-down position. The slant should be no more than 15 degrees. This will help trap any air bubbles that may have entered the bloodstream.
4. Provide care for shock.

First Bleeding from a large cut or severed neck veins usually cannot be controlled by pressure dressings. For such emergencies, you should (Figure 11.49):

1. Immediately apply direct pressure to the wound, using the palm of your gloved hand.
2. Apply an occlusive dressing of plastic wrap.

FIGURE 11.48
When possible, place the patient on the left side with the body slanted in a head-down position.

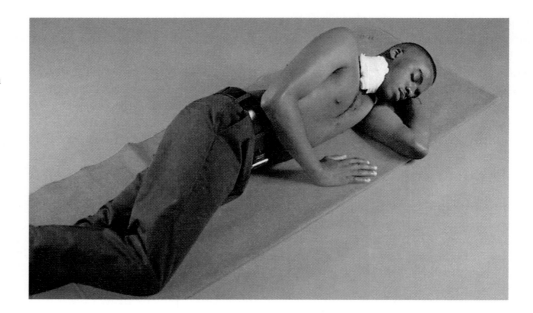

WARNING:

Do *not* attempt to reposition the patient if there are indications of spinal injury (very likely), if the bleeding was very difficult to control (usually the case), or if you had difficulty carrying out the dressing and bandaging procedures (true for most rescuers).

3. Use tape to seal this dressing on all sides. When complete, the dressing must be airtight.

4. Place the patient on the left side for transport, with the body slanted as described above (see WARNING). There is a greater chance of air entering the blood when a large vein is opened. Air bubbles may be sucked into open veins and carried to the heart. This situation can cause cardiac arrest. The greatest potential problem is with the large neck veins.

5. Care for shock by maintaining body warmth and providing oxygen.

If you do not have the materials to make an occlusive dressing, use any sterile or clean dressing material and attempt to control bleeding by direct pressure.

Some EMS systems have tried a new method for controlling profuse bleeding from the blood vessels in the neck. Their success indicates that other EMS systems may be adopting this method. Your instructor will tell you if this technique is approved for use in your state.

The newer method uses the same procedure for both arterial and venous bleeding. If the patient is bleeding from the neck, you should:

1. *Immediately* apply direct pressure over the wound, using the palm of your gloved hand.

2. Place a plastic occlusive dressing over the wound and continue to apply pressure, using the palm of your hand. Do *not* use a single layer of plastic wrap. It is too thin and may be sucked into the wound. Ideally, the occlusive dressing should extend 1 inch beyond the wound on all sides.

3. Place a roll of gauze dressing or dressing materials over the occlusive dressing and continue to apply pressure. Another roll can be placed between the wound and the trachea to help reduce pressure on the trachea.

4. While maintaining pressure, secure the entire dressing with a figure-eight wrap of self-adherent roller bandage. This eliminates the problem of trying to make adhesive tape stick to a bloody surface.

5. Place the patient on the left side for transport, with the body slightly slanted in a head-down position.

6. Care for shock by maintaining body warmth and providing oxygen.

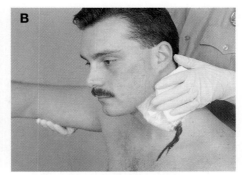

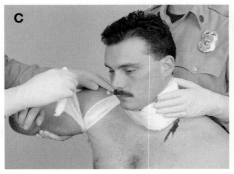

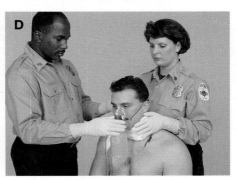

FIGURE 11.49
Use an occlusive dressing to help control bleeding from the neck.

All these methods take a great deal of practice and review if they are to be done correctly in the field.

Should your attempts to control the bleeding fail, a last-resort method would be to place your gloved finger or fingers into the wound and attempt to compress the vessel or pinch shut the ends. This a very difficult procedure that has little chance for success. If the vessel has been severed, the ends may have shifted or rolled away from the wound opening, making success even less likely. Again, this is a last resort to be used only when standard First Responder-level care procedures have failed to control life-threatening profuse bleeding.

Penetrating Chest Wounds

The results of most soft-tissue injuries to the chest are the same as those in other areas of the body and will receive the same basic type of care. Typically, these injuries are cuts, bruises, and puncture wounds.

Serious soft-tissue injuries to the chest include deep puncture wounds, penetrating wounds, and impaled objects. For puncture and penetrating wounds, apply dressings; impaled objects must be stabilized. Wounds from punctures and impaled objects may go through the chest, and if so, you will have to care for both an entrance wound and an exit wound. Deep punctures to the chest are generally serious because of the vital organs located there. This type of wound occurs when an object tears or punctures the chest wall and creates an open wound to the chest cavity. The object may remain impaled in the chest, or the wound may be completely open. As explained in Chapter 6, breathing causes pressure in the chest cavity. When the chest wall is open, this pressure balance is affected. The lung will collapse because air gets between the lung and the chest wall and extra pressure builds up inside the chest cavity. You must seal the wound on the outside to prevent air from entering the chest space and causing lung collapse. The seal will also allow the lungs to reexpand.

In some cases, the lung itself will be penetrated (Figure 11.50). As the patient inhales, air from this lung will leak out and enter the chest cavity from inside the chest. If the wound has been tightly sealed on the outside, pressure

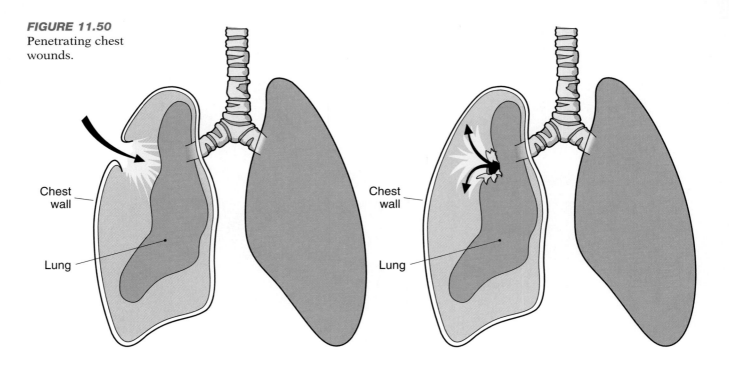

FIGURE 11.50
Penetrating chest wounds.

Note

Be very observant. The air may enter through the chest wall, from damaged lungs with the chest having an opening, or from damaged lungs with the chest wall remaining intact, as with damage caused by fractured ribs and/or sternum.

sucking chest wound an open chest wound in which air is sucked through the wound opening and into the chest cavity each time the patient breathes.

may still build from the inside as air continues to enter the cavity from the punctured lung during each breath. Unless this pressure is released, it may interfere with heart and lung actions.

First You will be able to tell if a puncture wound has penetrated the lung by noting:

- An open chest wound in which the chest wall is torn or punctured
- A sucking sound each time the patient breathes. This is why this type of wound is sometimes called a **"sucking" chest wound.**
- The patient is coughing up bright red, frothy blood

If you find that a penetrating chest wound has both an entrance and an exit wound, assume that at least one lung has been punctured.

First The following method is recommended for all penetrating chest wounds free of impaled objects (Figures 11.51 and 11.52). If there is no puncture to the lung, the method will work. If there is a punctured lung, this method will allow release of air trapped in the chest.

1. Have all dressing materials ready. Don personal protective equipment. Then seal the patient's wound with the palm of your gloved hand as the patient exhales (a forceful exhalation will push trapped air out of the chest cavity). Do not unseal the wound to prepare dressings. Have others at the scene help in preparing the dressings.

2. Place an occlusive dressing under your hand while the patient exhales, and hold it in place. Have someone seal it by placing tape on three edges.

   - Taping three edges produces a "flutter valve" effect. When the patient inhales, the free edge will seal against the skin. As the patient exhales, the free edge will break loose from the skin and allow any buildup of air in the chest cavity to escape.

   - Some EMS systems prefer that all four edges be taped. The last edge is taped as the patient exhales.

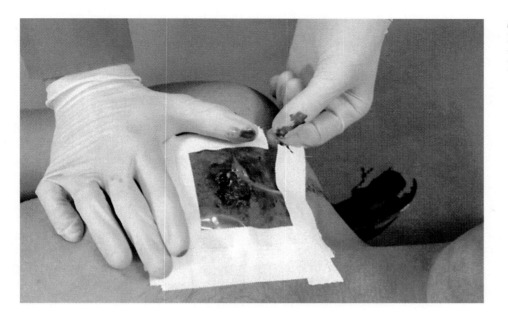

FIGURE 11.51
Penetrating chest wound—punctured lung.

With either taping method, the patient must be monitored. If the patient begins to have trouble breathing again, lift up one side of the plastic and have him forcefully exhale. Then quickly reposition the plastic to reseal.

3. Provide oxygen as soon as possible, and maintain body temperature to prevent shock.

A commercial occlusive dressing is the best choice for open chest wounds. Plastic wrap can be used, but it must be folded over several times so that it is thick enough to prevent air from seeping through it and so it will not be sucked into the wound. The occlusive dressing should extend 2 or more inches beyond the edge of the wound.

If blood or perspiration prevents the tape from sticking to the patient's skin, apply bulky dressings over the occlusive dressing and secure this in place with cravats (cloth ties). You must still monitor the patient and relieve pressure buildup if the patient develops difficulty breathing. In cases when the EMTs will not be delayed in their arrival and tape will not hold the dressing, hold the

Note

Closely monitor the breathing of all patients with penetrating chest wounds.

On inspiration, dressing seals wound, preventing air entry

Expiration allows trapped air to escape through untaped section of dressing

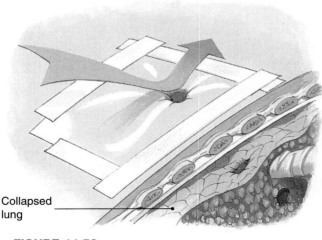

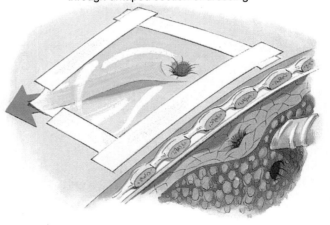

Collapsed lung

FIGURE 11.52
Create a flutter valve to release entrapped air.

occlusive dressing in place with the palm of your gloved hand. If the patient's condition declines, periodically release one edge of the seal in order to allow trapped air to escape as described above.

If there is an entrance wound and an exit wound, both wounds will need a dressing. You may have to wait for EMT assistance to roll the patient and apply a dressing to the patient's back.

Penetrating wounds of the chest may also penetrate the heart. When this occurs, there is little that the First Responder can do other than provide care for shock and for the open chest wound and provide basic life support as needed.

Impaled Objects

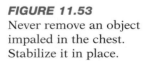 An impaled object must be left in place. Even though it created the wound, the impaled object is also sealing the wound. If it is removed, the patient may bleed profusely. The object must be stabilized with bulky dressings or pads (Figure 11.53). Begin by placing these materials on opposite sides of the object, along the vertical line (long axis) of the body. Place the next layer perpendicular (opposite direction) to the first. Use tape or cravats to hold all dressings and pads in place. If tape will not hold, carefully apply cravats according to local protocols.

Abdominal Injuries

In Chapter 4, we studied the locations of the various body organs. Before continuing with this section of Chapter 11, study Scan 4-1 (page 55) to review the locations of the major hollow and solid organs of the abdomen and pelvis.

Internal bleeding can be severe when an internal organ ruptures. In addition, hollow organs can rupture and drain their contents into the abdominal and pelvic cavities, producing a very serious and painful reaction. As a First Responder, you should be aware of the following signs that indicate injury to the abdominopelvic organs:

- Any deep cut or puncture wound to the abdomen, pelvis, or lower back
- Indications of blunt trauma to the abdomen or pelvis
- Pain or cramps in the abdominopelvic region
- The patient is protecting the abdomen (guarded abdomen)
- The patient is trying to lie still with legs drawn up
- Rapid, shallow breathing and a rapid pulse
- Rigid and/or tender abdomen

FIGURE 11.53
Never remove an object impaled in the chest. Stabilize it in place.

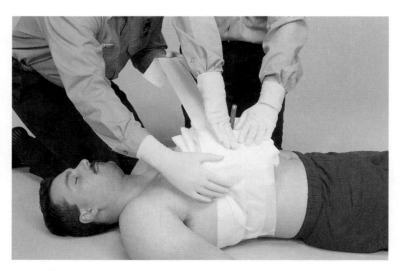

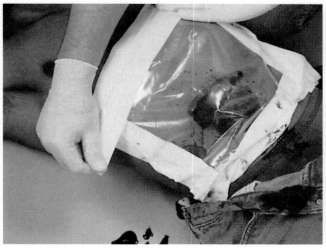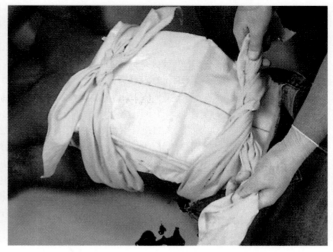

FIGURE 11.54
For open wounds of the abdomen, apply an occlusive dressing and cover to prevent heat loss.

First | Care for all possible abdominal and pelvic injuries by:

1. Dressing all open wounds.
2. Laying the patient back, with the legs flexed. Do not flex the legs if there are any signs of injury to the pelvic bones, lower limbs, or back.
3. Caring for shock and constantly monitoring vital signs.
4. Being alert for vomiting.
5. Being certain that you do not touch any exposed internal organs. Cover them with an occlusive dressing, such as plastic wrap. Maintain warmth to the organ by placing dressings or a towel over the occlusive dressing (Figure 11.54). (Some EMS systems provide sterile materials to allow the First Responder to apply a moist, sterile dressing in place of the occlusive dressing.)
6. Being certain that you do not remove any impaled objects. Stabilize the object with bulky dressings.

Many patients with abdominal pain find some relief by hugging a bulky, soft object such as a pillow against the abdomen.

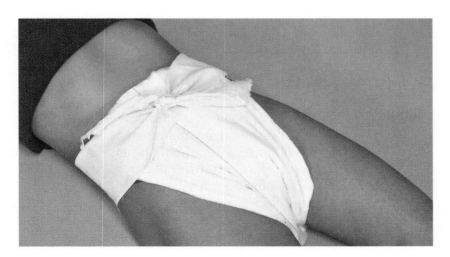

FIGURE 11.55
Dressings applied to the genitalia can be secured with a triangular bandage.

Injury to the Genitalia

genitalia (jen-i-TA-le-ah) the external reproductive organs.

First | Because of their location, the external reproductive organs are not a common site of injury. The pelvis and the thighs usually prevent injury to these organs, which are known as the external **genitalia.** When injury does occur, two types of soft-tissue injury are commonly seen:

- *Blunt trauma injury*—Such injury is very painful, but little can be done by the First Responder. An ice pack, if available, will help reduce the pain.
- *Cuts*—Bleeding should be controlled by direct pressure. A sterile dressing or a sanitary pad should be used. If either of these is not available, then use any clean, bulky dressing. Once bleeding is controlled, the dressing can be held in place with a large triangular bandage, applied in the same manner as a diaper (Figure 11.55).

Other soft-tissue injury care procedures also apply when treating injuries to the genitalia:

- Do *not* remove impaled objects.
- *Save* avulsed parts, wrapping them in plastic, sterile dressings, or any clean dressing.

First Responders are a part of the professional health care team. As such, you must carry out your role in a manner that will reduce embarrassment for the patient. Tell the patient what you are going to do. Tell the patient why you must examine and care for the genitalia. Protect the patient from the sight of onlookers by having them leave the scene. If this is not possible, have them turn their backs to the patient. Then, provide care without any hesitation. Conduct all procedures in the same manner as you would care for an injury to any other part of the body. This is essential if you are to provide proper total patient care.

Many genital injuries are self-inflicted or are the result of abuse. They may also be caused by an illegal abortion. If this is the case, the patient will also need emotional support, understanding, and sympathy. (See Chapter 10 for management of behavioral emergencies.)

CAUTION:
Provide emotional support and understanding for patients with genital injuries.

BURNS

First Responders should consider burns to be very complex soft-tissue injuries that can range from a simple upper skin surface (epidermis) injury to very serious deep injury that may involve nerves, blood vessels, muscles, and bones. Careful patient assessment is necessary to avoid missing injuries or medical problems that may be far more serious than obvious burns.

CLASSIFICATIONS OF BURNS

First | Burns can be classified in a number of ways. One approach is to categorize burns based on the agent that caused the injury or the source of the burn. This information should be gathered and forwarded to more highly trained personnel during transfer of care. Burns may be caused by:

- Heat (thermal)—This includes fire, steam, and hot objects.
- Chemicals—This includes caustics, such as acids, and alkalis.
- Electricity—This includes electrical outlets, frayed wires, and faulty circuits.
- Lightning—This includes injuries during electrical storms.

- Light—This includes burns to the eye caused by intense light sources and burns to the skin or eyes by ultraviolet light (including sunlight).
- Radiation burns—Usually from nuclear sources.

Always investigate the source of a burn carefully and never assume a source. The environment where the patient was burned may be hazardous and may contain hazardous materials. Talk with bystanders and the patient in addition to performing a patient assessment. This information will assist in finding out exactly what happened to cause the injury.

 Most often burns are categorized according to the depth of skin involved (Figure 11.56):

- **Superficial burns** involve the top layer of skin known as the epidermis. Also known as *first-degree* burns, they involve reddening of the skin and pain at the site. A common example is a sunburn.
- **Partial-thickness burns** involve both the epidermis and the dermis (the top two layers of skin). Also known as *second-degree* burns, they generally involve intense pain, white to red skin that is moist and mottled, and blisters. A classic example is a steam burn.
- **Full-thickness burns** extend through all dermal layers and may involve subcutaneous layers, muscle, bone, or organs. Also known as *third-degree* burns, they can be dry and leathery and may appear white, dark brown, or charred. Since there is often nerve damage present, there may be no sensation of pain present.

superficial burn a first-degree burn involving only the outer layer of skin (epidermis).

partial-thickness burn a second-degree burn in which the outer layer of skin is burned through and the second layer (dermis) is damaged.

full-thickness burn a third-degree burn involving all the layers of skin. Muscle layers below the skin and bones may also be damaged.

FIGURE 11.56
Burns classified by depth.

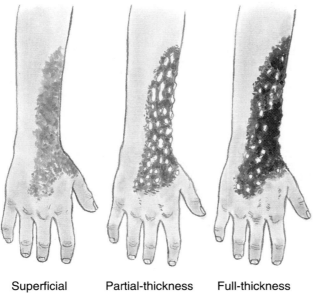

Superficial   Partial-thickness   Full-thickness

Epidermis
Dermis
Fat
Muscle

Skin reddened   Blisters   Charring

SEVERITY

First | An important aspect of treating burns is being able to assess the severity or extent of the damage. A system in place for determining the amount of skin surface burned is the **rule of nines** (Figure 11.57). A quick reference for learning the rule of nines is to keep in mind that a patient's palm is about 1% of his or her body surface area. You can apply this concept to yourself during study periods and in practice situations. When in doubt, your own palm can help you make a quick estimate, but burns often overlap different body regions. When in doubt, estimate to the higher percentage. As you go through this textbook, practice estimates and work up to typical body sizes in practical class exercises.

For adults, the head and neck, chest, abdomen, each arm, the front of each leg, the back of each leg, the upper back, and the lower back and buttocks are each considered equal to 9% of the total body surface area. This gives a total of 99%. The remaining 1% is assigned to the genital area.

For infants and children, a simple approach assigns 18% to the head and neck, 9% to each upper limb, 18% to the chest and abdomen, 18% to the entire back, 14% for each lower limb, and 1% to the genital area. This method adds up to a total of 101% but provides an easy way to make approximate determinations.

By using the rule of nines, you can add up the areas affected by burns to determine how much of the patient's body has been injured. For example, if an adult patient has third-degree (full-thickness) thermal burns to the chest and front of one leg, this 9% + 9% means that 18% of the total body surface area has been burned.

As a First Responder, you may not be required to learn the rule of nines. In most situations, knowing this information will not be necessary to carry out your duties. This information, however, may be useful when communicating patient information to more highly trained EMS personnel, such as EMT-Bs or Paramedics on the scene.

FIGURE 11.57
Rule of nines.

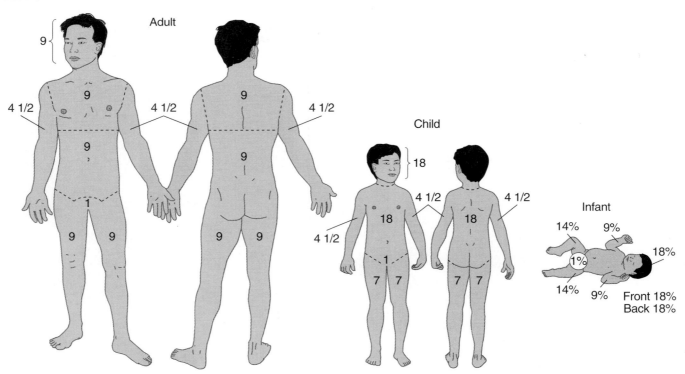

RULES FOR FIRST RESPONDERS

 Regardless of the system used to evaluate burns, follow these rules:

1. Always perform the initial assessment and the focused assessment. Provide basic life support as needed.
2. Provide care for all burns—even the most minor or superficial.
3. Any of the following burns should be considered critical and should be evaluated by someone in the EMS system above the level of First Responder:
   - hands, feet, face, groin, buttocks, thighs, major joints
   - any burn that encircles a body part
   - burns estimated at greater than 15% or more of the patient's body
4. When in doubt, overclassify. For example, consider a serious superficial burn to be partial thickness.
5. Always consider the effects of a burn to be more serious if the patient is a child, elderly, the victim of other injuries, or someone with a medical condition (for example, respiratory disease).

CARE OF BURNS

> **WARNING:**
>
> Do *not* attempt to rescue people trapped by fire unless you have been trained to do so. The simple act of opening a door or window could cost you your life. Do not endanger yourself and risk creating more patients.

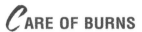 **Minor Burns:** A superficial or partial-thickness burn that involves less than 9% of the patient's total body surface area is a minor burn. The exceptions are if the burn involves the respiratory system, face, hands, feet, groin, buttocks, or major joint.

Major Burns: Any burn to the *face* (other than simple sunburn) is an example of a major burn. Other major burns include any superficial burns covering a large area of the body or burns involving the feet, hands, groin, buttocks, or major joint.

 First Responder care for burns includes:

1. **Complete a scene size-up before initiating care.** Your first action once a scene size-up is completed is to ensure that the burning process has been stopped. This may require the patient to stop, drop, and roll to extinguish the flames. You might also have to smother the flames and wet down or remove smoldering clothing.
2. **Alert dispatch.** In some EMS systems, First Responders are directed not to request EMT support for minor or superficial burns. In some systems, dispatchers will ask certain questions to determine if EMTs or ambulance transport will be needed. If you are ever in doubt, play it safe and request an EMT response.
3. **Perform an initial assessment.** Assuring that a patient's airway, breathing, and circulation are intact is a priority for the First Responder. If a burn involves the mouth, nose, throat, or airway, the burn should be considered critical, and an EMT-B or Paramedic response should be requested.

minor burn a superficial or partial-thickness burn (first- or second-degree) involving a small portion of the body with *no* damage to the respiratory system, face, hands, feet, groin, medial thigh, buttocks, or major joints. It does not encircle or cover an entire body part.

major burn any full-thickness (third-degree) burn, a partial-thickness (second-degree) burn involving an entire body area of crucial area, a superficial (first-degree) burn that covers a large area, any burn to the face, or any burn that involves the respiratory system.

4. **For minor burns:** Flush the burned area with cool or running water (or saline) for several minutes.

5. **For major burns:** Do *not* flush burns with cool water unless they involve an area of less than 9% of the total body surface area, indicating a minor burn.
   - Remove smoldering clothing and jewelry.
   - Continually monitor airway.

6. **Prevent further contamination.** Keep the burned area clean by covering it with a dressing. Infection is common with burns.

7. **Cover with dry, sterile dressing** (Figure 11.58). In some EMS systems, you may be instructed to moisten dressings before placing them onto the patient. Otherwise, place dry, sterile dressings onto the burned area. Follow local protocols.

8. **Do *not* use ointment, lotion, or antiseptic.** With the exception of simple sunburn, these items can increase the rate of infection and complication of a burn patient.

9. **Do *not* break blisters.** Breaking blisters will increase the risk of infection.

10. **Give special care to the eyes.** If the eyes or eyelids have been burned, place sterile dressings or pads over them. As mentioned earlier in this chapter, you should moisten these pads with sterile water if possible.

11. **Give special care to the fingers and toes.** If a serious burn involves the hands or feet, always place a sterile or clean pad between each toe or finger before completing the dressing.

12. **Any burns to the face or exposure to smoke in a fire may cause airway problems.** Make sure the airway is open and clear, care for shock, and provide oxygen as soon as possible.

FIGURE 11.58
First Responder supplies for care of burns.

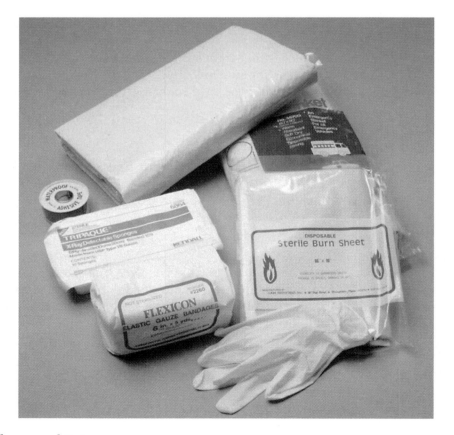

SPECIAL CONSIDERATIONS

Thermal Burns

See Scan 11-5 for a summary of caring for thermal burns.

Chemical Burns

Many chemicals exist that are harmless if they are used properly or remain contained; but if these chemicals come in contact with the human body, they can cause harm. Some chemicals irritate the skin and create burns very quickly, while others create a slow, painful burning process. In either case, it is crucial to stop the burning process and remove the irritant.

Some scenes involving patients with chemical burns can be very dangerous. Completing a scene size-up and ensuring scene safety is very important. There may be a pool of dangerous chemicals near the patient. Acids may be spurting from containers. Toxic fumes may be in the air. If you believe there are hazards at the scene that will place you in danger, do not attempt a rescue unless you have been trained to do so and have the necessary equipment.

Remember that body substance isolation is required on every patient contact. Wear latex or vinyl gloves and additional equipment if required by local protocol.

The primary method of caring for chemical burns is to wash away the chemical with water. A simple wetting of the burned area is not enough. Flood the area of the patient's body that has been exposed. Continue to **flush the area for at least 20 minutes.** Be sure to remove all contaminated clothing, shoes, socks, and jewelry from the patient during the wash.

Once you have flushed the area for at least 20 minutes, apply a dry, sterile dressing, care for shock, and make sure dispatch has been notified. If the patient begins to complain of increased burning or irritation once a dressing is in place, remove the dressing and flush the burned area with water for several minutes. Then, apply a new dry dressing.

Alert dispatch on all cases of chemical burns.

First | Remember, when treating chemical burns:

- Flush the burned area for at least 20 minutes.
- Apply a dry, sterile dressing.
- If burning continues, remove dressing and flush again.

First | If dry lime is the agent causing the burn, DO NOT begin by flushing with water. Instead, use a DRY dressing to BRUSH the substance off the patient's skin, hair, and clothing. Also have the patient remove any contaminated clothing or jewelry. Once this is done, you may flush the area with water (Figure 11.59).

Chemical burns to the eyes require immediate attention. Also assume that both eyes are involved. When caring for chemical burns to the eyes, you should:

1. Perform scene size-up. Ensure scene safety.
2. Assure BSI precautions.
3. Perform initial assessment/ABCs.
4. Immediately flood the eyes with water (Figure 11.60).
5. Keep the water flowing from a faucet, bucket, or other source into the eye. You may have to hold the eyelid open to ensure a complete washing.

> **WARNING:**
> Scenes involving chemical burns may be hazardous to emergency personnel.

> **WARNING:**
> Take appropriate BSI precautions on every patient contact.

> **Note**
> Brush dry lime from the patient's skin before applying water.

Care for Thermal Burns

Type of Burn		Tissue Burned			Color Changes	Pain	Blisters
		Outer Layer of Skin	Second Layer of Skin	Tissues Below Skin			
Superficial	(First degree)	Yes	No	No	Red	Yes	No
Partial-Thickness	(Second degree)	Yes	Yes	No	Deep red	Yes	Yes
Full-Thickness	(Third degree)	Yes	Yes	Yes	Charred black or white	Yes	Yes

MINOR: SUPERFICIAL AND PARTIAL-THICKNESS

❏ Have someone alert dispatch.
❏ Immerse in cold water 2–5 minutes.
❏ Cover entire burn with dry, sterile dressing.
❏ Moisten—only if burn is less than 9% of skin surface.

MAJOR BURNS: EXTENSIVE SUPERFICIAL, PARTIAL-THICKNESS, AND ANY FULL-THICKNESS BURNS

❏ Stop burning process.
❏ Have someone alert dispatch.
❏ Maintain open airway.
❏ Wrap area with dry, clean dressing.*
❏ Provide care for shock.

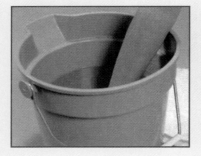 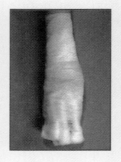

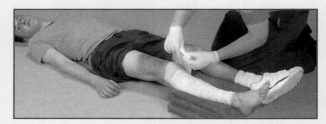

*Moisten dressing if less than 9% of skin surface is affected.

IF HANDS OR TOES ARE BURNED:

❏ Separate digits with sterile gauze pads.
❏ When appropriate, elevate the extremity.

BURNS TO THE EYES:

❏ Do not open eyelids if burned.
❏ Be certain burn is thermal, not chemical.
❏ Apply moist, sterile gauze pads to both eyes.

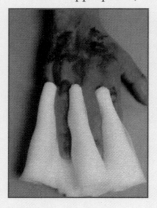 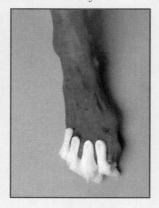

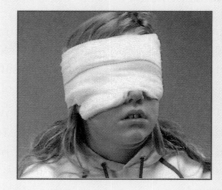

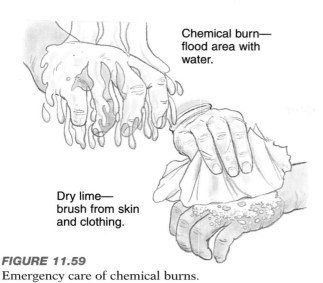

Chemical burn—flood area with water.

Dry lime—brush from skin and clothing.

FIGURE 11.59
Emergency care of chemical burns.

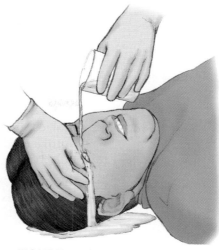

FIGURE 11.60
Care of chemical burns to the eyes.

6. Continue flushing for at least 20 minutes, continuing to flush after transport.

7. After flushing the eyes, cover both eyes with moistened pads.

8. Remove the pads and flush again if the patient begins to complain about increased burning sensations or irritation.

Electrical Burns

On the scene of an electrical injury, burns are not usually the most serious problem a patient sustains. Cardiac arrest, nervous system damage, and injury to internal organs may occur with these incidents (Figure 11.61).

Alert dispatch for *all* cases involving electrical burns.

The scene of an electrical injury is often very hazardous. Make sure that the source of electricity has been turned off before caring for the victim. If the electricity is still active, do *not* try to attempt a rescue unless you have been trained to do so and have the necessary equipment.

> **WARNING:**
>
> Always make certain the electricity is off before entering the scene of an electrical injury.

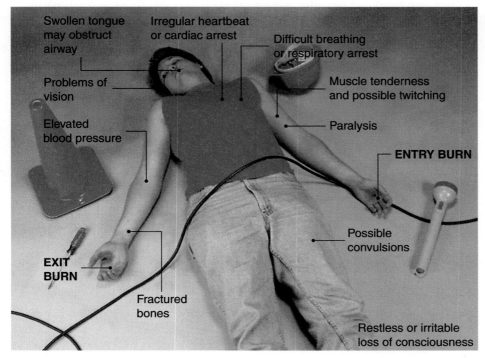

FIGURE 11.61
Injuries due to electrical accidents.

Swollen tongue may obstruct airway

Irregular heartbeat or cardiac arrest

Difficult breathing or respiratory arrest

Problems of vision

Muscle tenderness and possible twitching

Elevated blood pressure

Paralysis

ENTRY BURN

EXIT BURN

Possible convulsions

Fractured bones

Restless or irritable loss of consciousness

To provide care for a patient with an electrical burn, you should:

1. Perform scene size-up, including scene safety.

2. Assure BSI precautions.

3. Perform an initial assessment. Electricity passing through a patient's body will often cause cardiac arrest. Even if the victim appears stable, be prepared for complications involving the airway and heart. External injuries do not reflect the true nature of injury; all electrical injuries require medical attention.

4. Evaluate the burn. Look for two burn sites, the entrance and exit wounds. The entrance wound (often the hand) is where the electricity entered the body. The exit wound is where the electricity came into contact with a ground (often a foot). External injuries *do not* reflect the *true* nature of the injury; all electrical injuries require medical attention.

5. Apply dry, sterile dressings to the burn sites. You may apply moistened dressings if transport is delayed, the burn involves less than 9% of the body, and the patient will not be in a cold environment.

6. Provide care for shock.

7. Make certain dispatch has been notified.

Infants and Children

The extent of burns to young children and infants can be very difficult to assess because they may not understand why they hurt or may feel the hurt is a punishment for something they did wrong. They may be unable to explain how much or exactly where it hurts because of their fear and/or limited knowledge because of their age. You should remember that children will be afraid as well as in pain because of their injury. Also, remember that:

- Children have a greater skin surface area in relation to total body size. In other words, more areas can be burned.
- The greater the surface area is, the greater the fluid and heat loss will be.
- Keep the environment warm whenever possible.
- You may consider the possibility of child abuse. If the burns are suspicious, do not confront the parents. Report your suspicion to local authorities.

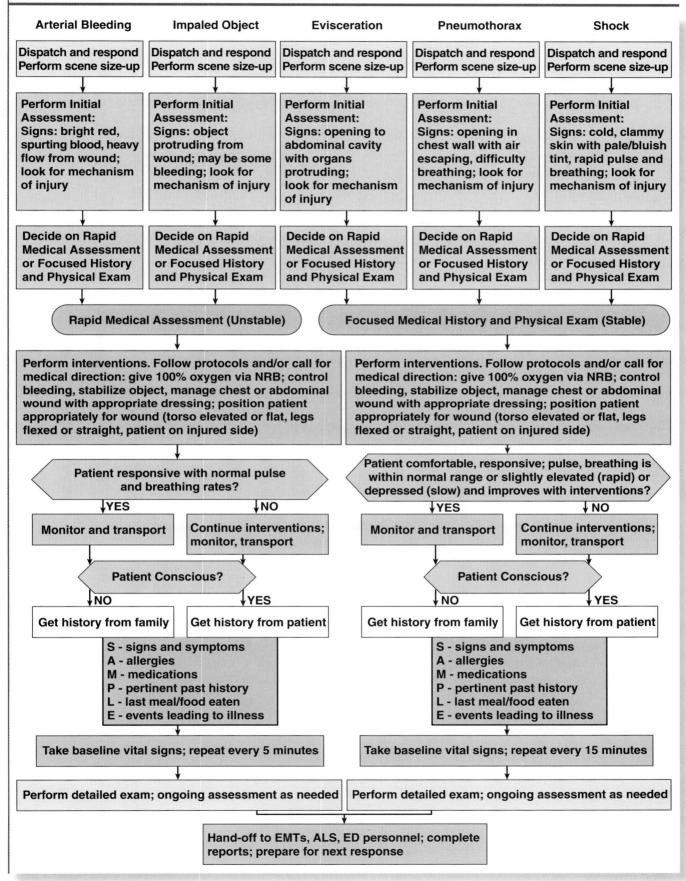

Arterial Bleeding	Impaled Object	Evisceration	Pneumothorax	Shock
Dispatch and respond Perform scene size-up	Dispatch and respond Perform scene size-up	Dispatch and respond Perform scene size-up	Dispatch and respond Perform scene size-up	Dispatch and respond Perform scene size-up
Perform Initial Assessment: Signs: bright red, spurting blood, heavy flow from wound; look for mechanism of injury	Perform Initial Assessment: Signs: object protruding from wound; may be some bleeding; look for mechanism of injury	Perform Initial Assessment: Signs: opening to abdominal cavity with organs protruding; look for mechanism of injury	Perform Initial Assessment: Signs: opening in chest wall with air escaping, difficulty breathing; look for mechanism of injury	Perform Initial Assessment: Signs: cold, clammy skin with pale/bluish tint, rapid pulse and breathing; look for mechanism of injury
Decide on Rapid Medical Assessment or Focused History and Physical Exam	Decide on Rapid Medical Assessment or Focused History and Physical Exam	Decide on Rapid Medical Assessment or Focused History and Physical Exam	Decide on Rapid Medical Assessment or Focused History and Physical Exam	Decide on Rapid Medical Assessment or Focused History and Physical Exam

Rapid Medical Assessment (Unstable)

Focused Medical History and Physical Exam (Stable)

Perform interventions. Follow protocols and/or call for medical direction: give 100% oxygen via NRB; control bleeding, stabilize object, manage chest or abdominal wound with appropriate dressing; position patient appropriately for wound (torso elevated or flat, legs flexed or straight, patient on injured side)

Perform interventions. Follow protocols and/or call for medical direction: give 100% oxygen via NRB; control bleeding, stabilize object, manage chest or abdominal wound with appropriate dressing; position patient appropriately for wound (torso elevated or flat, legs flexed or straight, patient on injured side)

Patient responsive with normal pulse and breathing rates?

Patient comfortable, responsive; pulse, breathing is within normal range or slightly elevated (rapid) or depressed (slow) and improves with interventions?

↓YES → Monitor and transport   ↓NO → Continue interventions; monitor, transport

↓YES → Monitor and transport   ↓NO → Continue interventions; monitor, transport

Patient Conscious?

Patient Conscious?

↓NO → Get history from family   ↓YES → Get history from patient

↓NO → Get history from family   ↓YES → Get history from patient

S - signs and symptoms
A - allergies
M - medications
P - pertinent past history
L - last meal/food eaten
E - events leading to illness

S - signs and symptoms
A - allergies
M - medications
P - pertinent past history
L - last meal/food eaten
E - events leading to illness

Take baseline vital signs; repeat every 5 minutes

Take baseline vital signs; repeat every 15 minutes

Perform detailed exam; ongoing assessment as needed

Perform detailed exam; ongoing assessment as needed

Hand-off to EMTs, ALS, ED personnel; complete reports; prepare for next response

$\mathcal{S}$ummary

Bleeding can be classified as external or internal. Both types of bleeding can range from minor to life-threatening.

The risk of infectious disease must be considered when treating bleeding patients. Use gloves, goggles, gowns, and masks to protect yourself from infectious bodily fluids.

Bleeding may be classified as:
- **Arterial**—profuse loss of bright red blood spurting from an artery
- **Venous**—mild to profuse loss of dark red blood flowing steadily from a vein
- **Capillary**—slow loss of red blood oozing from a bed of capillaries as seen in minor scrapes of the skin

The four major techniques for *controlling external bleeding* are: direct pressure and pressure dressing, elevation, pressure points, and tourniquet.

Direct pressure and pressure dressing is the first step in controlling bleeding.

Dressings cover wounds, and **bandages** hold dressings in place. Dressings can be single-layered or built up into bulky dressings. Occlusive dressings are used when an airtight seal is required.

To control bleeding, use sterile or clean materials and cover the entire wound. Do not remove any dressing once it is in place.

Secure a bandage so that it is not too loose or too tight. It should have no loose ends. Do not cover the patient's fingertips or toes.

Internal bleeding can be very serious. Look for mechanisms of injury that may cause internal bleeding. Look for wounds associated with internal bleeding, and examine the patient for signs and symptoms of shock. Care for internal bleeding is the same as for shock.

Shock, or **hypoperfusion,** is the *lack* of perfusion to all vital parts of the body. Unless the process is stopped, the patient will die. The symptoms of shock may include weakness, nausea, thirst, dizziness, and fear. The signs of shock may include restlessness, combativeness, profuse external bleeding, vomiting or loss of body fluids, shaking and trembling (rare), altered mental status, shallow and rapid breathing, rapid and weak pulse, pale skin (with the face often turning blue), cool and clammy skin, and lackluster eyes with dilated pupils.

To prevent or care for shock, you should keep the patient at rest, maintain an adequate airway, and maintain normal body temperature. Be sure to control external bleeding and splint major fractures. For most cases of shock, elevate the lower extremities.

Closed wounds and **open wounds** are soft-tissue injuries. Internal body organs may also be involved. **Bruises** (contusions) are the most common form of closed wound, while **scratches** and **scrapes** (abrasions) and cuts (lacerations and incisions) are the most common forms of open wounds.

Puncture wounds are open wounds, classified as penetrating or perforating. Perforating wounds have an entrance *and* an exit wound.

Avulsions occur when skin or a body part (tip of the nose, fingertip, external ear, tooth, lip) is torn loose or off the body. The cutting or tearing off of fingers, toes, hands, feet, arms, or legs is called an **amputation.**

Crush injuries can have open wounds with severe soft-tissue damage. Both internal and external bleeding are seen with these injuries.

When caring for closed wounds, assume there is internal bleeding. When providing care for open wounds, ensure personal safety, then expose the wound. Control bleeding by dressing the wound. Care for shock (hypoperfusion). Remember to care for the entire patient. Provide emotional support by reassuring the patient.

For puncture wounds, assume that there are internal injuries and bleeding. Remember to look for exit wounds.

Do *not* remove **impaled objects.** Control bleeding and stabilize the object. If the object is in the cheek wall, has passed though into the mouth, and causes an airway obstruction, remove the object.

Partially avulsed skin can be placed back in its normal position. If skin is torn loose, preserve the part. Do not try to replace an avulsed eye. Do not try to replace protruding organs. In cases of avulsion, control bleeding and be prepared to care for shock.

Attempt to control bleeding from **amputation** with direct pressure applied to a dressing held firmly over the stump. Elevate and apply pressure point techniques if needed. Your last resort is a tourniquet.

Specific care procedures require you to remember certain rules and exceptions. For example:

- *Scalp wounds*—Do not try to clean the wound; do not apply finger pressure if there is any chance of a skull fracture.
- *Facial wounds*—Maintain an open airway, control bleeding, dress and bandage the wounds. If there are no skull, neck, or spinal injuries, position the patient for drainage.
- *Eye wounds*—
    - Do not apply direct pressure to a cut eyeball.
    - Do not remove impaled objects; cover with dressing pads and a rigid shield (for example, a paper cup).
    - Do not replace an eyeball pulled from its socket.
    - Do not open the eyes of a patient with burns to the eyelids.
    - Wash foreign objects from the eye.
    - Care for chemical burns by washing the eyes for at least 20 minutes.
    - Keep the patient's eyelids closed.
    - Always cover both of the patient's eyes.
- *Ear wounds*—Do not probe into the ear; do not pack the ear canal. For cuts and bleeding from the ear, apply a dressing and bandage. Wrap avulsed parts in plastic.
- *Nose injuries*—Maintain an open airway; do not pack the nostrils. Control bleeding by pinching nostrils shut. Wrap avulsed parts in plastic.
- *Mouth injuries*—Maintain an open airway and position for drainage. Do not pack the mouth. Use dressings and direct pressure to control bleeding and hold the dressings in place.
- *Neck wounds*—Look for signs of neck wounds. Care for arterial bleeding with pressure dressings and venous bleeding with an occlusive dressing.

- *Penetrating chest wounds*—Place occlusive dressings on penetrating chest wounds. Apply and seal three or four edges of the dressing and monitor the patient for signs of pressure buildup in the chest. If you see signs of pressure buildup, release the seal and reseal it after the patient has exhaled.
- *Abdominal injuries*—Look for signs of abdominal injury, care for shock, be alert for vomiting. If there are no injuries to the pelvic bones or lower limbs, flex the patient's legs to reduce pain.
- *Genitalia injuries*—Conduct an examination and provide care in a professional manner. Control bleeding by direct pressure and pressure dressing. Save avulsed parts.

Burns can be caused by heat (thermal), chemicals, electricity, light, or radiation, and they may be classified as:

- **Superficial** *(first-degree)*—involve the top layer of skin known as the epidermis.
- **Partial-thickness** *(second-degree)*—involve both the epidermis and the dermis (the top two layers of skin).
- **Full-thickness** *(third-degree)*—extend through all dermal layers and may involve subcutaneous layers, muscle, bone, or organs.

For **minor burns,** flush the burned area with water (or saline) for several minutes. Do not flush **major burns** with water unless they involve less than 9% of the total body area, indicating a minor burn. Cover with dry, sterile dressings.

Remember and Consider...

Bleeding is a very common condition. All of us at some point in our lives have suffered a scraped knee, paper cut, or perhaps a laceration to the palm from a broken glass while washing dishes. The good news is that most wounds are relatively minor and can be controlled easily. Approximately 95% of the time, direct pressure and elevation can effectively control bleeding. The bad news is that even minor bleeding can, in some cases, become serious. Never assume that a condition is minor simply based on the absence of major bleeding.

In your First Responder classes, you will practice bandaging wounds, controlling bleeding, and treating patients for shock. Bandages do not have to be neat; they simply have to be functional. Think about the types of wounds you may encounter and how you will treat them.

✔ Do you have personal protective equipment readily available for use?

✔ What will you use to control bleeding?

✔ What equipment will you need to care for bleeding/shock victims?

You should feel comfortable answering these questions. Review what you have learned in this chapter and in class and try applying it to your life. How will these things be useful to you, your coworkers, family, friends, and others?

Remember, the purpose of the initial assessment is to detect and control life-threatening problems.

✔ Go back to Chapter 7 and review the steps involved in performing an initial assessment.

Relate the detection of developing shock to all stages of the patient assessment.

✔ What might you find during the initial assessment?

✔ What might your see that would indicate shock when you observe the entire patient?

✔ What will you find when taking vital signs (breathing, radial pulse, and skin temperature)?

✔ What should you notice about a patient's eyes if he or she is going into shock?

✔ What information related to shock is gained when you examine the head and face of a patient?

✔ What might have caused this patient to go into shock?

Investigate...

✔ Do public places keep emergency care supplies handy for public use?

✔ Does your employer have a first-aid kit stocked and ready to use?

Accidents and injuries can happen anywhere. They often occur in places when you least expect them. What would you do if you encountered someone who is bleeding or in shock in a public place or at work? Are bandages or dressings available that you could use? What would you do without supplies? What plan could you have in mind in case you run into such a problem?

You might choose to carry a personal first-aid kit in your car. This would allow you access to first-aid supplies and BSI equipment at any time. While some malls and shopping centers are beginning to have equipment available at a centralized location, many do not. Know where the equipment is or how to gain access to it. Be prepared to render aid at any time and any place.

CHAPTER 12

MUSCLE AND BONE INJURIES

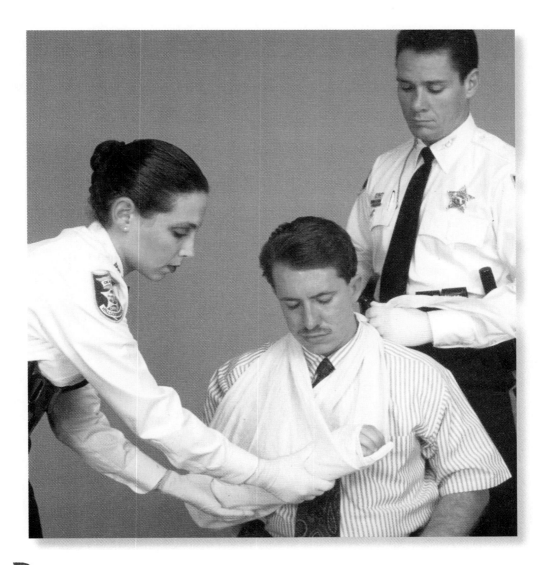

*B*ones are the foundation of our body. Like the steel girders that make the foundation of buildings and give the strength to their structure, bones provide the tough, internal structure and support for the daily demanding activities we put our bodies through. The difference between buildings and bodies, though, is that bodies are made of live tissue. They are able to move and bend by the actions of muscles and other tissues attached to bone structures and by the messages received from a system of nerves controlled by the brain.

   This chapter describes the structure and function of the muscles and bones and reviews the function of the nervous system that controls the actions of the muscles and bones. It explains how to recognize signs and symptoms of and care for injuries to muscles and bones and describes the purpose of splinting and stabilizing injuries and how to immobilize them with different types of splints.

National Standard Objectives

This chapter focuses on the objectives of Module 5, Lesson 5–3 of the U.S. DOT First Responder National Curriculum and serves as an instructional aid to help you meet any specific objectives added to the course by your local EMS system.

By the end of this chapter, you will know how to:
(from cognitive or knowledge information) . . .

5–3.1	Describe the function of the musculoskeletal system. (pp. 373–374)
5–3.2	Differentiate between an open and a closed painful, swollen, deformed extremity. (pp. 379–382)
5–3.3	List the emergency medical care for a patient with a painful, swollen, deformed extremity. (pp. 383–410)
5–3.4	Relate mechanism of injury to potential injuries of the head and spine. (pp. 414–415)
5–3.5	State the signs and symptoms of a potential spine injury. (pp. 420–421)
5–3.6	Describe the method of determining if a responsive patient may have a spine injury. (pp. 421–423)
5–3.7	List the signs and symptoms of injury to the head. (pp. 416–418)
5–3.8	Describe the emergency medical care for injuries to the head. (pp. 418–420)

Learning Tasks

Chapter 12 explains the functions of the muscles and bones and how they are controlled by the nervous system. You will need to understand the relationship between the system of muscles and bones (musculoskeletal system) and the nervous system and apply the knowledge you gain from this chapter to the assessment and care steps that you will provide to patients with trauma injuries. As you work through this chapter and meet the above objectives, you will also need to keep the following information in mind and be able to perform the skills listed.

You will learn the parts of the skeleton through the pictures in this chapter and from your instructor. As you practice your assessment skills, be able to:

✔ Locate and name the major bones of the extremities.

During your patient assessment steps, you will look and feel for signs and symptoms of injured extremities. Be able to:

Feel comfortable enough to (by changing attitude, values, beliefs) . . .	5–3.9	Explain the rationale for the feelings of patients who have need for immobilization of a painful, swollen, deformed extremity. (pp. 384, 389–390, 402, 406, 407, 408, 418, 440)
	5–3.10	Demonstrate a caring attitude towards patients with a musculoskeletal injury who request emergency medical services. (pp. 384, 389–390, 402, 406, 407, 408, 418, 440)
	5–3.11	Place the interests of the patient with a musculoskeletal injury as the foremost consideration when making any and all patient-care decisions. (pp. 380, 381, 383, 388, 389, 397)
	5–3.12	Communicate with empathy to patients with a musculoskeletal injury, as well as with family members and friends of the patient. (pp. 384, 389–390, 402, 406, 407, 408, 418, 440)

Show how to: (through psychomotor skills) . . .	5–3.13	Demonstrate the emergency medical care of a patient with a painful, swollen, deformed extremity. (pp. 383–410)
	5–3.14	Demonstrate opening the airway in a patient with suspected spinal cord injury. (p. 424)
	5–3.15	Demonstrate evaluating a responsive patient with a suspected spinal cord injury. (pp. 421–423)
	5–3.16	Demonstrate stabilizing of the cervical spine. (pp. 424–425)

✔ Define painful, swollen, deformed extremity.

✔ Demonstrate how to assess patients and identify injuries to extremities based on signs and symptoms.

You will also practice stabilizing and immobilizing or splinting injured extremities. Splinting helps reduce pain and control bleeding. Proper care through splinting can help make recovery less complicated. Be able to:

✔ List five complications related to extremity injuries.

✔ Define splinting and state its primary purpose.

You must handle extremity injuries carefully. There are several steps to follow when you immobilize or splint these injuries. Be able to:

✔ State the rules for splinting and the general steps to follow in all cases requiring splinting.

✔ Describe the splinting procedures for injuries to the bones of the extremities.

✔ Define manual traction and describe how it is applied to an extremity prior to splinting.

Sometimes the mechanism of injury is so severe its force causes the extremity to become deformed or bent out of its normal position. This "bent" position is also called "angulated." Be able to:

✔ Define angulated fracture and describe the procedures for straightening angulated closed fractures.

First Responders may not carry many, or even any, commercial splints. Painful, swollen, deformed extremities can be immobilized with a variety of rigid, semi-rigid, and soft items that will support and stabilize an injured extremity. Be able to:

✔ List objects that can be used as splints when commercial splints are not available.

✔ Perform splinting procedures on "patients" with simulated painful, swollen, deformed extremity injuries, using improvised or commercial splints provided for First Responders in your area.

Trauma accidents will often harm more than the extremities. Many vital organs are protected by bones that make up the center of the skeleton, the skull, the spine, and the chest or rib cage. This central part of the skeleton is the *axial skeleton*. Be able to:

✔ List the parts of the axial skeleton and describe its function.

Enclosed in the skull and spinal column is the central nervous system (brain and spinal cord), which sends messages to all parts of the body so it can move and function. You must be able to assess and recognize injury to the central nervous system by:

✔ Listing the parts of the central nervous system and describing its function.

✔ Describing common mechanisms of injury that can damage and affect the function of the axial skeleton and the central nervous system.

✔ Listing the signs and symptoms of head, spine, and chest injuries.

The mechanism of injury and the resulting traumatic injuries can cause you to focus on the injury before you do anything else. However, remember your patient assessment steps and what always comes first. Be able to:

✔ Describe the importance of airway management for patients with head, spine, and chest injuries.

✔ Describe and demonstrate airway management techniques for head and spine injuries.

Trauma patients with head injuries may be responsive or unresponsive. For either patient, airway management and the assessment steps must be performed carefully. Depending on the mechanism of injury, trauma patients may have multiple injuries. First Responders must know how to manage a variety of injuries. Be able to:

✔ Describe and demonstrate the steps for assessing responsive and unresponsive patients for head and spine injuries.

✔ Demonstrate the emergency care procedures for a patient with simulated open and closed head injuries.

✔ Describe and demonstrate how to stabilize and care for injuries to the head and spine.

✔ Describe and demonstrate the care and airway management techniques for patients with chest injuries.

✔ Demonstrate the emergency care procedures for a patient with simulated open and closed chest injuries.

✔ Describe the possible patient problems that may result from improper care to head, spine, and chest injuries.

---

*N*ote

First Responders are often busy with initial assessment and care for any life-threatening injuries, so they may not have time to begin splinting interventions before EMTs arrive. Usually, EMTs will bring the appropriate types and sizes of splints and will splint extremities when they arrive at the scene. EMTs may need First Responders to assist them with splinting. But First Responders who learn how to assess and recognize extremity injuries, and who can quickly and carefully splint them after stabilizing life-threatening problems, will be able to make the patient comfortable sooner. Your ability to use scene time wisely to assess and manage trauma patients while waiting for EMTs to arrive will also help shorten the time patients must spend on the scene.

---

*I*NTRODUCTION

The **musculoskeletal system** is made up of many muscles, bones, joints, connective tissues, blood vessels, and nerves. Trauma, whether minor or major, can cause a variety of injuries to the muscles, bones, and other tissues that make up the musculoskeletal system. When assessing these injuries, First Responders are not expected to determine whether an injury is a fractured bone, a joint dislocation, a ligament sprain, or a muscle strain. You will assess the patient and typically see common signs of trauma—swelling and deformity; and hear patients describe a common symptom of trauma—pain. Sometimes fractures and dislocations are obvious, but often the extremity just looks swollen and deformed. Because of this, an injury to the arms and legs is classified as a **painful, swollen, deformed (PSD) extremity,** which will have the common signs and symptoms noted above.

The extremities include the many bones and joints of the arms and legs. Surrounding the bones and joints are muscles and other soft tissues such as blood vessels and nerves. These other tissues work with the skeletal structures to nourish, support, and move them. Figure 12.1 shows the major blood vessels and a few of the major nerves found in the arms and legs. You do not need to remember every vessel and nerve, but you must remember that a large network of vessels and nerves weaves throughout the body. Injuries to the skeleton can also damage blood vessels and nerves and cause bleeding and loss of movement or function. Careful assessment and initial management is important for preventing or reducing blood loss and for minimizing or preventing nerve damage. Your actions can promote healing and help restore the function of the musculoskeletal system.

musculoskeletal system all the muscles, bones, joints, and related structures such as tendons and ligaments that enable the body and its parts to move and function.

PSD an abbreviation for painful, swollen, deformed extremity.

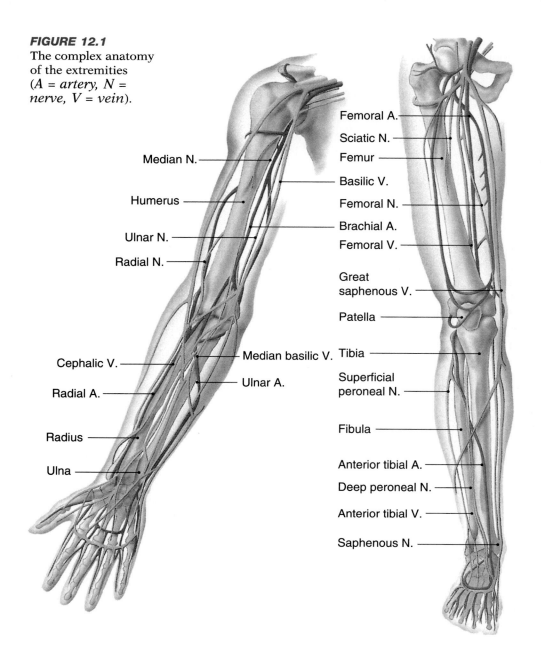

FIGURE 12.1
The complex anatomy of the extremities (*A = artery, N = nerve, V = vein*).

Median N.

Humerus

Ulnar N.

Radial N.

Cephalic V.

Radial A.

Radius

Ulna

Median basilic V.

Ulnar A.

Femoral A.

Sciatic N.

Femur

Basilic V.

Femoral N.

Brachial A.

Femoral V.

Great saphenous V.

Patella

Tibia

Superficial peroneal N.

Fibula

Anterior tibial A.

Deep peroneal N.

Anterior tibial V.

Saphenous N.

THE MUSCULOSKELETAL SYSTEM

FUNCTIONS OF THE MUSCULOSKELETAL SYSTEM

First | The musculoskeletal system has four major functions:

- The bones **support** the body, acting as a framework to give it form and to provide a rigid structure for the attachment of muscles and other body parts.
- Acting with muscles, the bones and joints allow for body **movement.**
- Many of the bones in the body provide **protection** for the vital organs: the skull protects the brain; the spine protects the spinal cord; the ribs protect the heart, lungs, liver, stomach, and spleen; the pelvis protects the urinary bladder and internal reproductive organs.
- Some bones have a special function of **producing blood cells.**

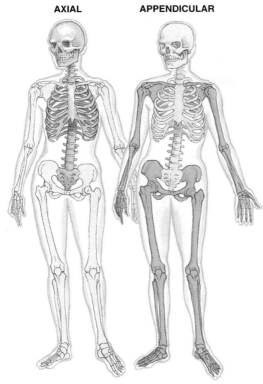

AXIAL APPENDICULAR

FIGURE 12.2
Two major divisions of the skeletal system are the axial skeleton and the appendicular skeleton.

Note

First Responders are not required to learn the medical names for each bone in the body. Common names are used in First Responder training so that you will spend more time learning how to recognize injuries and how to provide proper care. Medical names for bones are provided only for reference. You need to remember only the common names; but you will find that the medical terms become familiar as you go through the course and begin to work with EMTs in the field.

MAIN PARTS OF THE SKELETAL SYSTEM

First | The **skeletal system** has two major divisions (Figure 12.2):

- **Axial skeleton**—all the bones that form the upright axis of the body, including the skull, spinal column, **sternum** (breastbone), and ribs.
- **Appendicular skeleton**—all the bones that form the upper extremities including the collarbones, shoulder blades, arms, wrists, and hands; and the lower extremities, including the hips, legs, ankles, and feet.

The Upper Extremities

The upper extremities are made up of the shoulder girdle and both arms, down to and including the fingers (Figure 12.3). Table 12-1 lists the bones of the upper extremities and the number of bones that form each structure.

TABLE 12-1: BONES OF THE UPPER EXTREMITIES

COMMON NAMES	MEDICAL NAMES

Shoulder girdle
  collarbone (1/side)
  shoulder blade (1/side)
	Pectoral (PEK-tor-al)
	  clavicle (KLAV-i-kul)
	  scapula (SKAP-u-lah)

Upper arm bone (1/arm, from shoulder to elbow)	Humerus (HU-mer-us)
Forearm bones (2/arm, from elbow to wrist: 1 medial and 1 lateral)	Ulna (UL-nah)—medial Radius (RAY-de-us)—lateral
Wrist bones (8/wrist)	Carpals (KAR-palz)
Hand bones (5/palm)	Metacarpals (meta-KAR-palz)
Finger bones (14/hand)	Phalanges (fah-LAN-gez)

skeletal system all the bones and joints of the body. The skeletal system provides body support and organ protection, enables movement, and produces blood cells.

axial (AK-si-al) skeleton bones and joints that form the center or upright axis of the body. It includes the skull, spine, breastbone, and ribs.

sternum the breastbone.

appendicular (ap-en-DIK-u-ler) skeleton bones and joints that form the upper and lower extremities.

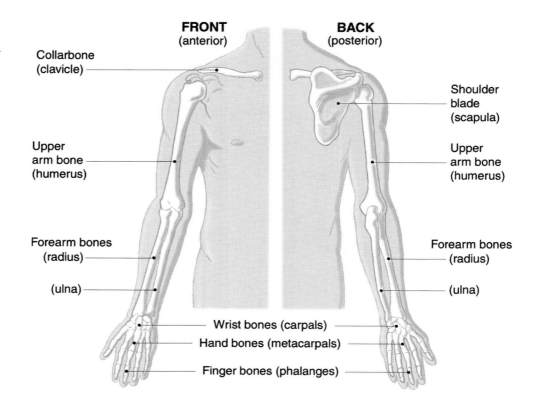

FIGURE 12.3
Bones of the upper
extremities.

FRONT
(anterior)

BACK
(posterior)

Collarbone
(clavicle)

Shoulder
blade
(scapula)

Upper
arm bone
(humerus)

Upper
arm bone
(humerus)

Forearm bones
(radius)

Forearm bones
(radius)

(ulna)

(ulna)

Wrist bones (carpals)
Hand bones (metacarpals)
Finger bones (phalanges)

The Lower Extremities

The lower extremities are made up of the pelvis and both legs, down to and including the toes (Figure 12.4). Table 12-2 lists the bones of the lower extremities and the number of bones that form each structure.

TABLE 12-2: ℬONES OF THE LOWER EXTREMITIES

COMMON NAMES	MEDICAL NAMES
Pelvic girdle (pelvis and hips)	Innominate (eh-NOM-eh-nat) or os coxae (os-KOK-se)
Thigh bone (1/leg)	Femur (FE-mer)
Kneecap (1/leg)	Patella (pah-TEL-ah)
Lower leg bones (2/shin: 1 medial and 1 lateral)	Tibia (TIB-e-ah)—medial Fibula (FIB-yo-lah)—lateral
Ankle bones (7/foot)	Tarsals (TAR-salz)
Foot bones (5/foot)	Metatarsals (meta-TAR-salz)
Toe bones (14–15/foot)	Phalanges (fah-LAN-jez)

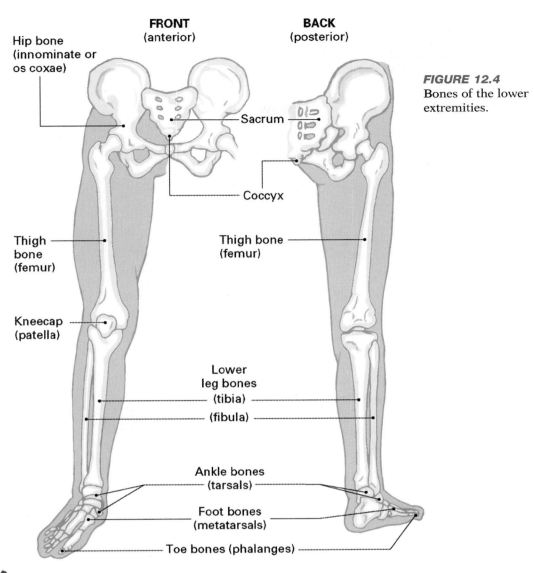

FRONT
(anterior)

BACK
(posterior)

Hip bone
(innominate or
os coxae)

Sacrum

FIGURE 12.4
Bones of the lower
extremities.

Coccyx

Thigh
bone
(femur)

Thigh bone
(femur)

Kneecap
(patella)

Lower
leg bones
(tibia)
(fibula)

Ankle bones
(tarsals)

Foot bones
(metatarsals)

Toe bones (phalanges)

INJURIES TO EXTREMITIES

CAUSES OF INJURIES

There are three major **forces** that cause musculoskeletal injuries. They are **direct force, indirect force,** and **twisting force** (Scan 12-1). Extremities are often injured because of the *direct force* applied to a bone when a person falls and strikes an object (the edge of a step or curb) or when a person is struck by an object (the bumper of a car). Sometimes the energy of the direct force may be transferred up or down the extremity and can cause an injury farther along the extremity. Such *indirect force* injuries can occur when one puts out the hand to break a fall and dislocates the shoulder instead of breaking the wrist. An example of an injury caused by a *twisting force* is when someone gets a hand or foot caught in a wheel or gear. The body may keep moving forward while the hand or foot is trapped in a turning mechanism; or the body remains stationary while the hand or foot turns in the wheel.

Aging and disease also can cause bone breaks. As we age, our bones can become weak and brittle, and they break more easily. People with certain medical conditions such as bone cancer or osteoporosis have fragile bones that even the mildest force can fracture.

*T*he *E*xtremities—*S*elect *M*echanisms of *I*njury

mechanism of injury
The force of an object and its intensity and direction that caused an injury to an area of the body.

direct force
Energy is transmitted directly to an extremity, causing an injury at the site. This energy may be from a fall and by striking an object, or by being struck by an object.

indirect force
Energy of a direct force blow is transferred along the arm or leg and causes an injury farther along the extremity.

twisting force
The energy transmitted to an extremity that is caught in a twisting or circular mechanism, while the rest of the extremity or the body is stationary or moving in another direction.

DOWNWARD BLOW
Clavicle
and
Scapula

LATERAL BLOW
Clavicle
Scapula
and
Humerous

FORCED FLEXION
OR
HYPEREXTENSION
Elbow
Wrist
Fingers
Femur
Knee
Foot

TWISTING FORCE
Hip
Femur
Knee
Leg bones
Ankle
Shoulder
Elbow
Forearm
Wrist

INDIRECT
FORCE
Pelvis
Hip
Knee
Leg bones
Shoulder
Humerus
Elbow
Forearm bones

LATERAL BLOW
Knee
Hip
Femur
(Very forceful)

TYPES OF INJURIES

There are two basic types of injuries—**closed** and **open** (Figure 12.5). An injury is considered closed when there is no break in the skin. In some cases, the surrounding soft tissue (skin and muscle) can be damaged extensively and internal bleeding can be profuse, even though the skin is unbroken, and the external signs of injury show only some reddening and swelling. An injury is considered open when soft tissues are damaged and the skin is broken. The mechanism of injury causes the ends or pieces of bone to tear through the skin from inside out; or, in some cases, something enters and opens the skin from the outside and also fractures the bone underneath (for example, a gunshot wound).

Any time a bone is broken, chipped, cracked, or splintered, it has what is called a **fracture.** But if the wound is closed and we cannot see underneath the skin, it is impossible to tell if the bone is actually fractured just by looking at it or by listening to the patient's description. Any strong force to the extremities can cause a fracture, a dislocation, a sprain, or a strain, and also damage to the soft tissues. All of these injuries will show typical signs of pain, swelling, and deformity (either from the swelling or from the angle of the injured extremity). Do *not* try to determine the specific type of injury. Do notice the **mechanism of injury (MOI),** or what caused the injury, which is very important (Figure 12.6). What types of injury would you look for in each of the following examples?

- *Falls:* you find a patient at the bottom of the steps or a ladder, near a high curb, or lying on wet, icy, or snow-covered streets.
- *Struck by or thrown against an object:* you find a patient against a steering wheel, lying beside a vehicle that has struck something or was struck, a fallen football player, or suspect the patient may have been struck by or thrown against an object.
- *Caught or twisted arms or legs, hands or feet:* you find a child whose foot was caught in the spokes of a moving bicycle, or a worker whose hand was caught in a machine.

Besides the fracture, crushing, or twisting type of injury caused by the three forces, another type of injury can occur. These forces may cause a joint to be dislocated. A **dislocation** occurs when one end of a bone that is part of a joint is pulled or pushed out of place. The dislocated bone also causes serious damage to muscles, nerves, and blood vessels that swell because of the injury to them and the pressure applied to them by the dislocated bone. Sometimes the force that caused the dislocation of a bone will also cause it or an adjoining bone to fracture.

closed injury an injury with no associated opening of the skin.

open injury an injury with an associated opening of the skin. The cause of the opening may be from bone ends or fragments tearing out through the skin or a penetrating injury that has damaged a bone and surrounding soft tissue.

fracture any break, crack, chip, split, or crumbling of a bone.

mechanism of injury (MOI) a force or forces that may have caused injury.

dislocation the pulling or pushing of a bone end partially or completely free of a joint.

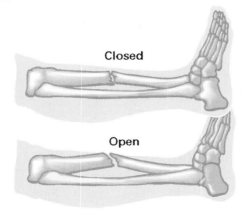

FIGURE 12.5
Closed and open injuries.

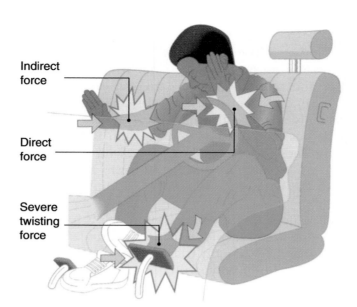

FIGURE 12.6
There are three basic types
of mechanisms of injury to
the musculoskeletal system.

Indirect
force

Direct
force

Severe
twisting
force

ligament fibrous
tissue that connects
bone to bone.

sprain a partial or
complete tearing of
a ligament.

strain the
overstretching or
tearing of a muscle.

angulated fracture
a fracture that causes
a bone or joint to take
on an unnatural shape
or bend.

At each joint, there are tough fibrous tissues called **ligaments** that hold bones together. Twisting forces cause ligaments to tear or stretch. The result is a **sprain.** Muscles are injured when we overexert, overwork, and overstretch or tear them. These types of injuries to muscles are called **strains.** Again, since you cannot see the ligament or muscle beneath the skin, you won't know for sure if the injury is a sprained ligament, a strained muscle, or a fractured bone. In many cases, the exact nature of the injury cannot be determined until X rays are examined. Still, the signs and symptoms are the same—painful, swollen, and deformed; care, which will be described later, will be the same.

Another type of injury to a bone is an **angulated fracture,** which describes an extremity injury that causes a bone to bend where it normally does not (Figure 12.7). Angulated fractures may be *slight*, which means you will still be able to feel a distal pulse and the patient will have sensation (be able to feel your touch) and motor function (will be able to move the limb). If angulated fractures are *extreme*, you will not feel a distal pulse and the patient will have no sensation or motor function. Angulated fractures may be open or closed injuries.

First | First Responders must carefully assess and treat all painful, swollen, deformed extremities.

*N*ote

Carefully assess
and treat all PSD
extremities.

FIGURE 12.7
Angulated fractures may
be closed or open.

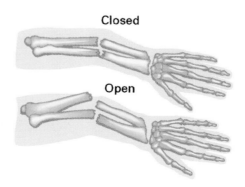

Closed

Open

SIGNS AND SYMPTOMS OF INJURY TO BONES AND JOINTS

First | The three main signs and symptoms to look for in an extremity injury include (Figure 12.8):

- **Pain**—Nerves surrounding the injury have been injured and are being pressed by swelling tissue or broken bone ends. Tissues near the injury site will be very tender. The patient often experiences severe and constant pain at the injury site. The patient can usually tell you where it hurts. As part of your focused assessment, you will gently examine (touch) the area along the injured site. Carefully look at, rather than feel, the area, if the bone is protruding through the skin.

- **Swelling**—The area around the injury will begin to swell because blood from ruptured blood vessels is collecting inside the tissues. The blood trapped under the skin may cause it to look reddish or discolored. Later, as these blood cells die, they cause the typical black-and-blue bruising, which may take 24 hours or longer to develop.

- **Deformity**—A part of a limb appears different in size or shape than the same part on the opposite side of the patient's body. (Always compare both arms and legs to one another.) If a bone appears to have an unusual angle, bulge, or swelling, consider this deformity to be a sign of possible fracture or dislocation. Feel gently along the patient's limbs, noting any lumps, swelling, discoloration, or ends of bones through the skin.

Other common signs and symptoms will include the following (Figure 12.9):

- *Loss of use or joint locked in place:* The patient will be unable to move a limb. Sometimes movement is possible but is very painful. If the patient can move an arm but not the fingers, or if a patient can move a leg but not the toes, a fracture may have caused severe damage to nerves and blood vessels. The patient will often cradle or "guard" an injured arm, or hold it close to the body to stabilize it in a comfortable position. An injured person will often ask you not to touch or move the injured extremity.

- *Numbness or tingling sensation:* This can be from pressure on nerves or blood vessels caused by swelling or broken bones.

FIGURE 12.8
Signs of a painful, swollen, deformed extremity.

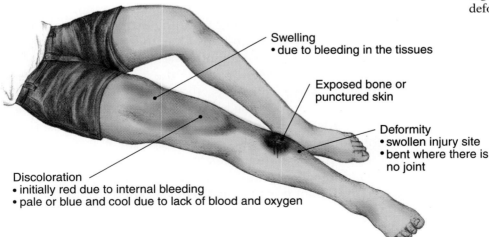

Swelling
• due to bleeding in the tissues

Exposed bone or punctured skin

Deformity
• swollen injury site
• bent where there is no joint

Discoloration
• initially red due to internal bleeding
• pale or blue and cool due to lack of blood and oxygen

FIGURE 12 9
Typical signs and symptoms
of extremity injury.

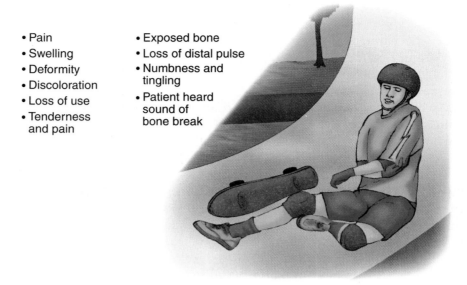

- Pain
- Swelling
- Deformity
- Discoloration
- Loss of use
- Tenderness and pain
- Exposed bone
- Loss of distal pulse
- Numbness and tingling
- Patient heard sound of bone break

■ *Loss of distal pulse:* Bone ends or bone fragments may have pressed against or cut through an artery. Swelling from internal bleeding may have pressed against an artery. The extremity may be pale and cold because of restricted blood flow, and then turn bluish (cyanotic) because of lack of oxygen.

■ *Slow capillary refill:* Capillary refill takes longer than 2 seconds (see explanation below).

■ *Grating:* When the patient moves, the ends of the fractured bones rub together, making a grating sound (referred to as crepitus [KREP-i-tus]). Do not ask a patient to move in order to confirm or reproduce this sound.

■ *Sound of breaking:* If the patient or bystanders tell you this, assume a fracture has occurred.

■ *Exposed bone:* In cases of open fractures, the fragments or ends of fractured bone may be visible where they break through the skin.

Several important signs described in the list above will tell you the state of circulation to the extremity: if the injury site is swollen and red, there is bleeding in the tissues; if there is no distal pulse and the extremity is pale and cool, there is lack of blood flow; if the extremity is blue, there is lack of oxygen.

To check circulation in pediatric patients, check *capillary refill*. To do this, press the nail bed or tip of the finger or toe on the injured extremity between your finger and thumb. When you press, the finger or toe turns white, or blanches, because you have pressed the blood out of it. When you release pressure, the blood should flow back into the area in less than 2 seconds. If it takes more than 2 seconds, then you must suspect that there is pressure on or damage to a blood vessel and that circulation is restricted in the extremity or that there is significant blood loss in the circulatory system. This procedure is more reliable in children than it is in adults. The blood-flow return time is also affected by cold temperature.

While you are checking **distal pulse,** you can also check **sensation** (feeling) and **motor function** (ability to move). Ask the patient to tell you if he can feel your touch and where you are touching. You can also ask the patient to try to move the fingers or grasp your hand. For the foot, ask the patient to wiggle toes or press a foot against your hand. Checking for sensation and motor function gives you information about the nervous system. A lack of feeling or the inability to move may indicate that there is pressure on or damage to a nerve. This nerve damage may be a result of injury to the spinal cord and not just an injury to the extremity. Later in this chapter, we will discuss the signs and symptoms of spinal injury and the precautions to take when managing a spine-injured patient.

TOTAL PATIENT CARE

In the scene size-up, quickly determine scene safety, don all personal protective equipment, and note mechanism of injury and number of patients. Then determine what additional assistance you may need. During your initial assessment, get an impression of the environment and the patient and determine how quickly the patient needs to be moved and transported; do *not* focus on obvious injuries but first assess responsiveness, then airway, breathing, and circulation. Look for and control all major bleeding. You must detect and correct these life-threatening problems as quickly as possible.

There is a certain order to caring for injuries. *After* correcting and stabilizing life-threatening injuries to airway, breathing, and circulation, *after* you have checked for and stabilized neck and spinal injuries, and *after* you have provided care for shock that develops from major bleeding or serious burns, then you can focus on extremity injuries. Always be sure to note the mechanism of injury as this will give you an idea of the possible extent, type, and location of injury.

In the order of care for injuries, *first priority is given to possible injury to the spine*. Next is care for possible injuries to the following areas:

- *Skull*—because it protects the brain and contains a portion of the airway.
- *Pelvis*—because it protects reproductive and urinary organs and major nerves and blood vessels.
- *Thigh*—because it takes major trauma to injure the largest, sturdiest bone (femur) in the body, which is surrounded by major nerves and blood vessels. Blood loss can be life-threatening.
- *Rib cage*—because it protects the heart and lungs and broken sections may damage the function of these organs. Priority rises to "first" if the patient develops difficulty breathing.
- *Any extremity injury*—where no distal pulse is detected during the initial assessment.
- *Injuries to the arm, lower leg, and individual ribs*—are considered and managed last.

Note the mechanism of injury and be concerned with major bleeding and possible shock whenever there are injuries to the pelvis and the thigh. A great amount of blood can be lost internally in these areas. Watch the signs and symptoms carefully. A slow pulse, pale or blue skin color, slow or no response or confusion, and cold extremities are signs and symptoms that will alert you to manage and transport this patient as soon as possible.

Patient Care Steps

It is easy to focus on an obvious deformed extremity. However, remember the following steps when you care for injuries:

1. Perform an initial assessment before you focus on a particular injury.
   - Manage life-threatening problems *first*.
   - Prioritize and manage other injuries.

Note

Medical direction may allow you to reposition an extremity if there is no distal pulse. Check local protocols to see if First Responders are allowed to straighten angulated injuries or reposition extremities if there is no distal pulse.

2. Carefully cut away clothing to expose the injury site.
   – Apply a dressing if there is an open wound.
   – Check for distal pulse, sensation, and motor function.
3. Immobilize the extremity.
   – Use soft or rigid splints and secure them appropriately.
   – To help reduce blood flow to the site, which causes swelling after you have immobilized the extremity, elevate it in the following manner: Use a sling and swathe for an arm to keep it elevated across the chest. Splinted, immobilized legs may be propped up on a folded blanket or pillow if there is no indication of spinal injury.
   – Recheck distal pulse.
4. Apply a cold pack to the injury site to help control bleeding and reduce the pain and swelling.
   – Never put a cold pack directly on the skin. Wrap it in a towel first. Then place it gently over the injury site.
   – If the patient experiences pain from this extra pressure on the injury, place the cold pack just above the site.
5. Give oxygen as soon as possible to prevent the effects of developing shock per local protocols (see Appendix 2).
6. Cover the patient to maintain body temperature and prevent the effects of developing shock.

Emotional support is important when caring for a patient with injuries. Tell the patient what you suspect may be wrong, how you will manage it, and what will be done by other emergency care providers on the scene and at the hospital. You may need to remind the patient that fractures can be set at the hospital and bones will heal. Talking with the patient provides simple emotional support that gives the patient confidence and relieves anxiety. It may also help lower blood pressure, pulse rate, and breathing rate.

CARE FOR MUSCULOSKELETAL INJURIES

Painful swollen deformed extremity → Expose injured site → Immobilize the extremity → Apply cold pack to control bleeding and reduce pain/swelling → Maintain body temp to prevent developing shock

Reposition with medical direction

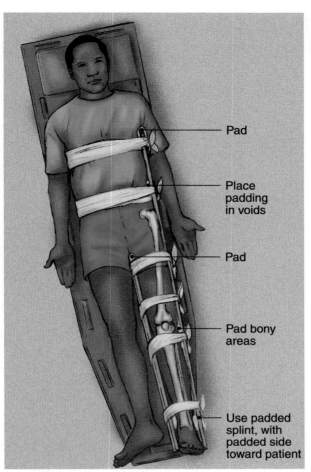

FIGURE 12.10
Splinting immobilizes and stabilizes painful, swollen, deformed (PSD) extremities.

Pad

Place padding in voids

Pad

Pad bony areas

Use padded splint, with padded side toward patient

SPLINTING

First | **Splinting** is a process of **immobilizing** and **stabilizing** painful, swollen, deformed (PSD) extremities (Figure 12.10). Any object that can be used for this purpose is called a splint. There are two types of splints: **soft** and **rigid.**

SOFT SPLINTS

When properly applied, **soft splints,** such as pillows, blankets, towels, cravats, and dressings, may be used to stabilize injuries to the extremity and are as effective as rigid splints. Soft splints can provide support to the injured extremity and help decrease patient pain. A commonly used soft splint is the **triangular bandage.** It can be folded to any width to fit any part of the body, to secure arms to the torso and legs to each other, or to secure extremities to board splints. A triangular bandage is frequently used for a sling and swathe.

The Sling and Swathe

A **sling** is a triangular bandage used to stabilize the shoulder and arm. The sling supports and maintains elevation of the lower arm, which will help blood flow return to the heart and possibly reduce or limit swelling. Once the arm is placed in a sling, a **swathe** is used to hold the arm against the side of the chest and restrict movement. A swathe is made from a triangular bandage, but it is folded

splinting to apply a device that will immobilize a painful, swollen, deformed (PSD) extremity.

immobilize to fix or hold a body part in place in order to reduce or eliminate motion.

stabilize to steady a body part in order to help reduce involuntary movement caused by pain or muscle spasm.

soft splint a device, such as a sling and swathe or a pillow secured with cravats, that can be applied to immobilize a painful, swollen, deformed (PSD) extremity.

triangular bandage a piece of triangular cloth material about 50″ to 60″ long at its base and 36″ to 40″ long on each of its sides. It can be folded and used as a sling, a swathe, or a cravat.

sling a large triangular bandage or other cloth device that is applied as a soft splint to immobilize possible injuries to the shoulder girdle and upper extremity.

swathe a large cravat, usually made of cloth, used to secure a sling or rigid splint and sling to the body.

Sling and Swathe

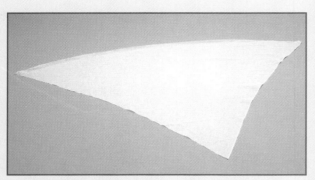

1. A sling and swathe starts with a triangular bandage 50–60" at its base and 36–40" on each side. Fold it to any width.

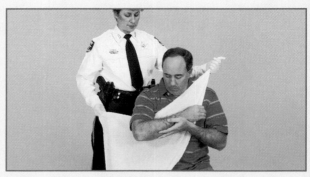

2. Check distal pulse, sensation, and motor function. Position sling over the chest. The point is toward the injured side and beyond the elbow. The upper end is over the shoulder.

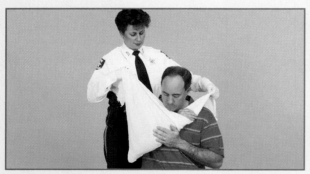

3. Bring the bottom end up and over the patient's injured arm. Keep the hand elevated above the elbow.

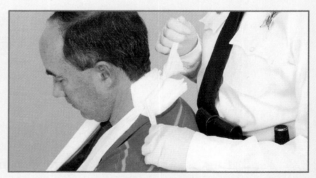

4. Tie the two ends together. Pad the knot and make sure it does not rest on the patient's neck. Reassess distal pulse and sensation.

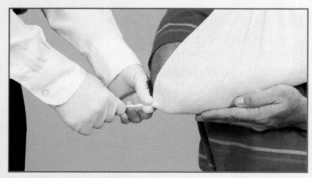

5. Secure the point of the sling to form a pocket for the elbow.

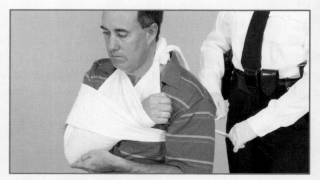

6. Fold another triangular piece of material to form a swathe. Tie it around the patient. Be sure it is positioned to support the arm and to maintain elevation.

to about a 4″ to 6″ width so it fits the area of the arm between the shoulder and elbow. (A triangular bandage folded to a width of 3″ or 4″ and used to tie soft or rigid splints in place is called a cravat.) Together, the sling and swathe immobilize the joints above and below the injury site. The sling and swathe are effective for support and immobilization of the following upper extremity injuries:

- Shoulder girdle
- Upper arm
- Elbow
- Lower arm
- Wrist, hand, and fingers
- Fractured ribs

Go over the following steps for applying a sling and swathe. After seeing demonstrations by your instructor, use Scan 12-2 to review and practice the process.

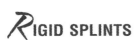 To make and apply a sling and swathe, you should:

1. Use a commercial sling, or make one from a piece of cloth or sheet. Fold or cut this material so that it is in the shape of a triangle. The ideal sling should be about 50″ to 60″ long at its base and 36″ to 40″ long on each of its sides.

2. Position the triangular material over the chest with the point towards the patient's injured arm and the long end draped over the opposite shoulder. The point of the triangle should extend beyond the elbow. Gently position the patient's arm over the material and the chest so the arm is above the elbow. If the patient cannot hold the arm, have your partner or a bystander support the arm while you prepare and secure the sling.

3. Take the bottom end of the triangle and bring it up and over the patient's arm and shoulder on the injured side.

4. Draw up on the ends of the sling to support the patient's hand about 4 inches above the elbow. Tie the two ends together and be sure to position the knot so it does not rest on the back of the patient's neck. Place a flat layer of cloth (gauze pads or handkerchief) under the knot for comfort. Leave the patient's fingertips exposed so you can check for color and temperature changes and any loss of sensation, which may indicate restricted circulation. Recheck radial pulse. If absent, support the arm while the sling and swathe is removed and gently reposition it until you can feel the pulse. (Follow local protocols.) Replace the sling and swathe.

5. Take the point of the sling at the patient's elbow and fold it forward. Then tuck it in or pin it in place, or twist and tie the point. (It may be easier to tie the knot before the sling is placed on the patient.) This will form a pocket for the patient's elbow.

6. Take a second piece of triangular cloth and fold it to a 4″ or 6″ width. Center the widest part on the patient's injured arm. Take one end across the patient's back and one end across the chest and tie on the opposite side under the other arm. Be sure that the swathe helps support the arm and maintains elevation by positioning it under the injured arm.

Roller bandages and wide Velcro fasteners can be used to form a sling and swathe. Any material can be used as long as it will not cut into the patient's skin and cause further damage.

RIGID SPLINTS

Rigid splints are stiff and usually made of plastic, metal, wood, or compressed cardboard and have very little give or flexibility. They are applied along an

Note
Some First Responder courses do not teach students how to use rigid splints. All First Responder courses will teach the basic steps of splinting, and you will learn in this chapter how to use improvised or noncommercial splints. You cannot learn splinting without proper instruction and supervised practice. You must be trained by a qualified instructor, and you must practice splinting procedures under the guidance of that instructor.

rigid splint a stiff device made of a material with very little flexibility (such as metal, plastic, or wood) that is long enough to immobilize an extremity and the joints above and below the injury site.

FIGURE 12 11
Severity of complications
associated with PSD
extremity injuries can be
prevented or decreased
with splinting.

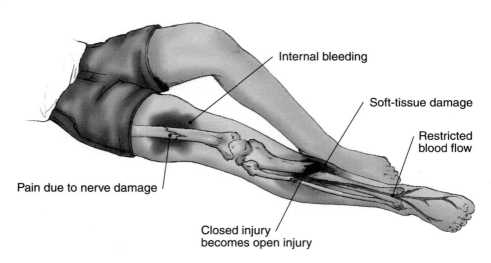

Internal bleeding

Soft-tissue damage

Restricted
blood flow

Pain due to nerve damage

Closed injury
becomes open injury

injured extremity to immobilize the entire limb and the joints directly above
and below the injury site. Used in this way, rigid splints stabilize the injured
extremity and prevent the patient from moving the injured part.

*W*HY SPLINT?

First | Applications of splints enable emergency care providers to reposition
and transfer the patient to other immobilization or carrying devices
without moving injured bones and joints or damaging soft tissues. Damage to
soft tissues can cause complications and prolong recovery (Figure 12.11).
Complications include:

- *Pain*—A splint can reduce much of the patient's pain because it secures
  the broken or dislocated bones in place and prevents them from
  compressing or damaging surrounding nerves and tissues.
- *Damage to soft tissues*—The mechanism of a PSD extremity injury may
  cause blood vessels, nerves, and muscles to be crushed, ruptured, pinched,
  or compressed. Splinting reduces movement of the injured part, the possibility of further damage to soft tissues, and the accompanying pain, internal bleeding, and swelling.
- *Bleeding*—Dislocated bones, ends of fractured bones, and moving bone
  fragments can damage blood vessels and cause internal and external
  bleeding. Splinting immobilizes the bone ends and reduces the possibility
  of their damaging blood vessels and causing bleeding. (The initial force
  of injury may have caused bone ends to damage soft tissues and blood
  vessels. Splinting will stabilize the injury and apply a steady pressure
  that can reduce and control bleeding.)
- *Restricted blood flow*—Dislocated joints and fractured bones and fragments also can press against blood vessels and shut off blood flow. Splinting can help relieve the pressure against blood vessels.
- *Closed injuries become open injuries*—The sharp edge of a broken bone can
  rip through skin to produce an open wound. Immobilizing the injured
  extremity by splinting it will prevent movement of the broken part and
  can help prevent a closed wound from becoming an open wound.

Note

Never delay the
transport of a
patient with life-
threatening
injuries in order
to splint a PSD
extremity.

FIRST RESPONDER RESPONSIBILITIES

The primary duties of a First Responder are to detect and control life-threatening patient problems first. In your assessment, you will find all injuries and care for the worst injuries first. Fractures are cared for after neck and spinal injuries, which you will stabilize; open head, chest, and abdominal wounds, which you will dress; shock (hypoperfusion), which you will manage with oxygen and warmth; and serious burns, which you will dress. EMTs will likely arrive before you have an opportunity to apply splints.

Some patients may have indications of neck or spinal injuries, and you will not be able to splint extremities until you have additional help and equipment from the EMTs. In the meantime, this patient must not be moved but should be kept still in position while you stabilize his head with your hands (explained later in this chapter). The process of splinting may cause you to move the patient or the injured limb and even slight movements, without appropriate help to stabilize the body and coordinate the move, could make a spinal injury worse.

 For all cases involving PSD extremities, alert dispatch so you may receive appropriate assistance from EMTs.

 When the mechanism of injury and the patient's signs and symptoms indicate PSD extremities and require that you apply splints:

- Use soft splints (blanket, towel, pillow, sling and swathe) if rigid splints are not available. Provide further rigid support by securing upper extremities to the torso with a swathe and lower extremities to each other with cravats.
- If available, apply rigid splints for injuries to the forearm (Figure 12.12) and the lower leg. Rigid splints may be used for injuries to the thigh, but traction splints are more effective.
- Use soft or rigid splints for injuries to the arm, the elbow, the wrist, and the hand.
- Use soft splints for injuries to the ankle or foot.

When in doubt, splint any PSD extremity.

RULES FOR SPLINTING

For all cases of splinting, you will (Scan 12-3):
- Assess and reassure the patient and explain what you plan to do.
- Splint PSD extremities before moving the patient. Move the patient before splinting *only* if the environment is life-threatening.
- Expose the injury site. Cut away clothing if it cannot be easily removed or folded back. Remove jewelry from the injured limb if it can be done without using force, causing pain, or repositioning the patient or the limb.
- Control all major bleeding. Do *not* apply pressure over the injury site. To control major bleeding, use bulky dressings secured snugly with a bandage.
- Dress open wounds. Do *not* push bone ends back into the wound. Do *not* try to pick bone fragments from the wound. If the bone ends withdraw into the wound as you care for it, report this to the EMTs or hospital staff so appropriate infection prevention can be given.
- Check distal pulse, sensation, and motor function before and after splinting.

Note

Not all EMS systems allow First Responders to apply manual traction when splinting. You may only be allowed to gently reposition a limb to allow for the application of a splint. Your instructor will inform you of your local guidelines.

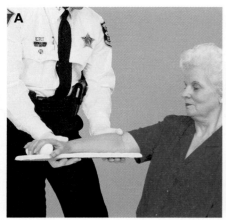
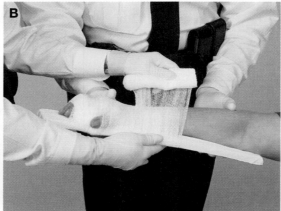
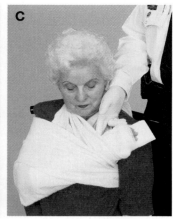

FIGURE 12.12
Applying a rigid splint.

- Have all materials ready and at hand before splinting. Use padded splints for patient comfort and improved contact between limb and splint. Wrap unpadded splints in dressings before applying them.
- If local protocols allow: gently attempt to realign an angulated limb in anatomical position before splinting; attempt to reposition the limb to regain a pulse if the limb is cold and blue and has no pulse.
- Apply gentle manual traction (see below), and secure the splint firmly but do not restrict circulation. Do not intentionally allow a protruding bone to reenter the skin.
- Immobilize the injured extremity and the joints above and below the injury site. (Secure upper extremities to the torso with a sling and swathe; secure lower extremities to each other and assist EMTs in transferring the patient to a spine board or orthopedic frame.)
- Secure splints with cravats or roller gauze, starting at the distal end of the extremity. Leave fingertips and toes exposed so you can monitor circulation.
- Check distal pulse, sensation, and motor function after splinting.
- Elevate the extremity. For an arm, use a sling and swathe to immobilize the arm against the chest in an elevated position. For a leg, prop it on a pillow or rolled blanket if there is no indication of spinal injury. (Otherwise, leave the patient lying flat.)
- Prevent the effects of developing shock by providing oxygen as soon as possible and by keeping the patient warm.

Applying Manual Traction

First | The effects of splinting are improved if you apply gentle tension to the PSD extremity during the splinting process. In First Responder care, this tension is applied by pulling *gently* on the injured limb. The process of applying this tension is called **manual traction,** and it helps stabilize fractured bones.

manual traction a stabilizing procedure that precedes the application of a rigid splint. Apply tension by pulling gently along the long axis of the injured limb. Maintain the tension until the splint is fully applied.

Most EMS systems do not allow First Responders to straighten angulated fractures. Do only what you have been trained to do and what is allowed in your EMS system. Check your local protocols to find out what you are allowed to do if there is angulation or no distal pulse. If you find no distal pulse, and the skin at the foot is pale or blue and cold, you need to take action immediately. Notify dispatch, the EMTs, or the hospital and let them know the patient's status. You may be directed to gently align the limb to restore distal pulse. Do *not* force the

$\mathcal{S}$plinting

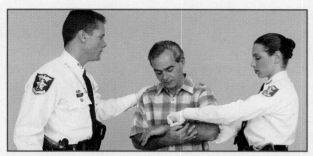

1. Perform initial assessment. Then, if appropriate, focus on injury.

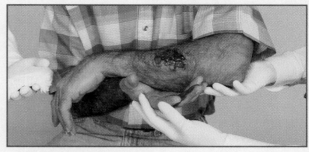

2. Expose the injury site.

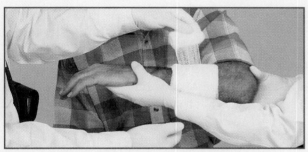

3. Control bleeding by dressing wounds.

4. Check distal pulse, sensation, and motor function *before* and *after* splinting.

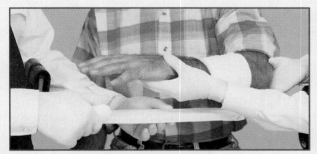

5. Reposition limb and apply a padded splint.

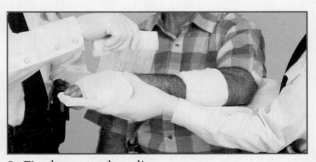

6. Firmly secure the splint.

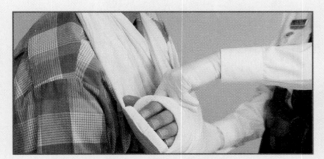

7. Reassess distal pulse and sensation.

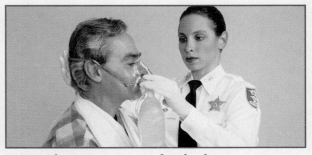

8. Provide emergency care for shock.

CHAPTER 12 ■ Muscle and Bone Injuries   **391**

WARNING:

Do only what
your training and
local protocols
allow when caring
for patients with
angulated
fractures.

limb if you meet resistance or if the patient complains of increased pain. Apply a soft splint and elevate the limb by propping it on a blanket roll or pillow. Provide oxygen and other appropriate emergency care interventions until the EMTs arrive.

When you start to apply manual traction, it may cause a temporary increase in pain for the patient. Explain this to the patient, but also explain that the pain caused by the injury will probably lessen once the traction and the splint are applied.

Traction is of little use if it is not maintained. A rigid splint helps maintain traction when it is secured to the patient. When you apply manual traction to an injured extremity, do *not* release it to apply a splint. It usually takes two people to properly apply a splint: one to hold and maintain manual traction, while the other applies the splint.

You can apply and maintain manual traction while another emergency care provider applies and secures the splint to the patient; or you may be able to direct a bystander to secure a splint while you maintain traction. (Follow your EMS system's guidelines.) If you are working alone, do *not* try to apply traction unless distal pulse is absent. Once you apply manual traction, you must maintain it until the extremity is secured to a splint.

To apply manual traction, you will:

1. Grasp the patient's limb by placing one hand above the injury site and the other hand below the injury site. Position your hands so that the splint can be applied without having to release manual traction (Figure 12.13).

2. Gently apply steady tension by pulling with your lower hand. The direction of pull should be along the long axis of the limb. If you feel resistance, stop the procedure.

3. Maintain manual traction throughout the splinting process.

Straightening Angulated Fractures

The main reason for straightening closed angulated fractures is to improve circulation. Straight limbs also make it easier for you to apply a rigid splint. If the limb cannot be straightened or if you are not allowed to do so by your state, use soft splints. The procedure for straightening closed angulated fractures is the same as for applying manual traction. If you are allowed to straighten closed angulated fractures, follow local protocols and generally:

■ Straighten closed angulated fractures of the elbow, knee, and ankle if there is no distal pulse. In these cases, do *not* apply manual traction to the limb. Simply align for splinting.

FIGURE 12.13
Applying manual traction will help to stabilize fractured bones.

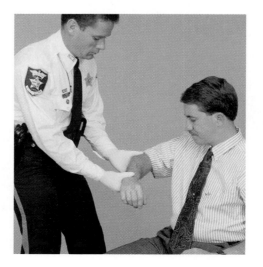

- Make only one attempt to straighten the angulation.
- Stop if you meet resistance or if the patient complains of severe pain.

Some jurisdictions and protocols do not allow for straightening angulated injuries under certain conditions or for certain extremities. Generally, your guidelines may say:

- Do *not* attempt to straighten open angulated fractures.
- Do *not* attempt to straighten angulated fractures and dislocations of the wrist and shoulder.
- Do *not* attempt to straighten angulations if the injury involves the shoulder, pelvis, hip, thigh, wrist, hand, foot, or a joint immediately above or below the injury site.

TYPES OF SPLINTS

Commercial Splints

A wide variety of commercial splints are available for emergency care. These splints are made of wood, aluminum, compressed wood fibers, cardboard, foam, wire, or plastic. Some come with their own washable pads. Others require padding to be applied before being secured. Most splints are either solid, rigid pieces, or air-inflatable plastic splints. Figure 12.14 shows some of the commercially available splints you might use in First Responder care. These include air or inflatable splints, vacuum splints, board-and-wire ladder splints, heavy duty cardboard splints, and flexible aluminum splints. All EMTs and many First Responders carry traction splints for splinting and stabilizing injuries to the pelvic girdle. Local protocols may provide guidelines for using a pneumatic anti-shock garment (PASG), a special device for pelvic and femur fractures. You must receive training and use the PASG only as protocols direct.

Inflatable Splints

First Responder units may not carry inflatable air splints. If you carry air splints and your jurisdiction allows you to use them, your instructor will teach you their application.

Typically, air splints are used for patients with injuries to the arm or lower leg bones. When using inflatable splints, slip the uninflated splint over your forearm, then grasp the patient's hand or foot and pull gentle traction while you slip the air splint onto the patient's limb. Smooth out the splint and inflate it. The splint is fully inflated and effective when you can make a slight surface indentation with your fingertip (see Scan 12-4).

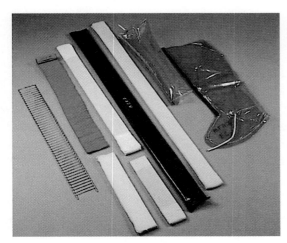

FIGURE 12.14
There are many types and sizes of commercial rigid splints.

*I*nflatable *S*plints

WARNING: Air splints may leak. When applied in cold weather, an air splint will expand when the patient is moved to a warmer place. Pressure will also change with different altitudes. Monitor the pressure in the splint by pressing with your fingertip. These splints may stick to the patient's skin in hot weather.

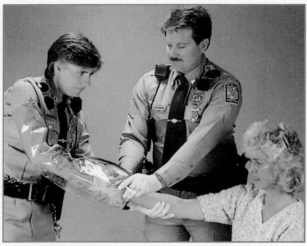

1. Check distal pulse, motor function, and sensation before and after splinting. Slide the uninflated splint onto your forearm, then grasp the patient's hand and pull manual traction.

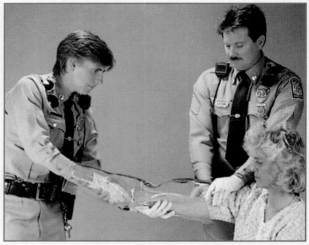

2. Slide the splint from your arm and onto the patient's arm. The lower edge of the air splint should be just above the second joints of the patient's fingers.

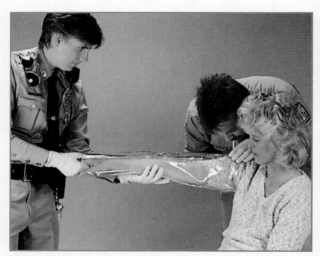

3. Maintain traction and support the arm while your partner inflates the splint. Inflate the splint to a point where you can make a slight dent when you press your thumb against the splint surface.

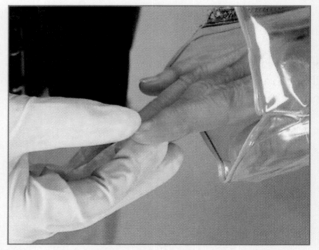

4. Monitor the splint pressure and the patient's fingertips and nail beds to assure continued circulation.

After inflating the splint, you must monitor the patient for changes in circulation and the splint for changes in pressure. If the patient is moved to a warmer or colder location, the air in the splint will expand or contract with the temperature change. You will have to recheck the pressure in the splint. You may have to remove increased pressure by deflating the splint slightly. The pressure in the splint also will change if the patient is moved to a different altitude. Always monitor the pressure in the splint. Precheck the condition of all air splints; old inflatable splints may leak.

Once an inflatable splint is applied, you will not be able to assess distal pulse. Instead, evaluate capillary refill—which is more reliable in pediatric patients—and skin color. The problems with inflatable splints—the inability to check distal pulse and the potential pressure changes—have led some EMS systems to drop inflatable splints from their approved equipment lists.

Making Emergency Splints

First Responders may arrive at the scene of an accident without any commercial or rigid splints, or they may use their supply of splints on one patient and have none for another patient. It is helpful to know how to make splints from materials found at the scene. Your improvised splints may be soft or rigid and may be made from a variety of materials.

First | Rigid splints can be made from pieces of lumber, plywood, compressed wood products, cardboard, rolled newspapers or magazines, umbrellas, canes, broom or shovel handles, sporting equipment (shin guards are an example), and tongue depressors for fingers (Figure 12.15). Soft splints can be made from towels, blankets, pillows, and bulky clothing like sweaters and sweat suits. Most of these items can be found at the scene of a typical accident. Many people carry some of these items in their cars. Ask people at the scene to help you find these items. Give them suggestions and ask if they have any ideas.

MANAGEMENT OF UPPER EXTREMITY INJURIES

Methods for splinting each type of upper extremity injury are summarized in Scan 12-5.

For injuries to the upper extremities, be sure to place the hand in the **position of function,** in which the fingers are slightly flexed and the wrist is cocked slightly upward, or dorsally. The position of function is a normal and comfortable position for the patient, especially if the extremity from forearm to hand is secured against a rigid splint. You may easily secure the hand in its

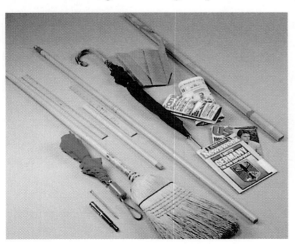

FIGURE 12.15
A variety of materials will serve as emergency splints.

> *Note*
> Make certain you describe the mechanism of injury (MOI) to the dispatcher, the EMTs, or the hospital. This information helps dispatch to determine appropriate equipment and field providers and helps other responders and hospital personnel prepare for and determine the extent and seriousness of the injury and plan appropriate care.

position of function the natural position of the body part. In the case of the hand, the natural position is slightly flexed.

> **WARNING:**
> Always wear latex or vinyl gloves when providing care for extremity injuries. Face and eye shields may be necessary if injuries are spurting blood.

Splinting: The Upper Extremity

Note: Place a roll of dressing in the hand to maintain position of function.

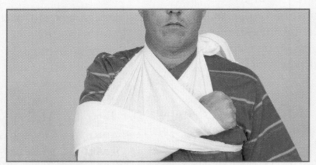

SHOULDER—Apply a sling and swathe. Elevate the wrist above the elbow and support it with the swathe.

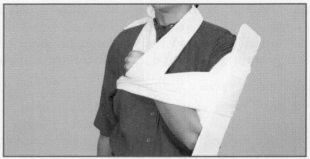

ARM—Immobilize with a rigid splint from shoulder to below the elbow. Apply a sling and swathe that will elevate and support the limb.

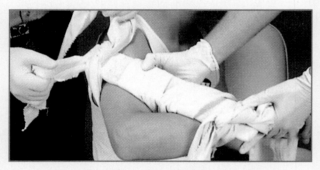

ELBOW (BENT)—Place the splint from shoulder to wrist. Secure the wrist first. Apply a sling and swathe to elevate and support the limb.

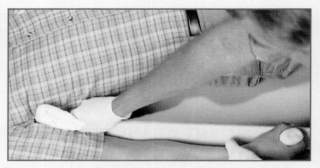

ELBOW (STRAIGHT)—Pad the armpit. Splint should extend from the armpit beyond the fingertips. Use roller bandages to secure the splint to the arm starting at the distal end. Secure the arm to body with cravats.

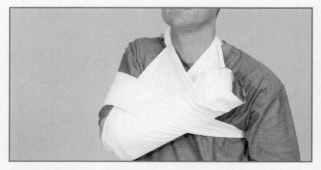

FOREARM, WRIST, HAND—The splint should extend from the elbow to beyond the fingertips. Use a sling and swathe for elevation and support.

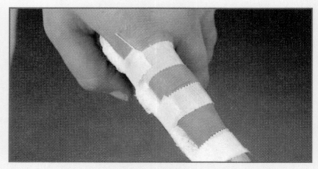

FINGER—Use a tongue depressor or tape finger to an uninjured finger.

position of function by placing a roll of gauze in the patient's hand before immobilizing an injured upper extremity in any kind of splint.

INJURIES TO THE SHOULDER GIRDLE

A common sign for shoulder girdle injuries is a condition known as "knocked down" shoulder or "dropped" shoulder. The patient's injured shoulder will appear to droop. The patient usually holds the arm up against the side of the chest (Figure 12.16).

Injuries to the shoulder joint often produce what is known as an "anterior (to the front) dislocation." The end of the upper arm bone that forms the shoulder joint can be felt, or even seen, bulging or protruding under the skin at the front of the shoulder.

It is not practical to use a rigid splint for injuries to the collarbone, shoulder blade, or shoulder joint. Place padding between any space between the patient's injured arm and chest, use a cravat to secure the padding in place, and use a sling and swathe to secure the arm to the chest. Remember to check for distal pulse, sensation, and motor function before and after splinting. If there is no pulse, attempt to reposition to gain pulse but do not force the arm.

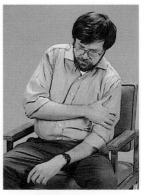

FIGURE 12.16
"Knocked down" or "dropped" shoulder.

 When you provide care for patients with shoulder injuries, you will:

1. Care for life-threatening problems and other injuries that have priority over fractures.

2. Check for a radial pulse (distal pulse at the wrist) and signs of restricted circulation on the injured arm. If there is no pulse, notify the EMTs or the hospital and arrange to transport as soon as possible. Note the time that you observed the absence of the distal pulse.

3. Check for sensation and motor function by testing for feeling and movement of the fingers on the injured arm. If the patient has no feeling or cannot move, then there is pressure on a nerve and the patient will need transport as soon as possible.

4. Apply a sling and swathe. If there appears to be an anterior dislocation, place padding (pillow, blanket, or towel) to fill any space between the patient's arm and chest on the injured side before applying the sling and swathe.

5. Reassess the distal pulse. If the pulse is absent, you may have to gently reposition the injured arm and reapply the sling and swathe. In such cases, follow your local protocols or contact the emergency department physician for directions before repositioning the limb. Sometimes a dislocated shoulder will correct (reduce) itself. If this happens or if you are told by the patient that this happened, you must still check the distal pulse, sensation, and motor function. You also should apply a sling and swathe. This patient still has to see a physician. Arrange for transport and make certain you tell the EMTs that the dislocation apparently corrected itself and the time it took place.

WARNING:

Do *not* try to realign or reposition angulations or dislocations of the shoulder. Movement in this area may cause damage to nearby blood vessels and nerves.

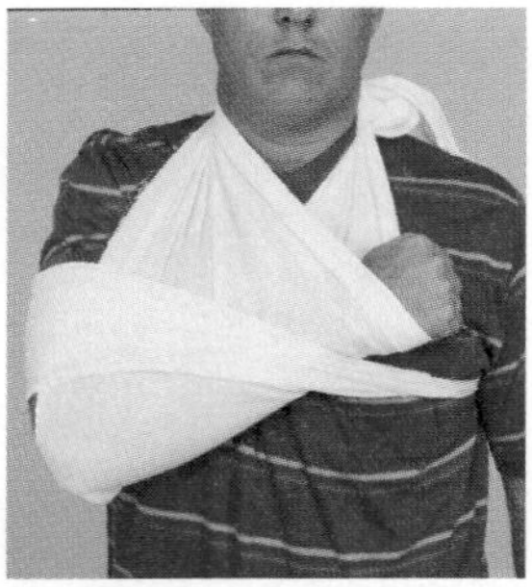

INJURIES TO THE UPPER ARM BONE

Injury to the upper arm bone (the humerus) can be at the upper end that forms the shoulder joint (proximal end), along the mid-shaft of the bone, or at the lower end that forms the elbow joint (distal end). Care for a patient with upper arm injuries is usually the same for all injury locations (Figure 12.17). Deformity is often a key sign of injury to this bone; but if you see no deformity, the patient will tell you the site is tender and painful when you examine it.

First Responders may use a soft splint (sling and swathe) or a rigid splint. If you use a sling and swathe on an injury that seems very close to the elbow, modify the full sling to a wrist sling, which will not place pressure on the elbow (Figure 12.18).

If the upper arm is angulated, check for a distal pulse. If it is present and the patient can tolerate movement, gently move the arm to the splinting position (bend the elbow with the hand elevated above the level of the elbow) and splint it. Do *not* force the arm to this position and do *not* try to straighten the angulation. Recheck for distal pulse.

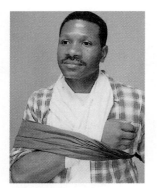

FIGURE 12.17
Use the sling and swathe for painful, swollen, deformed injuries to the shoulder and upper arm bone.

WARNING:

If you do not feel a pulse, attempt to straighten the angulation in the upper arm bone *if your EMS system allows you to do so*. Do *not* force the arm. You should attempt to straighten the angulation only once and stop if there is resistance or additional pain. If straightening the limb fails to restore a distal pulse, arrange to transport the patient *as soon as possible*. If the pulse is restored, splint the arm and recheck distal pulse again.

If you use a rigid splint, secure a padded board splint to the lateral (outside) part of the arm with roller gauze or folded cravats. Then apply a wrist sling and wide swathe. The swathe will secure the injured arm to the body and immobilize the joints above and below the injury site (Figure 12.19).

First When you apply a splint to an upper arm fracture, work with a partner. One of you will maintain manual traction, while the other applies the splint and the sling and swathe. To apply a splint for injuries to the upper arm bone:

1. Check for distal pulse, sensation, and motor function.
2. Select a padded splint long enough for the area between shoulder and elbow.
3. Apply manual traction to the injured extremity. If there is an angulation or no distal pulse, gently realign and recheck for pulse.
4. Place the splint against the injured extremity.
5. Secure the splint to the patient with a roller bandage, handkerchiefs, cravats, or cloth strips. Begin securing at the distal end of the splint.
6. Place the hand in position of function and apply a sling and swathe; recheck distal pulse, sensation, and motor function.
7. Provide oxygen as soon as possible and maintain body temperature to prevent the effects of developing shock.

FIGURE 12.18
For a painful, swollen, deformed upper arm injury near the elbow joint, gently apply a modified sling so it supports only the wrist.

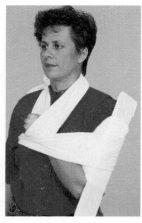

FIGURE 12.19
Splinting an injured upper arm.

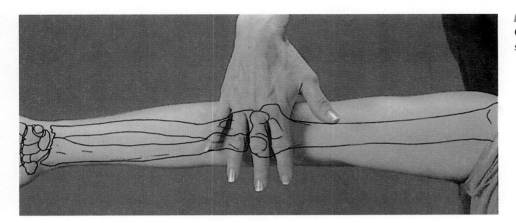

FIGURE 12.20
Consider this area to be the
site of elbow injuries.

INJURIES TO THE ELBOW

The elbow is a joint (not a bone) formed by the lower, or distal, end of the upper arm bone and the upper, or proximal, end of the forearm bones. You can determine if the injury is to the elbow area by placing your hand over the back of the elbow. The elbow includes all the structures that can be covered by the palm of your hand (Figure 12.20). If the injury is above this area, the injury is to the upper arm bone. If the injury is below this area, the injury is to one of the forearm bones.

When caring for elbow injuries, immobilize the elbow in the position in which it is found. Have your partner stabilize the arm while you apply and secure the splint. Check pulse, sensation, and motor function before and after splinting.

First | The following methods can be used in caring for a patient with an elbow injury:

■ If the elbow is found in a flexed (bent) position natural for the joint, rigid splinting is preferred; but a wrist sling and a swathe can be effective. Apply a splint as shown in Figure 12.21.

■ If the elbow is found in the straight position, and it cannot be placed in the natural flexed or splinting position, immobilize it in the straight position. Rigid splinting is preferred, but body splinting is effective. This is done by tying the injured arm along the side of the patient's torso. If you use a rigid splint, select a padded splint that will extend from the patient's armpit past the fingertips. Place a roll of dressing in the patient's hand to maintain it in the position of function and secure the splint with roller gauze or folded cravats starting at the distal end of the arm (fingertips) (Figure 12.22).

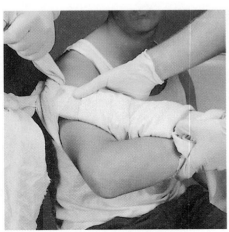

FIGURE 12.21
Splinting an
injured elbow
with the arm in
a flexed position.

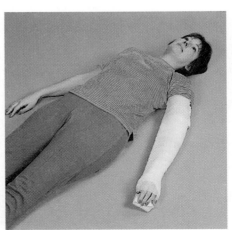

FIGURE 12.22
Splinting an
injured elbow
with the arm in a
straight position.

Some EMS systems allow First Responders to make one gentle attempt to reposition the limb when there is no distal pulse. Perform this move only if you are allowed to do so. Check with your instructor. Do not try to force the arm, and stop if the limb offers resistance or if the patient complains of increased pain.

WARNING:

If the injury is to the wrist, do *not* attempt to straighten it. Attempts to straighten the wrist may damage blood vessels and nerves. Apply the splint while keeping the wrist in the position in which it is found and place padding in any space between the wrist and the splint. Your jurisdiction may allow you to make an attempt to gently reposition the wrist if there is no distal pulse and the hand is cold and blue.

■ If the elbow appears to be dislocated and it is in an unnatural or awkward position and cannot be repositioned, place padding around the arm and between the arm and chest if necessary. Secure the arm to the body with a sling and swathe.

INJURIES TO THE FOREARM, WRIST, AND HAND

First | The most effective splint for a painful, swollen, deformed forearm, wrist, or hand is a rigid one. However, the patient can be made comfortable with a pillow splint (soft splinting, Figure 12.23) and a sling and swathe. A sling and swathe used alone is also effective for a forearm. Be sure to check distal circulation before and after immobilizing.

To use a rigid splint for any painful, swollen, deformed (PSD) extremity injury to the forearm, wrist, or hand, select a padded rigid splint that extends from beyond the elbow to past the fingertips (Figure 12.24). Place a roll of dressing in the patient's hand to maintain the hand in the position of function. The steps for splinting the forearm, wrist, and hand are the same as steps 3 through 7 listed above for the upper arm. Do *not* apply manual traction to wrist or hand injuries.

First | Rolled newspapers, magazines, and creased cardboard make effective rigid splints for injuries to the forearm or wrist (Figure 12.25), but they still should be padded. Apply a sling after splinting to keep the forearm elevated. Add a swathe to secure the forearm to the chest and immobilize the joint above and below the injury site.

INJURIES TO THE FINGERS

Not all injuries to the fingers require rigid splinting. You can immobilize a fractured finger by taping the finger to an adjacent, uninjured finger (Figure 12.26). You can tape the finger to a tongue depressor, an aluminum splint, or a pen or pencil. You can also make a soft splint by placing a roll of gauze in the patient's hand and wrapping more gauze around the hand and dressing. This soft-splint method immobilizes the hand and fingers and keeps them in the position of function. Some emergency department physicians prefer that this type of soft bandage be used rather than a finger splint or tape. Check to see if this may be part of your EMS system's care procedures.

FIGURE 12.23
Soft splinting for wrist and hand injuries.

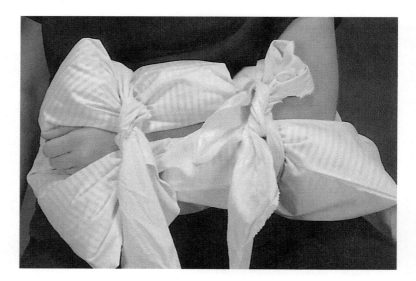

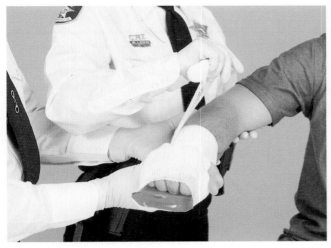

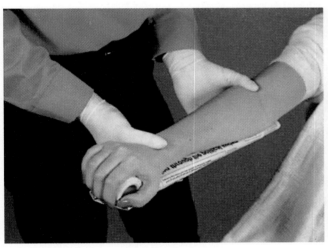

FIGURE 12.24
The rigid splinting of an injured forearm, wrist, or hand.

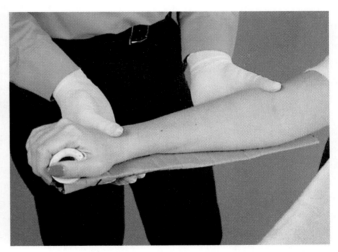

FIGURE 12.25
Rigid splints can be made from rolled newspapers, rolled magazines, or cardboard.
Note that the hand is in the position of function.

Apply a sling and swathe to keep the forearm elevated and a swathe to immobilize the joints above the injury site and to improve circulation and patient comfort.

Do *not* attempt to "pop" dislocated fingers back into their sockets. Immobilize dislocated fingers as you would an injured hand.

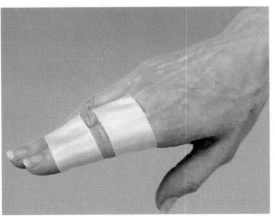

FIGURE 12.26
Immobilizing a fractured finger.

MANAGEMENT OF LOWER EXTREMITY INJURIES

REMEMBER:

Always assess distal pulse, sensation, and motor function before and after splinting. If there is no pulse, and your jurisdiction allows, gently realign an angulation or reposition the leg to regain pulse.

As in all First Responder care, providing emotional support to the patient is a significant part of total patient care.

Go over the following steps for immobilizing each of the injuries to the lower extremities. After seeing demonstrations by your instructor, use these steps to review and practice the process. Splinting the lower extremities is summarized in Scans 12.6, 12.7, and 12.8.

When the patient has multiple injuries, it may be best to totally immobilize the patient on a long spine board or a scoop (orthopedic) stretcher rather than try to immobilize each individual injury. Do not attempt to use these immobilization devices unless you are trained in your class to correctly move the patient onto them and to properly strap the patient to them. Before moving or rolling a patient with suspected spinal injury or with lower extremity injuries, be sure you have the proper equipment ready and a sufficient number of First Responders and EMTs on hand to assist.

INJURIES TO THE PELVIC GIRDLE

First The patient may have injuries to the pelvic girdle (pelvis and hip joints) if:

- The patient complains of pain in the pelvis, hips, or groin.
- The patient complains of pain when gentle pressure is applied to the sides of the hips or to the hip bones.
- The patient cannot lift the legs while lying face up. The patient will usually tell you that "it hurts" or "I can't move my legs." Do not insist that the patient try to lift the legs.
- The foot on the injured side turns outward.
- There is noticeable deformity of the pelvis or the hip joint.

Pelvic injuries are serious because they can also damage major blood vessels and reproductive and genitourinary organs. Injuries to these soft tissues can cause profuse internal bleeding, sterility, and infection. The trauma force that caused the pelvic injury may also have caused spinal injuries. Because of all these critical factors, it is best to wait for EMT assistance before attempting to immobilize a patient with pelvic injury. In the meantime, provide oxygen as soon as possible and maintain body temperature to prevent shock. Note the mechanism of injury so you may report it to EMTs or hospital staff.

The Ankle Hitch

NOTE: Make an ankle hitch from a cravat folded to about 3 inches. Use it with a single padded board splint to immobilize legs.

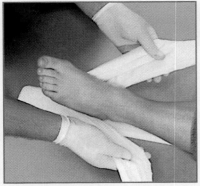

1. Kneel at the foot. Center the cravat in the arch.

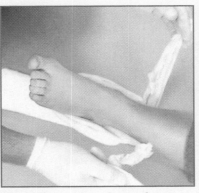

2. Bring cravat ends up along each side of the foot and cross the cravat behind the ankle.

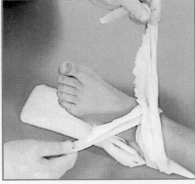

3. Cross the cravat ends over the top of the ankle.

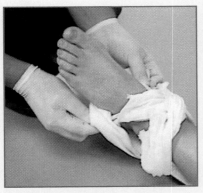

4. This has formed a stirrup.

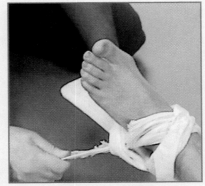

5. Thread the ends through the stirrup.

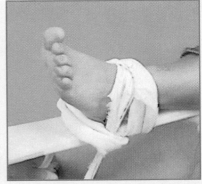

6. Gently pull the ends downward to tighten them.

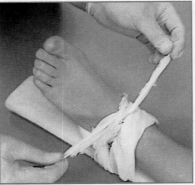

7. Pull the ends upward and tie them over the ankle.

Splinting: The Lower Extremity

NOTE: Pillows can be used to splint injured ankles and feet.

REMEMBER: Check for distal pulse, motor function, and sensation before and after splinting.

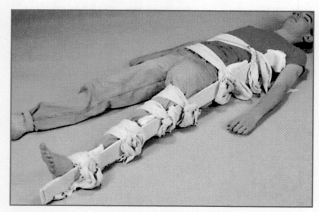

HIP—Tie the legs with a blanket roll or apply a long rigid splint:

- ❑ Use a splint from armpit to past the foot.
- ❑ Pad the splint and add extra padding at the armpit.
- ❑ Use two cravats to secure splint to trunk and four to secure the splint to the leg (two above knee and two below).

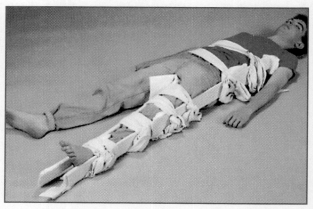

THIGH—Apply two splints, one long and one short:

- ❑ Long, from armpit to past foot.
- ❑ Short, from groin to past foot.
- ❑ Pad armpit, groin, voids between patient and splint, and bony areas.
- ❑ Secure the splints to trunk and limb with cravats.

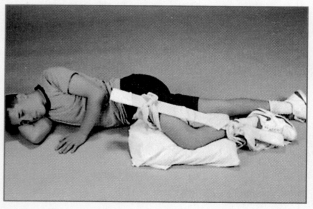

KNEE—

- ❑ If distal pulse present, then splint as found.
- ❑ If no distal pulse, attempt to gently realign or reposition to regain pulse (if your EMS system allows).
- ❑ Bent Knee: secure splints behind knee, at the thigh, and at the lower leg.
- ❑ Straight Knee: splint using same steps as "Hip" or "Thigh" above, or "Single-splint Method for Lower Leg."

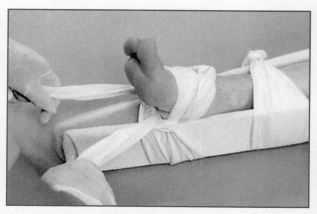

LOWER LEG—Apply two rigid splints, one lateral and one medial. A single splint can be applied to the back of the leg and secured with ankle hitch and dressing or cravats.

Single-Splint Method for Lower Leg

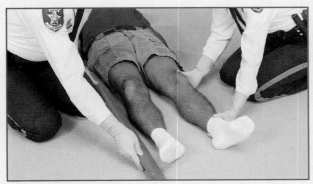

1. Measure the splint. It should extend from mid-thigh to about 4 inches below the ankle.

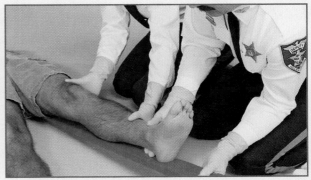

2. One First Responder applies and maintains manual traction. The other kneels at the patient's ankle and grips it while sliding the splint under the leg.

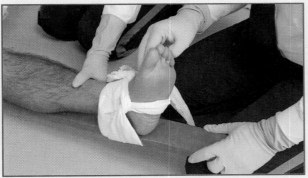

3. The First Responder holding traction grips the splint to the leg and elevates it about 10 inches. Another First Responder applies an ankle hitch.

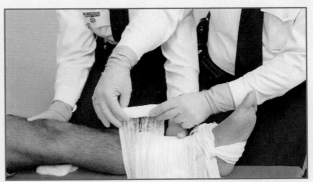

4. Secure the splint to the leg with a roller bandage starting at the distal end of the extremity.

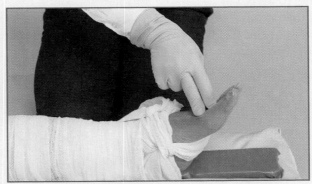

5. After the splint is secured from foot to thigh, check for distal pulse, motor function, and sensation.

With certain symptoms, pelvic girdle injuries may be managed at the scene with a specialized pressure garment called a pneumatic antishock garment (PASG). Your instructor will know if First Responders are trained and allowed to use or assist EMTs with PASGs in your jurisdiction. Follow your local protocols or medical direction when using a PASG. Other devices and materials that are effective for immobilizing injuries to the pelvic girdle include: long spine boards, scoop (orthopedic) stretchers, long board splints, and blankets. If you do not carry this equipment, you may continue your assessment and history while you are waiting for EMTs to arrive with the necessary equipment and additional personnel to help move and immobilize the patient.

First | As a First Responder, you can care for patients with fractures to the pelvic girdle by using a soft splint. Place a blanket roll between the patient's legs and tie them together with cravats (Figure 12.27). This simple and quick immobilization method will stabilize the injury and provide patient comfort before the EMTs arrive.

To immobilize a pelvic injury with a blanket roll, do the following:

1. Provide oxygen to the patient as soon as possible.

2. Place a folded blanket, large towel, or other thick padding material between the patient's legs from groin to feet.

3. Prepare four folded triangular bandages (cravats) or other strips of material.

4. Use a short splint or coat hanger and drape the ends of all four cravats over the splint or hanger. Slide them under the space behind the knees.

5. Gently slide two cravats above the knees and two below the knees.

6. Starting at the feet (distal end), tie one cravat at the ankles, one just below the knees, one just above the knees, and one just below the hips. Do not tie a cravat over or too near the injury site.

You may also use a rigid splint. Apply a long board that will extend from the patient's armpit to beyond the foot. (Add additional padding at the armpit.) Secure the splint to the patient with cravats tied around the splint and the patient's trunk and injured leg. Use a board splint or coat hanger to slide the cravats under the patient at the voids behind the back and knee (Figure 12.28). While your partner maintains manual traction, secure the splint in place by tying the cravats across the chest and hips and four places on the leg. This process may take several people. For this reason, it may be best to wait for EMTs to arrive or to use the simpler approach of securing the patient's legs with a blanket roll and cravats.

When the EMTs arrive, you can help them place the stabilized patient on a scoop (orthopedic) stretcher or spine board. Remember to provide oxygen to

FIGURE 12.27
For pelvic girdle fractures, place a blanket roll between the patient's legs. Then tie the legs together with cravats.

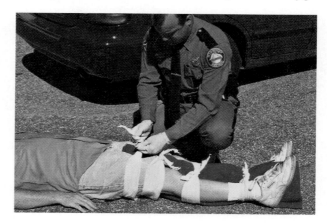

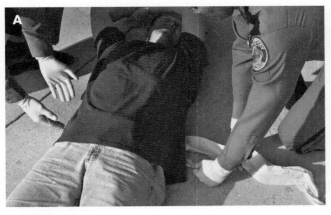
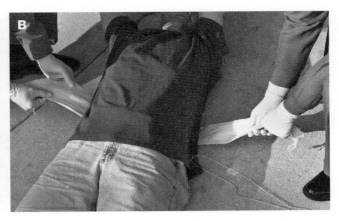

FIGURE 12.28
A Use a coat hanger or flat splint to push cravat under void.
B Then reposition cravat to proper side.

the patient as soon as possible and cover the patient to maintain body temperature to help prevent shock. If you suspect spinal injury, do not attempt to move the patient until the EMTs arrive with additional help. In the meantime, stabilize the patient's head and continue to talk with and reassure the patient.

Because the signs and symptoms of a fracture, a dislocation, a sprain, and a strain are so similar, you will not be trying to determine which type of injury the patient has. Even so, there are certain signs that indicate a possible hip dislocation, and you should look for them because you do not want to attempt to move the injured leg if there is a possible hip dislocation. If you suspect a hip dislocation, there may also be injury to the thigh bone (femur) because the trauma force to the hip may be severe enough to also damage the femur. Do not try to straighten an angulated femur if the hip also appears to be dislocated.

First | The following points describe two types of hip dislocation. Assume the patient has a dislocated hip if you find:

■ *Anterior hip dislocation*—The leg from hip to foot is rotated outward. Leg rotation also may be an indication of hip fracture. With hip fracture, the injured leg may appear to be shorter than the other leg. You will probably see or feel the bony end of the femur under the skin at the front or side of the leg where it joins the torso (Figure 12.29A).

■ *Posterior hip dislocation (most common)*—The leg is rotated inward and the knee is usually bent. You may see or feel the bony end of the femur under the skin at the back of the leg where it joins the buttocks (Figure 12.29B).

FIGURE 12.29
Classic signs of **A** anterior hip dislocation and **B** posterior hip dislocation.

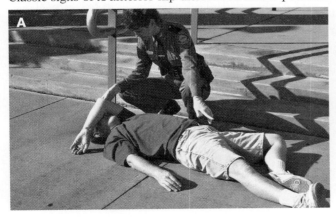
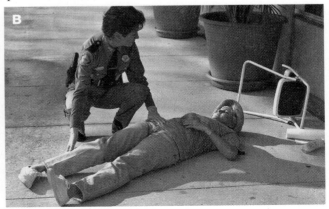

If the hip is dislocated, wait for EMTs to arrive. While waiting, provide oxygen as soon as possible and cover the patient to maintain body temperature and help prevent shock. You can immobilize the injured leg by placing and securing pillows or folded blankets or towels around the injured leg, which will support the leg and provide comfort to the patient. Do *not* reposition or move the patient's leg when you place or secure pillows or blankets.

INJURIES TO THE UPPER LEG OR THIGH

Injuries to the upper leg or thigh bone (femur) are often open. Even when the injury is closed, bleeding inside the tissues can be heavy and life-threatening. There may be a severe and obvious deformity with upper leg fractures. The leg below the injury site may be bent where there is no joint, or it will appear twisted.

To immobilize thigh injuries, use rigid splints or a special device called a "traction" splint. First Responder units may carry traction splints, and you may be trained and allowed to use them. (Your instructor will check your jurisdiction requirements.) Soft splints are not as effective as rigid or traction splinting, but they will stabilize the injury and provide some pain relief.

While waiting for EMTs to arrive, provide the patient some relief from pain by securing a blanket roll between the legs in the same way you would for injuries to the pelvic girdle. This is effective once the patient is secured to a spine board or scoop (orthopedic) stretcher, a form of rigid splinting. Provide oxygen as soon as possible and cover the patient to maintain body warmth to help prevent shock.

If you use a padded board splint, follow the same steps as you did for pelvic injury and remember to place padding between the board and the armpit. Never tie cravats over the injury site but position them just above and below the injury.

An alternative approach is to immobilize the leg with two splints: one long splint that extends from the patient's armpit to past the foot, and a shorter splint that extends from the groin to beyond the foot. Be certain to pad the armpit and groin. To secure the splints, use another splint or coat hanger to push cravats under the patient's trunk and legs at the natural voids (lower back and knees). Do not place a tie over the injury site but place one tie above and one tie below the injury.

INJURIES TO THE KNEE

In most cases, you will not be able to tell if the knee is fractured, dislocated, or both. Sometimes a dislocated kneecap (patella) will spontaneously reposition itself. The patient will probably be able to tell you if this happened. Because of the many nerves and blood vessels and the possibility that soft tissues were damaged, immobilize an injured knee in the position in which it is found. Do *not* attempt to reposition or straighten the injured knee. Some EMS systems allow First Responders to make one attempt to straighten the limb if there is no distal pulse. Your instructor will let you know the requirements of local protocols.

Rigid splinting is the most effective method to use when immobilizing an injured knee, but you can provide support to the leg and comfort to the patient with soft splints. Place and secure pillows or folded blankets around the knee, especially if it is found in the bent position. Do not reposition or move the patient's legs in order to place or secure pillows or blankets. If the injured knee is found in the straight position, you can effectively immobilize with a blanket roll between the legs and secure it with cravats, just as you would for hip and femur injuries.

REMEMBER:

Fractures to the thigh can bleed profusely. Provide oxygen as soon as possible and maintain body temperature to reduce the effects of shock. Monitor the patient's vital signs and comfort level.

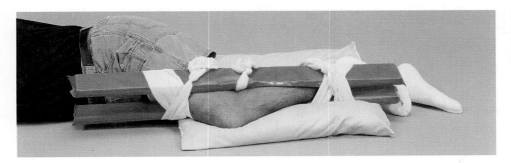

FIGURE 12.30A
Splint an injured knee in
the position in which it is
found.

For rigid splinting of an injured knee found in the straight position (or straightened because there was no distal pulse), secure a long splint from the patient's armpit to beyond the foot. If you cannot find a splint that long, use a splint that will extend from the patient's waist to beyond the foot. You may also use the method described below for splinting the lower leg. In cases where the patient's leg will remain flexed at the knee, you can secure one or two shorter splints at an angle across the thigh and lower leg (A-frame) with cravats (Figure 12.30A and Scan 12-7).

INJURIES TO THE LOWER LEG

You can provide care for injuries to the lower leg with either rigid or soft splints. A blanket roll between the legs is an effective soft splint. Secure it as you did for pelvic, thigh, and knee injuries described previously. Once you assist the EMTs in placing the patient on the spine board or scoop (orthopedic) stretcher, a form of rigid splinting, you have completed immobilizing all joints above and below the injury site.

If you use a rigid splint, you will need assistance. One person must maintain manual traction while you apply one or two splints. Splint the lower leg with one or two rigid splints. Use the two-splint method as described earlier for fractures of the thigh bone. A single-splint method also can be used to immobilize lower leg injuries. The procedure is shown in Scan 12-8.

After splinting, check for distal pulse, sensation, and motor function. If there is no pulse, remove the splint, realign or reposition the limb, and resplint.

If you live in an area where skiing is a popular sport, you may have to treat a certain kind of fracture, the boot-top fracture (Figure 12.30B). This is a fracture of the tibia and/or fibula (usually both) that typically occurs when a skier falls forward of the ski tips. The leg bends hard over the top of the ski boot, causing a transverse fracture (a break in the bone that is at a right angle to the long part of the bone) of one or both bones. The leg below the fracture is often angulated or rotated, and the fracture is quite painful. Dr. Warren Bowman, author of *Outdoor Emergency Care* and the Medical Director for the National Ski Patrol recommends the following:

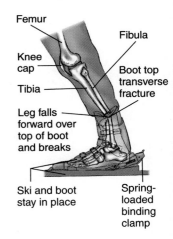

FIGURE 12.30B
Boot-top fracture.

Femur
Fibula
Knee cap
Boot top transverse fracture
Tibia
Leg falls forward over top of boot and breaks
Ski and boot stay in place
Spring-loaded binding clamp

- Notify the ski patrol immediately. (Send another skier to an emergency phone or lift shack.)
- Keep the patient warm with others' coats; place something between the skier and the snow.
- Leave the leg alone or in the position found until the ski patrol arrives; or
- Gently align the injury to see if that will reduce the patient's pain.
- Manually stabilize or splint the fracture. (A ski or ski pole will work, or use splints). Secure with scarves, handkerchiefs, or cravats.
- Do *not* apply snow to the fracture site to prevent swelling. (Swelling is due to bleeding from the fractured bone ends, and applying cold will *not* help but will hasten the development or frostbite and/or hypothermia.)

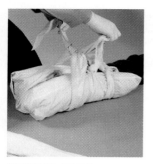

FIGURE 12.31
Emergency care procedures for an injured ankle or foot.

INJURIES TO THE ANKLE OR FOOT

First | Rigid splints may be used for injuries to the ankle or foot, but the soft splint is probably the most comfortable for the patient and the quickest for the First Responder to apply. If you apply a rigid splint, use one that extends from above the patient's knee to beyond the foot as described for the single-splint method for the lower leg.

For soft splinting an injury to the foot or ankle, immobilize it in the position found with a pillow or folded blanket. Secure the soft splint around the foot and ankle with several cravats or with roller gauze (Figure 12.31), then elevate it by propping it on a blanket roll or pillow.

RESPLINTING

After splinting, you will always recheck distal pulse, sensation, and motor function. If absent, your protocols may direct you to remove the splint, realign the extremity until distal pulse returns, then resplint. If you are allowed to realign an extremity, do not force the limb and stop immediately if the movement causes more pain. Resplint once the distal pulse returns. One reason for an absent pulse after splinting is because the gauze or cravats may have been applied too tightly. If there is still no distal pulse after removing the splint or realigning the limb, it may be that swelling and pressure have restricted circulation. Arrange for transport immediately if distal pulse does not return.

THE AXIAL SKELETON

Remember that the axial skeleton consists of the head (skull), spinal column, and chest (sternum and ribs) (Figure 12.32). It makes up the long axis of the body. Injuries to the axial skeleton can be very serious because trauma can also

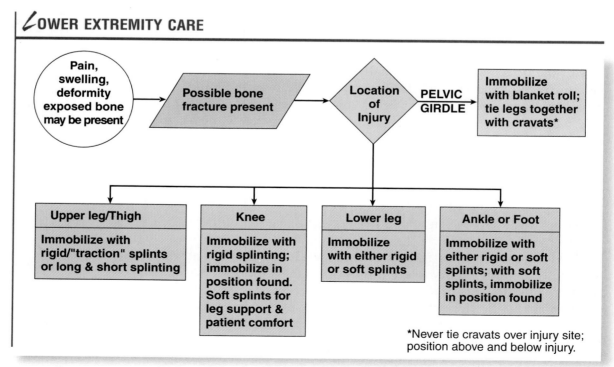

LOWER EXTREMITY CARE

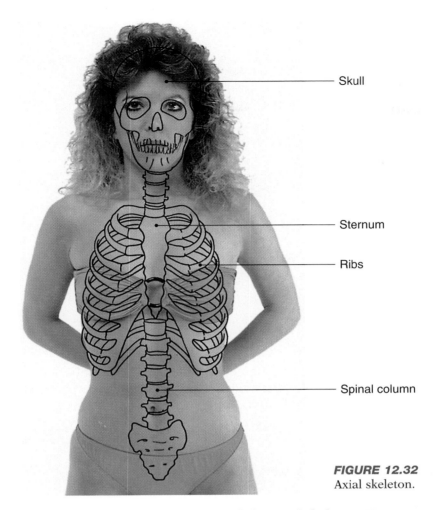

Skull

Sternum

Ribs

Spinal column

FIGURE 12.32
Axial skeleton.

injure the structures protected by the bones of the axial skeleton. Your concern is not just with the bones, but also with the brain, spinal cord, airway, lungs, and heart—all vital organs protected by the axial skeleton. When the head, spine, or chest is injured, also assess the patient for the signs and symptoms that indicate injuries to the protected vital organs.

THE HEAD

The head or skull is divided into two major structures, the **cranium** and the face (Figure 12.33). Flat, irregularly shaped bones make up the floor, back, top, and sides of the skull and the forehead. The bones are fused together into immovable joints, which form a rigid, protective case for the brain.

In infants, fusion of the head bones is not complete. Places called "soft spots" (fontanelles) can be felt at the top, sides, and back of the baby's skull. The smaller soft spots at the sides and back close in the first few months, but the largest soft spot at the top of the skull does not close completely until about 18 to 24 months. When caring for an infant with possible head injuries, avoid applying point pressure to the skull with your fingertips. Instead spread your fingers and hold or stabilize the head with your entire hand.

The face is made up of strong, irregularly shaped bones. The face bones include part of the eye sockets, the cheeks, the upper part of the nose, the upper jaw, and the lower jaw. These bones also are fused into immovable joints except for the lower jaw bone, or **mandible**, which is the only movable joint in the head.

cranium (KRAY-ne-um)—the bones that form the forehead and the floor, back, top, and upper sides of the skull. Usually the term *skull fracture* refers to a break in one or more of the cranial bones.

mandible (MAN-di-bl)—the lower jaw bone.

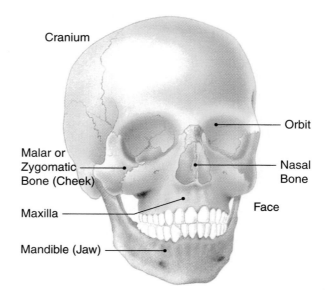

FIGURE 12.33
The skull.

Cranium

Orbit

Malar or
Zygomatic
Bone (Cheek)

Nasal
Bone

Face

Maxilla

Mandible (Jaw)

THE SPINAL COLUMN

cervical (SER-vi-kal) spine—the neck bones.

The spinal column includes the neck bones and the back bones (Figure 12.34). The neck bones are called the **cervical spine** and connect to the skull. The rest of the spine is commonly known as the backbone. The spine protects the spinal cord as it runs from the brain down through the back. Many of the body's major nerves run into and out of the spinal cord and connect most areas of the body to the brain. In addition, the spine supports the entire body. The skull, shoulder bones, ribs, and pelvic bones connect to the spine.

THE CHEST

There are 12 ribs on each side of the chest. All the ribs connect with the spine. Most of the ribs attach directly to the sternum (breastbone) by pieces of cartilage (Figure 12.35). Some of the ribs connect to other ribs by a common cartilage strip. The bottom two ribs on each side—sometimes called "floating" ribs—do not connect to the breastbone or to other ribs. They are held in place by muscles.

The lower ribs help protect the organs in the upper part of the abdomen: the liver, gallbladder, stomach, and spleen. The upper ribs and sternum help protect the organs in the center or middle part of the chest. These organs include the heart and major blood vessels leading into and out of the heart, the trachea (windpipe) leading to the lungs, and the esophagus leading to the stomach. The upper ribs also protect the lungs, which lie on each side of the heart. The muscles of the back and chest, along with the muscles found between the ribs, give added strength to the spine and the ribs and help protect the heart and lungs.

THE CENTRAL NERVOUS SYSTEM

Remember, injuries to the head and spine can involve much more than just the bones that make up these structures. Soft-tissue injuries to outer skin and to underlying muscles, organs, blood vessels, and nerves can occur as well.

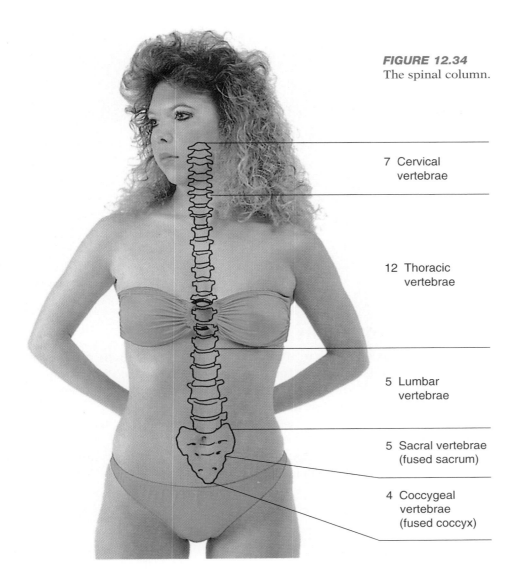

FIGURE 12.34
The spinal column.

7 Cervical
vertebrae

12 Thoracic
vertebrae

5 Lumbar
vertebrae

5 Sacral vertebrae
(fused sacrum)

4 Coccygeal
vertebrae
(fused coccyx)

The brain and spinal cord make up what is known as the **central nervous system (CNS).** The brain not only takes care of thinking, it also controls many of our most basic functions, including heart activity and breathing. The brain tells muscles when to contract and relax so that we can move. It receives messages from all over the body and decides how the body will respond to these messages. Any injury to the skull could injure the brain and cause vital body functions to fail.

The spinal cord carries messages along nerves from the brain to the body and from the body back to the brain. Injury to the spine could damage the spinal cord and prevent it from carrying messages to or from a part of the body. That part of the body would no longer have contact with the brain and would be unable to function. The damage could be temporary, caused by pressure or swelling that may be corrected with proper care, or the damage could be permanent so that part of the body would never again be able to move or function. In addition, the spinal cord is the site of many reflexes, which allow us to react quickly to such things as pain and heat (Figure 12.36). Damage to the spinal cord can take away these reflex abilities.

central nervous system—the brain and spinal cord. Sometimes referred to as the CNS.

FIGURE 12.35
The chest.

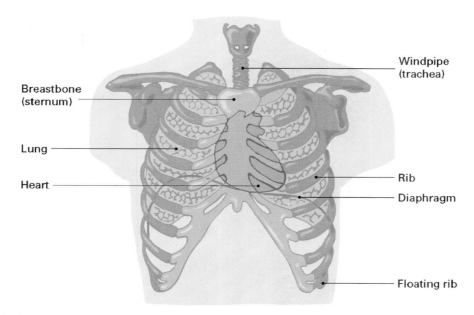

Windpipe (trachea)

Breastbone (sternum)

Lung

Heart

Rib

Diaphragm

Floating rib

MECHANISMS OF INJURY

You will not always be able to find and determine all patient injuries. Most of the time, you will assume that the patient is injured based on the mechanism of injury (MOI). Be highly suspicious of injury if the patient has been involved in or reports the following situations:

■ Falls, diving, and motor vehicle accidents that result in swelling or pressure on a body part
■ Direct or indirect forces that caused excessive flexion or extension or excessive bending or stretching of a body part
■ Twisting forces that caused rotation or excessive twisting of a body part

FIGURE 12.36
Reflexes allow for swift reactions to stimuli.

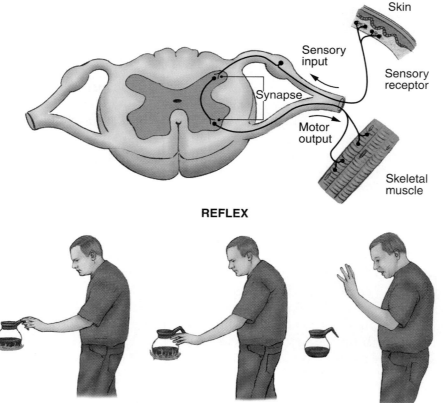

Skin

Sensory input

Sensory receptor

Synapse

Motor output

Skeletal muscle

REFLEX

- Pulling or hanging forces that caused spinal stretching
- Axial load to the top of the head
- Blunt trauma such as that caused by blows, a car striking a pedestrian, or a driver striking a steering wheel or windshield
- Penetrating trauma such as that caused by gunshots or stabbings
- Blows in assault and battery or abuse incidents and the rapid forceful shaking of infants and children
- Any trauma situation where the patient is unconscious or unresponsive

INJURIES TO THE HEAD

TYPES OF INJURIES

Injuries to the head can be caused by a variety of mechanisms that result in pain, swelling, and deformity similar to what was described for extremity injuries. In addition, the mechanism of injury (MOI) may be forceful enough to cause a patient to be unresponsive. Because the skull surrounds or encases the brain, the force of the mechanism of injury can also be transmitted to the brain. Injury to the brain can affect the patient's ability to breathe. Because of this, airway management is always the first consideration in the care of any patient who has a head injury. Keep the airway open. In addition to skull and brain injury, there can be cuts to the scalp and other soft tissues.

There are certain signs and symptoms that will help you determine if a head injury is an **open head injury** or a **closed head injury.**

In an *open head injury*, you may be able to see or feel that the skull is cracked (fractured) or depressed (deformed), that there is blood and clear or yellow watery fluid leaking from the ears or nose, and that the eyelids are swollen shut and beginning to discolor or bruise. The fluids that protect the brain and are normally contained within the skull are leaking out into the tissues through the crack in the skull. The brain may also be injured in open head injuries. Broken bones or foreign objects forced through the skull can cut, tear, or bruise the brain. There may be no evident soft-tissue damage in some cases of open head injury.

In a *closed head injury*, the skull is not damaged or cracked, but the brain can still be injured by the force of something striking the skull. Though the force does not crack the skull, it does cause the brain to bounce off the inside of the skull. The resulting injuries to the brain include (Figure 12.37):

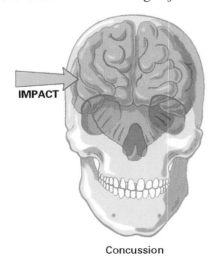

Concussion

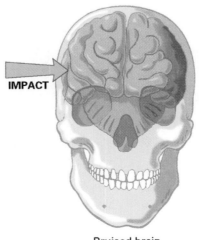

Bruised brain
(contusion)

FIGURE 12.37
Closed head injuries.

concussion (kon-KUSH-un)—injury to the brain that results from a blow or impact from an object but does not cause an open head injury.

contusion (kon-TU-zhun)—a bruising of the brain caused by a force of a blow great enough to rupture blood vessels on the surface or deep within the brain.

■ **Concussion**—when a blow to the head does not cause an open head injury but does cause damage to the brain. The injury may be so minor it does not cause unconsciousness; or it may be mild, causing headache after brief loss of consciousness; or it may be severe, causing lengthy unconsciousness and abnormal vital signs. Sometimes short-term memory is lost. Any signs and symptoms of concussion are an indication of brain injury.

■ **Contusion** (bruising)—when the force of a blow is great enough to rupture blood vessels on the surface or deep within the brain. In a closed head injury, the blood has no opening from which to drain. The blood builds up inside the skull, presses on the brain, and affects or impairs its function or ability to send messages to the body.

Signs and Symptoms of Head Injury

First | Many injuries to the skull are obvious. Also consider the possibility of head injury when the mechanism of injury suggests it and when you find the following in your focused assessment (Figure 12.38):

■ Unresponsiveness or unconsciousness
■ Deep cuts or tears to the skin
■ Exposed brain tissue
■ Penetrating injuries such as gunshot wounds and impaled objects
■ Swelling ("goose eggs") and discoloration of the skin
■ Edges or fragments of bones seen or felt through the skin
■ Deformity of the skull, such as depressed or "sunken-in" areas
■ Swelling and discoloration behind the ears—Battle's sign (late sign)
■ Swelling or discoloration of the eyelids or the tissues under the eyes
■ Unequal pupils or both pupils are dilated; one or both eyes appear sunken
■ Bleeding from the ears and/or the nose
■ Clear or bloody fluid flowing from the ears and/or nose. This fluid—called *cerebrospinal* (ser-e-bro-SPI-nal) *fluid* (CSF)—surrounds the brain and spinal cord and cannot flow from the ears or nose unless the skull has been fractured.
■ Weakness or numbness on one side of the body

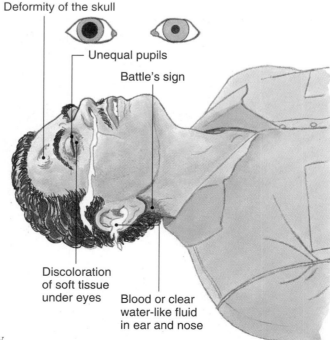

Deformity of the skull

Unequal pupils

Battle's sign

Discoloration of soft tissue under eyes

Blood or clear water-like fluid in ear and nose

FIGURE 12.38
Signs of head injury.

- Deterioration of vital signs. Each time you assess the patient's pulse and respirations, the results are progressively worse.

Note

Since many of the signs of head and brain injury can be produced by drug or alcohol abuse, take great care in assessing the patient. *Never assume alcohol or drug abuse, and always assess and care for possible injuries.*

Signs and Symptoms of Brain Injury

First | In cases of head injury, consider the possibility of a brain injury if you find the following in your focused assessment:

- Headache (mild to severe) following the accident
- Any sign of head injury
- Loss of consciousness, unresponsiveness, or altered mental states
- Confusion or personality changes
- Unequal or unresponsive pupils
- Paralysis or loss of function, usually to one side of the body and opposite the side of head injury (also an indication of spinal-cord injury)
- Loss of sensation, which may be to one side of the body (also an indication of spinal cord injury)
- Bilateral weakness or numbness, an indication of spinal cord injury
- Paralysis of facial muscles (may interfere with airway and speech)
- Disturbed or impaired vision, hearing, and/or sense of balance
- Nausea and/or vomiting
- Any changing patterns in respiration that include cycles of rapid, slow, shallow, and stopped breathing, and efforts to breathe with the diaphragm but no other chest movement
- Seizures

Signs and Symptoms of Facial Injury

Facial injuries can be very serious because of the potential for airway obstruction. Blood and other fluids, blood clots, bone, and teeth may cause partial or full airway obstruction. The force that caused injury to the face can also be transferred to the base, or floor, of the skull and cause an open head injury. If this has happened, you will see cerebrospinal fluid (CSF) leaking from the ears and nose.

Consider the possibility of facial injuries when you find the following in your focused assessment (Figure 12.39):

- Blood in the airway (nose or mouth)
- Facial deformities
- Swelling and discoloration of the eyelids or discoloration of the tissues below the eyes

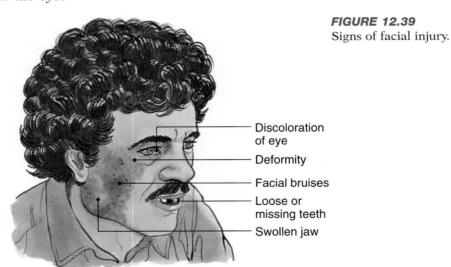

FIGURE 12.39
Signs of facial injury.

Discoloration of eye

Deformity

Facial bruises

Loose or missing teeth

Swollen jaw

- Swelling or discoloration of any part of the face
- Swollen lower jaw, poor function of or inability to close jaw
- Deformity or depression of any part of the face
- Teeth that are loose or have been knocked out, broken dentures
- Any mechanism of injury that indicates a blow to the face

CARE FOR HEAD INJURIES

Injuries to the Cranium

First When caring for patients with injuries to the cranium, assume that neck or spinal injuries also exist. Always don personal protective equipment, then take the following steps:

1. Maintain an open airway. Use the jaw-thrust maneuver and stabilize the head.

2. Provide resuscitative measures as needed.

3. Keep the patient still. This can be a critical factor. *Do not let the patient move or change position.*

4. Control bleeding. Do *not* apply direct pressure over the injury site, because you may cause further damage to the brain or soft tissues. Use a bulky dressing. Do *not* attempt to stop the flow of blood or cerebrospinal fluid (CSF) from the ears or nose—it needs to flow out, not build up pressure inside the skull. Secure a loose dressing to absorb flow and prevent this now contaminated fluid from flowing back into the brain.

5. Talk to the conscious patient. Try to keep the patient alert.

6. Dress and bandage open wounds and stabilize penetrating objects. Do *not* remove any objects or bone fragments.

7. Provide care for shock. Maintain body warmth but avoid overheating. Provide 100% oxygen and give nothing to eat or drink.

8. Monitor and record vital signs. Watch for and record changes.

9. Monitor level of consciousness.

10. Provide emotional support.

11. Be prepared for vomiting.

12. Arrange to transport as soon as possible.

Do *not* reposition any patient with an open head wound or any other possible serious injury to the skull unless you must do so to provide CPR or assist ventilations. If the mechanism of injury and the patient's responsiveness level indicate the possibility of spinal injury, do *not* reposition the patient. Assume that any patient who is unconscious or unresponsive and has trauma above the collarbones has spinal injury. Stabilize the head and open the airway with the jaw-thrust maneuver.

WARNING:

It is a serious sign when an unconscious patient regains consciousness and then loses consciousness again. Make certain you report this to the EMTs.

Note

The two most important factors in determining the outcome in head injury are:

1. hypoxia (low oxygen level in blood)
2. hypotension (low blood pressure)

FIGURE 12.40
Head and shoulders elevated for patients with mild head injuries.

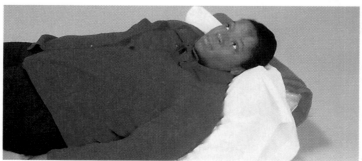

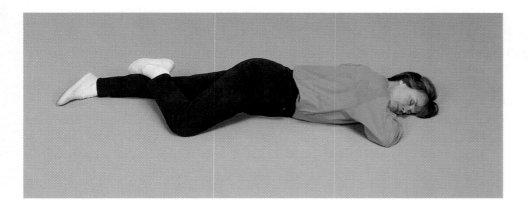

For conscious, responsive patients with minor closed head injuries and **no signs of spinal injuries,** you have two choices for positioning the patient. Both methods are suitable for patients with facial fractures. The methods are:

1. Elevate head and shoulders (Figure 12.40). Place the patient's upper body at a 45-degree angle, using several pillows or a blanket roll as needed.

2. Place the patient in the recovery position (on the side) as shown in Figure 12.41. Position the lower shoulder behind the patient and the hand of the upper shoulder under and supporting the cheek. Tilt the head slightly back and the face downward to allow for drainage of fluids.

Injuries to the Face

First | As in all cases of facial injury, make certain that the patient has an open airway. If you must assist ventilations, use the jaw-thrust maneuver and stabilize the head in case there is injury to the spine. Do not apply direct pressure to bleeding wounds; use a bulky dressing to care for soft-tissue injuries.

The lower jaw can be dislocated or fractured. Because it is a movable joint, dislocations occur where the lower jaw attaches to the skull just in front of the ears. Look for the mechanism of injury—a force that could have struck the jaw from the front or side. The signs and symptoms to look for include:

- Pain and tenderness
- Swelling and discoloration
- Deformity or facial distortion or disfigurement
- Loss of use or inability to control jaw movement or to open or close mouth
- Difficulty in speaking
- Bleeding from the nose, mouth, or around the teeth
- Missing or broken teeth or broken dentures

To care for possible fracture or dislocation of the lower jaw:

1. Maintain an open airway.

2. Control bleeding and dress any open wounds. Do not tie the patient's mouth shut since there may be vomiting.

3. Keep the patient at rest and provide care for shock.

4. Closely monitor the patient and stay alert for vomiting.

5. Monitor and record vital signs.

Injuries to the face can damage teeth, crowns (caps), bridges, and dentures. Always look for and remove avulsed (dislodged) teeth and parts of broken dental appliances. Be careful not to push these down the patient's airway.

When a tooth is avulsed, there is bleeding from the socket. Have the responsive, conscious patient bite down on a pad of gauze placed over the socket, but leave several inches of gauze outside the mouth for quick removal. For the unresponsive or unconscious patient, hold the gauze over the socket. This will control the bleeding and prevent the airway from becoming obstructed with blood.

Wrap the avulsed tooth in a dressing. If you have a source of clean water, keep the dressing moist. (Milk can also be used.) Do *not* attempt to clean the tooth. Your efforts could damage microscopic structures needed to replant the tooth.

INJURIES TO THE SPINE

TYPES OF INJURIES

Soft tissues of the neck can be injured by a number of mechanisms of injury. The forces that cause soft-tissue injury can also injure underlying bones of the spinal cord in the neck (cervical) spine. Injuries to and improper care of cervical spine injuries can impair breathing and lead to paralysis or death. Injuries along the rest of the spinal column also can cause paralysis and reduce normal body movement and function.

Spinal injuries are caused by forces to the head, neck, back, chest, pelvis, or legs. Often, you will find patients with head injuries who also have cervical spine injuries. Fractures to the upper leg bones or to the pelvic bones may also cause spinal injury. (Remember the earlier explanation of how indirect forces send the energy along the bone to injure another part.) Accidents from certain activities such as motor vehicle crashes (including those causing whiplash), falls, diving, and skiing often cause spinal injuries.

If a patient has numbness, loss of feeling, or paralysis in the legs with no problems in the arms, the injury to the spine is probably below the neck. If numbness, loss of feeling, or paralysis involves the arms and the legs, the injury is probably in the neck. Numbness, loss of feeling, and paralysis may be limited to only one side of the body, but usually both sides are involved.

Injuries to the spine can include fractured or displaced spinal bones (vertebrae) or swelling that presses on nerves. These injuries can produce the same signs and symptoms. In some cases, the loss of function associated with spinal injuries may be temporary if the loss is caused by pressure or swelling that will recede. But if the spinal cord was cut, even the best surgery and care cannot restore function.

SIGNS AND SYMPTOMS OF SPINAL INJURY

First | In general, the signs and symptoms of spinal injury include:

- Weakness, numbness or tingling sensations, or loss of feeling in the arms or legs
- Paralysis to arms and/or legs
- Painful movement of arms and/or legs (or no pain or sensation)
- Pain and/or tenderness along the back of the neck or the backbone
- Burning sensations along the spine or in an extremity
- Deformity of the spine; the angle of the patient's head and neck may appear odd to you. You may feel pieces of bone that have broken off the spine, though such findings are rare.

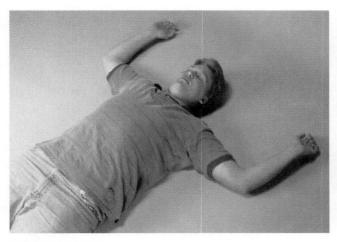

FIGURE 12.42A
Patients found face up with arms stretched above the head may have spinal injuries.

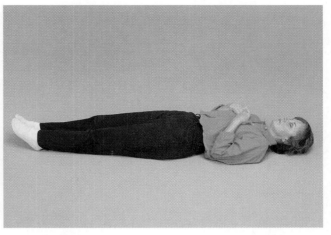

FIGURE 12.42B
Patients with severe head and spinal injuries may be found with arms and hands curled onto the chest in a decorticate (toward the center) position.

- Loss of bladder and bowel control
- Difficult or labored breathing with little or no movement of the chest and slight movement of the abdomen
- Positioning of the arms. You may find the patient lying face up with arms stretched out above the head or with arms and hands curled to the chest (Figure 12.42).
- Persistent erection of the penis called *priapism* (PRY-ah-pism), which indicates spinal injury affecting nerves to the external genitalia.

THE FOCUSED ASSESSMENT

The methods of assessing a patient for spinal injuries were presented in Chapter 7.

First | For the conscious and responsive patient, remember to conduct a patient interview in your focused assessment. You may learn things about the accident that will help determine the mechanism of injury. When focusing your assessment on the patient's injury, you should (Scan 12-9):

1. Question the patient. Do his arms or legs feel numb? Can the patient feel you touch his hands and feet? Can he squeeze your hand or push your hand with his foot? Do *not* ask the patient to repeat any movement that causes pain.

2. Look and feel gently for injuries and deformities.

3. See if the patient can move his arms and legs. Do not do this if you have noted any mechanism of injury or other signs that indicate possible injury to the spine.

First | For the unconscious and unresponsive patient, remember to:

1. Ask bystanders for information on how the accident happened and what they saw happen to the patient. This may help you to determine the mechanism of injury.

2. Look and feel for injuries and deformities.

3. See if the patient responds to pressure on or pinching of the feet and hands. Never probe palms and soles with sharp objects.

Assessing Patients for Spinal Injuries

SIGNS AND SYMPTOMS

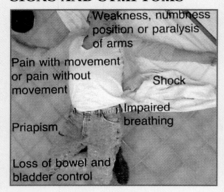

Weakness, numbness position or paralysis of arms

Pain with movement or pain without movement

Shock

Priapism

Impaired breathing

Loss of bowel and bladder control

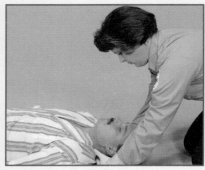

Cervical point tenderness and deformity

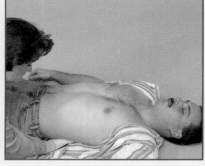

Spinal column tenderness and deformity

CONSCIOUS: LOWER EXTREMITIES ASSESSMENT

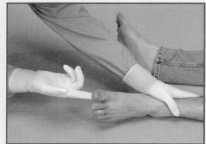

Touch toe

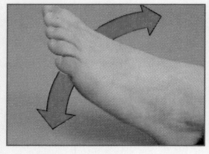

Foot movement

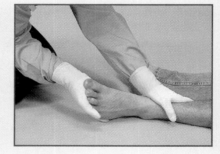

Foot push

RESULTS: If the patient can perform these tasks, there is little chance of injury to the spinal cord, but EMS systems prefer that you immobilize the spine since this test does not rule out all types of injuries, including spinal fractures. If the patient can perform only to a limited degree and with pain, there may be pressure somewhere on the spinal cord. When a patient is not able to perform any of the tests, assume that there is spinal injury.

CONSCIOUS: UPPER EXTREMITIES ASSESSMENT

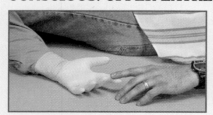

Touch finger

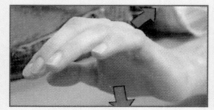

Hand movement

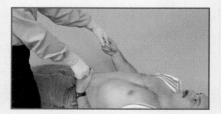

Hand squeeze

RESULTS: If the patient can perform these tests, there is little chance of damage in the cervical area, but you cannot rule out all injuries. Limited performance and pain: pressure on spinal cord in cervical area. Failure to perform any: assume severe spinal cord injury in neck.

(continued)

Unconscious patients: Test the responses to painful stimuli (pinching) applied to the foot or ankle. Removing shoes may aggravate injuries.

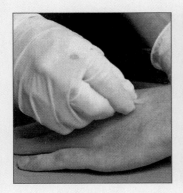
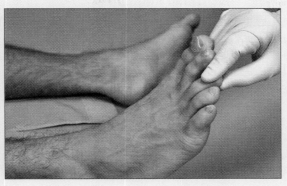

REMEMBER: It is difficult to accurately assess the unconscious patient. A deeply unconscious patient will not pull back from a painful stimulus. If the mechanism of injury indicates possible spinal damage, or if the patient is unconscious, assume and care for a spinal injury.

RESULTS: Slight pulling back of foot: spinal cord usually intact. No foot reaction: possible damage anywhere along the spinal cord. Hand or finger reaction: usually no damage to spinal cord. No hand or finger reaction: possible damage to the spinal cord. Assume damage to the spinal cord if you find no reactions, failure to perform any test, limited performance, or performance with pain.

SUMMARY OF OBSERVATIONS AND CONCLUSIONS

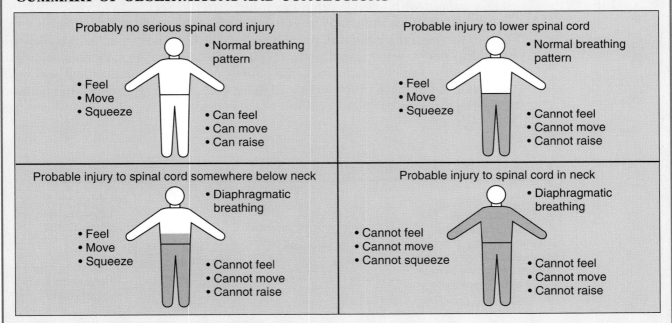

WARNING: If the patient is unconscious or the mechanism of injury indicates spinal injury, assume and care for spinal injury.

REMEMBER:

Consider every unconscious, unresponsive injured patient to have spinal injuries. Stabilize the patient's head and open the airway with the jaw-thrust maneuver.

CARE FOR INJURIES TO THE SPINE

Rules for Care

First | Always follow these rules for First Responder care for patients with possible spinal injuries.

- **RULE 1:** Make certain the airway is open and assist ventilations or perform CPR as needed, even though the patient may have spinal injuries. Use the jaw-thrust maneuver for mouth-to-mask resuscitation.
- **RULE 2:** Attempt to control serious bleeding. Avoid moving the injured part of the patient and any of the limbs when applying dressings.
- **RULE 3:** Always assume that an unconscious accident patient has spinal injuries.
- **RULE 4:** Do not attempt to splint fractures if there are indications of spinal injuries until you have appropriate help.
- **RULE 5:** Never move a patient with spinal injuries unless you must do so to provide CPR or assist ventilations, need to reach and control life-threatening bleeding, or must protect yourself and the patient from immediate danger at the scene.
- **RULE 6:** Keep the patient still. Tell him or her not to move. Position yourself to stabilize or immobilize the patient's head, neck, and as much of the body as possible.
- **RULE 7:** Continuously monitor patients with possible spinal injury. These patients will often go into shock. Sometimes, their chest muscles will be paralyzed and they will go into respiratory arrest.

Stabilizing the Patient's Head and Neck

Assume that a patient with head injuries also has spinal injuries. Also assume that a patient with chest trauma has injuries to the neck.

Work carefully and gently as you immobilize the patient. Do *not* apply traction to the patient's head and neck; just grip the head with your hands like you would to perform the jaw-thrust maneuver. Do *not* try to place an extrication collar on the patient or position the patient on a spine board unless you have had training in these procedures and there is enough help to move the patient. (The Department of Transportation has not designated application of cervical

SPINAL INJURY ASSESSMENT

Patient has numbness, loss of feeling in legs and arms, paralysis to arms and legs Pain/tenderness in neck or along backbone → Possible spinal injury → Patient conscious

YES → Lower extremity assessment / Upper extremity assessment

NO → Any unconscious patient assume spinal injury

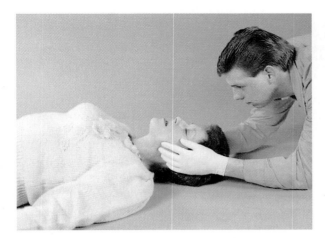

FIGURE 12.43
When necessary, in-line stabilization may be applied to the patient's head and neck.

collars and spine boards as a part of First Responder training programs. Your instructor will teach you techniques required by your EMS system's protocols.)

A patient with spinal injuries may be able to move the head, neck, arms, trunk, or legs but movement can cause more injury. For this reason, keep the patient from moving by verbally reassuring him and by physically stabilizing the head and neck.

When you must stabilize a patient's head and neck, (Figure 12.43):

1. Kneel at the top of the patient's head.

2. Place your hands on each side of the head and position your fingers under the lower jaw.

3. Keep the patient's head and neck steady (stable) in this position. Do not allow the patient to move his head and neck. Explain your actions to the patient and offer reassurance while you are keeping his head stable. Do not apply traction or turn or lift the patient's head.

4. Maintain your position until a rigid cervical or extrication collar is applied. (See Chapter 5, Scans 5-8 and 5-9, for application steps, but do not attempt to apply a collar to a patient until you have received proper training from your instructor.)

First | It is best to just stabilize the patient's head and neck and wait for the EMTs to arrive before trying to proceed any further in immobilizing the patient. Immobilizing a patient on a backboard is not a required First Responder skill; however, your jurisdiction may require that you learn this skill. If so, your instructor will teach you the proper techniques. Do *not* attempt to place a patient on a backboard without proper training.

> **WARNING:**
> Stabilize the patient's head and neck and wait for EMTs to arrive before attempting to immobilize him further.

HELMET REMOVAL

Helmets are designed to absorb energy forces and prevent injury to the head. However, even well-fitting helmets cannot prevent the brain from striking the interior of the skull in extreme or high-speed crash forces. When the brain rapidly and repeatedly strikes the inside of the skull, brain tissue is bruised and blood vessels tear and bleed. The patient can suffer a concussion, a contusion, or develop a hematoma (blood clot) in the brain tissue or under one of the layers of tissue that protect the brain. First Responders must monitor their patients for changes in mental status, airway and breathing, seizures, vomiting, blood or fluid draining from the nose and/or ears, and changes in pupil size and

Types of Helmets

To be effective, all helmets must fit the wearer properly, must be worn correctly, and must meet helmet criteria based on testing by the Snell Memorial Foundation, the only helmet testing lab accredited to ISO 25 in the United State by the American Association for Laboratory Accreditation. Snell also tests helmets for removability. Emergency care providers must be able to quickly remove headgear from accident victims in order to check for vital signs and to perform emergency procedures. See the Snell Memorial Foundation web page at *http://www.smf.org/testing.html*.

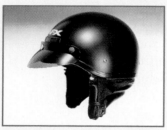

HALF-SIZE MOTORCYCLE HELMET Provides head protection from impact but may not provide face and eye protection, even with a face shield; easier to remove than a full helmet.

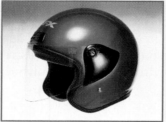

THREE-QUARTER-SIZE MOTORCYCLE HELMET Provides head protection from impact and may provide face and eye protection; somewhat easier to remove than the full size helmet.

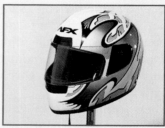

FULL-SIZE MOTORCYCLE HELMET Provides a measure of facial protection with a face shield in place in addition to head impact protection. Properly fitting helmets have room beneath the chin bar for a hand to slide under and check for airway breathing.

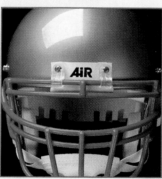

FOOTBALL HELMET Provides a measure of facial protection with a face shield in place as well as head impact protection.

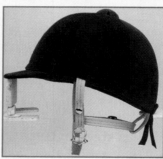

HORSEBACK RIDING HELMET Provides head protection from impact but may not provide face and eye protection.

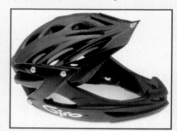

MOUNTAIN BIKE HELMET Provides head protection and, with a chin bar, some face protection.

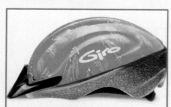

YOUTH'S BICYCLE HELMET Provides head protection if it fits properly and is worn correctly.

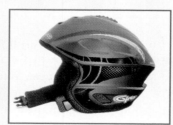

SNOWBOARDING HELMET Provides head protection and, with a chin bar, some face protection.

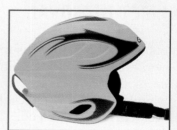

DOWNHILL SKIING HELMET Provides head protection and, with a chin bar, some face protection.

equality. More recently made helmets are designed with padding and made to fit snugly. Most have very durable, protective outer shells. Regardless of all the safeguards now built into helmets, they cannot offer a guarantee against injury in a severe crash, whether it is on the football field, the race track, or the road.

Many states have helmet laws for bicycle and motorcycle riding. Many sports and competitions require helmet use, such as football, bicycle and motor cross racing, and auto racing. Many other sports activities are recommending helmet use, such as skiing and snowboarding, harness racing, horseback riding, and go-cart racing. Many of these activities have specially designed helmets, which all offer the best head and face protection for the type of sport. Each of these activities has its dangers, and those who participate in these activities may need special care if injured. First Responders will focus treatment on maintaining the airway and assuring that Responders can perform initial assessment and evaluation steps on the patient with the helmet in place. The general recommendation is to leave the helmet in place, but this will depend on the type of helmet and whether or not the First Responders can assess the airway and assist breathing.

The American College of Sports Medicine (ACSM) has made recommendations for managing sports injuries, particularly football. For injured or unconscious athletes, the college advises against removing the helmet. For an unconscious athlete (or any injured patient wearing a helmet), suspect a spinal injury, properly immobilize the spine, and provide safe transport to the hospital. When it is necessary to assess the patient's face to manage the airway, to assist breathing, or to provide CPR, the ACSM advises removing only the face guard of the football helmet. Removing the face guard gives emergency care providers access to the face and airway and allows them to assess vital signs, provide care for face injuries, or begin resuscitation. The ACSM emphasizes that the helmet should be removed only if the rescuers are unable to gain access to the airway by any other means.

For football players who are wearing shoulder pads, the helmet left in place keeps the cervical spine in a midline position. Removing the helmet with shoulder pads in place causes the head to hyperextend or fall back in an overextended position, which pulls the spinal column out of alignment. Helmets do not prevent neck injuries. Sports related helmet injuries are caused by extended flexing of the neck either too far forward (hyperflexion) or too far backward (hyperextension) or by a sudden compressing force to the top of the head, which compacts the spinal column.

There are many types of helmets (Scan 12-10). They are made in half-size, a three-quarter-size, and a full size. Full-size helmets cover the mouth and sometimes part of the nose and usually have a face shield. Bicycle helmets are usually half-size and open in the front—have no face shield or face guard. Football helmets are full-size and have face guards. Motorcycle helmets are available in all three sizes, with the full-size helmets having a clear face shield or visor that moves up and down and is easy to remove. Motorcyclists who wear the half-size or three-fourths-size helmets will usually wear glasses or goggles to protect their eyes. If the helmet has a face guard or face shield, remove it to gain access to the patient's airway. If any patient *who is not breathing* is wearing a helmet with a face guard or face shield that cannot be removed, remove the helmet to gain access to the airway. If a helmet is removed, it must be done cautiously and by two people. Before removing the helmet, perform the following steps:

1. Remove the face piece or face shield while your partner stabilizes the head. Do not cut the chin strap. Remove glasses or goggles.

2. Check to see if the patient is breathing by placing your ear and/or hand in front of the nose and mouth. Even with full-size, snug fitting helmets, there is room to slip your hand under the protective face portion to check breathing.

3. If the patient is breathing, check the helmet for fit. A First Responder can stabilize the head by grasping the patient's lower jaw under the helmet while a partner gently pulls on the helmet. (For an example of *stabilizing* the head as described, see Figure 3 in Scan 12-11, in which the rescuers are preparing to *remove* the helmet.) An alternative method is to have a partner stabilize the head by placing her hands on either side of the helmet while you slide both hands under the helmet on either side of the jaw to check the helmet for fit and snugness. A well-fitting helmet can stay in place as long as the patient is breathing.

4. Determine if you can gain access to the patient's airway without removing the helmet if airway care and breathing assistance are necessary (opening the airway, suctioning, providing oxygen by mask or nasal cannula [see Appendix 2], inserting an airway, checking for and sweeping obstructions).

5. If you cannot gain access to the airway and you must clear the airway or assist the patient with breathing, remove the helmet. If the patient is wearing shoulder pads, leave them in place. While your partner is maintaining the head in line with the body, place a similar amount of padding under the patient's head to help your partner keep the patient's head in line with the body while you perform airway, ventilation, or resuscitation measures.

Check local protocols for helmet removal procedures. Work with local coaches to learn and practice their steps for removing helmets, which will be based on sports medicine programs and recommendations. Check with helmet vendors to become familiar with the types of helmets and their fit. The current recommendation for injured helmeted patients is to leave the helmet in place. Note that the half-size and three-quarter-size helmets give easy access to airway and breathing, but if they are left in place, their position may require you to place extra padding behind the patient's shoulders. If the patient is conscious, get the patient's history. If the patient is unconscious, treat as if there is a spinal injury.

When you find any helmeted patient face down or on one side, log roll him on to his back (supine). Your instructor will show you how to log roll a patient if First Responders are allowed to do this in your jurisdiction.

Leave the helmet in place if you find the following:

1. The helmet fits well, and the patient's head does not move (or moves very little) inside the helmet. A well-fitting helmet keeps the head from moving and should be left on if there are no airway or breathing problems and the helmet does not interfere with assessment and managing the airway and assisting breathing.

2. The patient is breathing adequately and has no airway problems (fluids, obstructions).

3. You may cause further injury if you attempt to remove the helmet.

4. You are able to stabilize the head with the helmet in place until additional, appropriate help arrives to immobilize the patient on a spine board.

5. The patient can be placed in a neutral, in-line position for immobilization on a spine board.

6. The helmet does not interfere with your ability to reassess and maintain the patient's airway or assist breathing.

Helmet Removal

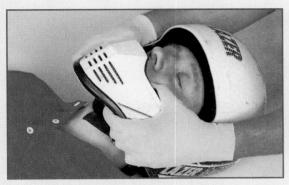

1. First Responder #1: kneel at the head of the patient; stabilize the patient's head.

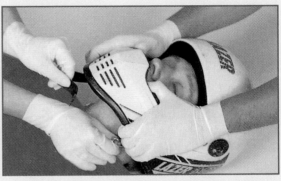

2. First Responder #2: kneel at the side of the patient's shoulders; unfasten the chin strap, remove the face guard, face shield, goggles, or glasses if present.

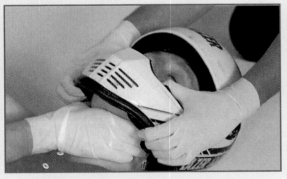

3. First Responder #2: place one hand on the mandible at the angle of the jaw and the other hand behind the neck at the base of the skull to stabilize the patient's head.

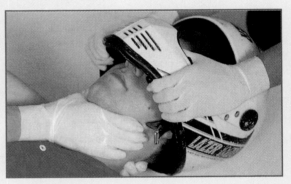

4. First Responder #1: pull sides of helmet apart and carefully slip helmet halfway off.

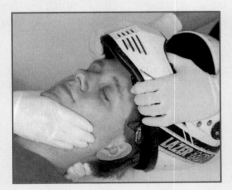

5. First Responder #2: maintain position of hand stabilizing the jaw; reposition at the back of the neck slightly higher on the back of the head to maintain in-line stabilization.

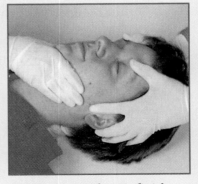

6. First Responder #1: finish removing the helmet and then place hands on either side of the patient's head to take over in-line stabilization.

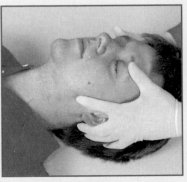

7. First Responder #2: check and clear airway, provide ventilations, and apply a collar.

Helmet Removal—Alternate Method

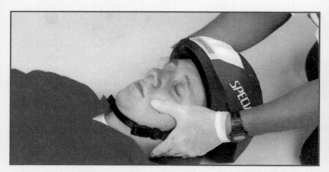

1. Apply steady stabilization to the neck in neutral position.

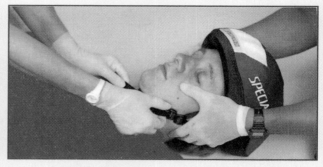

2. Remove the chin strap.

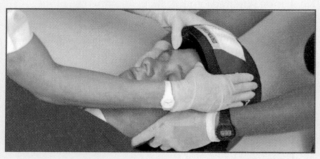

3. Remove helmet by pulling the sides apart (laterally).

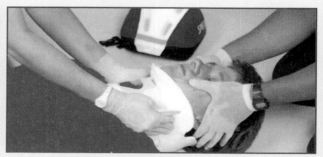

4. Apply a suitable cervical spine immobilization collar and secure the patient to a long board.

7. The patient is wearing shoulder pads. If the helmet is removed, place a similar amount of padding under the head, or remove the shoulder pads also. Removing the shoulder pads may cause further harm to the patient.

Remove the helmet if you find the following:

1. The helmet interferes with your ability to assess or manage the patient's airway and breathing.

2. The helmet does not fit snugly, and the patient's head moves inside the helmet.

3. The helmet interferes with placing the patient on a spine board in a neutral, in-line position. When the helmet rests on the spine board, its size may force the patient's head forward (hyperflexion) and close the airway. Padding can be placed under the patient's shoulders to prevent hyperflexion and maintain an in-line position.

4. The patient is in cardiac arrest. Quickly remove the helmet while a partner stabilizes the head. Proceed with CPR steps, using the jaw-thrust maneuver.

If you must remove the helmet, consult with medical control, remove it according to your local protocols, and perform the steps listed below, which generally provide directions for removal of full-size helmets (Scans 12-11 and 12-12). Your instructor will demonstrate all steps. Practice with all three sizes of helmets.

1. First Responder #1 will kneel at the head of the patient and stabilize the patient's head by placing his hands on each side of the helmet with fingers on the patient's jaw to prevent movement.

2. First Responder #2 will kneel on one side of the patient at the patient's shoulders, unfasten the chin strap, remove the face guard or face shield (if not yet done), and remove the patient's glasses or goggles if present.

3. First Responder #2 will place one hand on the mandible at the angle of the jaw and the other hand behind the neck at the base of the skull and stabilize the head while First Responder #1 removes the helmet.

4. First Responder #1 will pull sides of the helmet apart and slowly and carefully slip the helmet halfway off the patient's head until First Responder #2 can reposition the hand behind the head and neck.

5. First Responder #2 will maintain the hand position that is stabilizing the jaw. Reposition the hand at the back of the neck a little higher on the back of the head to maintain stabilization of the head and its in-line position of the body, particularly if the patient is wearing shoulder pads.

6. First Responder #1 will finish removing the helmet, place padding under the patient's head if needed (the patient is wearing shoulder pads), and then place his hands on either side of the patient's head to take over in-line stabilization.

7. First Responder #2 will check and clear the airway, provide ventilations with supplemental oxygen, and apply a collar.

Remember, you do not have to remove a helmet from a patient if the patient has an airway and is breathing, if the helmet is snug, and if the patient can be secured to a spine board with the helmet on and the head in a neutral, in-line position with the spine.

INJURIES TO THE CHEST

Chest injuries may damage the lungs, heart, major vessels, and upper abdominal organs protected by the ribs. Ribs can be fractured or crushed or the sternum may become fractured or completely separated from the ribs. Broken and crushed ribs and sternum can cause punctures and tears to organs and vessels underneath. The force of the trauma may also directly or indirectly damage the section of the spine where the ribs are attached. Because of these problems, it is important to stabilize the head and neck of a chest trauma patient. Wounds to the chest need immediate attention and care (see also Chapter 11).

FRACTURED RIBS

First | The signs and symptoms of fractured ribs include (Figure 12.44):

- Pain and tenderness at the site of the fracture
- Deformity at the site of the fracture, which may be slight swelling or obvious rib displacement
- Increased pain at the site upon moving or inhaling

FIGURE 12.44
A Guarding;
B Signs of rib fracture.

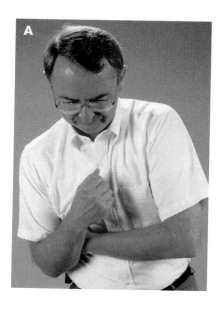

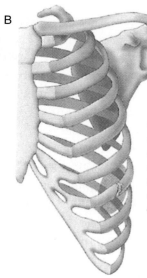

- Tenderness
- Local pain
- Deformity
- Shallow breathing
- Coughing
- Painful movement
- "Crackling" sensation in skin if lung is punctured

- Shallow breathing, sometimes with the patient reporting a crackling sensation at or near the site of fracture
- Characteristic stance. Often, the patient will lean toward the side of the fracture, with a hand or forearm pressed over the injury.
- Guarding the injury site. Often the patient will hold his hand across the injured side to help support and stabilize the injury. This is called "self-splinting."

If only one or two ribs are fractured, which you may be able to determine by palpating (gently feeling) the injury site, mechanism of injury, and patient signs and symptoms and history, you do not need to take any immediate action other than keeping the patient at rest in a comfortable position. But if there are signs that the lungs have been damaged by the fractured rib (for example, frothy blood in the mouth) or several ribs are apparently fractured, you must provide additional care for the patient.

 The care for fractured ribs requires you to wear personal protective equipment and:

1. Assure an airway; suction or clear the mouth if necessary; keep the patient at rest and monitor breathing.

2. Provide oxygen as soon as possible and maintain body temperature to minimize the possibility of shock.

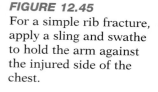

FIGURE 12.45
For a simple rib fracture, apply a sling and swathe to hold the arm against the injured side of the chest.

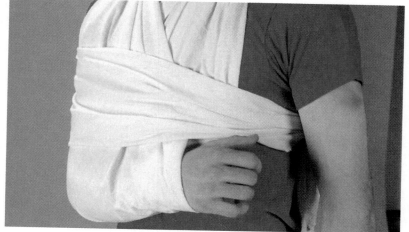

3. Place the forearm of the injured side in a sling so that it rests across the patient's chest and apply a swathe to provide additional support (Figure 12.45).

4. Alert dispatch and have the patient transported to the hospital to be examined by more highly trained personnel.

FLAIL CHEST

When three or more consecutive ribs on the same side of the chest are fractured in two places, this creates a section of chest that moves in the opposite direction of the rest of the chest wall during breathing. The same opposite-direction motion is seen when the breastbone is broken away from the ribs. Both of these conditions are called **flail chest** (Figure 12.46). First Responders see flail chests most often at motor vehicle accidents. The mechanism of injury is usually the steering wheel. The patient, who is not wearing a seat belt, is thrown against the steering wheel during the sudden deceleration (stop).

> **flail chest** the condition in which multiple rib fractures, or the breastbone separating from the chest, produces a loose segment of the chest wall. This segment will move in the opposite direction of the chest during breathing.

First | The signs and symptoms of flail chest include (Figure 12.48):

■ The same signs and symptoms of fractured ribs
■ A section of the chest wall that moves in the opposite direction of the rest of the chest when the patient is breathing. This motion may be slight and can be seen as you watch the patient inhale (the chest expands); the flail section will slightly depress or sink inward; as the patient exhales (chest relaxes), the flail section will slightly push out from the rest of the chest wall.

A flail chest must be cared for differently than simple rib fractures. Rather than using cravats to stabilize the loose segment as you would with simple rib fractures, you must hold the flail section in place.

First | To care for a flail chest and stabilize the loose segment, wear personal protective equipment, assure an airway, and (Figure 12.47):

1. Locate the flail section by gently feeling the injury site. In the majority of cases, the injury will be on the side of the chest.

2. Apply a bulky pad of dressings, several inches thick, over the site or use a small pillow. Whatever is used should be soft and lightweight.

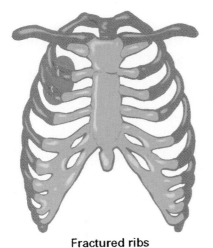
Fractured ribs

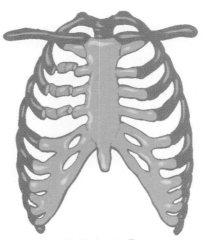
Flail chest ribs

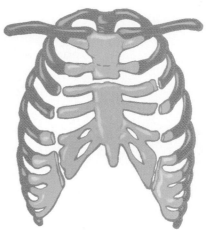
Flail chest sternum

FIGURE 12.46
Rib fractures and flail chest.

FIGURE 12.47
Emergency care for
flail chest.

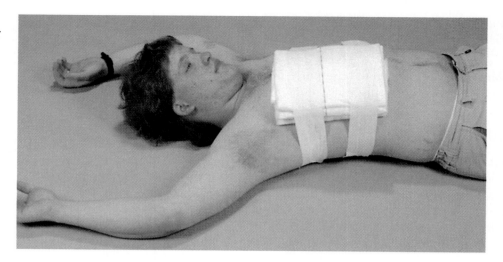

3. Use large strips of tape to hold the pad in place. Do *not* tape entirely around the chest—this will restrict breathing efforts. If you do not have tape:

   – Position the patient on the injured side—body weight against the surface will help splint the injury. (Do *not* do this if spinal injuries are suspected.) Or . . .

   – Hold the pad in place by hand. When doing so, position your body so that you will not have to shift your weight and move the pad.

4. Provide 100% oxygen via nonrebreather mask as soon as possible and maintain body temperature to reduce shock.

5. Monitor the patient to assure adequate breathing and look for signs of heart and lung injury.

The lungs and the heart also can be injured in accidents involving the ribs and breastbone. Always look for frothy blood in the patient's mouth and signs of difficult or labored breathing, which indicate injury to the lungs. In cases of flail chest, make certain to examine the patient for the following (Figure 12.49):

■ Distended (bulging) neck veins
■ Blue coloration of the head, neck, and shoulders
■ Bulging, bloodshot eyes
■ Blue coloration and swelling of the lips and tongue
■ Obvious chest deformity

These signs indicate that the heart has been injured and that blood has been forced back out of its right side and up through the major veins that lead to the heart from the neck. These patients need oxygen as soon as possible and must be transported immediately.

MECHANISMS OF INJURY

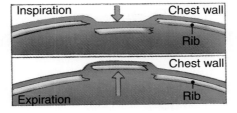

FIGURE 12.48
Flail chest.

SIGNS OF FLAIL CHEST

- Pain
- Shallow breathing
- Deformity
- Painful movement

- Tenderness
- Crackling sensation
- Irregular chest movement

Inspiration	↓	Chest wall
		Rib
		Chest wall
Expiration	↑	Rib

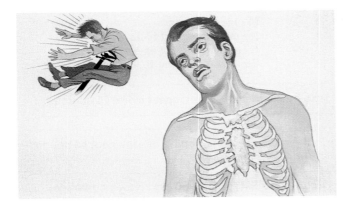

FIGURE 12.49
Chest injuries may involve the heart.

- Distended neck veins
- Head, neck, and shoulders appear dark blue or purple.
- Eyes may be bloodshot and bulging.
- Tongue and lips may appear swollen and blue.
- Chest deformity may be present.

MUSCULOSKELETAL INJURY EMERGENCY CARE

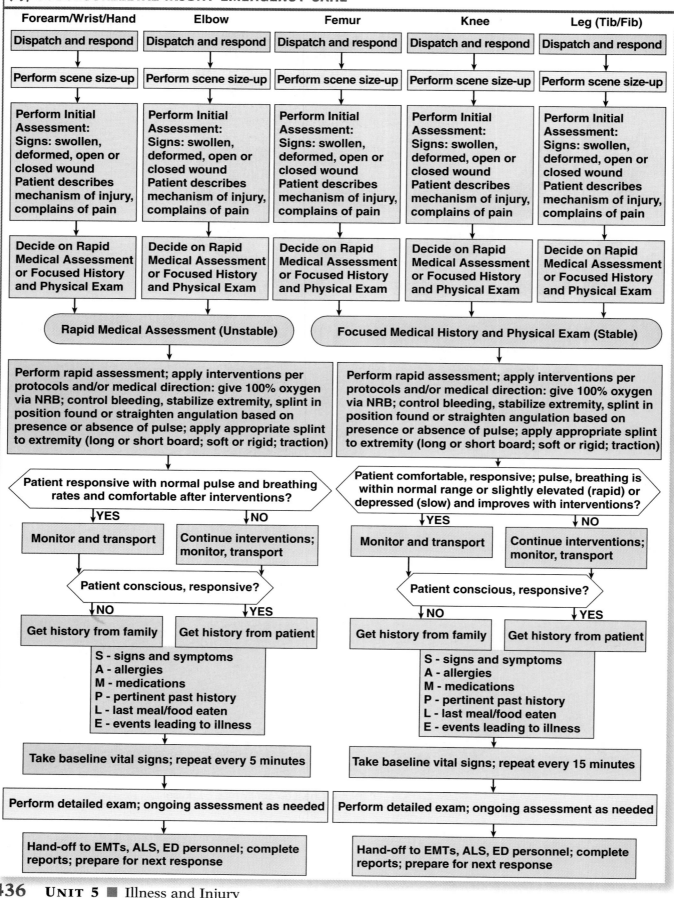

Forearm/Wrist/Hand	Elbow	Femur	Knee	Leg (Tib/Fib)
Dispatch and respond	Dispatch and respond	Dispatch and respond	Dispatch and respond	Dispatch and respond
Perform scene size-up	Perform scene size-up	Perform scene size-up	Perform scene size-up	Perform scene size-up
Perform Initial Assessment: Signs: swollen, deformed, open or closed wound Patient describes mechanism of injury, complains of pain	**Perform Initial Assessment:** Signs: swollen, deformed, open or closed wound Patient describes mechanism of injury, complains of pain	**Perform Initial Assessment:** Signs: swollen, deformed, open or closed wound Patient describes mechanism of injury, complains of pain	**Perform Initial Assessment:** Signs: swollen, deformed, open or closed wound Patient describes mechanism of injury, complains of pain	**Perform Initial Assessment:** Signs: swollen, deformed, open or closed wound Patient describes mechanism of injury, complains of pain
Decide on Rapid Medical Assessment or Focused History and Physical Exam	Decide on Rapid Medical Assessment or Focused History and Physical Exam	Decide on Rapid Medical Assessment or Focused History and Physical Exam	Decide on Rapid Medical Assessment or Focused History and Physical Exam	Decide on Rapid Medical Assessment or Focused History and Physical Exam

Rapid Medical Assessment (Unstable)

Focused Medical History and Physical Exam (Stable)

Perform rapid assessment; apply interventions per protocols and/or medical direction: give 100% oxygen via NRB; control bleeding, stabilize extremity, splint in position found or straighten angulation based on presence or absence of pulse; apply appropriate splint to extremity (long or short board; soft or rigid; traction)

Perform rapid assessment; apply interventions per protocols and/or medical direction: give 100% oxygen via NRB; control bleeding, stabilize extremity, splint in position found or straighten angulation based on presence or absence of pulse; apply appropriate splint to extremity (long or short board; soft or rigid; traction)

Patient responsive with normal pulse and breathing rates and comfortable after interventions?

Patient comfortable, responsive; pulse, breathing is within normal range or slightly elevated (rapid) or depressed (slow) and improves with interventions?

↓YES — Monitor and transport
↓NO — Continue interventions; monitor, transport

↓YES — Monitor and transport
↓NO — Continue interventions; monitor, transport

Patient conscious, responsive?

Patient conscious, responsive?

↓NO — Get history from family
↓YES — Get history from patient

↓NO — Get history from family
↓YES — Get history from patient

S - signs and symptoms
A - allergies
M - medications
P - pertinent past history
L - last meal/food eaten
E - events leading to illness

S - signs and symptoms
A - allergies
M - medications
P - pertinent past history
L - last meal/food eaten
E - events leading to illness

Take baseline vital signs; repeat every 5 minutes

Take baseline vital signs; repeat every 15 minutes

Perform detailed exam; ongoing assessment as needed

Perform detailed exam; ongoing assessment as needed

Hand-off to EMTs, ALS, ED personnel; complete reports; prepare for next response

Hand-off to EMTs, ALS, ED personnel; complete reports; prepare for next response

Summary

For any trauma, always perform a scene survey and the steps of the initial assessment. Remember that scene safety, mechanism of injury, and patient environment are important factors to consider before patient care begins. Check for and treat all life-threatening problems first. Before focusing on extremity injuries, check and care for injuries to the head and spine; look for and treat open injuries to the chest and abdomen; and care for all serious burns. Provide oxygen, and maintain body temperature to help prevent shock (hypoperfusion).

Soft tissues such as muscles, nerves, and blood vessels, are damaged when bones are injured, and they will be managed as part of total patient care.

The **musculoskeletal system** provides body support and movement, protects organs, and produces blood cells. There are two major divisions to the skeletal system, the **axial skeleton** and the **appendicular skeleton.** The upper and lower extremities are part of the appendicular skeleton.

Each upper extremity consists of the shoulder blade (scapula), collarbone (clavicle), upper arm (humerus), forearm bones (ulna and radius), wrist bones (carpals), hand bones (metacarpals), and finger bones (phalanges).

Lower extremities consist of the pelvic girdle (innominate or os coxae), thigh bone (femur), kneecap (patella), lower leg bones (tibia and fibula), ankle bones (tarsals), foot bones (metatarsals), and toe bones (phalanges). Each leg connects to the pelvis.

If a bone tears through the skin or the mechanism of injury causes a puncture to the outer skin and damages the bone inside, it is an **open injury.** If the bones do not tear through the patient's skin, the injury is called a **closed injury.** Apply sterile dressings to all open injuries.

A bone that is broken and bends at a place other than a joint is called an **angulated fracture.**

Any break in a bone is a **fracture. A dislocation** is a joint that is pulled or pushed out of its normal position. Ligaments that are torn or stretched are **sprains;** muscles that are overstretched are **strains.** It is difficult to determine the difference among these, and since the signs and symptoms are similar, injuries to extremities will be called **painful, swollen, deformed** extremities, or **PSD** extremities.

Typical signs and symptoms for musculoskeletal injuries include pain, swelling, and deformity. Other signs and symptoms include discoloration, loss of use, tenderness, guarding, loss of distal pulse, slow capillary refill (in pediatric patients), numbness, tingling, grating, the sound of breaking bone, and exposed bone.

Some special signs to look for with injured extremities include:

- Patient guarding or position of the injured extremity
- A bulge where there is a joint or where the extremity joins the torso
- Pelvic pain on compression of the patient's hips
- Leg rotating outward or inward

Emergency care procedures for PSD extremities are **rigid** or **soft splinting.** When in doubt about the extent of the injury, splint. All splinting must immobilize the injured extremity and the joints directly above and below the injury site.

Soft splinting can effectively immobilize a painful, swollen, deformed extremity without rigid splints.

Use a sling and swathe for:

- Injuries to the collarbone or shoulder blade
- Dislocation of the shoulder with padding in the space between the arm and the chest and a sling and swathe
- Injuries to the upper arm bone and forearm; modify full sling to wrist sling if the injury is in the elbow area and add a swathe.
- Injuries to the elbow, using a wrist sling and a swathe
- Injuries to the wrist, hand, or fingers

NOTE: Always place the hand in the position of function.

Use padding such as folded blankets or towels for:

- Injuries to the pelvis or hip
- Injuries to the thigh
- Injuries to the knee
- Injuries to the leg

Secure the blanket or towels with four cravats, two above and two below the knees. Then, with EMT assistance, place the patient on a spine board or scoop (orthopedic) stretcher.

Use a pillow for:

- Injuries to the ankle or foot—secure pillow with cravats and elevate.

Applying a splint can prevent or reduce complications, such as pain, soft-tissue damage, bleeding, restricted blood flow, and can prevent closed injuries from becoming open injuries.

Cut away or remove clothing from the injury site before splinting. Control bleeding and dress open wounds. Check for a distal pulse, sensation, and motor function *before* and *after* splinting. If there is no distal pulse, realign angulated fractures or reposition extremities until pulse is regained, if allowed to do so by your EMS system.

Pad all rigid splints before they are secured to the patient. **Manual traction** is applied by pulling gently on an injured limb along its long axis. If manual traction is applied, maintain it until the rigid splint is secured.

First Responders can use noncommercial splints, such as lumber, plywood, rolled newspapers and magazines, compressed wood products, sporting equipment, canes, umbrellas, cardboard, and tool handles.

The skull, spinal column, ribs, and breastbone (sternum) form the axial skeleton. The skull is made up of the **cranium** and the face. The spine connects to the skull. The portion of the spine that runs through the neck is called the **cervical spine.** The ribs are attached to the thoracic spine.

The skull protects the brain, and the spinal column protects the spinal cord. The brain and spinal cord are parts of the central nervous system.

Injuries to the skull include **open** and **closed** head injuries. If the cranium remains intact or unbroken, the injury is a closed head injury.

$\mathcal{S}$ummary,

continued

Open head injuries involve fractures of the cranium (skull fractures). There can be direct injury to the brain in open head injuries such as cuts, tears, and bruising. In closed head injuries, the skull is not damaged but injuries to the brain can occur and include **concussions** (brain shaking or bouncing), **contusions** (brain bruises), and **hemorrhage** (bleeding inside skull).

Head injuries may be obvious, or they may be difficult to detect. Always look for wounds to the head, deformity of the skull, bruises behind the ear, black eyes, sunken eyes, unequal pupils, and blood or clear fluids flowing from the ears and/or nose.

Brain injury can occur with head injuries. Look for signs of skull fracture, loss of awareness, confusion, unequal pupils, and paralysis.

When caring for a patient with injuries to the cranium, maintain an open airway, using the jaw-thrust maneuver, and stabilize the head. Assist ventilations or provide CPR if needed.

Keep the head-injury patient at rest and talk to the patient. Control bleeding but avoid pressure over the site of a fracture. Do not remove impaled objects, bone fragments, or other objects from head wounds.

Facial injuries often cause airway obstruction. Maintain an open airway with the jaw-thrust maneuver. The mechanism of injury that causes facial fractures can also cause spinal injury. Be sure to stabilize the head when managing the airway.

Spinal injuries can be very serious and can result in permanent paralysis or disability. Keep the patient from moving. The focused assessment is very important in determining if the patient has spinal injuries. Always look for weakness, numbness, loss of feeling, pain, or paralysis to the limbs of a patient. Remember to press or pinch the feet and hands of the unconscious patient and look for reactions. Assume that all unconscious injury patients have spinal injuries. If the mechanism of injury indicates possible spinal injuries, assume the injuries are present.

Follow certain rules when caring for a patient who may have spinal injuries. Even though a patient has spinal injuries, provide ventilations or CPR, if needed, and control bleeding. Do not attempt to splint fractures without help. Never move a patient with spinal injuries without help unless absolutely necessary. Stabilize the patient's head and neck and as much of the body as possible. Continuously monitor the patient.

Injuries to the chest can include soft-tissue injuries, crushing injuries, and penetrating injuries that can cause fractured ribs, flail chest, spinal injuries, lung injuries, and heart injuries.

Pain at the site may indicate rib fractures; apply a sling and swathe, placing the forearm of the injured side across the chest. Opposite motion in the ribs or breastbone may indicate **flail chest;** apply a thick pad over the site and tape it in place.

Remember and Consider...

When you are at the scene of any injury, listen to what other care providers are saying and how they consider the emotions of their patients. When people are injured, they are concerned with the pain and how soon you can relieve it. Children want to stop hurting and want you to make the pain go away.

✔ Think about what you will tell your injured patients as you provide care for their injuries.

Sometimes when you have to move a patient during the assessment or while you dress a wound or splint an extremity, the movement will cause additional pain. You must let your patients know what you are doing and why, if it will hurt and for how long, and what the result will be when you are finished.

✔ Keep in mind that most patients will cooperate with your care if they know what to expect. You must respect their concerns, answer their questions, and provide them with as much information about their injury as possible.

Investigate...

If you have not had a chance to look through your First Responder unit and see what equipment and supplies are carried, take some time to do so. Ask another department member to work with you to show you where splinting items are kept, or to suggest to you what items can be used as improvised splints.

✔ What materials for securing splints are carried on the unit?

✔ Are the splinting materials in places where they are easily reached, or will you have to take a few minutes to access them?

Practice using items in your unit for splinting. Work with other department members or with friends.

✔ As you hold traction, can you direct your friends to properly apply a commercial or an improvised splint?

✔ As you work with more experienced department members, can you follow their directions to hold traction or to splint while they hold traction?

> **CHAPTER 10** **MEDICAL EMERGENCIES, APPENDIX 4**
> **CHAPTER 11** **BLEEDING AND SOFT-TISSUE EMERGENCIES**
> **CHAPTER 12** **MUSCLE AND BONE INJURIES**

Study the following scenarios. Place check marks in the columns below as appropriate to indicate which skills you would perform for each scenario. You will use skills from previous units in these scenarios. Refer to text pages 1–81, 85–123, 129–178, and 183–236. Write the skill number of any skills you would use from Units 1–4 after each scenario. Also write these skill numbers in the columns under "Units." Discuss answers with other students and your instructor.

SCENARIO 1: Mr. Grayson had been working in his garden on a muggy summer morning. He thought he'd better take a break when his left shoulder and arm started to ache and he found it hard to breathe. When he sat down to have a glass of water, he thought he felt a little pressure in his chest, so he called 911. When you arrive, he is sitting in the shade and tells you about his continued pain and difficulty breathing.

(Skills from Unit 1: _____   Skills from Unit 2: _____)

(Skills from Unit 3: _____   Skills from Unit 4: _____)

SCENARIO 2: After a hard set of tennis, 15-year-old Carla complains of dizziness and faints. Her friends call 911. While waiting for the ambulance to arrive, Carla revives, but she is angry with her friends for calling the ambulance, complaining that now she'll have to go to the hospital, her dad will have to leave work to get her, and she'll have to stay home for the rest of the day. Your First Responder unit arrives before EMTs. As you approach, you hear Carla's tirade to her friends. You notice her speech is slurred and see that her skin is pale and clammy. As you get her history, you learn that she is a diabetic, took her insulin this morning, but only ate a banana for breakfast before running out to play tennis.

(Skills from Unit 1: _____   Skills from Unit 2: _____)

(Skills from Unit 3: _____   Skills from Unit 4: _____)

SCENARIO 3: You and your partner are on the first arriving unit at a reported shooting. The bartender tells you and your partner that the brawl started inside, but he made the guys leave. When he heard a shot, he called 911 and intended to stay inside until the police got there. He tells you that the guy who was shot staggered in with his hand pressed to a bloody place on his chest, and he's now in the back booth. As you approach, you see that the victim's shirt is soaked with blood from a wound on his upper left chest and his skin is pale. He watches you approach and says he feels weak and can't breathe.

(Skills from Unit 1: _____   Skills from Unit 2: _____)

(Skills from Unit 3: _____   Skills from Unit 4: _____)

SCENARIO 4: At a house fire, one of the firefighters brings you a 20-year-old man who was sleeping in an upstairs bedroom. The man tells you he awoke and smelled smoke, and when he opened his bedroom door, he saw flames downstairs. He ran to other bedrooms to make sure no one else was upstairs before he tried to leave the burning home. By then, the flames were higher and hotter. He ran through a part of the fire to get to the front door and outside, where firefighters grabbed him and rolled him on the ground to put out the fire on his T-shirt and shorts. He has some small charred areas on his back and blistering on his shoulders and the back of his thighs.

(Skills from Unit 1: _____ Skills from Unit 2: _____)

(Skills from Unit 3: _____ Skills from Unit 4: _____)

SCENARIO 5: Your rescue team has been called to bring a hiker off the mountain. There are reports he fell from some rock ridges and may have some fractures. When you arrive at the scene, you find him on a broad, rock-cluttered ledge about six feet below you. He calls up to you in obvious pain. "Please help me. I think my leg is broken." When you climb down to him, you see that his left lower leg is bent at a slight angle mid-shin; it is a little swollen at the break site, but he still has a distal pulse.

(Skills from Unit 1: _____ Skills from Unit 2: _____)

(Skills from Unit 3: _____ Skills from Unit 4: _____)

Instructors will demonstrate all skills and will give you time to practice them while they coach you.

Skills	Scenarios					Units			
	#1	**#2**	**#3**	**#4**	**#5**	**#1**	**#2**	**#3**	**#4**
Chest pain, possible heart attack: Scans 10-1, A3-4 1. Assess patient 2. Assist patient in taking nitroglycerin (per local protocol) 3. Perform CPR (adult, child, infant, neonate—See skills from Unit 4.) **Respiratory emergencies: Scans 10-2, A3-3** 4. Assess patient 5. Assist in taking Albuterol (per protocol) 6. Open airway, assess breathing, clear airway (see skills from Unit 2).									

Skills	Scenarios					Units			
	#1	#2	#3	#4	#5	#1	#2	#3	#4
Diabetic emergencies/altered mental status: Scans 10-3, 10–4, A3-2									
7. Assess patient									
8. Give patient oral glucose (per local protocol)									
Allergies: Scans 10-2, A3-3									
9. Assess patient									
10. Assist patient with epinephrine by auto-injector (per local protocol)									
Poisoning/overdose: Scan A3-1									
11. Assess patient									
12. Describe steps of/need for giving activated charcoal (per local protocol)									
13. Describe steps of/need for giving ipecac (per local protocol)									
Heat emergencies: Scan 10-5									
Describe the steps for heat exhaustion									
14. Assess patient									
15. Move patient to cool place; loosen/remove clothing									
16. Give water to responsive patient									
17. Position patient per responsive or unresponsive									
18. Apply moist towels to cramped muscles									
Describe the steps for heat stroke									
19. Rapidly cool patient and move to cool place									
20. Place wrapped cold packs in armpits, wrists, ankles, neck; immerse in water if necessary									
21. Monitor vital signs									
Provide oxygen by nonrebreather mask									
Cold emergencies: Scan 10-6									
Describe the steps for hypothermia, pages 280–281									
22. Assess patient and remove from cold environment									

Skills	Scenarios					Units			
	#1	#2	#3	#4	#5	#1	#2	#3	#4
23. Protect patient from further heat loss, remove wet clothing, cover with blanket									
24. Handle patient gently; do not allow patient to walk									
25. Do not give patient anything by mouth									
26. Comfort and reassure patient									
27. Monitor vital signs									
Describe the steps for local cold injuries, pages 281, 283									
28. Assess patient and remove from cold environment									
29. Protect patient from further cold exposure									
30. Remove wet/restrictive clothing									
31. Provide care steps for early or late cold injury									
32. Comfort and reassure patient									
33. Monitor vital signs									
Behavioral emergencies:									
Describe the steps for emotional emergencies, pages 284–285									
34. Assess patient, acknowledge problem, assure help									
35. Explain your actions; make no quick moves; avoid unnecessary physical contact; maintain eye contact									
36. Talk in calm, reassuring voice; encourage patient to discuss problem									
37. Answer questions honestly									
38. Do not threaten, challenge, argue, "play along"									
39. Involve trusted family member or friend									
40. Be prepared for extended scene time									
Describe the steps for violent emergencies, page 286									
41. Perform careful scene size-up; assure there are no weapons									
42. Get history from family, neighbors; be aware of past violent incidents									

Skills	Scenarios					Units			
	#1	#2	#3	#4	#5	#1	#2	#3	#4
43. Note patient posture, body language; maintain safe distance									
44. Consider abusive language a warning to violence									
45. Consider physical activity may escalate to violence									
Before restraining patient									
46. Decide to do so for protection of patient, self, others									
47. Talk and listen to patient and divert focus									
48. Remain passive but alert to patient actions									
49. Avoid actions that may alarm patient									
50. Wait for law enforcement assistance									
51. Use reasonable force in self-defense									
Alcohol and drug emergencies:									
Describe the steps for alcohol emergencies, pages 287–288									
52. Assess patient									
53. Monitor vital signs; be alert for respiratory problems									
54. Keep patient alert									
55. Be alert for vomiting and assist patient									
56. Protect from further injury									
57. Call for appropriate assistance									
Describe the steps for drug emergencies, page 289									
58. Assess patient; provide basic life support as needed									
59. Call for appropriate assistance									
60. Monitor vital signs and be alert for respiratory arrest									
61. Gain patient's confidence; maintain level of consciousness									
62. Protect from further harm; continue to reassure									
63. Provide care for shock									

Skills	Scenarios					Units			
	#1	#2	#3	#4	#5	#1	#2	#3	#4
Bleeding, shock, soft-tissue injuries: External bleeding: Scan 11–1, pages 304, 306–311									
64. Apply direct pressure (Figure 11.4)									
65. Elevate extremity if there is no suspected fracture (Figure 11.7)									
66. Apply appropriate pressure dressing and bandage (Figures 11.5, 11.6)									
67. Apply pressure point (Figures 11.8, 11.9, 11.10)									
68. Apply tourniquet (Figure 11.11)									
Shock Management: Scan 11–3									
69. Properly position and maintain body temperature (Figures 11.23, 11.24)									
70. Control external bleeding									
71. Give nothing by mouth									
72. Monitor vital signs									
Specific wounds:									
Demonstrate care steps for the following wounds									
73. Abdominal evisceration (Figure 11.54)									
74. Impaled object in body (Figure 11.53)									
75. Impaled object in cheek (Figure 11.42)									
76. Impaled object in eye (Figure 11.45)									
77. Sucking chest wound (Figures 11.51, 11.52)									
78. Flail chest									
79. Wounds to large blood vessels of neck (Figures 11.48, 11.49)									
80. Burns—thermal (Scan 11–5)									
81. Burns—chemical (Figures 11.59, 11.60)									
Fracture management:									
Demonstrate care/splinting of fractures									
82. Humerus—short board, sling and swathe (Scans 12–2, 12–5, Figures 12.18, 12.19)									

Skills	Scenarios					Units			
	#1	**#2**	**#3**	**#4**	**#5**	**#1**	**#2**	**#3**	**#4**
83. Elbow—short board, cravats, sling and swathe (Scan 12–5, Figure 12.21, 12.22)									
84. Forearm/wrist/hand/finger—secure splint, hand position of function, sling and swathe (Scans 12–3, 12–5, Figures 12.22, 12.23, 12.24, 12.25)									
85. Hip/pelvis—blanket roll, cravats (Figure 12.27)									
86. Femur—long board splints (Scan 12-8)									
87. Knee, bent—1 or 2 long board splints, cravats (Scan 12–8, Figure 12.30)									
88. Tibia/fibula, straight knee—long board splint, cravats (Scans 12–7, 12–8)									
89. Ankle/foot—pillow, cravats (Scan 12–6, Figure 12.31)									
Head, neck, and spine management:									
Head immobilization									
90. Stabilize seated, supine, and standing patients (Figure 12.43)									
91. Measure and apply collar to sitting, supine, and standing patients									
Helmet removal									
92. Stabilize head as partner unfastens									
93. Transfer stabilization during helmet removal									
94. Retake stabilization									

Special axial skeleton injuries:

Work with a group of classmates to create scenarios that will use listed skills. Exchange scenarios with other class groups to check your knowledge and to practice your decision-making skills.

CHAPTER 13

CHILDBIRTH

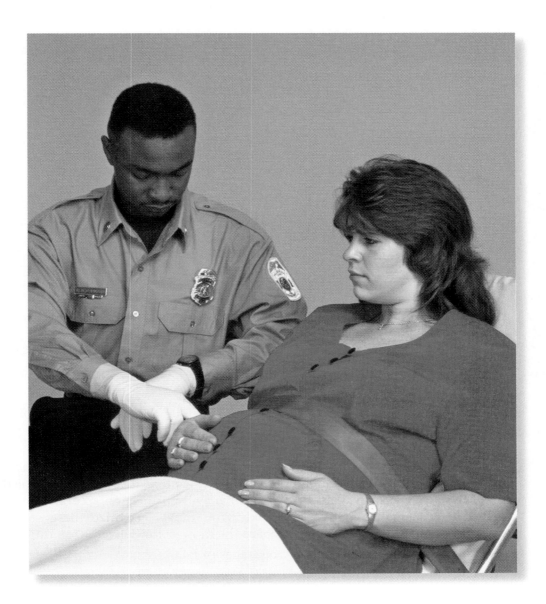

*M*ost expectant mothers know they need to care for themselves and for their unborn infants during the time of pregnancy. Usually, expectant mothers are under the care of a physician so they do not often have to call for emergency services to deliver their babies. Sometimes, though, physiological or environmental situations cause birth to occur unexpectedly and before the mother can get to the hospital. When the unexpected happens, the First Responder must know what to do. This chapter will introduce you to the terms, events, stages, and steps of pregnancy and childbirth.

National Standard Objectives

This chapter focuses on the objectives of Module 6, Lesson 6–1 of the U.S. DOT First Responder National Standard Curriculum and serves as an instructional aid to help you meet any specific objectives added to the course by your local EMS system.

By the end of this chapter, you will know how to (from cognitive or knowledge information) . . .

6–1.1	Identify the following structures: birth canal, placenta, umbilical cord, amniotic sac. (p. 453)
6–1.2	Define the following terms: crowning, bloody show, labor, abortion. (pp. 453, 469–470)
6–1.3	State indications of an imminent delivery. (pp. 453, 456)
6–1.4	State the steps in the predelivery preparation of the mother. (pp. 455–458)
6–1.5	Establish the relationship between body substance isolation and childbirth. (pp. 455, 458)
6–1.6	State the steps to assist in the delivery. (pp. 458–461)
6–1.7	Describe care of the baby as the head appears. (pp. 459–460)
6–1.8	Discuss the steps in delivery of the afterbirth. (pp. 466–467)
6–1.9	List the steps in the emergency medical care of the mother post-delivery. (p. 467)
6–1.10	Discuss the steps in caring for a newborn. (pp. 461–465)

Learning Tasks

Emergency care providers deliver thousands of babies each year in the United States. You must be able to remember the steps involved in childbirth and be able to assist in delivery. The mother will go through several stages of labor, which may happen very quickly. You must recognize these stages and, if needed, in the meantime, prepare the mother for delivery. You must be able to:

✔ List and describe the three stages of labor.

✔ List and explain the use of the materials needed for preparation and delivery.

The mother is not the only patient. If the baby arrives before you can get the mother to the hospital, you must also know what to do for the infant. Be able to:

✔ Describe assessment steps for the newborn and how to determine the need for resuscitation.

Sometimes the mother will go through a prolonged birth process, which not only is distressing to the mother, but also to the infant. One of the signs of a stressful birth is meconium. You must be able to:

Feel comfortable enough to (by changing attitude, values, beliefs) . . .	6–1.11	Explain the rationale for attending to the feelings of a patient in need of emergency medical care during childbirth. (p. 452)
	6–1.12	Demonstrate a caring attitude towards patients during childbirth who request emergency medical services. (pp. 456, 458, 460, 466, 467)
	6–1.13	Place the interests of the patient during childbirth as the foremost consideration when making any and all patient care decisions. (p. 457)
	6–1.14	Communicate with empathy to patients during childbirth, as well as with family members and friends of the patient. (pp. 458, 460)
Show how to (through psychomotor skills) . . .	6–1.15	Demonstrate the steps to assist in the normal cephalic delivery. (pp. 458–461)
	6–1.16	Demonstrate necessary care procedures of the fetus as the head appears. (pp. 459–460)
	6–1.17	Attend to the steps in the delivery of the afterbirth. (pp. 466–467)
	6–1.18	Demonstrate the postdelivery care of the mother. (p. 467)
	6–1.19	Demonstrate the care of the newborn. (pp. 461–465)

✔ Recognize meconium staining in the birth fluids, understand its seriousness, and know what to do for the baby.

✔ Discuss the significance of a stressful birth in which meconium is present.

Because of medical or trauma situations, the mother may also show signs of stress, illness, or injury. You will care for most medical and trauma situations as you do in other emergencies, but you must be aware of special problems related to expectant mothers. Be able to:

✔ List basic care procedures for predelivery emergencies including seizures, vaginal bleeding, and trauma.

Most mothers will progress through the birth process without any problems. Some mothers will have medical or physical problems that will cause an unusual or complicated birth. Be able to:

✔ List common delivery complications such as prolapsed cord, breech birth, limb presentation, premature births, miscarriages, and stillbirths and state the care for each.

Even more rare than delivering an infant in the field is delivering two. Once you have delivered one baby, you need to recognize the signs of another delivery, which are slightly different from a delivering afterbirth, and be prepared to deliver another infant. Be able to:

✔ Describe First Responder actions in cases of multiple births.

Trauma is critical for anyone, but especially for an expectant mother. Not only is she an injured victim, but so is the fetus. In the event of a trauma or any type of assault, be able to:

✔ Describe the care and considerations for patients who have been victims of trauma or sexual assault.

In Chapters 6 and 8, you learned about resuscitating infants. As you work with classmates on your skills, continue to practice the steps for neonatal resuscitation. You must practice these skills frequently so that you can perform them automatically and effortlessly when needed. Be able to:

✔ Demonstrate resuscitation steps for a newborn with slow or no respiratory and/or heart rate.

UNDERSTANDING CHILDBIRTH

You may have noted that this chapter is called "Childbirth" and not "Emergency Childbirth." As a culture, we have arrived at the point where any birth away from a hospital delivery room is considered an emergency, which is just not true. In many parts of the world, babies are born away from medical facilities. Birth is a natural process. The anatomy of the human female, unborn child, and the structures formed during pregnancy enable the birth process to occur with few problems. Assistance from the medical community reduces the chances of problems for mother and child, but in most deliveries, high-tech medical skills and equipment are not needed.

First | Mothers do all the work of delivering their babies; First Responders assist. Your role, then, will be one of helping the mother as she delivers her child.

The presence of a First Responder at the scene of a birth that takes place away from a medical facility can prove to be the key factor in a baby's survival if something should go wrong. First Responder-level skills may be needed **during** the birth process to ensure safe delivery if there are complications. The care provided **after** delivery is just as important. The first hour of life after birth can be a difficult time for some babies and for some mothers. Your participation in the delivery process and in the care you provide to a newborn infant can make a difference.

ANATOMY OF PREGNANCY

fetus (FE-tus) the developing unborn child. The fertilized egg is an embryo until the eighth week after fertilization, when it becomes a fetus.

uterus (U-ter-us) the womb. The muscular structure in which the fetus develops.

A baby is called a **fetus** as it develops and grows inside of its mother. The average period of development for the fetus is from 36 to 40 weeks, or from 9 to 10 months. This development period is divided into 3-month segments called *trimesters*. The fetus develops inside a muscular organ called the **womb,** or **uterus** (Figure 13.1). The mother and the developing fetus are normally physiologically ready to deliver sometime after 37 weeks of pregnancy. Then labor will begin.

During labor, the muscles of the uterus contract and push the baby down through the neck of the uterus, which is called the **cervix.** As the cervix expands to allow the head of the fetus through, a slight staining of blood or blood-tinged mucus may be noticed by the mother. This is called "bloody show" and is normal. The fetus passes through the cervix and enters the *birth canal,* or **vagina,** through which it moves to the outside world to be born. During your assessment of the mother, you must examine her to check for **crowning.** Once the infant passes into the birth canal, you will be able to see the crown of the baby's head grow larger with each contraction. This means that birth is imminent.

The fetus grows inside a special sac of fluids, the **amniotic sac,** which surrounds and protects the baby. Although it may rupture earlier, this sac usually breaks during labor, and the fluid or "water" flows out of the vagina. This is called the "rupture of membranes" and is an important milestone of active labor. When you are assessing the mother, you will ask her if her "water has broken." She will know and be able to tell you if it has or not. Sometimes the sac will break very early in the labor process; sometimes it will break much later. The fluids help lubricate the birth canal for the passage of the baby.

During pregnancy, a special organ called the **placenta** develops in the womb. Oxygen and nourishment from the mother's blood pass through the placenta and enter fetal circulation through the **umbilical cord.** Fetal wastes pass back through the umbilical cord and the placenta to the mother's circulation to be excreted.

STAGES OF LABOR

Usually, the process of labor lasts about 16 hours for the first-time mother. In some cases, labor may take longer, or it may take a much shorter time. The time will vary with each mother. You may also expect that, typically, the labor process will be shorter with each successive birth. There are three stages of labor:

1. *First stage*—begins with contractions and ends when the cervix is fully dilated so the baby can enter the birth canal.

2. *Second stage*—begins when the baby enters the birth canal and ends when the baby is born.

3. *Third stage*—begins when the baby is born and ends when the afterbirth (placenta, umbilical cord, some tissues from the amniotic sac, and some tissues from the lining of the uterus) is delivered.

There will be vaginal discharges throughout labor. During the first stage of labor, the first type of discharge to appear should be a watery, bloody mucus. Later, the discharge will appear as a watery, bloody fluid. This is normal and not the same as bleeding. If there is bleeding from the vagina prior to delivery rather than the normal bloody fluids, then something is wrong. This could be a serious problem and requires assistance from a higher level of EMS provider and transport as soon as possible.

Contractions of the uterus cause labor pains, and they occur in cycles of contraction and relaxation. At first, contractions are far apart. As the fetus is pushed into the birth canal, and the time of birth gets closer, the time between contractions becomes shorter. The first contractions are about 30 minutes apart and become closer and closer until they are 3 minutes apart or less. Pain during labor is normal and usually starts as an ache in the lower back. The pain

cervix (SUR-viks) the neck of the uterus. The lower portion of the uterus, where it enters the birth canal (vagina).

vagina (vah-JI-nah) the birth canal.

crowning the bulging-out of the vagina and eventual exposing of the baby's head during successive contractions.

amniotic (am-ne-OT-ik) sac the fluid-filled sac that surrounds the developing embryo and fetus.

placenta (plah-SEN-tah) an organ of pregnancy that is composed of maternal and fetal tissues. Exchange between the circulatory systems of the mother and fetus can take place without the mixing of blood. Main component of "afterbirth" that must be delivered after baby.

umbilical (um-BIL-i-kal) cord the structure that connects the body of the fetus to the placenta. It contains fetal blood vessels.

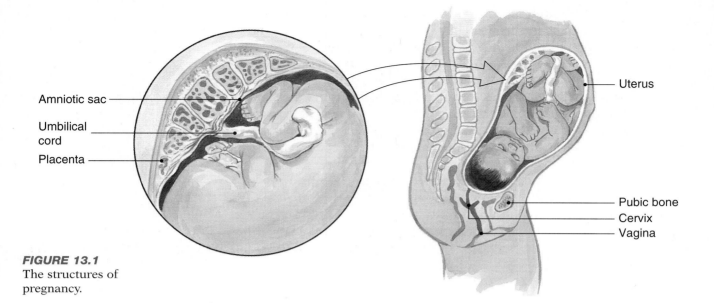

FIGURE 13.1
The structures of pregnancy.

is then felt in the lower abdomen as contractions progress. The intensity of the pain increases as labor progresses. As the muscles of the uterus contract, the pain begins. When the muscles relax, the pain is usually relieved. During the relaxation time, the mother rests. Labor pains will normally come at regular intervals and last for about 30 seconds to 1 minute. It is not unusual for these pains to start, stop for a period of time, and then start again.

First Responders can time labor pains for two characteristics:

■ **Contraction time:** how long it takes from the time the uterus begins to contract until it relaxes; and

■ **Interval time:** the time from the start of one contraction to the beginning of the next.

contraction time the period of time a contraction of the womb lasts during labor. It is measured from the start of the uterus contracting until it relaxes.

interval time during labor, this term means the time from the start of one contraction until the beginning of the next.

Sometimes the mother will experience light, painless, irregular contractions throughout her pregnancy, which may increase gradually in intensity and frequency during the third trimester. About four weeks prior to delivery, as the uterus begins to change its size and shape, some women begin to experience these types of contractions and have the sensation that labor has begun. This is known as *false labor,* also referred to as Braxton Hicks contractions. False labor pains are not as regular and rhythmic as true labor contractions.

It may be difficult for you and the mother to tell false labor pains from true labor. In most cases, before you have completed your assessment to determine if the mother is in false labor, the EMTs have arrived. Even when you are certain that the patient is having false labor, it is still recommended that transport be arranged for the patient. Any pregnant woman having contractions should be evaluated by her obstetrician or midwife.

Remember that your primary role is to help the mother deliver the baby if birth is imminent. You will need to make sure that you have the necessary supplies and materials to do this.

SUPPLIES AND MATERIALS

The items you will need for preparing the mother for delivery and initial care are provided in a commercial obstetric (OB) kit (Figure 13.2). If your response unit does not carry a commercial OB kit, assemble and store the required items in a special kit and keep it on your unit. Some of these items are available at the patient's home, but during the emergency is not the time to find supplies. The items you will need include:

- Personal protective equipment for body substance isolation such as vinyl or latex gloves, face and eye shields, and gowns
- Towels, sheets, and blankets for draping the mother, for placing under her, and for drying and wrapping the infant
- Gauze pads for wiping mucus from the infant's mouth and nose
- Rubber bulb syringe for suctioning the baby's mouth and nose
- Cord clamps and ties for use on the cord before cutting
- Sterile scissors or a single-edged razor for cutting the cord
- Sanitary pads or bulky dressings for vaginal bleeding
- Basin and plastic bags for containing and transporting the afterbirth and other body tissues
- Red plastic "medical hazard" bag for storage and disposal of soiled linens and dressings

Your initial and focused assessments will help you to determine if the mother is ready to deliver. If birth appears likely before a hospital can be reached, place supplies so they are within reach during the delivery process, don your personal protective equipment, and prepare the mother for delivery. It is important to use full personal protective equipment since we assume that blood and other body fluids of all persons (including newborn infants) are potentially infectious. This is called taking *universal precautions,* and you are practicing body substance isolation for your protection and that of the mother and infant.

DELIVERY

PREPARING FOR DELIVERY

Always begin by introducing yourself to the mother and letting her know that you are a trained First Responder. Have someone alert the dispatcher. Let the

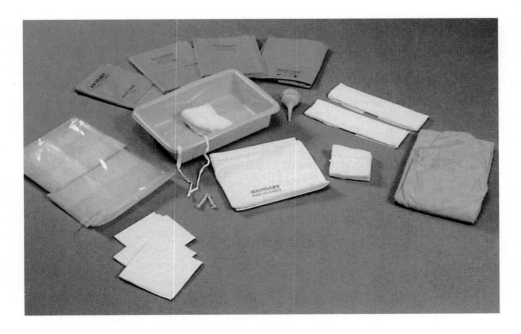

FIGURE 13.2
Contents of a disposable obstetric (OB) kit.

mother know that this has been done and that you will stay with her to help if she starts to deliver the baby. Provide emotional support throughout the entire process of birth. Talk with the mother to help her remain calm and, if needed, remind her that birth is a natural process. If she complains that she feels as if she needs to go to the bathroom, tell her that this is normal and that it is caused by pressure on her bladder and intestine. *Do not let her get up or leave to find a bathroom.* Explain that her body is reacting normally to all the changes taking place. It is important that you keep her calm and begin assessing her status as soon as possible. Place layers of newspaper covered with layers of linens under her. If she does have a bowel movement or urinates, tell her that this is normal. Remove soiled linens and replace them with fresh ones.

Fear of delivering away from a hospital can lead some people to try to delay the process. The mother and/or onlookers may suggest the mother hold her knees together, which you should *not* allow. This will not slow delivery, and it may complicate the birth or harm the fetus. Have unneeded onlookers call for help and find supplies so you may reassure the mother and begin your assessment and appropriate care.

First | Begin to evaluate the mother by asking:

- Her name, age, and expected due date.
- If she has been seeing a doctor during her pregnancy and how the doctor can be contacted. The doctor's knowledge of the patient's history will help you make the decision to transport.
- If this is her first pregnancy. The typical first delivery lasts about 16 hours. Labor time is usually shorter for subsequent babies.
- If she has any known complications, particularly multiple births.
- If she has discharged any watery or bloody mucus.
- How long she has been having labor pains.
- If her water has broken and when.
- If she feels strain in her pelvis or lower abdomen, if she feels as if she needs to move her bowels, and if she can feel the baby beginning to move into her vaginal opening.
- If she has any significant medical information such as a history of seizures, diabetes, or vaginal bleeding during the pregnancy.

If the mother says she feels the baby trying to be born, birth will probably occur before a higher level of EMS personnel arrive. If the mother is having contractions about 2 minutes apart, birth is near. Should she also be straining, crying out, and complaining about having to go to the bathroom, prepare to deliver very shortly.

Even a first-time mother will have some understanding of what is going on. When she says she feels the baby coming, believe her.

Find out if she has taken a childbirth preparation class or natural childbirth class. Tell her that you will work with her to help her follow the procedures she learned in her class with her coach or partner. Though you must follow standard EMS system practices for assisting with the delivery and for providing care afterwards, you can help the mother with breathing and timing contractions as she was taught in her classes. In addition, you can also offer the encouragement and support she will need throughout labor. If you know the procedures of natural childbirth but the mother does not, this is not the time to try to teach her. You can make suggestions on how she can breathe and how she can reduce strain, but do *not* try to give her a "crash course."

First After evaluating and examining the mother and finding that birth may occur shortly, prepare her for delivery immediately. You will:

1. Control the scene so that the mother will have privacy. Ask unneeded bystanders to leave. If you are outdoors, request that they turn their backs to help shield the mother. If she appears to be in early labor, this is her first child, and labor pains are typical, you may choose to move her a short distance to a more private place. It is best to avoid moving her if possible. By now you will have put on your personal protective equipment.

2. Position the mother on her back with her knees bent, feet flat, and legs spread wide apart. If this position causes her to feel dizzy and faint, it is because the weight of the baby is pressing on the inferior vena cava, the vessel that returns blood from the lower part of the body to the heart, and restricting blood flow back to the heart. Some EMS areas will allow you to place her slightly on her left side with one knee bent and foot flat, the other leg extended, and legs spread wide apart. If you position her on her side, place pillows or blankets under her back to support her during birth.

3. Feel on the abdomen for contractions when the patient says she is having labor pains. If the mother says that she can feel the baby coming, skip this step. Explain what you are going to do and place the palm of your hand on her abdomen above the navel. This can be done without removing any of the patient's clothing. Do not delay other procedures to wait for a contraction. Feel for and time contractions and repeat as necessary to help determine if birth is near. As birth nears, you will feel the uterus and the abdomen become more rigid.

4. Prepare the mother for examination. Tell the mother that you need to see if her baby has entered the birth canal. Remove clothing or underclothing that obstructs your view of her vaginal opening. Use clean sheets, towels, or tablecloths to cover the mother as shown in Figure 13.3. If you have an obstetrical pack (OB kit), use the materials provided. Make sure you have enough light to see what you are doing. It may be necessary to supply portable lighting or to move lamps in the home to permit adequate evaluation and delivery.

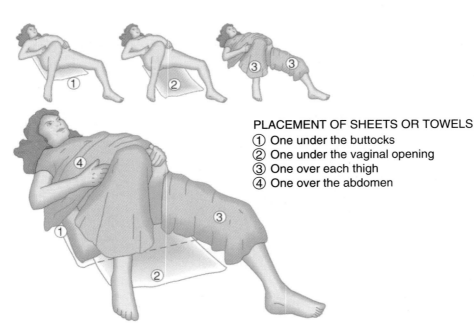

FIGURE 13.3
Preparing the mother for delivery.

PLACEMENT OF SHEETS OR TOWELS
① One under the buttocks
② One under the vaginal opening
③ One over each thigh
④ One over the abdomen

5. Check for crowning. See if any part of the baby is visible at the vaginal opening. In a normal cephalic, or head-first birth, you will see the top of the baby's head. As you learned earlier, this is called crowning. The area of the head that is seen on your first inspection may be less than the size of the new dollar coin. If more of the baby's head becomes visible with each contraction, birth is occurring. The mother is now in the second stage of labor because the baby is in the birth canal. Assume that the birth is in progress. Do not try to transport the mother yourself or in your first response unit; wait for the EMTs or ALS to respond.

   The mother, father, or anyone assisting may be embarrassed when you examine her for crowning. You can minimize this embarrassment by maintaining your professional manner and by explaining what you are going to do and why before you begin. Your professional appearance and approach will generate confidence and trust.

6. Do not attempt any type of internal or vaginal exam. Touch the vaginal area only as necessary during the delivery process.

During the entire process of assessment and delivery, you should be wearing the necessary items supplied for personal protection. Latex or vinyl gloves should be worn to avoid contact with blood or other body fluids and mucous membranes. Wearing a gown is recommended to help reduce the chance of your arms coming into contact with blood and other body fluids. Wear eye protection and face shields since blood and fluids inevitably splash during the birth process. It is essential that you understand the high potential for infectious exposure if you do not protect yourself with personal protective equipment while assisting in childbirth.

NORMAL DELIVERY

During delivery, talk to the mother. Ask her to relax between contractions. If her water breaks, remind her that this is normal. Consider the delivery to be normal if the baby's head appears first.

NORMAL DELIVERY ASSESSMENT

Normal Delivery

A Support the head

B Aid in the birth of the head

C Support the trunk

D Support the feet

E Position for drainage

Assist the mother by supporting the baby throughout the entire birth process.

First | Steps for assisting the mother with a normal delivery are (Scan 13-1):

1. Drape the mother and place her on top of layers of newspapers and clean sheets or towels (Figure 13.3). Place a folded blanket, towels, or sheets under her buttocks so that her pelvis is lifted about 2 inches above the supporting surface. You may also place a pillow under her head and shoulders for comfort.

2. If you have not done so, don the sterile gloves from the OB kit. Wash your hands with soap and water first if it is available at the scene, or use one of the commercially available hand washes.

3. Place someone near the mother's head to reassure and offer her encouragement and to turn her head in case she vomits. If no one is on hand to help, talk with the patient during the delivery process and be alert for vomiting.

4. Place one hand below the baby's head as it delivers. Spread your fingers evenly around the head to support it but avoid pressing the soft areas at the top, back, and sides of the baby's skull. Apply a slight pressure on the baby's head as it emerges to control the delivery speed. Sometimes the head "explodes" from the birth canal quickly, which can badly tear the skin at the vaginal opening. (Some stretching and tearing is normal.) Use your other hand to help cradle the baby's head. **Do not pull on the baby.**

   As the baby's head emerges, you may notice that it has caused the skin area between the vaginal and rectal openings (called the *perineum*) to tear. This is normal and will be treated at the hospital. After the delivery, place a sanitary pad at the vaginal opening, which will also help control bleeding from torn tissues. Replace sanitary pads as needed.

5. If the umbilical cord is wrapped around the baby's neck, place your finger under the cord and gently pull it over the baby's head. If the amniotic sac has not yet ruptured, use a cord clamp to tear the membrane and pull it away from the baby's mouth and nose. Tear the bag with your fingers if necessary. An unbroken sac will prevent the baby from breathing.

6. Most babies are born face down as the head emerges, and then they rotate to the right or left. The upper shoulder (usually with some delay) delivers next, followed quickly by the lower shoulder. Continue to support the baby throughout the entire birth process. If you can gently guide the baby's head downward, you will assist the mother in delivering the baby's upper shoulder. Scan 13-1 illustrates hand placement during delivery.

7. Once the baby's feet are delivered (the end of the second stage of labor), lay the baby on the side with the head slightly lower than the body. This position will enable blood, other fluids, and mucus to drain from the mouth and nose. Wipe the baby's mouth and nose with gauze pads. Suction the mouth first, then the nose.

   Standard procedures call for clearing the baby's airway once the head is delivered, but most First Responders do not carry the rubber bulb syringe needed for this procedure. Even if you have the syringe, do not try to stop the birth process or release your support of the baby in order to clear the airway. Since you will not be delivering babies every day, it will be normal to find you lack the confidence needed to try to assist with the birth and clear the airway at the same time. The majority of babies can wait the few more seconds of delivery to have their airways cleared.

Note

Tearing of the perineum is normal.

Note

Maintain support of the baby throughout the birth process.

8. Note the exact time of birth. In many systems, this is done by notifying dispatch or medical direction and having them record it manually or electronically.

9. Keep the baby at the level of the vagina until the cord is cut.

10. Clamp or tie the cord. Then cut the cord between the ties (described in detail later). If you do *not* have sterile equipment, do not cut the cord; simply clamp it.

11. Monitor and record the ABCs of the infant and the mother.

12. Watch for more contractions, which signal the delivery of the afterbirth (the third stage of labor). After the afterbirth delivers, wrap it in a towel and place it in a plastic bag. Transport it to the hospital for examination.

13. Place a sanitary pad over the vaginal opening. Lower the legs, and place them together.

CAUTION: Babies in the process of being born are slippery. Make certain you have a good but gentle grip and provide proper support throughout the delivery process. Some deliveries are explosive. Do not squeeze or counter-push the baby too much. Remember that an explosive delivery can be controlled by using one hand to maintain a slight pressure on the baby's head.

*C*ARING FOR THE NEWBORN

First | Each step of newborn care is important to the well-being of the infant. Remember from the CPR chapter, the newborn is considered a neonate and you may have to perform some special care steps. As you assist the mother with the delivery of her baby:

1. Clear the baby's airway. Position the baby on his side and keep the head slightly lower than the body to allow for drainage. Use a sterile gauze pad or a clean handkerchief to clear mucus and blood from around the baby's nose and mouth (Figure 13.4). If it is available, use a rubber bulb syringe. The proper method for using the bulb syringe is to squeeze the bulb first,

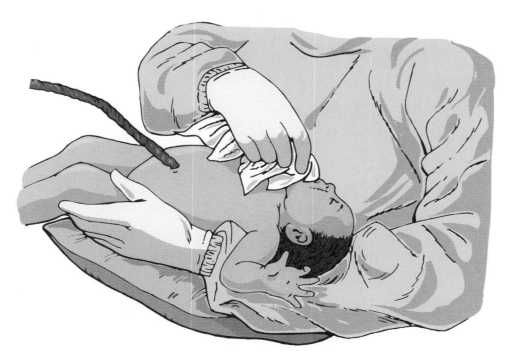

FIGURE 13.4
Use a sterile pad or clean handkerchief to wipe blood and mucus from around the infant's mouth and nose.

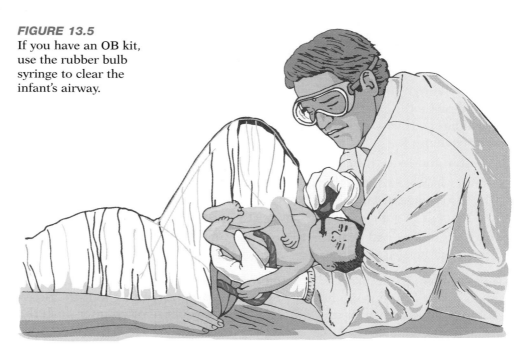

FIGURE 13.5
If you have an OB kit, use the rubber bulb syringe to clear the infant's airway.

then insert the tip about 1 inch into the baby's mouth. Gently release the pressure to allow the syringe to take up fluids from inside the baby's mouth (Figure 13.5). Remove the tip of the filled syringe from the baby's mouth and squeeze out any fluids onto a towel or gauze pad. Repeat this process two or three times in the mouth and then once for each nostril. Throughout the rest of your care steps, be sure that the baby's nose is clear because babies are nose breathers. Plugged nostrils will prevent adequate breathing.

2. Make certain that the baby is breathing. Usually the baby will be breathing on his own by the time you clear the airway, which will take about 30 seconds. If the baby is not breathing, then you must "encourage" him

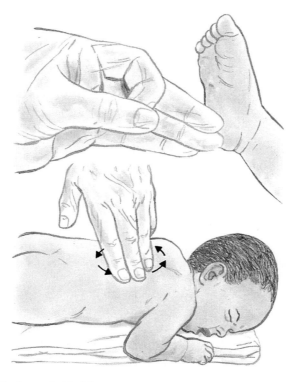

FIGURE 13.6
It may be necessary to stimulate the newborn to breathe.

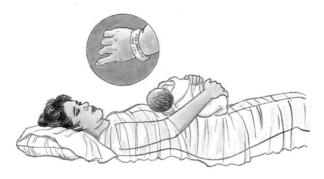

FIGURE 13.7
Wrap the infant and place him on the mother's abdomen. Make an ID bracelet of tape for the infant. Write on it the mother's last name and time of delivery.

to do so. Begin by vigorously but gently rubbing the baby's back. If this fails to stimulate breathing, snap one of your index fingers against the soles of the baby's feet (Figure 13.6). Do *not* hold the baby up by his feet and slap his bottom. (Care for the nonbreathing newborn will be covered later in this chapter.)

3. Clamp or tie off the cord. (Directions will be given later in this chapter.)

4. Keep the baby warm. Dry the baby, then discard the wet material. Wrap the baby in a clean, dry towel, sheet, or baby blanket and place him on the mother's abdomen (Figure 13.7). Keep the baby's head covered. This will help reduce heat loss. The mother may wish to nurse the baby. You may suggest and encourage nursing as this helps contract the uterus and control bleeding.

5. If tape is available, write the mother's last name and the delivery time on a long piece of tape. Place a slightly shorter piece of tape on the back so the adhesive does not come in contact with the baby's skin. Leave an end exposed to tape to itself in a loop. Place it loosely around the baby's wrist.

The Nonbreathing Newborn

The newborn is considered a neonate (see Chapter 8). If you fail in your efforts to "encourage" the baby to breathe, provide two gentle but adequate breaths, preferably by mouth-to-mask. Then assess breathing and heartbeat. Remember,

NEWBORN ASSESSMENT

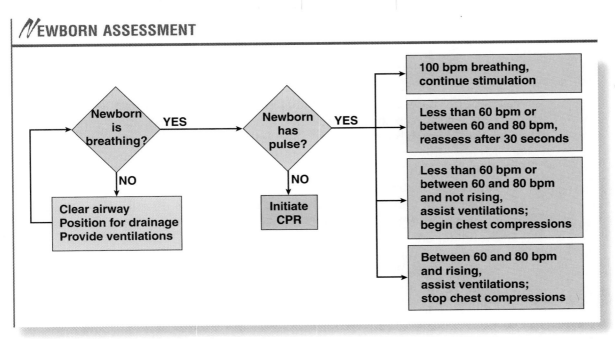

for a neonate, check the heartbeat by listening at the chest with your ear or a stethoscope over the heart or feel for a pulse by lightly grasping the base of the umbilical cord. If you use a breathing adjunct, such as an airway or bag-valve mask, make sure it is approved for neonates. Do *not* use a bag-valve mask or airway adjuncts designed for older children or adults in neonatal resuscitation. Be careful not to hyperextend the head and neck, which will close off the airway. Provide ventilations if breaths are:

- Shallow
- Slow
- Absent

Ventilate at 40 to 60 breaths per minute and reassess breathing after 30 seconds. Watch for the chest to rise, which is the best indication of adequate ventilation. If there is no improvement, continue to provide artificial ventilations.

After giving adequate ventilations for 15 to 30 seconds, the next step depends on the heart rate. If you cannot feel a pulse at the base of the umbilical cord or hear a heartbeat through the chest wall, begin CPR. Remember, this is infant CPR, performed with fingers, not whole hands.

If **there is a pulse** but you

See This	Do This
Heart rate at least 100 beats per minute and spontaneous breathing is present . . .	stop ventilations but continue to gently stimulate the baby by rubbing the skin.
If breathing rate is inadequate . . .	continue ventilations at 40 to 60 breaths per minute and reassess after 30 seconds.
Heart rate less than 60 beats per minute or between 60 and 80 beats per minute . . .	reassess after 30 seconds.
Heart rate less than 60 beats per minute or between 60 and 80 beats per minute and *not* rising (increasing) . . .	continue to assist ventilations and begin chest compressions.
Heart rate is between 60 and 80 beats per minute, and rising (increasing) . . .	continue to assist ventilations but stop chest compressions.

Continue resuscitation until the infant has spontaneous heart and lung actions or you are relieved by a higher level of EMS providers. Alert dispatch to the status of the baby so they may contact appropriate assistance.

Check with your instructor to find out if your protocols allow you to provide oxygen to the newborn. If so, take the following steps:

- Do *not* blow a stream of oxygen directly into the baby's face. This may cause the baby to react by holding her breath, and the rich oxygen supply can cause medical problems.
- Make a tent above the infant's head, using aluminum foil. Direct the flow of oxygen into the tent above the baby's head. Use a humidifier source if available, or
- Direct a stream of oxygen towards the baby's face either through a face mask or through a cup with an oxygen tube placed through the bottom. Hold the mask or cup several inches from the baby's face (see Chapter 14, Figure 14.4).

Research has shown that withholding oxygen may be more damaging than delivering too much. Follow your local protocols for oxygen delivery to the newborn, but *never* withhold oxygen from a sick newborn or one who is struggling to breathe in the prehospital setting. If your response unit does not carry oxygen, notify EMT or ALS providers that it will be needed on their arrival.

These few steps of ventilation and chest compression will usually revive the newborn, but it is still important to have the infant and mother transported as expeditiously as possible to a medical facility. If you are unable to contact dispatch or if the EMS system is unable to respond, transport the mother and child. If the afterbirth has not delivered yet, you will have to carefully move and transport the mother and child as a unit. Keep the mother on her back and the infant between her legs. Coordinate your moves so you do not have to stop resuscitation while moving the mother and infant. Continue to monitor the infant's breathing and pulse during transport and continue resuscitation as needed. Do *not* stop resuscitation to tie and cut the umbilical cord; someone else can do this while you continue monitoring and resuscitating the infant.

If you are transporting, keep in mind that the mother may still be in labor if she has not delivered the afterbirth. She still carries the placenta, which has the other end of the umbilical cord attached to it. Monitor both ends of the cut cord for bleeding. Move the mother carefully. If you have not tied and cut the cord, both mother and infant are a unit that has to be moved with great care so the afterbirth is not torn from the uterine wall.

Most first response units are not designed for transport. First Responder transport of mother and child is not advised unless there is no other choice. If EMT or ALS transport units can respond, the First Responder should provide basic life support until they arrive.

Umbilical Cord Care

In most cases, if dispatch has been alerted, EMTs or ALS should arrive before the cord needs to be clamped or tied. Your instructor will tell you if local protocols allow First Responders to tie and cut the cord. Some EMS systems recommend that First Responders only tie the cord. Cutting the cord may not be recommended unless a medical facility is more than 30 minutes away. If you are to cut the cord, you will need a sterile pair of scissors or single-edged razor blade. Soak these items in isopropyl alcohol for 20 minutes if no sterile items are available.

There may be special cases (for example, the cord was around the baby's neck during delivery) when First Responders will have to tie the cord. First, slip one or two fingers under the cord and try to remove it from around the neck. If this cannot be done, quickly place clamps or ties on the cord and cut it. If the cord is not removed or cut, it will choke the baby. In a normal delivery, take the following steps to clamp and cut the cord (Figure 13.8):

1. Tie or clamp the cord within 30–45 seconds after birth. Use sterile clamps or umbilical tape found in the OB kit. If you do not have a kit, then clean shoelaces may be used. Never use wire or string because it is too narrow and will slice the cord rather than clamp it. Tie the tape or shoelace in a square knot.

2. Apply one tie or clamp to the cord about 10 inches from the baby's belly.

3. Place a second tie or clamp about 3 inches closer to the baby.

4. If you also need to cut the cord, cut between the two ties or clamps. Never untie or unclamp a cord once it is cut. Examine the cut ends of the cord.

Note

A newborn who is sick or struggling to breathe should always be given oxygen.

Note

Transport childbirth patients only as a last resort.

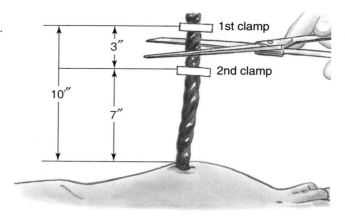

FIGURE 13.8
Cutting the umbilical cord.

1st clamp

3"

2nd clamp

10"

7"

After trapped blood drains, bleeding should stop if the clamps or ties are secure. If bleeding continues, apply another tie or clamp as close to the original as possible.

If the afterbirth delivers while you are still providing care for the infant and you are not allowed to cut the cord, then place the afterbirth at the same level as the baby, or slightly higher. The placenta is still the infant's blood source, and this will allow blood to continue to flow to the infant. Once the afterbirth is delivered, the cord should be tied or clamped and cut. Let dispatch and medical direction know of the delivery status.

CARING FOR THE MOTHER

Care for the mother includes helping her deliver the afterbirth, controlling vaginal bleeding, making her as comfortable as possible, and providing reassurance.

Delivering the Afterbirth

Delivery of the afterbirth, the third stage of labor, takes place a few minutes after the baby is born. In some cases, it may take 20 minutes or longer. Some women wish to get up or assume a seated position after they deliver their babies. You may have to remind some mothers that they will have to remain at rest until they deliver the afterbirth. Make the mother as comfortable as possible and wait for the delivery. You will both know that delivery will be soon because she will begin to have more contractions. They will be milder with little discomfort.

First The afterbirth must be saved. It is critical that the afterbirth be examined by a physician. Try to position a basin or container at the vaginal opening so the afterbirth will deliver into it (Figure 13.9). It may be

FIGURE 13.9
Collect the afterbirth and transport it with the mother and infant.

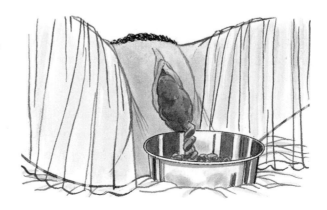

very difficult to position the container you have selected for use. After collecting the afterbirth, wrap the container in a towel, newspaper, or plastic wrap. If no container is available, allow the afterbirth to deliver onto a towel or newspaper, or into a plastic bag. Wrap this in additional towels, newspaper, or plastic wrap.

Control of Vaginal Bleeding After Delivery

Bleeding from the uterus, which is discharged through the vagina, is normal after the mother has delivered the afterbirth and is seldom a problem.

First | To help control vaginal bleeding after delivery, you should:

1. Place a sanitary pad or clean towel over the vaginal opening. Do not place anything in the vagina.
2. Have the mother lower her legs and keep them together. (She does not have to squeeze them.) Elevate her legs.
3. Feel the mother's abdomen until you find a grapefruit-size object. This is the uterus. Gently, but firmly rub this area of her abdomen in a circular motion (Figure 13.10).
4. If bleeding continues, provide oxygen and maintain normal body temperature to reduce the effects of shock (hypoperfusion). Arrange transport as soon as possible and continue to massage the uterus. If the mother wishes to nurse, allow her to do so. Nursing stimulates contraction of the uterus and helps control bleeding.

Providing Comfort to the Mother

First | Talk with the mother throughout the entire birth process and after she has delivered. Once you have completed your duties with the afterbirth, replace any soiled towels or sheets with clean, dry ones. If possible, wipe and dry the mother's face and hands. Make sure that both she and the baby remain warm and comfortable.

Remember, birth is an exciting and joyous event. Talking to the mother and attending to her and her new baby are important First Responder roles.

COMPLICATIONS AND EMERGENCIES

Prebirth bleeding and other predelivery emergencies, miscarriages, prolonged labor, abnormal deliveries, premature deliveries, multiple births, and stillbirths are some of the more common complications in childbirth. Keep in mind that most births are normal. Those births that produce complications often do not

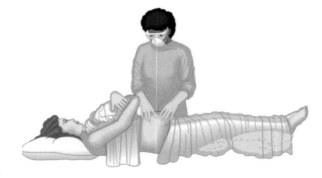

FIGURE 13.10
Control vaginal bleeding that follows delivery of the afterbirth by massaging the mother's abdomen over the top of the uterus.

present with immediate problems at the scene. First Responders can often care for some of the difficulties that arise with unusual deliveries. However, some severe complications must be handled by advanced life support and immediate transport to a medical facility.

The risk of complications before, during, and after delivery increases when the patient has one or more of the following factors:

- Age under 18 or over age 35
- First pregnancy or more than five pregnancies
- Swollen face, feet, or abdomen from water retention
- High or low blood pressure
- Diabetes
- Illicit drug use during pregnancy
- History of seizures
- Predelivery bleeding
- Infections
- Drug or alcohol dependency
- Injuries from trauma
- Premature rupture of membranes (water broke more than a few hours before delivery)
- Using medications such as lithium carbonate, magnesium, or reserpine

You will determine this information while taking a history during the patient interview. As you assess the patient, ask her the questions necessary to see if she is in a high-risk group.

First | Some pregnant patients develop medical problems long before they are ready to deliver. Some patients will require care for these problems before they show any outward signs of pregnancy. You may improperly assess the patient if you do not know she is pregnant. Be certain to ask the patient if she is pregnant when you note or the patient tells you of any of the following:

- Any *new* medical complaint in females of childbearing age
- Unusual vaginal bleeding or missed menstrual period(s)
- Swelling of the face, hands, and feet
- Headache, visual problems, apprehension, and shakiness along with upper abdominal pain
- Nausea, vomiting, or severe abdominal pain that had a sudden onset

Other pregnancy-related medical emergencies may present as:

- Chest pain
- Difficulty breathing
- New seizure

Your instructor will tell you which of these signs are critical and require immediate EMT or ALS response, and which signs indicate pregnancy and are normal reactions to the changes in the body.

With complications present, the woman may experience a stressful or difficult delivery, which also affects the fetus. When the baby is stressed during delivery, it may defecate (empty the bowel). The infant's fecal material is called *meconium.* When this material mixes with amniotic fluid, the normally clear fluid is stained green or brownish-yellow and is called **meconium staining.** If the baby inhales this fluid on her first attempt to breathe, the lungs will become infected. Look for meconium staining when assessing the mother after the membranes have ruptured (water has broken). Be prepared to wipe the baby's mouth and nose and to suction. Sometimes the membranes will rupture many

---

Note

Always assess for meconium staining during the focused history and physical exam.

meconium staining
amniotic fluid that has a green or brownish-yellow color due to fetal fecal contamination.

hours before delivery. You will have to rely on information from the mother to determine if the fluids were clear or stained.

Infections of the reproductive organs, especially infection by sexually transmitted diseases (STDs), may be transmitted to the baby and to you during birth. Remember to wear all personal protective clothing and use universal precautions for body substance isolation. Personal protective equipment will protect you as well as the mother and infant. Report to the hospital any information you receive from the mother on history of infection.

Note

Protect yourself and the baby from STDs during childbirth.

PREDELIVERY EMERGENCIES

Prebirth Bleeding

First When a pregnant woman has vaginal bleeding early in pregnancy, it may be due to a miscarriage. Light, irregular discharges of blood, called "spotting," are normal in early pregnancy but may cause the patient to be concerned. If bleeding occurs late in pregnancy or while the patient is in labor, the problem may be with the placenta. Regardless of the cause of bleeding or stage of pregnancy, you will:

1. Make certain that someone alerts dispatch, telling them of the excessive bleeding. Don personal protective equipment.

2. Place the patient on her left side, but do not hold her legs together (Figure 13.11).

3. Provide care for shock and monitor the patient's airway.

4. Place a sanitary pad or bulky dressings over the vaginal opening.

5. Replace pads or dressings as they become soaked. Do not place anything in the vagina.

6. Save all blood-soaked pads and dressings and any tissues that are passed. Place them in a plastic bag for transport to the hospital and examination by a physician.

7. Monitor and reassure the patient while you wait for EMTs or ALS.

If First Responders in your jurisdiction are trained to provide oxygen, place the mother on a high concentration of oxygen.

Miscarriage and Abortion

If the fetus delivers before it can survive on its own (before the twenty-eighth week), it is considered a **miscarriage.** The correct term for a miscarriage is a *spontaneous abortion.* However, since the word **abortion** has other meanings in our society, never use the word with a woman who is having a miscarriage or premature signs of labor.

miscarriage the natural loss of the embryo or fetus before the twenty-eighth week of pregnancy. Also called a spontaneous abortion.

abortion spontaneous miscarriage or induced loss of the embryo or fetus.

FIGURE 13.11
Position the patient to control excessive prebirth bleeding.

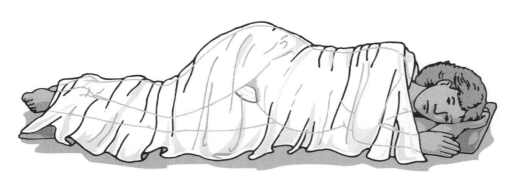

When special procedures are performed to end a pregnancy, the term *induced* or *therapeutic abortion* is used. This may be done legally by a physician as a medical procedure, or it may be attempted illegally by the woman or someone else. The woman may attempt an illegal abortion by taking large doses of medicines or other chemicals that will require care for an overdose or poisoning. Some women may have others help her abort the fetus by having them insert objects into the uterus through the vagina. These women may have major internal and external bleeding, infection, and shock.

First | The miscarriage and the abortion patients typically have abdominal cramps and pains. Vaginal bleeding is to be expected and ranges from mild to severe. In many cases, there will be vaginal discharges of bloody mucus and tissue particles.

When caring for a woman having a miscarriage or following an abortion, first get a general impression of the environment and the patient, perform your initial assessment, then focus on the physical exam and patient history. Then take the following steps to care for the patient:

1. Take an initial set of vital signs and repeat every few minutes.
2. Provide care for shock and place the patient on her side.
3. Place a sanitary pad or bulky dressing over the opening to the vagina. Do not place anything into the vagina.
4. Save all blood-soaked pads and any tissues that are passed.
5. Provide emotional support.
6. Arrange for transport immediately.

Regardless of the cause of the emergency, the patient will be in need of emotional support. Provide professional care, show concern, and reassure the patient.

Note

Provide emotional support to all miscarriage or abortion patients.

*A*BNORMAL DELIVERY

Breech Birth

In a **breech birth,** the buttocks or both feet (not just one leg) present and deliver first. Even in this position, the baby can be born without complications. As the infant's buttocks and trunk deliver together, place one hand and forearm under the baby for support. Also support the head as it delivers.

First | In cases where the baby's head does not deliver within **3 minutes** of its buttocks and trunk, you must:

1. Create an airway for the baby because the umbilical cord has been compressed between the infant and vaginal wall and blood flow has been shut off. Tell the mother what you must do and why. Insert your gloved hand into the vagina, with your palm toward the baby's face. Form a "V" by placing one finger on each side of the baby's nose (Figure 13.12). Push the wall of the birth canal away from the baby's face. If you cannot complete this process, then try to place one fingertip into the infant's mouth and push away the birth canal wall with your other fingers.
2. Maintain the airway. Once you have created an airway for the baby, keep this airway open. **Do not pull on the baby.** Allow delivery to take place while you maintain support for the baby's body and head.
3. Allow 3 minutes for delivery after you have established an airway. If delivery of the head does not take place, immediate transport to a medical

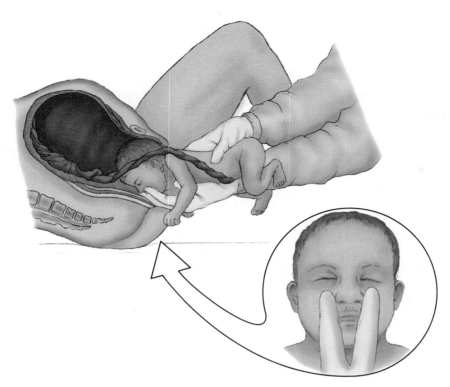

facility is necessary. Maintain the airway throughout *all* stages of care until you are relieved by higher-level EMS personnel.

4. The mother needs to be on a high concentration of oxygen. If you do not carry oxygen, arrange for EMT or ALS response immediately.

The presentation of just an arm or a leg is *not* a breech birth. This is a limb presentation and requires immediate transport to a medical facility. Call for EMT or ALS response. Do *not* pull on the limb or try to place your gloved hand into the birth canal. Do *not* try to place the limb back into the vagina. Place the mother in the knee-chest position (Figure 13.13) to help reduce pressure on the fetus and the umbilical cord. You may be instructed to keep her in the typical delivery position. Follow local protocols.

Prolapsed Cord

First When you examine the mother for crowning, you may find the umbilical cord protruding from the vaginal opening. When the umbilical cord delivers first, this is called a **prolapsed cord** and is common in a breech birth. Immediate transport to a medical facility is required because this situation endangers the life of the baby. As the baby emerges through the vaginal opening, the umbilical cord is squeezed between the vaginal wall and the baby's head. Blood flow and oxygen are reduced or cut off completely. When oxygen flow through the cord is obstructed, the baby will try to breathe. But since the baby's face is pressed against the wall of the birth canal, the mouth and nose cannot take in air. To help the baby breathe, provide an airway for the infant, using the same methods described for breech birth.

Do *not* try to push the cord back into the birth canal. Place the mother in a knee-chest position to reduce pressure on the cord. (Your EMS system guidelines may call for the mother to remain in the normal delivery position.) Place wet dressings (use sterile water or saline if available) over the cord to keep it moist. Then wrap the cord in a towel or dressings to keep it warm. The mother will need a high concentration of oxygen as soon as possible. Monitor vital signs and arrange for transport as soon as possible.

Note

All limb presentations require immediate ALS assistance and transport.

breech birth a birth in which the buttocks or both feet are delivered first.

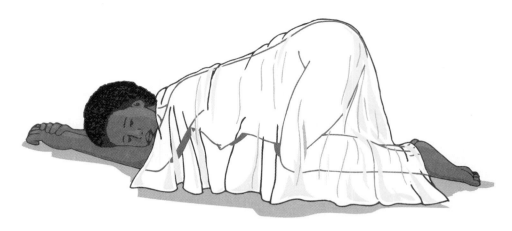

NOTE: The baby's chances for survival improve if you can keep the head from pressing on the umbilical cord. Check with your instructor to see if you are allowed to insert several fingers into the mother's vagina and gently push up on the baby's head to keep pressure off the cord.

Multiple Births

In cases of multiple births, contractions will start again shortly after the birth of the first child, and these contractions may deliver the afterbirth of the first newborn or another newborn. If more than one baby is in the uterus, the mother's abdomen will remain rather large. Ask the mother if she has been told to expect twins (or more). The procedures for assisting the mother remain the same. Normally, you will tie or clamp the cord of the first baby before the second baby is born if the umbilical cord has stopped pulsating. Check with your instructor for protocols or procedures in your area for caring for the cords of multiple newborns. Once they are delivered, assess each baby and resuscitate if necessary. Document time of birth of each infant. Call for assistance as soon as possible.

Premature Births

prolapsed cord
umbilical cord that presents through the vaginal opening before the baby's head.

Any baby weighing less than 5½ pounds at birth is considered **premature.** Any baby born before the thirty-seventh week (prior to the ninth month) of pregnancy is considered premature. If the mother tells you the baby is early by more than 2 weeks, play it safe and consider the baby to be premature.

In addition to the procedures for normal births, you must take special steps to keep a premature baby warm. It is important to dry the baby. Wrap the newborn in a blanket, sheet, towel, or aluminum foil (fold the edges to avoid cutting the baby). A blanket covered with foil is ideal. Cover the baby's head, but keep its face uncovered. Transfer the baby to a warm environment (90°F to 100°F), but do *not* place a heat source too close to the baby. Premature infants often need resuscitation. If you have a mask that will fit the newborn, provide mouth-to-mask resuscitation. If not, provide mouth-to-mouth-and-nose resuscitation, which may be done through a gauze pad or handkerchief for some protection. Wipe or suction blood and mucus from the mouth and nose first before ventilating.

Stillborn Deliveries

Some infants are born dead or die shortly after birth. Such events are very sad. You should be prepared for stillbirths so that you can act professionally and be able to provide comfort to the mother, father, and other family members who may be present.

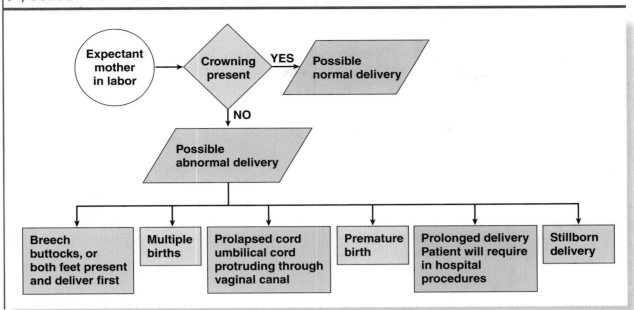

If a baby appears lifeless when born or goes into respiratory or cardiac arrest, provide the resuscitation measures described earlier in this chapter and in Chapter 8. Do *not* stop resuscitation until the baby regains respirations and a heartbeat, until you are relieved, or until you are too exhausted to continue.

There are cases when a baby has died hours or longer before it is born. Do not attempt to resuscitate a stillborn baby that has large blisters and a strong unpleasant odor. There may be other indications that the infant died earlier in the uterus such as a very soft head, swollen body parts, or obvious deformities.

OTHER EMERGENCIES

Trauma

When a pregnant woman is involved in a trauma, she and her fetus can be injured. In your initial assessment, get an impression of the environment and the patient. Look for the mechanism of injury and try to determine what injuries it might have caused. The pulse rate of a pregnant patient is 10 to 15 beats per minute faster than the average woman who is not pregnant. The pregnant woman also has a greater blood volume and may lose more blood before showing the effects of shock.

Injuries to the abdomen will often be due to blunt force from falls, automobile accidents, or physical assaults. Penetrating injuries may be caused by gunshot wounds, stabbings, or punctures from the debris of the auto wreckage.

During the early months of pregnancy when the fetus is small, it is very well protected by the fluids in the amniotic sac. As the fetus grows, and especially in the last two months of pregnancy, its size and location cause it to be easily injured in a trauma situation. Trauma can cause other injuries to the internal organs of both the mother and fetus. You will be able to provide direct care only for the mother and, as a result, will provide indirect care for the fetus.

The greatest danger to both the mother and the baby is bleeding and shock. Based on the mechanism of injury, provide appropriate care such as immobilization for possible spinal injuries, splinting for possible fractures, dressing wounds, and most importantly, providing a high concentration of oxygen to the mother as soon as possible. Maintain body temperature but do not overheat the patient. The steps that prevent or care for shock will assist the fetus also. Arrange for transport as soon as possible. In advanced pregnancies, the larger fetus can press on the mother's inferior vena cava and restrict blood return to the heart. If you immobilize an injured pregnant woman on a spine board, you may have to tilt it slightly to the left (raise the right side). After she is secured, this position will allow better blood flow (venous return) to the heart.

Vaginal Bleeding

There are many reasons for excessive vaginal bleeding during pregnancy. Included among them are trauma, intercourse, sexual assault, reproductive organ problems, and abnormal pregnancy. In another type of serious pregnancy-related condition, the placenta sometimes lies low in the uterus and covers the opening of the cervix. In this position, the placenta will tear when the cervix dilates during labor. In a similar condition, sometimes parts of the placenta will tear away from the wall of the uterus and cause internal bleeding that is contained between the placenta and the uterine wall. The only indication that shock is developing is through changes in vital signs and a hard, painful uterus. Get an initial set of baseline vital signs as soon as possible in your assessment and monitor the vital signs by retaking them every few minutes. Arrange to provide high-concentration oxygen as soon as possible and maintain body temperature to help reduce the effects of shock.

Place a sanitary pad or bulky dressings over the vaginal opening. Replace pads or dressings as they become soaked. Do not place anything in the vagina. Save all blood-soaked pads and dressings. Place them in a plastic bag for transport to the hospital and examination by a physician.

Sexual Assault

Sexual assault or rape is always a psychologically and physically traumatic experience. The First Responder's professional manner, attitude, and emotional support are important steps in the care of the expectant mother who has been assaulted.

As the woman struggles or resists the attacker, and as the attacker uses force to make her submit, she can receive many types of injuries to the external soft tissues, internal organs and vaginal canal, and the musculoskeletal system. The fetus is also a victim in the assault. The injuries that the fetus receives may be direct from blows to the abdomen, or indirect as a result of injuries to the mother. The emotional trauma to the woman may be greater initially than the physical trauma.

You may have multiple roles to perform as a First Responder who is caring for a pregnant woman. You may have to provide care for injuries, including spinal immobilization, extremity splinting, and wound dressing. In cases of sexual assault, you will need to provide emotional support and protect the patient from embarrassment from onlookers. Do *not* clean the vaginal area or let the patient wash; however, collect clothing and any items used during the assault for examination and future legal needs. Transport evidence in paper container or towel, never in plastic. For any emotional or traumatic injury and for complicated deliveries, provide care that will prevent or treat shock and arrange transport as soon as possible. Promote patient confidence and provide emotional support and comfort by listening to your patient and talking to her throughout all procedures. You will find that some roles come easily; other roles will take knowledge, practice, and skill.

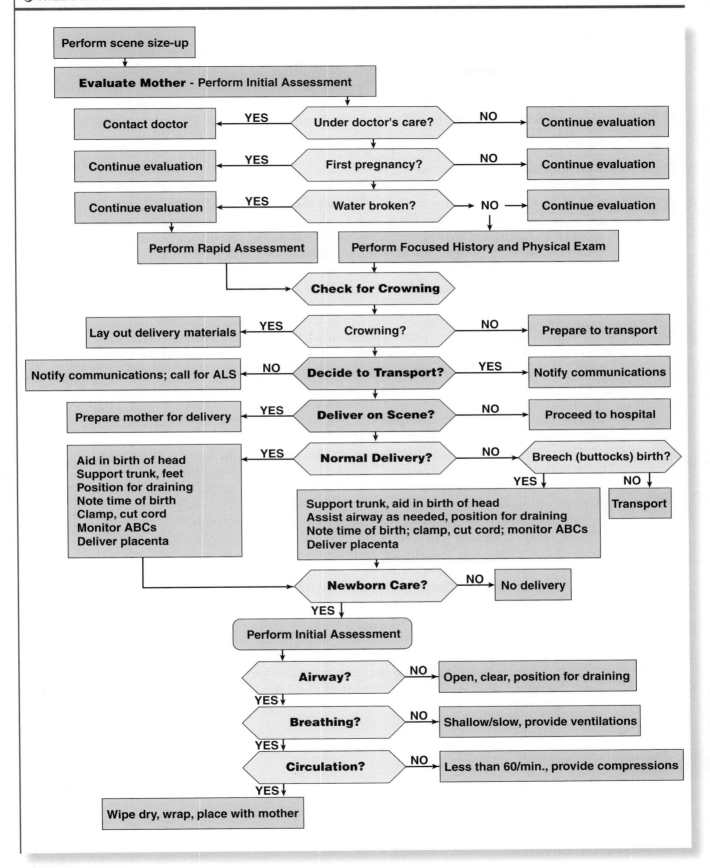

Summary

Begin caring for the pregnant mother by letting her know that you are a First Responder. Alert dispatch and gather all supplies and materials needed for delivery and for postdelivery care of the mother and baby.

Perform an initial and focused assessments and determine if the mother is about to deliver. Ask if this is her first labor and how far apart the contractions are. Ask if she feels pressure or if she has to move her bowels. Ask if her water has broken and look to see if there is **meconium staining.** Ask if she feels the baby moving into her vagina.

If you believe that birth may occur before the mother can be safely transported to the nearest hospital, provide the mother with as much privacy as possible. Position her on her back with her knees bent, feet flat, and legs spread apart. If this position makes her feel dizzy, position her slightly on her left side. Ensure your own protection by wearing gloves, eye and face shields, and a gown. Remove any clothing obstructing your view of the vaginal opening. See if any part of the baby is visible or becomes visible **(crowning)** during contractions.

Assist the mother as she delivers her baby. It is normal if the skin between the vaginal and rectal openings **(perineum)** tears during delivery. Carefully support the baby's head as it is born. Spread your fingers flat around the baby's head. A slight, evenly distributed pressure will prevent an "explosive" birth. Provide support for the baby's entire body and head as birth proceeds.

If the umbilical cord is around the baby's neck, gently loosen the cord with your fingers. If the membranes have not ruptured, puncture the sac and pull it away from the baby's mouth and nose.

For newborn care, clear the airway and be sure that the baby is breathing. If he is not breathing, "encourage" him to breathe by rubbing his back or by snapping your index finger on the soles of his feet. For nonbreathing babies, provide ventilations at 40 to 60 breaths per minute. If using a bag-valve mask, be sure to use only an infant-sized bag. Assess after 30 seconds. If there is no improvement, continue ventilations. Check for a heartbeat by listening over the chest or by feeling the base of the umbilical cord. If the heartbeat is at least 100 beats per minute and spontaneous breathing is present, stop ventilations but continue to gently stimulate the baby by rubbing the skin. If the breathing rate is less than 40–60 breaths per minute, continue ventilations and reassess after 30 seconds; if the heart rate is less than 60 beats per minute or between 60 and 80 beats per minute and the rate is not rising, continue to assist ventilations and begin chest compressions. If the heart rate is between 60 and 80 beats per minute, and the rate is rising, continue ventilations but stop chest compressions. Continue resuscitation until the infant has spontaneous heart and lung actions.

Your local protocols may require you to tie or clamp the cord. Do not tie, clamp, or cut the cord until the baby is breathing on her own (unless you must start CPR).

Assist the mother as she delivers the afterbirth and save all tissues for transport. Control vaginal bleeding by placing clean pads over the vaginal opening and massaging her abdomen over the site of the uterus. Allow the mother to nurse her baby. Replace wet towels and sheets with clean, dry ones. Wipe clean the mother's face and hands.

REMEMBER: Throughout the birth process, provide emotional support to the mother.

Be ready for complications during a delivery. Look for meconium staining. Provide an airway with your fingers in cases of breech birth. Maintain this airway until the baby is born or until you turn the mother over to more highly trained professionals. The EMS system should transport all mothers when there are emergencies that pose immediate life-threats to the baby (prolapsed umbilical cord or limb presentations). If there is severe bleeding before delivery, pad the vaginal opening, provide care for shock (hypoperfusion), and arrange for transport as soon as possible.

Expect a multiple birth if contractions of the same intensity continue after a first baby is born. When possible, tie or clamp the umbilical cord of the first baby before the next baby is born.

Keep all babies warm. It is especially critical that premature babies be kept warm. Be prepared to resuscitate premature babies.

In cases of miscarriage, provide emotional support to the mother. Place pads at her vaginal opening if there is bleeding. Save all blood-soaked pads and any passed tissues. Provide care for shock.

In cases of stillborns, remain professional and provide emotional support to the mother, father, and other family members.

When the mother is involved in trauma, sexual assault, or is bleeding heavily from the vagina, care for injuries and provide emotional support. The greatest danger to both mother and baby is bleeding and shock. Provide a high concentration of oxygen and maintain body temperature. Transport as soon as possible.

IMPORTANT: EMS personnel will want to reduce and avoid the risk of infection by taking appropriate body substance isolation (BSI) precautions when caring for patients. Wear appropriate personal protective equipment including latex or vinyl gloves and, when necessary, eye shields, face mask, and gown to avoid contact with the patient's blood, body fluids, wastes, and mucous membranes. Don gloves and face protection before checking for crowning in a woman in active labor; put on a gown to assist delivery.

Remember and Consider...

✔ Does your response unit carry any supplies for assisting in childbirth?

Check your station and unit and find out where the supplies are kept. Do you have a commercial package or have company members created a special "jump bag" for childbirth incidents? What would you put into a childbirth jump bag? Find out how many childbirth incidents your unit has responded to in this past year. Why do you think there are so few, or so many, in your area? Will obstetric patients go to the local hospital or to a specialized one? Are there separate birthing centers in your area? Do they handle only normal deliveries or complicated ones as well? Visit a birthing center and obtain additional information on childbirth and delivery.

Investigate...

✔ After you have checked your unit for childbirth supplies, check with your supervisor or supply officer to find out the procedure for replacing used items. Many childbirth items, such as gauze pads and trauma dressings, are used for wound care and trauma management as well. Ask if it would be practical to keep childbirth items in a separate cabinet or jump bag. Offer to set up, stock, monitor supplies, and replace them as needed. When extra dressings are needed for trauma emergencies, the childbirth dressings will be put into service, and supplies that were "set aside" for childbirth may get overlooked when personnel replace items after an incident.

✔ Assisting childbirth in the field is rare, but First Responders must be ready for the event. If you have a training officer, ask if he or she is planning a drill or refresher class on childbirth. Find out what you can do to help prepare for or present the program. County and state training agencies will have films you can borrow; health departments will have materials and information for handouts; obstetricians from local hospitals will be interested in speaking to emergency personnel who will be responsible for assisting childbirth in the out-of-hospital situation.

CHAPTER 14

/NFANTS AND CHILDREN

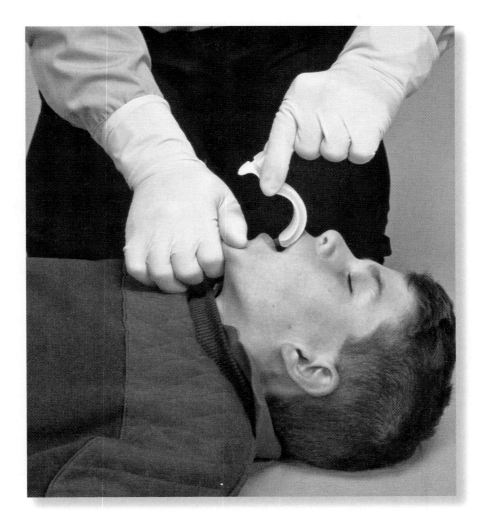

*C*hildren can be the most difficult patients for First Responders to assess and care for. They are not small adults; they must be managed and cared for differently than adults because of the differences in their age, physical and mental development, personalities, and experiences. Children's lack of life experiences results in accidents and events that cause injuries and illnesses. Children respond well to the "familiar" and to normal routines. They have difficulty handling strange situations such as dealing with unfamiliar adults, including First Responders, who suddenly arrive in their environment to look at and handle them while offering to help and make them feel better. Seriously ill and injured children also provoke strong emotions in emergency responders. But through training and practice, First Responders can increase their confidence and manage the pediatric incident calmly and professionally. As a result, child patients will find an empathetic care provider to respond to during emergencies. In addition, First Responders will decrease the effects for themselves and for the patients. This chapter introduces methods used in providing care for pediatric medical and trauma emergencies.

National Standard Objectives

This chapter focuses on the objectives of Module 6, Lesson 6–2 of the U.S. DOT First Responder National Standard Curriculum and serves as an instructional aid to help you meet any specific objectives added to the course by your local EMS system.

By the end of this chapter, you will know how to (from cognitive or knowledge information) . . .

6–2.1   Describe differences in anatomy and physiology of the infant, child, and adult patient. (pp. 488, 490–491)

6–2.2   Describe assessment of the infant or child. (pp. 494–496)

6–2.3   Indicate various causes of respiratory emergencies in infants and children. (pp. 496–499)

6–2.4   Summarize emergency medical care strategies for respiratory distress and respiratory failure/arrest in infants and children. (pp. 485, 486, 492–493, 496–498)

6–2.5   List common causes of seizures in the infant and child patient. (p. 500)

6–2.6   Describe management of seizures in the infant and child patient. (p. 500)

6–2.7   Discuss emergency medical care of the infant and child trauma patient. (pp. 506–511, 512–513)

6–2.8   Summarize the signs and symptoms of possible child abuse and neglect. (pp. 514–516)

LEARNING TASKS

This chapter describes some of the many characteristics of children. The text and your instructor will help you understand how to handle children in many types of emergency situations. No emergency is routine, but with some experience you become confident with what to do. With child patients, though, you will find you may have to adjust your approach and care. As you read about and discuss children, think about and be able to:

✔ State the special problems that may arise when caring for the child patient.

✔ Describe the changes in the approach to care when dealing with infants and children.

As children develop, their physical and emotional characters change. As they grow and get older, they also want to be treated differently, but may often regress when faced with a frightening emergency. Think about children you know and how they act in different situations. Then talk with classmates and

	6–2.9	Describe the medical-legal responsibilities in suspected child abuse. (pp. 514, 515, 516)
	6–2.10	Recognize the need for First Responder debriefing following a difficult infant or child transport. (pp. 482–483, 516)
Feel comfortable enough to (by changing attitudes, values, beliefs) . . .	6–2.11	Attend to the feelings of the family when dealing with an ill or injured infant or child. (pp. 484, 487)
	6–2.12	Understand the provider's own emotional response to caring for infants or children. (pp. 482–483, 516)
	6–2.13	Demonstrate a caring attitude towards infants and children with illness or injury who require emergency medical services. (pp. 483–484, 489)
	6–2.14	Place the interests of the infant or child with an illness or injury as the foremost consideration when making any and all patient-care decisions. (pp. 483–484, 487–488, 514–516)
	6–2.15	Communicate with empathy to infants and children with an illness or injury, as well as with family members and friends of the patient. (pp. 483–484, 487, 489, 514–515)
Show how to (through psychomotor skills) . . .	6–2.16	Demonstrate assessment of the infant and child. (pp. 485–486, 489, 494–496)

members at your station about the response of children in different age groups and how to handle them. Be able to:

✔ List the age categories of infants and children.

✔ List some methods to use that will help in interacting with infant and child patients.

First Responder units may or may not carry oxygen. If your unit carries oxygen equipment, you will want to learn how to use it. Your instructor will show you the equipment, demonstrate how to use it, and let you practice using it. A part of your responsibility for using oxygen equipment includes knowing how to operate it and when to use it. Once you have learned how to operate the equipment, also be able to:

✔ Describe the methods and devices used for delivering oxygen to infant and child patients.

The steps of infant and child patient care are generally the same as those for an adult. But we know that many children are afraid of strangers, and they can be most uncooperative when frightened by an emergency. Think about how children might respond, recall your patient assessment steps, and discuss how you could approach children to gain their confidence. Be able to:

✔ List the steps for performing a scene size-up, initial assessment, focused history and physical exam, detailed physical exam, and ongoing assessment for infant and child patients and describe the steps that are managed differently from those for adult patients.

Infant and child emergencies include injuries and illnesses, and you will provide much the same care as you do for an adult. Recall some emergency situations and be able to:

✔ List assessment and care concerns for the child patient who has signs and symptoms of fever, hypothermia, vomiting and diarrhea, and suspected neglect and abuse.

✔ Describe the care you will provide to the patient in suspected child abuse situations.

✔ List the signs and symptoms of shock and describe emergency care.

✔ List the causes and signs of altered mental status.

✔ Describe the steps to take with the infant and the parents when managing a sudden infant death syndrome (SIDS) incident.

By the time you finish reading the chapter and working with your instructor and other classmates, you will feel comfortable with what you know. In class, you will begin to practice the skills you need to perform when responding to infant and child emergencies. Take every opportunity to practice in and out of class so you can:

✔ Demonstrate on an infant or a child manikin the emergency care for trauma emergencies including caring for shock, burns, and spinal injuries.

✔ Demonstrate on an infant or a child manikin the emergency care for medical emergencies, including airway obstruction, respiratory infection, seizures, altered mental status, poisoning, near-drowning, and sudden infant death syndrome (SIDS).

INTRODUCTION

Responding to a call for a child's illness or injury can be stressful for the First Responder. Some situations will make you feel sad or angry. You will not be able to express your emotions in front of the child or parent. When faced with the assessment and care of an infant or a child, you may at first feel that you do not know what to do or where to start. Remember that many of the assessment and care techniques used for adults are the same for children, with some modifications. These adjustments will help make the child feel more at ease with you.

After caring for the child and dealing with the parents, be aware of how you feel. Do not hesitate to talk with other care providers, support groups, or your family about your feelings. Knowing that others have gone through the same emotions can help you feel more comfortable with your own. Do not feel that you have to get through the tough stressful calls by yourself. First Responders who are unsure of what to do in pediatric emergencies are likely to have a stronger emotional response during and after an incident than those who are prepared and confident in their actions. By training, practicing, and drilling to prepare for pediatric incidents, First Responders will not only improve their confidence and decrease their stress but improve patient outcome as well.

The procedures listed in this chapter are different from procedures used on an adult because they consider the child's age, physical development, and emotional response. A severe illness or injury is a new and unknown experience for children, and it is an experience that increases their anxiety if parents are not there. An anxious, fretful, or frightened child who cannot be comforted further adds to your stress level and reduces your confidence. Following are some methods that will help you understand and care for infant and child patients.

CHARACTERISTICS OF INFANTS AND CHILDREN

Everyone has some fear of the unknown. Since so many things are unknown to a child, it is easy to see why emergencies can be so frightening for them. For most children, security comes from their parents. Wanting the parents may be a child's first priority, even above having you offer help, comfort, or relief of pain.

First When you are dealing with children, you need to gain their trust. You can attempt to calm and reassure them by:

- Approaching them slowly, establishing contact from a safe distance, and asking permission to get closer. Offering them something (a toy of their own or one you brought) will help to prevent them from feeling threatened by your approach. (Many first response units carry teddy bears for their child patients.)
- Letting them know that someone will call their parents.
- Sitting down with them so you are at their level. Standing makes you appear large and frightening.
- Letting them see your face and expressions. You want to appear friendly, yet concerned and willing to listen. Speak directly to them. Speak clearly and slowly so that they can hear and understand you. Keep your voice gentle and calm even when you need to be firm. Try not to raise your voice or talk loudly to a crying or screaming child. Some children are bashful or uncomfortable with strangers and may not look at you. Try to maintain eye contact (Figure 14.1).
- Pausing frequently to find out if they understand what you have said or asked. Even if you communicate easily with your own children, never assume that other children understand you. Find out by asking questions.
- Quickly determining if there are any life-threatening problems and caring for them immediately (Scan 14-1). If there are no life-threatening problems, continue with patient assessment at a relaxed pace. Avoid moving children if possible. Movement may cause additional injury or severe responses to certain medical problems. Children may be frightened by a rapid-pace exam and a lot of "meaningless" questions that are asked by a stranger. Alert young children may become frightened if you start your exam with their head and face. If children show fear as you reach out to touch them, begin the physical examination at the feet and slowly work your way up to the head if they are not critically injured. While you are performing this "toe-to-head" assessment, you can look for the same signs of illness and injury as you do when assessing the adult patient. Take

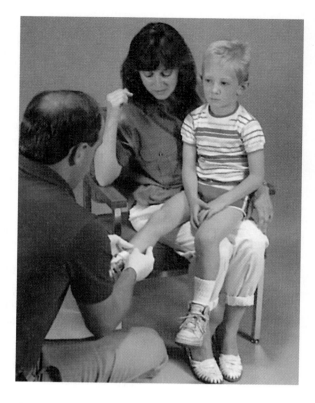

FIGURE 14.1
Let the child see your face and speak directly to him. Try to maintain eye contact.

time, though, to consider special assessment needs based on the anatomy of the child (Figure 14.2).

- Always telling children what you are going to do before each step of the patient assessment. Do *not* try to explain the entire procedure at once. Explain one step, do it, then explain the next step.
- **Never lying to children.** Tell them if it will hurt when you are examining them. If children ask if they are sick or hurt, tell the truth; but reassure them by saying that you are there to help, and other people also will be helping. While you talk and work with them, smile; it carries a lot of weight with most children.
- Offering comfort to children by stroking their foreheads or holding their hands. Children will let you know if they do not want to be touched. Most children have learned from parents and teachers that they should not let strangers touch them. Special child safety programs make children aware of what kind of touching is allowable and what is a "good touch" or a "bad touch." Children will show their acceptance of you by their reactions to your touch. Do not expect rapid acceptance; use your smile and gentle words to provide comfort.

If the parents are present, do *not* direct all your conversation to them. Talk to the child. If you are at the scene of an accident in which the parents are also injured, let the child know that people are caring for them.

While assessing and caring for children, you also will have to consider and work with the reactions of the parents or other adults who care for the child. Usually parents' or guardians' responses are positive and helpful even while they are concerned. Sometimes parents will react with strong emotional responses that can hinder your care of the child. Both types of reactions are natural. Ask the parent or guardian to help you with tasks, such as holding and reassuring the child, holding the dressing in place, holding the oxygen mask, or assisting with any other device you need to use in your care of the child. If this

Pediatric Emergencies–Initial Assessment and Basic Life Support

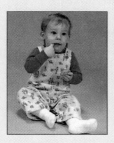

INFANTS
Birth to 1 Year

- Perform a scene size-up. In your initial assessment, get a general impression from a distance.
- Control your emotions and facial expressions to help reduce the child's fear.
- Protect the head and spine. Head and neck injuries are common because the infant's head is large and heavy.
- Ensure an adequate airway. If needed, provide ventilations as you watch for the chest to rise.
- Provide care to prevent shock. (A small amount of blood loss can cause shock.)

Establishing responsiveness: The infant should move or cry when gently tapped or shaken. Is he alert, responsive to voice or to pain stimulus, or unresponsive?

Opening the airway: Use slight head-tilt, chin-lift. (Use the jaw-thrust for possible spinal injury.)

Evaluating breathing: If the infant is conscious but cyanotic, struggling to breathe, or has inadequate breathing, arrange for immediate transport. If the infant is unconscious, look, listen, and feel for breathing. If there is no breathing, provide breaths.

Providing breaths

- Provide two ventilations while watching the chest rise. Ventilate with the mouth-to-mask technique, using an appropriate pediatric-size mask or a pediatric bag-valve mask.
- If there is evidence of airway obstruction, clear the airway.

Clearing the airway

- Make certain that you have not overextended or underextended the neck. Place a folded towel under shoulders to keep the head in a neutral position. If this does not open the airway . . .
- Place the infant over the length of your arm face down with the head lower than the trunk. Support the head with your hand placed around the jaw. Support your forearm by placing it on your thigh.
- Deliver five back blows between the shoulder blades with the heel of your free hand.
- Place your free arm on the infant's back and support the back of his head with that hand. Sandwich him between your arms and hands and turn him over. Support your arm on your thigh. Keep the head lower than the trunk and deliver five chest thrusts. If the airway remains obstructed, but the patient is conscious, continue back blows and chest thrusts.
- If the airway remains obstructed, but the patient is unconscious, wrap your fingers around the lower jaw, place your (gloved) thumb inside the mouth, and pull the mouth open to look for an obstruction.
- Do not attempt blind finger sweeps. You must see the object before you sweep the mouth. Use your little finger to sweep the mouth.
- Even if you did not see or dislodge an obstruction, give two breaths and repeat: reposition the head, attempt to ventilate, give back blows and chest thrusts, look for and remove visible obstructions, and attempt to ventilate again.

Continuing rescue breathing

- If patient is still not breathing but you gave two successful breaths, check for a brachial pulse (infant); or listen for the heartbeat with your ear or a stethoscope over the chest or feel for a pulse at the base of the umbilical cord (neonate).

- If there is a pulse, but no breathing, continue to breathe giving 20 breaths a minute (one every 3 seconds) for the infant and 40 to 60 breaths a minute (one every 1 to 1½ seconds) for the neonate. If there is no pulse, start CPR.

Performing CPR

- If the patient is unresponsive and not breathing, open the airway and look, listen, and feel for breathing. If there are no breaths, provide two initial breaths. (Assure the chest rises.) If there is no indication of obstruction, but the patient is unconscious and is not breathing, check pulse.
- Check brachial pulse (infant) or listen for heartbeat with your ear or a stethoscope over the chest or feel the base of the umbilical cord (neonate). If there is no pulse and no breathing, start CPR. Have someone call dispatch for EMTs or ALS. If you are alone, do CPR for 1 minute before calling dispatch.
- Start compressions. For the infant, the compression site is one finger width below an imaginary line drawn across the nipples. Compress with the tips of two or three fingers ½ to 1 inch deep at a rate of at least 100 per minute. For the neonate, use overlapping or side-by-side thumbs and compress on the middle third of the sternum just below the nipple line. The remaining fingers encircle the chest and support the back. Compress ½ to ¾ inch deep at a rate of at least 120 per minute.
- Deliver a ventilation once every five compressions for the infant and once every three compressions for the neonate.
- Check for a pulse after the first minute, then every few minutes (at the appropriate site for the infant or neonate).

Controlling bleeding

- Use direct pressure as a primary method to control bleeding.
- If bleeding is not controlled, use elevation combined with direct pressure. If bleeding is still not controlled, use pressure points combined with elevation and direct pressure.
- A small amount of blood loss (25 milliliters) is serious. The smaller the child, the less he or she can afford to lose. Treat for shock.

Caring for shock

- Ensure adequate breathing and circulation.
- Provide oxygen.
- Control bleeding and keep the infant warm.
- Place a pillow or folded blanket under the legs if there is no indication of spinal or leg injury.
- Splint painful, swollen, and deformed extremity injuries.
- Handle the child gently, give emotional support, give nothing by mouth.
- Arrange for transport and monitor vital signs.

(continued)

CHILDREN
1 to 8 Years

- Perform a scene size-up. In your initial assessment, get a general impression from a distance.
- Control your emotions and facial expressions to help reduce the child's fear.
- Protect the head and spine. A child's head is proportionately larger than her body.
- Ensure an adequate airway. If needed, provide ventilations as you watch for the chest to rise.
- Evaluate blood loss. Provide care to prevent shock. (A small amount of blood loss can cause shock.)

CAUTION: The child's size and weight may be more important than age when providing care.

Establishing responsiveness: The child should move or cry when gently tapped or shaken.

Opening the airway: Use the head-tilt, chin-lift or the jaw-thrust maneuver to provide an adequate airway.

Evaluating breathing: If the child is conscious but cyanotic or struggling and failing at attempts to breathe, arrange transport immediately. If the child is in respiratory arrest, open the airway and look, listen, and feel for breathing. If there is no breathing, provide breaths.

Providing breaths

- Provide two initial ventilations as you watch the chest rise. Ventilate with the mouth-to-mask technique, using an appropriate pediatric-sized mask or a pediatric bag-valve mask.
- If there is evidence of airway obstruction, clear the airway.

Clearing the airway

- Make certain that you have the proper head-tilt for an unconscious child. Place a folded towel under the shoulders to keep the head in a neutral position. If this does not open the airway . . .
- Rapidly deliver five abdominal thrusts for the unconscious child.
- If the airway remains obstructed, but the patient is conscious, continue with abdominal thrusts.
- If the airway remains obstructed, but the patient is unconscious, place the child on her back on a hard surface. Wrap your fingers around the lower jaw and pull the mouth open to look for an obstruction.
- Do *not* attempt blind finger sweeps. You must see the object before you sweep the mouth. Use your little finger.
- Even if you did not see or dislodge an obstruction, give two breaths and repeat: reposition the head, attempt to ventilate, provide abdominal thrusts, look for and remove visible obstructions, and attempt to ventilate again.

Continuing rescue breathing

- If the patient is still not breathing but you gave two successful breaths, check for a carotid pulse.
- If there is a pulse, but no breathing, continue to provide breaths at 20 breaths a minute. If there is no pulse, start CPR.

CPR

- If the patient is unresponsive and not breathing, open the airway and look, listen, and feel for breathing. If there are no breaths, provide two initial breaths. (Assure the chest rises.) If there is no indication of obstruction, but the patient is still unconscious and is not breathing, check pulse.
- Check the carotid pulse. If no pulse and no breathing, provide CPR. Have someone alert dispatch. If you are alone, do CPR for 1 minute before calling dispatcher.
- Apply compressions to the CPR compression site with the heel of one hand.
- Depress the sternum 1 to 1½ inches.
- Deliver compressions at a rate of 100 per minute.
- Provide one ventilation by mouth-to-mask every five compressions.
- Check for a carotid pulse after the first minute, then every few minutes.

Controlling bleeding

- Use direct pressure as a primary method to control bleeding.
- If bleeding is not controlled, use elevation combined with direct pressure. If bleeding is still not controlled, use pressure points combined with elevation and direct pressure.
- A blood loss of ½ liter (about 1 pint) is serious. Treat for shock.

Caring for shock

- Ensure adequate breathing and circulation.
- Provide oxygen.
- Control bleeding and keep the child warm.
- Place a pillow or folded blanket under the legs if there is no indication of spinal injury or leg injury.
- Keep the child warm.
- Splint painful, swollen, and deformed extremity injuries.
- Handle the child gently, give emotional support, give nothing by mouth.
- Arrange for transport and monitor vital signs.

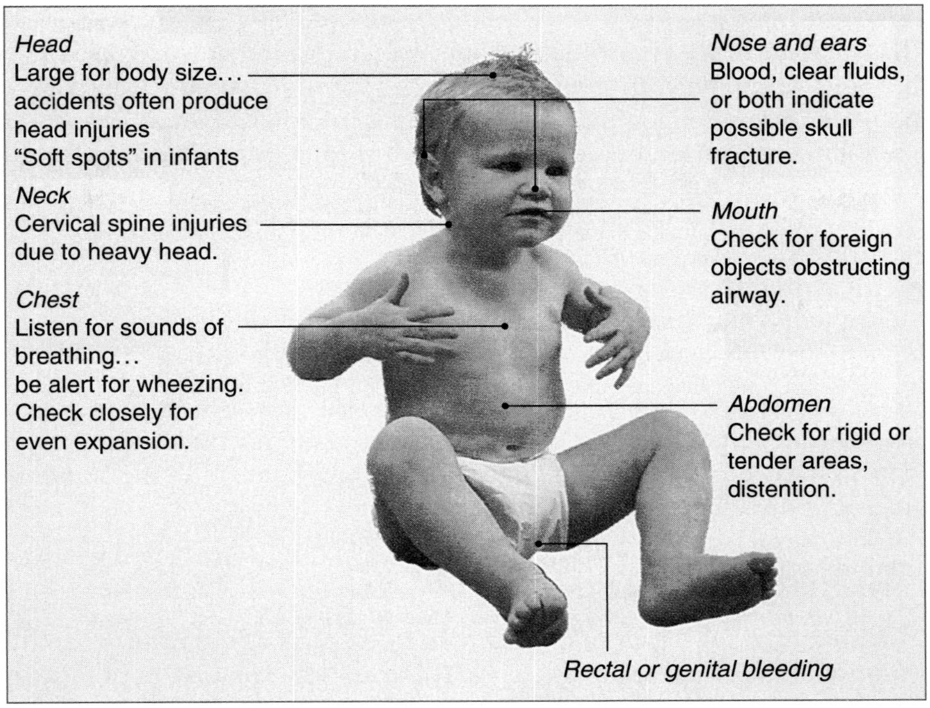

FIGURE 14.2
Special assessment considerations.

Head
Large for body size... accidents often produce head injuries
"Soft spots" in infants

Neck
Cervical spine injuries due to heavy head.

Chest
Listen for sounds of breathing... be alert for wheezing. Check closely for even expansion.

Nose and ears
Blood, clear fluids, or both indicate possible skull fracture.

Mouth
Check for foreign objects obstructing airway.

Abdomen
Check for rigid or tender areas, distention.

Rectal or genital bleeding

does not work to calm the parent, have a friend, neighbor, or other First Responder distract the parent with questions of the child's history or with getting the child's toy, favorite blanket, or clean clothes. Lastly, have someone gently and tactfully guide the parent away from the scene while you evaluate the child.

Some children who are seriously ill or injured are recuperating or being cared for at home while hooked up to technical medical equipment. These children may be on special monitors, have special tubes in their throats or abdomens, have intravenous drips containing medications, or be in special traction units. The parents have been trained by the child's doctors and nurses to care for the child's special equipment, but these children still have emergencies, and the parents will call EMS for help. You do not have to learn how to operate all the different types of special equipment, nor are you expected to. The parent will know how to manage the equipment; your concern will be how to help the child, and the parent can likely guide you in that. Ask the parents what they need you to do and how, then help the parents in doing it. Call for EMTs or ALS to transport if necessary.

Take advantage of public education or public relations opportunities to encourage families to notify local emergency responders of special patients in the community. Arrangements can then be made to ensure proper personnel and equipment are dispatched to them when emergencies occur.

AGE, SIZE, AND RESPONSE

First You will find that you instinctively treat infants and children differently from adults. You will automatically know that an infant needs to be handled and cared for differently than a toddler, and that a toddler is spoken to and cared for differently than a school-age child or a teenager. When you determine the age of a pediatric patient for CPR, recall that babies from birth to 1 month are classified as neonates and up to 1 year are classified as infants. Patients from 1 to 8 years are classified as children, and over 8 years they are considered adults. In your training and with experience, you will become familiar with the age ranges, mental and physical development, personality, and experience levels of child patients so you can assess and care for them appropriately. Keep the following categories in mind when assessing and caring for infants and children (Table 14-1):

- Newborns and infants: birth to 1 year
- Toddlers: 1 to 3 years
- Preschool: 3 to 6 years
- School age (usually in elementary school): 6 to 12 years
- Adolescent (usually in middle and high school): 12 to 18 years

Sometimes you will be unable to determine the age of the infant or child. Some are large or small for their age, and parents may not be there to tell you ages. You will have to estimate age based on the physical size, emotional responses, interaction with you, and language skills.

SPECIAL CONSIDERATIONS

You already realize that infants and children are not the same as adults in size, emotional maturity, and responses. You need to be aware that there are important anatomical differences as well. Because of these differences, your care will sometimes be somewhat different than it is for adults. Consider the following important differences and comparisons.

The Head and Neck

A child's head is proportionately larger and heavier than his or her body. The body will catch up with the size of the head at about age 4. Because of the size and weight of the head, the child can be considered "top heavy," and is likely to land head first in sudden falling or stopping situations. Common examples include falls from shopping carts and unrestrained children who are propelled head first through windshields in motor vehicle collisions. Both of these incidents result in severe head injuries to pediatric patients. Be especially suspicious of a mechanism of injury that suggests a possible fall from a height taller than the child.

Remember to handle the head of the newborn with caution because of the soft spots (fontanelles). The largest soft spot, the one on top of the head, does not close completely until about 18 months of age. This soft spot is flat when the child is quiet, and you may see it pulsate with each heartbeat. If the soft spot is sunken, the child may have lost a lot of fluids (*dehydration*) because illness has caused inadequate fluid intake and/or diarrhea and vomiting. If the soft spot is bulging, it may indicate that there is increased pressure inside the skull. This can be due to brain swelling from trauma or from an illness such as *meningitis*. Since the fontanelles can also bulge when the infant is agitated and crying, they should be assessed when the infant is quiet. Again, consider the mechanism of injury or nature of the illness during your assessment and care.

In any head injury, look for and suspect skull fractures if you see blood and clear fluids leaking from the nose and ears, just as you would in adults. **Children are more vulnerable to spinal injuries than adults are because of the larger, heavier head and the underdeveloped neck muscles and bone structure.**

The Airway and the Respiratory System

The airway and respiratory systems of the infant and child have not developed fully. The tongue is large for the oral cavity (mouth) and the airways (nasal,

Note

When infants and small children suffer head injuries that present with shock, also suspect internal injuries. A head injury itself is seldom a cause of shock.

TABLE 14-1: *D*EVELOPMENTAL CHARACTERISTICS OF INFANTS AND CHILDREN

AGE GROUP	CHARACTERISTICS	ASSESSMENT AND CARE STRATEGIES
Newborns and infants—birth to 1 year	■ Infants do not like to be separated from their parents. ■ There is minimal stranger anxiety. ■ Infants are used to being undressed but like to feel warm, physically and emotionally. ■ The younger infant follows movement with his or her eyes. ■ The older infant is more active, developing a personality. ■ They do not want to be "suffocated" by an oxygen mask.	■ Have the parent hold the infant while you examine him or her. ■ Be sure to keep the infant warm—warm your hands and stethoscope before touching the infant. ■ It may be best to observe the infant's breathing from a distance, noting the rise and fall of the chest, the level of activity, and the infant's color. ■ Examine the heart and lungs first and the head last. This is perceived as less threatening to the infant and therefore less likely to cause crying. ■ A pediatric nonrebreather mask may be held near the face to provide blow-by oxygen. ■ Have a parent hold the child while you examine him or her.
Toddlers— 1 to 3 years	■ Toddlers do not like to be touched or separated from their parents. ■ Toddlers may believe that their illness is a punishment for being bad. ■ Unlike infants, they do not like having their clothing removed. ■ They frighten easily, overreact, have a fear of needles, pain. ■ Toddlers may understand more than they communicate. ■ They begin to assert their independence. ■ They do not want to be "suffocated" by an oxygen mask.	■ Assure the child that he or she was not bad. ■ Remove an article of clothing, examine the toddler, and then replace the clothing. ■ Examine in a trunk-to-head approach to build confidence. (Touching the head first may be frightening.) ■ Explain what you are going to do in terms the toddler can understand. (Taking the blood pressure becomes a squeeze or a hug on the arm.) ■ Offer the comfort of a favorite toy. ■ Consider giving the toddler a choice: "Do you want me to look at your belly or your feet first?" ■ A pediatric nonrebreather mask may be held near the face to provide blow-by oxygen.
Preschool— 3 to 6 years	■ Preschoolers do not like to be touched or separated from their parents. ■ They are modest and do not like their clothing removed. ■ Preschoolers may believe that their illness is a punishment for being bad. ■ Preschoolers have a fear of blood, pain, and permanent injury. ■ They are curious, communicative, and can be cooperative. ■ They do not want to be "suffocated" by an oxygen mask.	■ Have a parent hold the child while you examine him or her. ■ Respect the child's modesty. Remove an article of clothing, examine the preschooler, and then replace the clothing. ■ Have a calm, confident, reassuring, respectful manner. ■ Be sure to offer explanations about what you are doing. ■ Allow the child the responsibility of giving the history. ■ Explain as you examine. ■ A pediatric nonrebreather mask may be held near the face to provide blow-by oxygen.
School age— 6 to 12 years	■ This age group cooperates but likes their opinions heard. ■ They fear blood, pain, disfigurement, and permanent injury. ■ School-age children are modest and do not like their bodies exposed.	■ Allow the child the responsibility of giving the history. ■ Explain as you examine. ■ Present a confident, calm, respectful manner. ■ Respect their modesty.
Adolescent— 12 to 18 years	■ Adolescents want to be treated as adults. ■ Adolescents generally feel that they are indestructible but may have fears of permanent injury and disfigurement. ■ Adolescents vary in their emotional and physical development and may not be comfortable with their changing bodies.	■ Although they wish to be treated as adults, they may need as much support as children. ■ Present a confident, calm, respectful manner. ■ Be sure to explain what you are doing. ■ Respect their modesty. You may consider assessing them away from their parents. Have the physical exam done by a First Responder of the same sex as the patient if possible.

oral, and laryngeal pharynx, and trachea) are more narrow than the adult airway and thus more easily obstructed. The muscles in the neck are not fully developed or as strong as those of the adult, and it may be more difficult for a child to hold his head in an open-airway position when sick or injured. Also, the large head may cause the airway to flex forward and close when the child is lying on his back (supine). Place a folded towel under the shoulders to help keep the head in line with the body (a neutral position) and the airway open (Figure 14.3). Fold the towel flat to a thickness that will keep the airway aligned and the head in a neutral position. For infants and small children, use a slight head-tilt. *Do not perform blind finger sweeps when trying to clear an airway obstruction.* You may unintentionally force and wedge the obstruction farther into the narrow pharynx and trachea.

There are some unique points to remember about children's breathing. An infant or a small child will automatically breathe through the nose as infants are obligate nasal breathers. If the nose is obstructed, the infant will not open the mouth to breath as an adult would. Make sure the nostrils are clear of secretions so the patient can breathe freely. Remember that the child's windpipe (trachea) is also softer, more flexible, and narrower than an adult's windpipe, and it will obstruct easily. For this reason, you must be careful when opening the airway. The chest muscles are not fully developed, so the child is more dependent on the diaphragm for breathing.

The child's normal breathing rate is faster than an adult's: 12 to 20 per minute in an adolescent, 15 to 30 per minute in a child, 25 to 50 per minute in an infant, and 40 to 60 per minute in a neonate (birth to 1 month).

The Chest and Abdomen

Since the diaphragm is the major breathing muscle for normal respirations in the infant and child, you will see more respiratory movement in the abdomen than in the chest. But the chest cage is more elastic, so when the child's breathing is labored or distressed, chest movement is obvious in all the muscles between the ribs and in the muscles above the sternum around the neck and shoulders. The use of these "accessory" muscles for breathing is important to note and indicates the child is in urgent need of medical care.

The child's less-developed and more elastic chest cage may have an advantage over an adult's chest. In a crushing trauma, the bones of the child's chest may not break but will flex. The disadvantage of this is that the more flexible chest cage offers less protection to the vital organs underneath—the heart and lungs. In your physical assessment, the mechanism of injury is important and will help you determine possible internal injury, especially if there is no obvious external injury. Some signs to look for are loss of symmetry (unequal appearance on both sides), unequal chest movement with breathing, and bruising over the neck and/or ribs.

FIGURE 14.3
Use a folded towel to keep the infant's head in a neutral position, neither hyperflexed nor hyperextended.

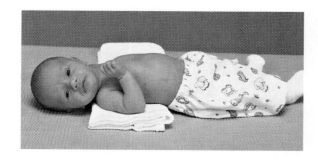

Injury to the abdomen can result in tenderness, distention, and rigidity just as it can in adults. The abdominal muscles are not as well developed as they are in the adult and provide the child less protection. The abdominal organs (especially the liver and spleen) are large for the size of the cavity and are more susceptible to trauma. A child who has a blunt abdominal injury can "bleed out" within minutes. Injury that causes distention or swelling can restrict movement of the diaphragm muscle and make it difficult for the child to breathe.

The Pelvis

The child can lose a large amount of blood into the pelvic cavity as a result of trauma to the pelvic girdle. If you suspect hip or pelvis injury, monitor vital signs for shock just as you would in the adult. Check for bleeding or bloody discharge from the genital area. Do *not* rock the hips to check for instability. Arrange for transport as soon as possible to a medical facility, following local trauma guidelines.

The Extremities

Check for pain and motor and sensory response at the distal ends of all extremities. Also check for pulse and capillary refill. Check capillary refill by pressing briefly and gently on the hand, foot, forearm, or lower leg. You do not have to press the tiny nail bed. Pressing on the skin will push blood out of the area and cause it to briefly whiten or blanch and then suddenly refill when pressure is released. Capillary refill time should be less than 2 seconds; and the refill time gives you an idea of circulatory status.

Injuries that cause soft-tissue swelling or that cause bones to be displaced, bent, or splintered can restrict circulation. Always check both pulses and capillary refill in injured extremities. If splinting or other immobilization are performed by the First Responder, the pulse must be rechecked after the splint is in place and regularly en route to the hospital.

Adults' bones may fracture in a trauma situation; children's bones are less developed and more flexible and will bend and splinter before they break, like new green growth on trees. Treat injury sites where there are signs and symptoms of painful, swollen, and deformed extremities.

Body Surface Area

Infants and children have a large amount of total surface area (skin) in proportion to total body mass. This large amount of skin surface can easily lose heat and cause the pediatric patient to become chilled or *hypothermic*, even in an environment in which an adult feels comfortable. It is important to keep infants and children covered and warm, especially if there is trauma and blood loss or illness and fluid loss. Burns on infants and children are also assessed differently than for adults because of the child's larger surface area, larger heads, and smaller extremities (see Chapter 11).

Blood Volume

Smaller patients have less blood volume. The newborn may have slightly less than 12 ounces, or about a cup and a half of blood, and cannot afford to lose many drops. Children will have from ½ liter to 2 liters (roughly 1 pint up to ½ gallon) of blood, depending on their size. Moderate blood loss in an adult may not concern you if it is easily controlled, but the same amount of blood loss in an infant or small child can be life-threatening.

PROVIDING EMERGENCY CARE

MANAGING THE AIRWAY

The airway is your first concern in the care of any patient. Always assure that the airway is open and clear and that the patient is breathing adequately or is receiving appropriate ventilations and supplemental oxygen when necessary. Review the airway care techniques for infants and children in Chapters 6 and 8.

Opening the Airway

First | When a child lies on his or her back, the tongue will fall to the back of the throat as it does in adults. Remember, though, that the infant's or child's tongue is larger and can more easily obstruct the airway. Also, when lying on the back, the larger head of the infant may cause the head to flex or bend too far forward and close off the airway. In small children, if you are not careful when opening the airway, you may cause *hyperextension* or bend the head too far back, which also can close off the airway. You must be sure to align the head and neck or place it in a neutral position so that the airway is open. As noted earlier in this chapter, you can easily position the infant or small child correctly by placing a towel under the shoulders. Check for breathing before repositioning the head. Then, if necessary, perform a slight head-tilt or a jaw-thrust maneuver (for trauma) to assess breathing and provide ventilations.

Clearing and Maintaining the Airway

If air does not enter easily or the chest does not rise when providing artificial ventilations, reposition the head and try again. If you still have no success in ventilating the patient, give back blows and chest thrusts on an infant less than 1 year of age and abdominal thrusts for children over 1 year. Then check the mouth to see if there is an obstruction. If you see one, sweep the mouth with the little finger of your gloved hand. Do *not* perform blind finger sweeps. Review techniques for infants and children in Chapters 6 and 8. If there are fluids in the airway, clear them by sweeping the mouth with a gauze pad or by suctioning (see Appendix 2). Check with your instructor to see if First Responders are allowed to use suctioning equipment in your area. If so, your instructor will provide you with training. You also may be able to use nasopharyngeal and oropharyngeal airways in the infant and child patient. Again, your instructor will let you know and give you appropriate training.

Providing Oxygen

In some jurisdictions, and for some emergency services agencies, training for First Responders in oxygen delivery is optional. If you are allowed to provide oxygen to patients, your instructor will have the appropriate equipment and train you how and when to use it.

EMS jurisdictions have debated the use of oxygen for infants and children over the years. Some EMS areas believed that infants and children did not need the high concentration of oxygen that we normally give adults. This attitude is rapidly changing as a result of studying the outcomes of pediatric patients in various medical and trauma emergencies. EMS systems now agree that oxygen delivery is just as important for children as it is for adults. Your instructor will instruct you in proper oxygen delivery methods for newborns.

Children must receive a high concentration of oxygen—just as adults do—when they are in respiratory distress, have inadequate respirations, or have blood loss that can result in shock. A low oxygen level (*hypoxia*) causes serious physical reactions in children. It can affect the heart rate, slowing the pulse and reducing oxygen circulating to tissues. This in turn affects the brain, decreasing oxygen to cells and causing altered mental status and tissue death. Always follow the rule "If they are blue, give O_2."

Oxygen is vital to children, but it may be difficult to deliver it to them. Many adults are not comfortable wearing an oxygen mask because it feels confining and suffocating. Children also will fear having a mask placed over the face, and the flow of oxygen may even cause children to hold their breath. The First Responder can still provide enriched oxygen to children who need it by using a technique called blow-by. Hold the oxygen tubing or the pediatric nonrebreather mask about 2 inches from the child's face so the oxygen will enrich the area in front of the face as it blows by and is inhaled (Figure 14.4). Oxygen tubing can be "plugged" into the bottom of a colorful paper cup and can provide oxygen just as effectively. The advantage to this method is that the child will likely be curious about the cup and hold it to his face to examine it or try to drink from it. At the same time the child is receiving oxygen, he will also calm down because he has something of interest to keep his attention. You have provided a toy and gained confidence so your exam can proceed more smoothly. (Note: Use a paper cup. A foam cup will crumble and particles can be blown into the child's face, eyes, and airway.) Allowing a child to hold a nonrebreather mask next to his face is frequently effective as well.

If the patient is not breathing, provide artificial ventilations at the rate of 40 to 60 per minute for the neonate and 20 per minute (once every 3 seconds) for both the infant and child under 8 years of age, using a pediatric-size pocket face mask or bag-valve-mask ventilator of the correct size. Remember the following steps when ventilating:

- Breathe less forcefully through the pocket face mask. Watch for the chest to rise. Ventilate slowly so as not to cause stomach distention.
- Excessive force is not needed with the bag-valve-mask ventilator. Watch for the chest to rise.
- Use properly sized face masks to get a good mask-to-face seal.
- Do *not* use flow-restricted, oxygen-powered ventilation devices.
- If ventilations are not successful, perform the procedures for clearing an obstructed airway. Then try to ventilate again.

Review the procedures for artificial ventilations and airway obstruction in Chapter 6.

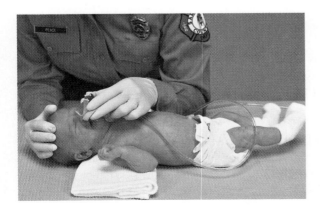

FIGURE 14.4
You can deliver oxygen by using the blow-by method.

First | PATIENT ASSESSMENT

Scene Size-up

Just as you check the scene as you approach an incident involving an adult, you will do a scene size-up for incidents involving pediatric patients. Approach slowly so you do not frighten the child. Determine scene safety and the number of patients, get an impression of the mechanism of injury or the nature of illness, and prepare for patient care by putting on appropriate personal protective equipment. If you think you may need additional resources, call for them immediately.

Initial Assessment

Perform an initial assessment to quickly get a general impression of the child and determine mental status. To get a general impression, look at the child and the environment as you approach. Quickly gather critical information that will help you decide whether to hurry or take your time. From a short distance or from across a room, you can see if the child is alert, struggling to breathe, crying, quiet and listless, or unresponsive to your approach. Is the skin pale, bluish, or flushed? How is the child interacting with the environment, with those around him, and to you as you approach? What is the child's body position? From these clues, you can get a general impression, or idea, of the child's status. In children, the general impression is an important indicator of the severity of illness.

Once you reach the child, you can quickly determine mental status. In Chapter 7, you learned about AVPU. Is the child alert? Is he responsive to your voice or only to a painful stimulus like squeezing his shoulder? Or is he unresponsive?

Next, quickly assess ABCs. The *crying* child has airway, breathing, and circulation. For the quiet or unresponsive child, check the airway: Is it open? Check breathing: Is the child breathing normally or with effort? What is the rate? Is chest expansion present and equal? Are there noises like grunting or high-pitched "stridor" associated with the child's respiratory efforts? Is the skin blue (cyanotic), indicating low oxygen levels? Check circulation: Is the pulse strong and regular? Is there any bleeding? For all children, you will want to find out: Is the skin warm and dry, indicating normal circulation? Or is it cool and clammy, suggesting blood loss and shock? What skin areas are most accessible for you to determine cool and clammy skin? Is capillary refill time less than 2 seconds? Care for the life-threatening conditions that affect airway, breathing, and circulation first. Remember: The unresponsive child needs immediate care.

When you determine priority of transport, you have a high-priority patient if the infant or child:

- Gives a poor general impression
- Is unconscious, unresponsive, or listless
- Has an airway problem
- Is in respiratory arrest, or has inadequate breathing or respiratory distress
- Has a possibility of developing shock
- Has evidence of uncontrolled bleeding that may soon result in shock

Focused History and Physical Exam

After getting critical information from your initial assessment, focus on getting a history and doing a physical exam. These steps may be done at the scene with the responsive patient and while you are waiting for the EMTs to arrive, or they may be done en route to the hospital. Normally, infants or very young children will not respond to your questions, but older children will be able to answer questions that require a yes or no answer, and they can tell you or point to where it hurts. Otherwise, parents or other responsible adults, such as baby-sitters or teachers, will have to give you information about the child's history and how she became sick or hurt.

While you are getting a general impression of the child, decide if the child is seriously injured or sick. For any child who is critically injured or sick, perform a rapid assessment, just as you learned in Chapter 7, and as you would do for adults:

- Rapid trauma assessment and physical exam (patient with significant mechanism of injury [MOI]): check ABCs first, with in-line stabilization of the head and spine; inspect and palpate each body area; get baseline vital signs; and, if possible, get a history.
- Rapid medical assessment and physical exam (unstable): perform any medical interventions, such as open and clear airway, ventilate, start CPR; inspect and palpate the complaint area; get a history or as much information as possible about the events leading to the illness; get baseline vital signs.

If you decide from your general impression of the child that she is responding or acting normally, then perform the following types of focused assessment:

- Focused history and physical exam (trauma patient with no significant MOI): find out the chief complaint, or what hurts; inspect and palpate the area; get baseline vital signs; get a history that focuses on events that caused the injury and the injury itself.
- Focused history and physical exam (stable medical patient): find out the chief complaint, or the nature of illness (NOI); get a history of or information on the events leading up to the illness and the illness itself; focus your physical exam on the area of complaint, or inspect and palpate the part of the body involved; get baseline vital signs.

To help you remember all the questions to ask while you are getting a history, use the SAMPLE memory aid that you learned in Chapter 7.

Detailed Physical Exam

Now that you know from the focused assessment what is wrong with the child, you may have time during transport (or while waiting for EMTs or ALS) to perform a more detailed physical exam. This exam will be very similar to what you do for the adult. The head-to-toe assessment that you perform on adults is usually reversed, though, and performed in toe-to-head order when you examine the alert but frightened or crying infant or young child. This reverse order will give the child an opportunity to get used to you and your touch if he or she has not done so during the short focused assessment.

In a medical situation, the child can be examined in more detail from toe-to-head while in the parent's lap or while being held by someone else the child knows well. In a nonsignificant trauma situation, you can again let the parent or other known adult help comfort the child while you begin your detailed toe-to-head physical exam. Always explain to the child and parent what you are doing and make sure that both understand. Most young children are used to being dressed and undressed and examined by their doctors and will not be embarrassed. As they get older, children are more modest and have learned that strangers should not touch them. Adolescents are concerned about body changes and wonder if they are normal. Remove or rearrange only the necessary clothing during your exam. Then replace it when you have examined that part of the body.

For significant trauma or medical situations that require a rapid assessment, the child is usually unresponsive, unconscious, or too critically injured or ill to know or care where you start your assessment. Stabilize the head and neck before you reposition the head to check ABCs in a trauma case, then follow the steps described above.

The Ongoing Assessment

You are never finished with your patient until she or he has been turned over to an equal or higher level of medical care. This means that when you finish your detailed assessment, you will start again. This is called the ongoing assessment, and it will continue until the EMTs arrive or until you reach the hospital. The status of a child can change rapidly and frequently, so you will need to reassess mental status, maintain airway, monitor breathing, check pulse, and reevaluate skin color, temperature, and moisture. Take and record vital signs every 5 minutes for unstable patients and every 15 minutes for stable patients. Continue to monitor effects of interventions, provide appropriate care, and give emotional support.

MANAGING SPECIFIC MEDICAL EMERGENCIES

Many of the specific medical emergencies listed here have been described in detail in other chapters. Much of the care you will provide to infants and children is similar to what you would provide to adults.

Respiratory Emergencies

Airway Obstruction You learned the signs and symptoms and the management of partial and complete airway obstruction for pediatric patients in Chapter 6. You should continue to review and practice recognizing the signs and symptoms of airway problems and performing the steps of airway care during and after your training. This will enable you to act quickly to assure an open airway and adequate breathing for all patients. Since the steps of relieving an obstructed airway in infants are different than for adults, you should practice the steps of back blows and chest thrusts frequently so that you can perform them quickly and effectively. Remember the following important points: *Never* perform a blind finger sweep on an infant or a child and *never* perform abdominal thrusts on an infant.

Difficulty Breathing A simple cold can cause swelling of the respiratory tract or blocking by mucous secretions. These conditions make it difficult for infants and children to breathe. There are also many more serious types of airway and respiratory infections and conditions that cause airway and breathing problems. Some infants can also have periods in which they do not breathe while sleeping. This condition is called **apnea** and occurs because the respiratory center in the brain does not stimulate adequate respiration during sleep.

Respiratory Infections Two common respiratory infections in infants and children include *croup* and *epiglottitis*. Any infant or child with noisy respiration and a hoarse cough may have croup. **Croup** is an infection caused by a virus and affects the larynx (voice box), trachea, and bronchi. It usually causes the tissues in the upper airway to become swollen, which restricts air flow. In **epiglottitis,** the epiglottis (the flap that closes over the trachea while swallowing) becomes inflamed. The child has difficulty swallowing and will drool. Children

Note

First Responders do not usually receive the indepth training for determining different respiratory illnesses and causes of airway and breathing problems in pediatric patients. This section will list some common causes, cover general signs and symptoms, and describe management of respiratory emergencies in pediatric patients.

apnea (ap-ne-ah) absence of breathing.

croup (CROOP) acute respiratory condition found in infants and children, which is characterized by a barking type of cough or stridor.

epiglottitis (ep-ih-glot-I-tis) swelling of the epiglottis that can be caused by a bacterial infection. It can obstruct the airway and can be potentially life-threatening.

with epiglottitis will also sit upright in a tripod position (leaning forward with arms braced on the edge of the bed or chair) with the chin thrust out and the mouth wide open. You will notice that they will use the muscles in their upper chest and those around their shoulders and neck to breathe. This effort to breathe is very tiring for the child. The First Responder must act quickly; epiglottitis is considered life-threatening.

Because it may be difficult to determine what type of respiratory distress an infant or a child has, consider any airway problem or breathing difficulty an urgent emergency and arrange transport quickly. Provide oxygen as soon as possible by blow-by technique if you cannot get the child to accept a face mask or a nasal cannula. **Do *not* place anything in the mouth, such as a tongue depressor, in an attempt to examine the airway.** Probing the mouth can cause spasms that will further close the airway. Avoid any actions that might agitate or stimulate the child.

First | Signs and symptoms of respiratory distress include the following:

- Wheezing or a high-pitched harsh noise, or grunting
- Exhaling with effort
- Breathing that is faster or slower than normal is inadequate and requires assisted ventilations and oxygen (normal respiratory rates: adolescent—12 to 20; child—15 to 30; infant—25 to 50)
- Straining to use (retraction of) the chest muscles, especially around the neck and shoulders
- The child sitting up and supporting himself in a tripod position
- Drooling
- Nasal flaring
- Cyanosis (late sign)
- Capillary refill of more than 2 seconds (late sign)
- Slow heart rate (late sign)
- Altered mental status (late sign)

Asthma A respiratory condition common to children that can become life-threatening if untreated is asthma. Most children who have asthma are being treated for it and are using a medication or inhaler prescribed by their doctors. Parents or caregivers call for assistance for a child with asthma if the signs and symptoms are new and unfamiliar and do not respond to at-home care, or the children are not responding to the usual prescribed treatment. The signs and symptoms of asthma occur when the small airways in the lungs go into spasm and constrict, or become too narrow for air to pass through. Something the child eats or breathes or some unusual excitement may trigger the attack.

Signs and Symptoms:
- Loud wheezing and breath sounds in a mild attack, becoming less audible as the attack worsens
- Shortness of breath
- Obvious respiratory distress with easy inhalation and forced expiration
- Cough
- Faster than normal breathing rate
- Increased heart rate; faster, weaker pulse
- Sleepiness or slowed response
- Bluish (cyanotic) tint to the skin, especially around the lips and eyes

FIGURE 14.5A
For respiratory distress, provide oxygen with a correctly sized pediatric nonrebreather mask placed on the child or position the mask in front of the child's face for the blow-by technique.

FIGURE 14.5B
For severe distress and respiratory arrest, provide assisted ventilations with a pediatric-sized bag-valve-mask ventilator and supplemental oxygen.

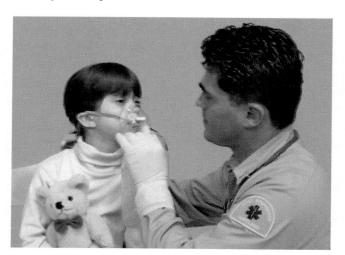

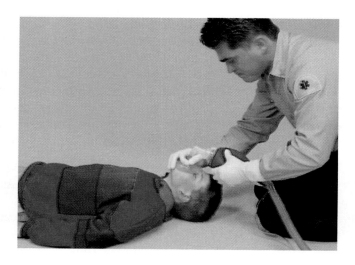

First Responder Care:

- Act calmly and with assurance, which will help calm and reassure the child and the parents or caregiver. For mild attacks, the child will be agitated; for severe attacks, the child will be exhausted and unable or unwilling to move. Signs of sleepiness and slow response mean low oxygen levels.

- Place the child in a sitting position. The child will likely have taken a position of comfort that makes it easy for him to breathe, usually a *tripod* position, leaning forward and bracing himself on his forearms.

- Provide humidified oxygen (follow local protocols). Ask the child to breathe in normally but to blow out air forcefully, as if blowing out the candles on a birthday cake or blowing up a balloon. Show the child how and breathe with him.

- If you are allowed to assist in giving medications, help the parents or caregiver administer the child's medication. Check local protocols and always call for medical direction before assisting a patient with medications (see Appendix 3).

- Have the parents or caregiver contact the child's doctor.

- Transport or arrange for transport by EMT-Bs or ALS. If the signs and symptoms are not relieved with your care steps and the child continues to worsen, call for ALS assistance immediately. A severe and ongoing asthma attack that is not relieved by medication and oxygen may be *status asthmaticus,* a very serious and life-threatening condition.

All respiratory disorders in children must be taken seriously and acted upon immediately. Respiratory distress and low oxygen levels in children are the primary causes of cardiac arrest not related to trauma. In cases of cardiac arrest, call for help. For respiratory distress, provide oxygen by a pediatric-sized nonrebreather mask (Figure 14.5A) or by using the blow-by technique. For severe distress and respiratory arrest, provide assisted ventilations with a pediatric-sized bag-valve-mask ventilator and supplemental oxygen (Figure 14.5B). Always allow the child to assume a comfortable position. The alert child will naturally find the position in which it is easiest to breathe.

Respond to an 11 year-old-boy who is in the school nurse's office with trouble breathing

→

Signs: responsive, rapid pulse and breathing, sitting up-right, leaning forward on his arms, agitated; blood pressure slightly elevated

→

Scene size-up; Initial Assessment; Rapid Medical Assessment

Rapid Medical Assessment (Unstable)

Perform interventions. Follow protocols and/or call for medical direction: provide 100% oxygen (humidified, if possible or as soon as possible) via bag-valve-mask; keep patient as calm as possible; call dispatch for ALS assistance; transport quickly

Pulse and breathing stabilize (within normal range)? Emotional state improves?

NO ↓   ↓ YES

Continue interventions transport by ALS

Is child able to give history?

NO ↓   ↓ YES

Get history from nurse/family   Get history from patient

S - signs and symptoms (How long has child been wheezing?)
A - allergies (Any known allergies to drugs, food, pollens, inhalants, pet dander?)
M - medications (Does he have an inhaler for asthma attacks, has he used it, how frequently?)
P - pertinent past history (Has he had a recent cold or respiratory infection?)
L - last meal/food eaten (Has he had any fluids since this attack started?)
E - events leading to calling 911 (What was he doing or exposed to that may have caused the attack?)

Take baseline vital signs; repeat every 5 minutes

Perform detailed exam (toe-to-head, if necessary) and ongoing assessment

Hand off to EMTs, ALS, ED personnel; complete reports; prepare for next response

Seizures

First | We usually think of a seizure as an episode of uncontrolled shaking that a person with epilepsy will have. A seizure will cause a sudden change in sensation, behavior, or movement. The more severe forms of seizure cause violent muscle contractions called *convulsions*. Seizures may be the result of high fever, epilepsy, infections, poisoning, hypoglycemia, head injury. They may also occur when the brain does not receive enough oxygen because of inadequate blood circulation (shock) or inadequate oxygen in the blood. In some cases, there is no known cause. Many children suffer seizures, but they are rarely life-threatening. Seizures caused by fever (febrile seizures) should be taken seriously.

In many cases, a patient's seizures have stopped before the emergency responders arrive. After a seizure, it is normal for children to be either lethargic (drowsy) and difficult to arouse, or they may be agitated and combative. Look for signs of illness or injury and question the child or family about symptoms. Also get the following information. Ask:

- Has the child had prior seizures? How long did they last? What part of the body was affected?
- Has the child had a fever?
- Has the child had an injury or fall in which the head may have been struck?
- Is the child taking any medications, specifically medication for seizures?

Any child who has had a seizure must have a medical evaluation. Arrange to transport as soon as possible. In the meantime, provide the following emergency care steps:

1. Maintain an open airway and insert nothing in the mouth.
2. Look for evidence of injury suffered during the seizure.
3. If you do *not* suspect spinal injury, position the child on his side.
4. Be alert for vomiting.
5. Provide oxygen or assisted ventilations with supplemental oxygen.
6. Monitor breathing and altered mental status.

Altered Mental Status

Any medical or trauma emergency that affects the brain can cause altered mental status. Some emergencies that can cause altered mental status include hypoglycemia, poisoning, infection, head injury, decreased oxygen levels, shock, or the period after a seizure. As you assess the child, note the mechanism of injury or nature of illness, which will give clues to causes of the child's mental status. Look for signs of poisoning (ingested, inhaled, or absorbed) and ask family members or teachers if there is a history of diabetes or seizure disorder. Take and monitor vital signs, which indicate shock as a cause. While observing and examining the child, you may notice signs of sleepiness, confusion, agitation, or listlessness.

As you gather information, begin the following emergency care steps:

1. Assure an open airway, but protect the spine in cases of trauma; ventilate, if necessary, with a pocket face mask.
2. Provide oxygen as soon as possible by nonrebreather mask, or assist ventilations with a bag-valve-mask ventilator and supplemental oxygen.
3. Place the patient in the recovery position.
4. Treat for shock.
5. Arrange to transport as soon as possible.

Shock

Shock is discussed in Chapter 11. Common causes of shock in infants and children include losing large amounts of fluid from diarrhea and vomiting, blood loss, and abdominal injuries and other trauma. Though not as common, shock can also be caused by allergic reactions and poisoning and, rarely, by cardiac related problems.

The child's body can compensate for shock for a long time, but the body's compensating mechanisms can suddenly fail. This failure is called *decompensated shock*. It occurs when the body can no longer try to function or compensate for low blood volume or lack of perfusion. When a child goes into the decompensated shock stage, signs and symptoms of shock can develop rapidly. In the adult, shock typically develops more gradually, and the signs tend to be easier to recognize. In the child, you must suspect and anticipate shock and begin caring for it immediately, even before you see definite signs of it (Figure 14.6).

First | Following are signs and symptoms of shock:

- Rapid heart and respiratory rate (Both heart rate and respiratory rate will reflect the course of shock.)
- Weak or absent pulse
- Delayed capillary refill
- Decreased urine output (information from parents), which indicates dehydration
- Altered mental status
- Pale, cool, clammy skin

Provide the following care in your management of the sick or injured infant or child who has evidence of shock:

1. Assure an open airway, but protect the spine in cases of trauma; provide ventilations through a pocket face mask if necessary.
2. Provide oxygen by nonrebreather mask or assist ventilations by bag-valve-mask ventilator with supplemental oxygen.
3. Control any bleeding and dress wounds.
4. Elevate the legs if there is no trauma or spinal injury.

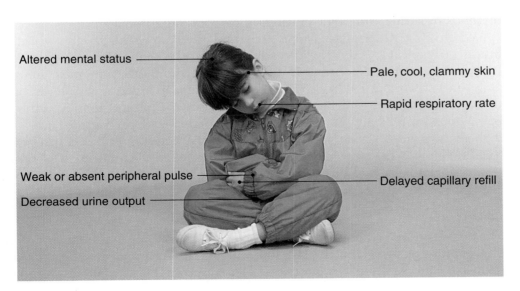

FIGURE 14.6
Signs of shock in an infant or a child.

Altered mental status

Pale, cool, clammy skin

Rapid respiratory rate

Weak or absent peripheral pulse

Decreased urine output

Delayed capillary refill

CARE FOR DEVELOPING SHOCK—PEDIATRIC PATIENTS

```
        Signs                          ┌─────────────────────────┐
        and          YES               │ Ensure open airway      │
      symptoms  ─────────────────┐     └───────────┬─────────────┘
      of shock                   │                 ▼
          │                      │     ┌─────────────────────────┐
          │ NO                   └────▶│ Protect spine—stabilize │
          ▼                            │ head                    │
┌──────────────────┐                   └───────────┬─────────────┘
│ Care for shock;  │                               ▼
│ monitor vital    │                   ┌─────────────────────────┐
│ signs            │                   │ Provide oxygen; assist  │
└────────┬─────────┘                   │ ventilations as needed  │
         ▼                             └───────────┬─────────────┘
┌──────────────────┐                               ▼
│ Arrange for      │                   ┌─────────────────────────┐
│ transport ASAP   │                   │ Elevate legs only if no │
└──────────────────┘                   │ spinal injury or trauma │
                                       └───────────┬─────────────┘
                                                   ▼
                                       ┌─────────────────────────┐
                                       │ Maintain body           │
                                       │ temperature             │
                                       └───────────┬─────────────┘
                                                   ▼
                                       ┌─────────────────────────┐
                                       │ Arrange for transport   │
                                       │ ASAP                    │
                                       └───────────┬─────────────┘
                                                   ▼
                                       ┌─────────────────────────┐
                                       │ Monitor ABCs and vital  │
                                       │ signs                   │
                                       └───────────┬─────────────┘
                                                   ▼
                                       ┌─────────────────────────┐
                                       │ Continue any care       │
                                       │ procedures              │
                                       └─────────────────────────┘
```

5. Maintain body warmth but do not overheat.

6. Arrange to transport as soon as possible.

7. While waiting for EMTs to arrive or en route, continue to monitor airway, breathing, and vital signs and continue any treatments.

Sudden Infant Death Syndrome (SIDS)

Sudden infant death syndrome (SIDS) is the sudden unexplained death during sleep of an apparently healthy baby in his or her first year of life. SIDS, which claims thousands of infants each year, can happen to infants who are receiving proper care and have just passed physical exams. Possible causes and theories are still being investigated. It is known that SIDS is not caused by external methods of suffocation, by vomiting, or by choking.

When First Responders arrive, they may see distraught parents with their infant in respiratory and cardiac arrest during the scene size-up. Since First Responders cannot determine if the infant suffered SIDS, they must immediately start treatment as they would for any patient in arrest. Provide resuscitation and arrange transport to the hospital. Assure the parents that everything is being done for the baby. Normally, First Responders will not begin resuscitation if there is obvious *rigor mortis* (stiffening of the body) or if blood has pooled (*lividity*) along whatever side of the child was lying on the mattress. Check with your instructor to find out what your protocols suggest for this situation. In either case, be sure to provide emotional support to the parents.

Fever

The body's normal response to many childhood diseases and infections is a high temperature or fever. But the rise in body temperature may also be caused by heat exposure or by a noninfectious disease problem. The parents probably monitored their child's temperature and can report the temperature readings taken before you arrived. Try to find out what caused the fever, how high it is, and how rapidly it rose. Most people think a fever is dangerous and a high fever will cause a seizure. Children can usually tolerate high fevers well. Increased temperature is not necessarily what causes a seizure; it is the rapid rise in body temperature that does.

A fever with a rash, with long bouts of diarrhea and vomiting, with little intake of fluids, or one that rose rapidly with or without seizure are all indications that a potentially serious medical condition may be present. Call for EMTs or ALS and arrange for transport as soon as possible.

It is not necessary to try taking a temperature. It will take time on the scene and likely agitate the child. An agitated child can be injured by an oral or a rectal thermometer. You may use one of the skin thermometers if you carry them. If the skin feels very warm to touch, report this finding along with skin color and condition. A child with a high fever will likely be flushed and dry. A mild fever may quickly elevate to a high fever and become a life-threatening problem. Arrange to transport immediately.

PEDIATRIC PATIENT WITH FEVER

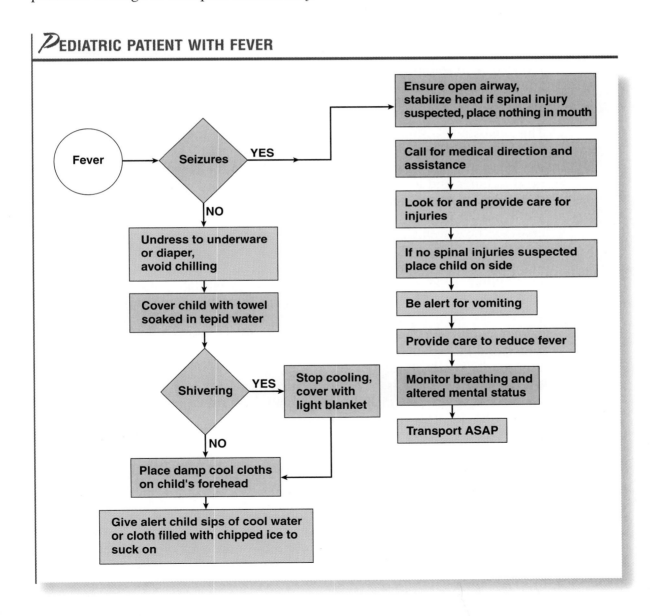

While you are waiting for the EMTs or en route to the hospital, take the following steps if your local protocols allow:

- **DO** undress the child down to underwear or diaper but do *not* allow him to become chilled. Many parents still believe that feverish children must be bundled up so they will not become chilled or so they will sweat out the fever. All this clothing retains the heat of the fever. Place a light blanket around the undressed child if he starts to shiver.
- **DO** cover the child with a towel soaked in tepid (not cold) water if the fever is the result of heat exposure. If the child starts to shiver, stop the cooling process and cover with a light blanket.
- **DO** place damp, cool cloths on the fevered child's hot forehead.
- **DO** give sips of cool water, but *only* if the child is alert and cooperative. Let the child suck on a cloth filled with chipped ice, or, if old enough, suck directly on chipped ice.
- **DO** transport any child who has had a seizure. If the child is seizing, monitor airway and breathing.
- **NEVER** submerge the child in cold water.
- **NEVER** use rubbing alcohol for cooling. It can be absorbed in toxic amounts through the child's skin.

Be cautious about cooling a fevered child. You can cause hypothermia or reduced body temperature. Wet towels and sheets cool rapidly and become cold, which causes the child to shiver and become chilled.

Hypothermia

The opposite extreme of fever (hyperthermia) is total body cooling (hypothermia). Children lose a lot of body heat through their heads. The surface area of the child's head is proportionately larger than the rest of the body. The large head radiates and loses heat when it is uncovered. When the head is exposed, the body will make every effort to keep the brain warm and functioning, so it sends heat from other parts of the body to the head. Since the child cannot conserve heat well, it will not take long to use up any reserves and develop hypothermia. Keep the head covered to prevent heat loss when caring for infants and children in cool environments.

Children have a proportionately larger body surface area for their weight than adults do, and their bodies are unable to regulate temperatures as adult bodies can. Most children do not have much fat stored under their skin and cannot conserve heat. They can become chilled through the environment, injury, and illness such as:

- Exposure to cool weather and water
- Damp or wet clothes, or removal of clothes for medical evaluation
- Alcohol or drugs, which dilate peripheral vessels
- Low blood sugar (hypoglycemia)
- Brain disorders or head trauma that affect the temperature regulation mechanism of the body
- Severe infection
- Shock

When you look for mechanism of injury or try to determine nature of illness, also think about conditions that may cause overheating or overcooling of the child. In a hot environment, cool the child by undressing or using damp cloths; in a cold environment, warm the child by stripping off wet clothes and by wrapping him in a blanket. Be sure the head is covered.

Diarrhea and Vomiting

The child can lose large amounts of needed body fluids through vomiting and diarrhea, which are normal reactions to illness (and sometimes to certain ingested poisons). This fluid loss is called **dehydration.** Infants are more susceptible to dehydration than adults are because the infant has such a small circulating blood volume to start with. For example, think about losing one cup of fluid during an illness. This would be insignificant to an adult, whereas the total circulating blood volume in a newborn is only a cup and a half.

dehydration excessive loss of body water.

Suspect that a child is dehydrated if he has been feverish for some time, if he has been vomiting without taking in any fluids, or if he has had diarrhea for several days. As the child loses fluids through vomiting and diarrhea and cannot replace them, the fluid balance in the body is disturbed. A balance of fluids in to fluids out is needed to maintain muscle and organ function. Shock can result when large amounts of fluids are lost, even if the fluid is not blood.

If you suspect a child is dehydrated, do the following:

1. Monitor the airway.
2. Position the child so the airway will not be obstructed if the child vomits. (Positioning can also prevent vomitus from getting in the lungs.) Children who are alert will generally protect the airway regardless of position.
3. Monitor respirations and provide blow-by oxygen.
4. Check vital signs. If they indicate shock, arrange to transport immediately.
5. If protocols permit and the child is conscious and alert, allow the child to sip water or suck on chipped ice.
6. If possible, save some vomitus for hospital personnel to examine.

Poisoning

Part of a child's learning experience includes exploring and tasting things. This can sometimes lead to exposure to or ingestion of poisonous substances. Poisons can affect any or all of the body's systems and can rapidly threaten the life of the child. Review the material on poisoning in Chapter 10. Much of your assessment and care will be the same as for an adult. Know your local protocols for contacting medical direction or the poison control center if there is any indication or suspicion that a child has been exposed to a poison. Be aware that some poisons may be considered hazardous materials, and these situations will require response by personnel trained to handle these materials—a hazmat team. The hazmat team will perform decontamination procedures.

Near-Drowning

The child who has been submerged in water may still be alive or clinically dead (no breathing and heartbeat), but not biologically dead (brain cells are still alive). The child has not drowned but is considered a near-drowning victim. Many patients have been revived after over 30 minutes of submersion in cold water. Children have been successfully revived more often than adults in these situations. Review management of the water emergency patient in Appendix 4. When caring for a near-drowning patient:

1. Make sure the airway is clear and free of fluids.
2. Provide artificial ventilations or CPR as necessary.
3. Protect the spine in cases where the near-drowning was the result of a diving or boating accident.
4. Get the patient to a warm and dry environment away from wind to prevent or care for hypothermia. Remove wet clothing.

5. Place the child in the recovery position to prevent aspiration; provide high-concentration oxygen (follow local protocols).

6. Arrange to transport all near-drowning patients even if they have recovered and are breathing on their own. It is possible that they will deteriorate hours after they have "recovered."

*M*ANAGING TRAUMA EMERGENCIES

General Care of the Child Trauma Patient

Because of their size, curiosity, and a lack of fear due to their inexperience, infants and children are frequent victims of trauma. It is the number-one cause of death in people 1–18 years of age, usually as the result of motor vehicle accidents, drowning, burns, firearms, falls, blunt and penetrating trauma, abuse, entrapment, crushing, and various other mechanisms of injury.

When performing the physical exam on the responsive child who is stable, you can reverse your assessment order and do a toe-to-head physical exam. For unresponsive patients, perform the head-to-toe assessment. For unstable patients, focus on the ABCs and determine priority of transport.

When managing injuries in children, keep in mind that their larger head size and weight will make them more prone to head and neck trauma in motor vehicle collisions, especially if unrestrained. This is also true of bicycle mishaps if children are not wearing helmets, in accidents in which they are struck, in swimming and diving accidents, and in sports accidents. First Responders should suspect abdominal and pelvic injuries in vehicle accidents in which the child is restrained, and extremity injuries in falls of three times their height or greater. Consider differences in child anatomy and adult anatomy when assessing and caring for children.

 General emergency care steps for the infant or child trauma patient include the following steps:

1. Assure an open airway. Stabilize the head and use a jaw-thrust maneuver to protect the spine.

2. Assure that the airway is clear. Suction if local protocols allow. Provide ventilations with a pocket face mask if necessary.

3. Provide oxygen by nonrebreather mask or assist ventilations with a bag-valve-mask ventilator with supplemental oxygen.

4. Control bleeding by applying appropriate dressings.

5. Stabilize injuries to painful, swollen, deformed extremities.

6. Immobilize the spine if you have the equipment and are trained to use it; otherwise, stabilize the patient (keep him still) until EMTs or ALS arrive.

7. Arrange for transport as soon as possible.

8. While waiting for the EMTs to arrive or en route, perform your detailed and ongoing assessments.

Safety Seats

Based on crash result studies over recent years, it has been determined that removing children from their safety seats and immobilizing them on spine boards is the best procedure for children involved in vehicle crashes. The National Safe Kids Campaign is working to promote this change for the following reasons based on crash studies:

- Too many safety seats are not installed properly, and children are often not secured properly by the safety straps and harnesses. Any movement of the seat or the child in the seat throws both forward in a crash. The child receives internal injuries, which emergency care providers may not be able to initially detect. The child compensates for these internal injuries and bleeding, which lulls the rescuers into thinking the child is unharmed and stable. On the way to the hospital, the child suddenly gets worse, or rapidly decompensates.

- First Responders and other emergency care providers cannot adequately provide airway management care, maintain an open airway, or provide bag-valve-mask resuscitation on a child who is immobilized in a safety seat.

- The child's torso in a safety seat is in a flexed position because the seat is designed that way. Spinal immobilization straightens and extends the spine from the cervical spine (the neck) to the sacrum (the part of the spine between the hip bones). Leaving the child in a safety seat continues to stretch the spine in a curved position rather than in a straight, extended position.

- If the infant or small child of any age is riding in the forward-facing position, the crash forces likely caused the child's body to flex forward extremely (hyperflexion), especially if the seat was installed improperly or the harness securing the child was too loose. This sudden forward flexion causes injury to the cervical spine.

- Children up to age 4 and up to 40 pounds may be too large for their child safety seat to support the head and protect them properly. If the child's head extends above the top edge of the seat back, the head may hyperextend (be forced extremely backward) in a crash. At the same time, the body is thrust forward. All this sudden and extreme motion stretches the ligaments and muscles of the spinal column, causing severe injuries.

- The safety seat involved in a vehicle crash (especially an improperly installed one) is likely to be damaged, though the damage may not be noticed even on close inspection. A damaged seat will not adequately immobilize and support the child. Further, manufacturers state that child safety seats *are not designed to be used as immobilizing devices*. Using the safety seat for purposes other than the manufacturer intended places the liability for further patient injury on emergency care providers.

- Safety seats cannot be properly secured in the ambulance. Further, if the ambulance is involved in a collision en route to the hospital, the safety seat cannot endure the forces of another crash. There are enough reports of ambulance crashes while en route to the hospital with patients to cause concern. A second crash may further weaken the effectiveness of the safety seat and leave the child, who is immobilized in it, unprotected.

The mechanism of injury, the vehicle involved in a crash, should lead you to suspect that the child has been injured, even if you do not see any damage to the safety seat. Carefully extricate the child from the safety seat onto a spinal immobilization device if local protocols allow First Responders to do so (and if you have been trained in the procedures). If not, then until other EMS providers arrive, maintain manual stabilization of the child's head in neutral alignment and assure an open airway.

There are many types of child safety seats, but each provides the same safety functions if properly used. First Responders should not hesitate to act to

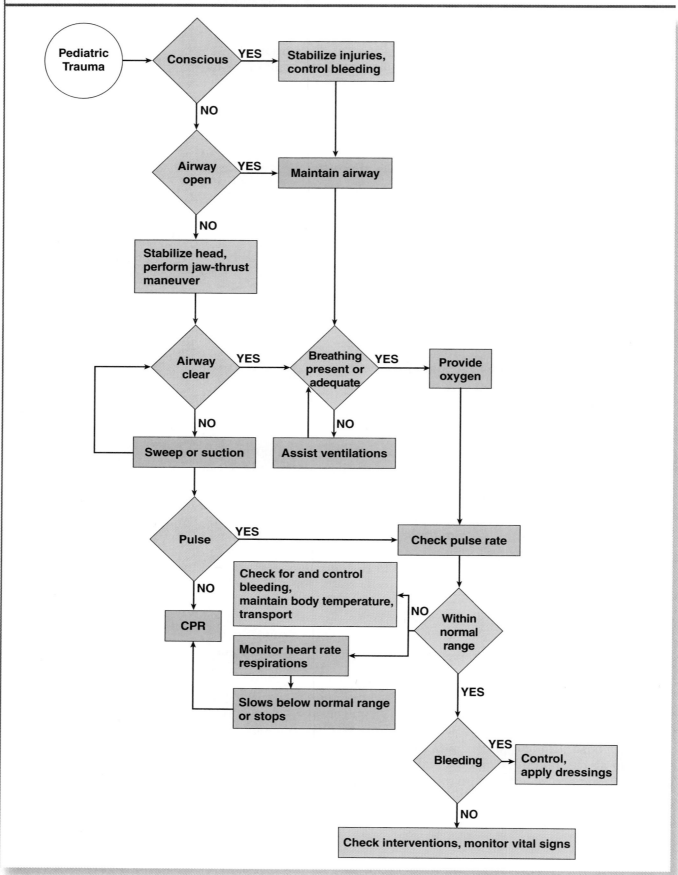

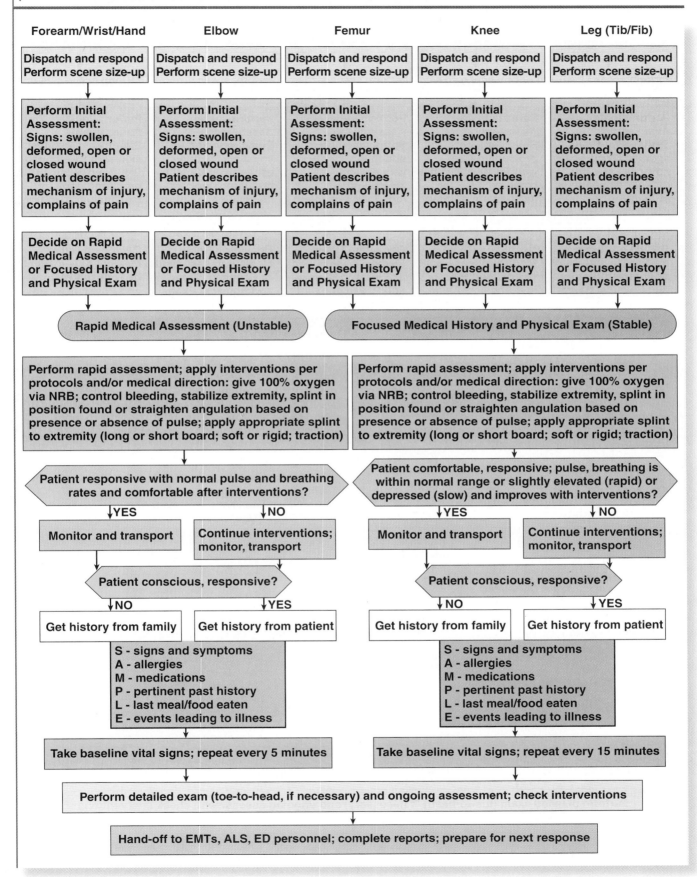

Forearm/Wrist/Hand	Elbow	Femur	Knee	Leg (Tib/Fib)

Dispatch and respond Perform scene size-up

Perform Initial Assessment: Signs: swollen, deformed, open or closed wound Patient describes mechanism of injury, complains of pain

Decide on Rapid Medical Assessment or Focused History and Physical Exam

Rapid Medical Assessment (Unstable) — **Focused Medical History and Physical Exam (Stable)**

Perform rapid assessment; apply interventions per protocols and/or medical direction: give 100% oxygen via NRB; control bleeding, stabilize extremity, splint in position found or straighten angulation based on presence or absence of pulse; apply appropriate splint to extremity (long or short board; soft or rigid; traction)

Patient responsive with normal pulse and breathing rates and comfortable after interventions?

↓YES — **Monitor and transport**
↓NO — **Continue interventions; monitor, transport**

Patient conscious, responsive?
↓NO — **Get history from family**
↓YES — **Get history from patient**

S - signs and symptoms
A - allergies
M - medications
P - pertinent past history
L - last meal/food eaten
E - events leading to illness

Take baseline vital signs; repeat every 5 minutes

Patient comfortable, responsive; pulse, breathing is within normal range or slightly elevated (rapid) or depressed (slow) and improves with interventions?

↓YES — **Monitor and transport**
↓NO — **Continue interventions; monitor, transport**

Patient conscious, responsive?
↓NO — **Get history from family**
↓YES — **Get history from patient**

S - signs and symptoms
A - allergies
M - medications
P - pertinent past history
L - last meal/food eaten
E - events leading to illness

Take baseline vital signs; repeat every 15 minutes

Perform detailed exam (toe-to-head, if necessary) and ongoing assessment; check interventions

Hand-off to EMTs, ALS, ED personnel; complete reports; prepare for next response

PEDIATRIC BLEEDING, SOFT-TISSUE INJURIES, AND SHOCK

Arterial Bleeding	Impaled Object	Evisceration	Pneumothorax	Shock
Dispatch and respond	Dispatch and respond	Dispatch and respond	Dispatch and respond	Dispatch and respond
Perform scene size-up	Perform scene size-up	Perform scene size-up	Perform scene size-up	Perform scene size-up
Perform Initial Assessment: Signs: bright red, spurting blood, heavy flow from wound; look for mechanism of injury	Perform Initial Assessment: Signs: object protruding from wound; may be some bleeding; look for mechanism of injury	Perform Initial Assessment: Signs: opening to abdominal cavity with organs protruding; look for mechanism of injury	Perform Initial Assessment: Signs: opening in chest wall with air escaping, difficulty breathing; look for mechanism of injury	Perform Initial Assessment: Signs: cold, clammy skin with pale/bluish tint, rapid pulse and breathing; look for mechanism of injury
Decide on Rapid Medical Assessment or Focused History and Physical Exam	Decide on Rapid Medical Assessment or Focused History and Physical Exam	Decide on Rapid Medical Assessment or Focused History and Physical Exam	Decide on Rapid Medical Assessment or Focused History and Physical Exam	Decide on Rapid Medical Assessment or Focused History and Physical Exam

Rapid Medical Assessment (Unstable)

Focused Medical History and Physical Exam (Stable)

Perform interventions. Follow protocols and/or call for medical direction: give 100% oxygen via NRB; control bleeding, stabilize object, manage chest or abdominal wound with appropriate dressing; position patient appropriately for wound (torso elevated or flat, legs flexed or straight, patient on injured side)

Perform interventions. Follow protocols and/or call for medical direction: give 100% oxygen via NRB; control bleeding, stabilize object, manage chest or abdominal wound with appropriate dressing; position patient appropriately for wound (torso elevated or flat, legs flexed or straight, patient on injured side)

Patient responsive with normal pulse and breathing rates?

Patient comfortable, responsive; pulse, breathing is within normal range or slightly elevated (rapid) or depressed (slow) and improves with interventions?

YES → Monitor and transport
NO → Continue interventions; monitor, transport

YES → Monitor and transport
NO → Continue interventions; monitor, transport

Patient Conscious?

Patient Conscious?

NO → Get history from family
YES → Get history from patient

NO → Get history from family
YES → Get history from patient

S - signs and symptoms
A - allergies
M - medications
P - pertinent past history
L - last meal/food eaten
E - events leading to illness

S - signs and symptoms
A - allergies
M - medications
P - pertinent past history
L - last meal/food eaten
E - events leading to illness

Take baseline vital signs; repeat every 5 minutes

Take baseline vital signs; repeat every 15 minutes

Perform detailed exam (toe-to-head), if necessary) and ongoing assessment; check interventions

Hand-off to EMTs, ALS, ED personnel; complete reports; prepare for next response

immobilize and provide initial airway care for a child, even if they are not familiar with the safety seat they find at a crash site. Use the following guidelines if you must extricate an infant or a child from a safety seat, but do *not* perform these steps unless you have learned and practiced them under the supervision of your instructor:

- Throughout the assessment and immobilization process, be sure that someone maintains manual stabilization of the infant's or child's head.
- Assess the infant or child for airway, breathing, and circulation. Assess for injuries.
- If the safety seat has a protection plate over the infant's chest, remove it (cut the straps securing it if necessary) so you can assess the chest area and provide care, such as lung assessment and chest compressions.
- As you assess the patient, also check for loose straps, which would have provided little protection. Do a quick visual inspection of the vehicle interior: Did the crash force the safety seat from its position, even slightly? Was the safety seat in the rear or front vehicle seat? Was the safety seat a rear-facing or forward-facing seat? Is there structural damage to the seat?
- Extricate the child onto an immobilization device, which can then be secured to the ambulance stretcher (see Scan 14-2).

Pneumatic Antishock Garments

Check with your instructor to see if your jurisdiction allows First Responders to become trained in using pneumatic antishock garments (PASGs) for stabilizing pelvic injuries in pediatric patients. If so, your instructor will provide you with the equipment and training. Be aware that the use of PASG in pediatrics is controversial regarding both proper fit and respiratory compromise; check your local protocols.

Burns

Refer to the information in Chapter 11. Pay particular attention to the *rule of nines* for estimating body surface area burned in infants and children. The figures are slightly different for children than adults. If you find it is hard to figure body surface area burned with any accuracy while you are trying to quickly care for and stabilize the patient, do not worry about precision. The safest procedure is to estimate quickly and overestimate rather than underestimate the body surface area burned. The younger the child, the more important it is that he or she is seen in a burn center because of concerns about abuse and long-term morbidity.

Carefully and quickly care for the burned area with dry, sterile, and nonadherent dressings or sheets. Dry dressings will keep air and foreign materials or dirt off the burn and will help keep the child warm, which will help in preventing shock. Moist dressings may chill the child and could speed the shock response. Follow local protocols for burn management. Arrange to transport the burned child as quickly as possible. Check local protocols for determining the type of cases (degree of seriousness, respiratory burns) that should be transported to a burn center. Burns are excruciatingly painful, and children are likely to be frantic. Rapid transport is important for obtaining pain relief for the child as well as for care of the burns.

Rapid Extrication from a Child Safety Seat

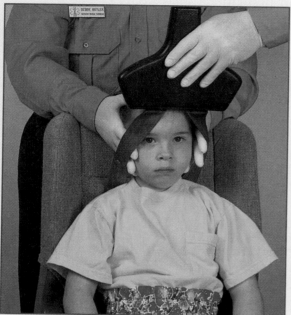

1. First Responder #1 stabilizes car seat in upright position and applies manual head/neck stabilization. First Responder #2 prepares equipment, then loosens or cuts the seat straps and raises the front guard.

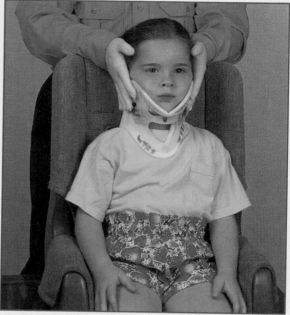

2. Cervical collar is applied to patient as First Responder #1 maintains manual stabilization of the head and neck.

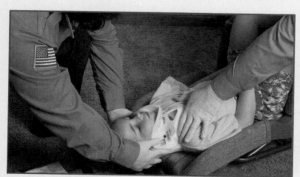

3. As First Responder #1 maintains manual head/neck stabilization, First Responder #2 places child safety seat on center of backboard and slowly tilts it into supine position. Both First Responders are careful not to let the child slide out of the chair. For the child with a large head, place a towel under area where the shoulders will eventually be placed on the board to prevent head from tilting forward.

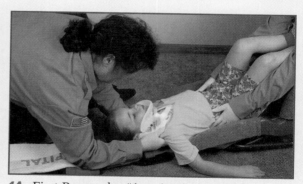

4A. First Responder #1 maintains manual head/neck stabilization and calls for a coordinated long axis move onto the backboard.

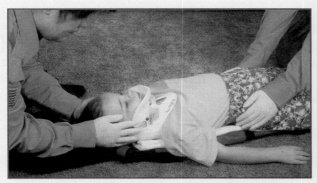

4B. First Responder #1 maintains manual head/neck stabilization as move onto board is completed, with the child's shoulders over the folded towel.

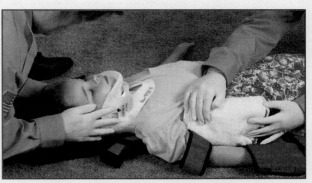

5. First Responder #1 maintains manual head/neck stabilization. First Responder #2 places rolled towels or blankets on both sides of the patient.

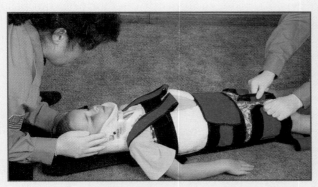

6. First Responder #1 maintains manual head/neck stabilization. First Responder #2 straps or tapes patient to board at level of upper chest, pelvis, and lower legs. **Do not strap across abdomen.**

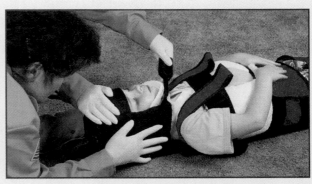

7. First Responder #1 maintains manual head/neck stabilization as First Responder #2 places rolled towels on both sides of head, then tapes head securely in place across forehead and maxilla (jaw bone) or cervical collar. **Do not tape across chin to avoid putting pressure on neck.**

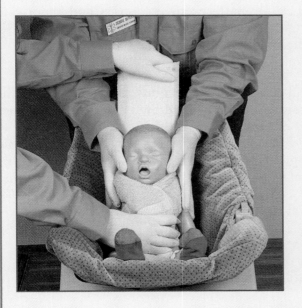

The infant procedure is exactly the same as for a child, except that an armboard is inserted behind the infant in step 2. If the infant is very small, the armboard may actually be used as the spine board.

SUSPECTED NEGLECT AND ABUSE

The news media have been reporting more stories of child neglect and abuse in recent years. These events are not something new; rather, they have always existed but are now more recognized and reported. A child abuse or neglect situation is one of the most difficult emergency situations for the First Responder to handle. It is normal to experience some very strong emotions that you must control in order to assess and care for the child. After the call, it is important to talk out your feelings with those who can offer support and understanding. Remember to maintain patient confidentiality. You cannot name the child or family to anyone but medical or juvenile authorities or the police.

First There are several different forms of child abuse, and these frequently occur in combination:

- Psychological or emotional abuse ("You're stupid," or "no good," or "not like your sister.")
- Neglect (withholding supervision, food, or appropriate clothing; not assuring that the child attends school or receives appropriate medical care)
- Physical abuse (beatings, shakings, burns with cigarettes or other hot objects)
- Sexual abuse (usually from a parent or other relative, sometimes from a neighbor, teacher, or other "trusted" individual)

Emergency response is usually for the obvious physical traumas that occur in physical and sexual abuse, although long-term neglect may result in physical injury or medical problems. On arrival, your scene size-up may reveal obvious signs of neglect, which you should report to EMTs providing transport, to the hospital staff, or to medical direction. In most jurisdictions, there is an obligation to report suspected child abuse. Be aware of your local laws regarding such reporting.

You must collect information, make your assessments, and provide care without making a judgment or expressing your suspicion, distaste, or disbelief. Keep in mind that the abuser also needs help. Also keep in mind that your suspicions may be unfounded and that not every injury to a child is the result of abuse. You will need to check for patterns in responses and reports to confirm your suspicions. Report your concerns to the appropriate authorities, but do not convey them to the family or onlookers at the scene.

Sexual Abuse

Do not expect that the abuser will admit that sexual abuse is the reason for the call. Many excuses and reasons are given for the child who has genital injuries or who has signs and symptoms of sexually transmitted diseases. Continue to act professionally and control your emotions. When providing care, avoid embarrassing the child or making him or her feel guilty. Let the child know that you and the people at the hospital will help. Some signs indicating sexual abuse include:

- Obvious injuries to the genital area, including burns, cuts, bruising, abrasions
- Rashes around the genitals, discharges (such as seminal fluid), bleeding from the genital openings or on underclothing
- Information from the child that indicates he or she was assaulted

First | Be sure to report your suspicions and findings to EMTs or ALS when they arrive or to the medical staff at the hospital. Use these emergency care steps:

1. Dress wounds and provide other appropriate care for injuries.

2. Save any evidence of sexual abuse, such as soiled or stained clothing. Do not let the child use the bathroom to urinate or defecate. If the child must go to the bathroom, try to collect it in a container for hospital examination. Do not let the child drink any fluids or eat anything. Do not wash the child or let the parent wash the child or change clothes.

3. Minimize embarrassment by covering the child with a blanket if necessary.

4. Arrange for transport as soon as possible.

5. Provide emotional support and reassurance. Remember, you are still caring for a child. Try to engage him or her with toys or age-appropriate conversation or games.

PHYSICAL ABUSE

In physical abuse cases, look for the following signs:
- The outline of marks or bruises that are the size or shape of the object used to strike the child, such as the hand, a belt, strap, rope, or cord
- Areas of swelling, black eyes, loose or missing teeth, split lips
- Lacerations, abrasions, incisions

Injuries listed above are often found on the back, legs, and arms and may be in various stages of healing. Also look for:
- Broken bones, signs of old fractures healing incorrectly (misshaped limbs), or a history of numerous fractures
- Head injuries, skull fractures, or indications of closed head injuries that could be the result of violent shaking (bulging fontanelles, unconsciousness), especially in infants and small children
- Bruises—old and new—in various stages of healing
- Abdominal injuries with signs of bruising, distention, rigidity, or tenderness that could be the result of punching or kicking
- Genitalia injuries with lacerations, avulsions, or bleeding
- Bite marks showing the teeth pattern and size of an adult mouth
- Burn marks or patterns from cigarettes, hot irons, stove burners; water burns or scalding marks on the legs (stocking burns from dipping in hot water) or a hand mark on the buttocks where the skin was protected from immersions when being held while dipped. The creases at the knees and thighs are also protected when the child flexes while being dipped.

The child's relationship with the parents or the parents' attitude toward the situation may be a clue to abuse. Responses will vary and will not always be a reliable indicator of the family relationship. Look for the following:
- A story of how the injury occurred that does not match the injury found
- The child who seems afraid to say how the injury happened
- The child who is obviously afraid of a parent or other person at the scene
- The child who seems to expect no comfort from the parent
- The child who has no apparent reaction to pain
- The parent who does not wish to leave you alone with the child
- The parents who tell conflicting stories or change explanations
- The parent who blames the child for being clumsy or accident-prone

- The parent who seems inappropriately concerned or unconcerned
- The parent who is angry and is having trouble controlling it
- The parent who appears depressed or withdrawn while the other parent is expressing anger or giving explanations
- Any signs of alcohol or drug abuse
- Any expression of suicide or seeking mercy for their children
- The parent who is reluctant to give the child's history or to permit transport or who refuses to go to the nearest hospital

You must be the child's advocate and convince the parents that the child needs to be seen by a doctor because of "the difficulty of determining the seriousness of injuries in the field." Do *not* accuse the parent.

You may respond to a call for an injured child and have no idea that the injury is abuse related. The child and parents relate well and there appears to be a strong bond among them. There are still abuse indications that will make you suspicious over time. Be alert for:

- Repeated responses for the same child
- Signs of past injuries during your assessment
- Signs of poorly healing wounds or fractures
- Signs of burns that are fresh or in various stages of healing
- Many types of injuries on numerous parts of the body

Keep in mind that obvious abuse situations can trigger strong emotions in you. Most people feel it is their duty to protect young children. Your first reactions to an abuse situation may be anger and disgust. However, you should not display these feelings while caring for the child or dealing with the parents or other caregivers. Providing necessary care for the child and alerting the proper authorities about your suspicions are appropriate actions. It also may be necessary for you to get help in dealing with the aftereffects of dealing with child abuse cases.

Summary

Assessment and treatment of infants and children is basically the same as for adults. However, you must consider the special characteristics of the infant's or child's anatomy, physiology, and emotional responses when assessing and caring for children.

For example, to help keep an infant or a child calm, reverse the order of the physical assessment: begin at the toes and work toward the head. Infants and children may also be examined while sitting on a parent's lap.

One example of the child's different anatomy compared to that of the adult's is the head, which is larger and heavier in proportion to the rest of the body in infants and children. Be suspicious of mechanisms of injury that have the potential to cause head and spinal injury. Also, carefully handle the head of an infant up to 18 months so you do not apply any pressure to the soft spots (fontanelles).

Infants will automatically breathe through their nose, and if it is obstructed, they will not open their mouths to breathe. Be sure to clear the nostrils of secretions. Remember also that because the tongue is larger in an infant and a child, it can cause airway obstruction. When managing the airway of an infant, make sure the large head is in a neutral position, neither hyperflexed nor hyperextended.

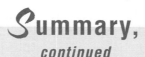

Care for respiratory distress in infants and children immediately. For respiratory distress, provide oxygen with a pediatric-sized nonrebreather mask or by using the blow-by technique. For severe distress and respiratory arrest, provide assisted ventilations with a pediatric-sized bag-valve-mask ventilator and supplemental oxygen. Do not place anything in the mouth of the infant or child unless you see an obstruction. Transport immediately.

Children tolerate high fevers better than adults do, but a fever that rises rapidly can cause seizures. Arrange to transport the feverish child as soon as possible. Also transport the child who is vomiting and has diarrhea.

The surface area of the infant's or child's body is large in proportion to weight. This makes infants and children more vulnerable to hypothermia. Covering the patient, especially the head, will help maintain warmth.

Treat for shock early. Signs and symptoms of shock mean it has progressed and is in late stages in an infant or a child. If you suspect that shock may result from the mechanism of injury or nature of illness, provide emergency care immediately. An infant or a child has less blood than an adult; a relatively small blood loss can be life-threatening.

Because of their size, curiosity, and a lack of fear due to their inexperience, infants and children are frequent victims of trauma. When performing the physical exam on the responsive child who is stable, reverse the assessment order and do a toe-to-head exam. For unresponsive patients, perform the head-to-toe assessment.

Provide care for physical and emotional needs of the child who is suffering from abuse or neglect. Be calm and professional and be discreet about suspicions in the presence of the possible abuser. Be an advocate for the child and remember your obligation to report any suspicions to the proper authorities.

Remember and Consider...

Children are everywhere. We may have our own children or brothers and sisters at home. We see children of all ages going to and coming from school, the playground or ball fields, the mall or movies. They are out in the street chasing balls, or riding bikes and skateboards, or just hanging around. They do chores for their parents and neighbors such as mowing grass, shoveling snow, washing cars; and they help around the house with baby-sitting, cooking, cleaning, and caring for pets. They are curious and daring, and they like to explore, have fun, make fun, taunt, tease, and sometimes get into fights or into situations in which they get hurt. Many falls result in bumps and scrapes that are easy for a parent to care for, but sometimes an illness or injury is serious enough, or frightening enough to the child or parent, that emergency services are needed.

✔ What are some of the types of injuries you expect to see in certain age groups?

✔ What can you do to help calm a crying and frightened child?

Think about the many activities that children are involved in today. How do they compare with what you did as a child? Do children have more opportunities, freedom, and choices of activities today? Do these activities bring a higher potential for illness or injury?

✔ Find out how many pediatric calls your agency had this past year and what types they were. Did the company respond to more illness or injury calls?

With this information, you can get an idea of where you will want to concentrate your learning and practice.

Many emergency care responders are nervous about treating children. It may be because children appear small and helpless, and the care provider is afraid of causing more pain while trying to help. Many children are afraid of strangers, and the care provider will find it hard to communicate with them. This may make you uncomfortable and, as a result, you may not know what to do. This is normal, but you cannot allow it to interfere with your ability to care for these patients. If you never have the opportunity to work with or be around children, of course it is harder to work with them in an emergency. If you have the time to work with children as a baby-sitter, a coach, a camp counselor, or a tutor, you will learn more about their personalities and feel more comfortable working with any child.

Investigate...

✔ Locate the schools and day-care centers in your area.

Find out if the schools have health rooms and school nurses. Are the nurses on duty every day? What does the school or day-care center do when a child is taken seriously ill or is injured? Are parents or emergency services called first? Will you be able to treat or transport a child without a parent present? (Review legal and consent issues in Chapter 3.) Ask other company members to tell you about their experiences.

✔ Locate the ball fields, parks, and playgrounds in your area.

During what seasons are these areas the most populated by children? What sports do they play, who supervises them, and what policies are followed if a child is hurt at an organized game? What injuries would you expect to find at a baseball or softball game; at a field- or ice-hockey game; at a soccer, basketball, or football game? Are the coaches trained in treating sports injuries? If the parents are not at the game, how can they be contacted? Will you care for the child without consent?

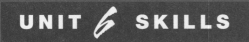
Study the following scenarios. Place check marks in the columns below as appropriate to indicate which skills you would perform for each scenario. You will use skills from previous units in these scenarios. Refer to text pages 1–81, 85–123, 129–178, 183–236, and 241–440. Write the skill number of any skills you would use from Units 1–5 after each scenario and in the column under "Units." Discuss answers with other students and your instructor.

SCENARIO 1:   Ahead on the interstate, you see a car pulled over to the shoulder. As your units gets closer, a man jumps out and frantically waves you down. When you stop, he runs up to the window and says his wife is having a baby. You have your partner notify dispatch while you follow the man to the car. You do a quick scene survey and ask a few questions of the mother: When is your baby due? (Two weeks ago.) How long have you been having labor pains? (Only an hour.) Has your water broken? (Yes.) You notice that her ankles are swollen and she is having trouble breathing. You have your partner call for ALS assistance. ETA in traffic is about 10 minutes. You move the mother to the back seat and prepare for delivery.

(Skills from Unit 1:   _____   Skills from Unit 2:   _____)

(Skills from Unit 3:   _____   Skills from Unit 4:   _____)

(Skills from Unit 5   _____)

SCENARIO 2:   You are behind two cars that are slowing down to carefully maneuver around a boy of about 12 years old who is riding his bike on the shoulder of the road. The boy seems to be having trouble steering over the rough shoulder and suddenly loses control of his bike. He swerves in front of one of the cars, the driver slams on his brakes, but the vehicle still strikes the front wheel of the bike and throws the boy to the rough ground on the side of the road. You position your vehicle to protect the scene, turn on your emergency lights, and report to dispatch. You run up to the child to do an initial assessment and a rapid assessment before calling in for further assistance.

(Skills from Unit 1:   _____   Skills from Unit 2:   _____)

(Skills from Unit 3:   _____   Skills from Unit 4:   _____)

(Skills from Unit 5   _____)

Instructors will demonstrate all skills and will give you time to practice them while they coach you.

Skills	Scenarios		Units				
	#1	#2	#1	#2	#3	#4	#5
Patient assessment (review Unit 1 skills)							
1. Demonstrate the use of BSI; taking vital signs as appropriate; taking SAMPLE history as appropriate							
CPR and airway management (review Unit 2 skills)							
2. Demonstrate CPR techniques on child, infant, neonate							
3. Demonstrate techniques for opening airway, managing airway obstruction, and suctioning							
4. Demonstrate measuring/inserting oropharyngeal and nasopharyngeal airways							
5. Demonstrate ventilation with pocket face mask and bag-valve-mask ventilator							
6. Demonstrate blow-by techniques							
Patient Assessment (review Unit 3 skills)							
7. Demonstrate scene size-up, patient assessment, communication and documentation requirements							
Medical							
8. Demonstrate assistance/administration of Albuterol, epi-pen injector, activated charcoal, ipecac							
Trauma							
9. Demonstrate management of bleeding, shock, soft-tissue injuries							
10. Demonstrate management of fractures							
11. Demonstrate management of head, neck, and spine injuries/immobilization techniques							

Work with a group of classmates to create scenarios that will use listed skills. Exchange them with other class groups to check your knowledge and to practice your decision-making skills.

CHAPTER 15

GAINING ACCESS AND TRIAGE

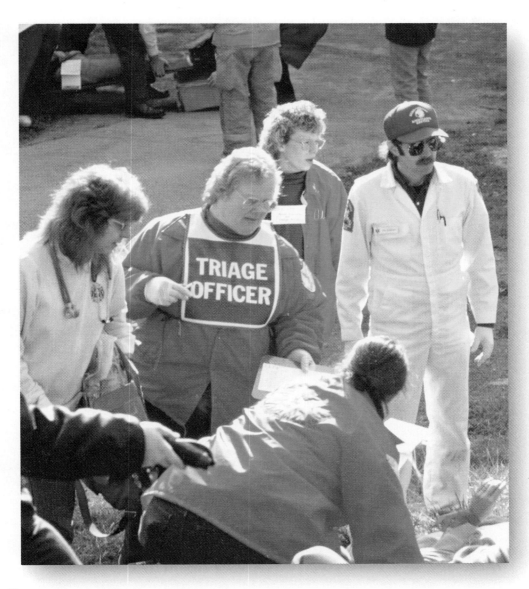

*F*irst Responders are part of a system of emergency services operations that function and respond 24 hours of every day. These continuous operations include a range of services. First Responders provide basic services such as responding to minor illness and injury. As an important part of EMS operations, First Responders are also prepared for more serious medical and trauma incidents. They help EMTs and ALS personnel in monitoring and providing care for critically injured patients at vehicle crashes, building fires and other hazardous scenes, and multiple-casualty incidents. Learning what steps to take, what care to provide, what assistance to give, and performing these tasks in cooperation with other personnel and services in the system are all part of EMS operations.

National Standard Objectives

This chapter focuses on the objectives of Module 7, Lesson 7–1 of the U.S. DOT First Responder National Curriculum and serves as an instructional aid to help you meet any specific objectives added to the course by your local EMS system.

By the end of this chapter, you will know how to (from cognitive or knowledge information) . . .

7–1.1	Discuss the medical and nonmedical equipment needed to respond to a call. (pp. 524–525)
7–1.2	List the phases of an out-of-hospital call. (pp. 524–526)
7–1.3	Discuss the role of the First Responder in extrication. (pp. 527–535)
7–1.4	List various methods of gaining access to the patient. (pp. 529–533, 535–536)
7–1.5	Distinguish between simple and complex access. (p. 529)
7–1.6	Describe what the First Responder should do if there is reason to believe that there is a hazard at the scene. (pp. 536–541)
7–1.7	State the role the First Responder should perform until appropriately trained personnel arrive at the scene of a hazardous materials situation. (pp. 538–541)
7–1.8	Describe the criteria for a multiple-casualty situation. (p. 541)
7–1.9	Discuss the role of the First Responder in the multiple-casualty situation. (pp. 542–543)
7–1.10	Summarize the components of basic triage. (pp. 542–545)

Feel comfortable enough to (by changing attitude, values, beliefs) . . .

7–1.11	Explain the rationale for having the unit prepared to respond. (pp. 524–526)

Show how to (through psychomotor skills) . . .

7–1.12	Given a scenario of a mass-casualty incident, perform triage. (pp. 542–548)

Learning Tasks

Chapter 15 explains the operations of the EMS system and how all system services and personnel coordinate their activities to rescue and provide care in critical or disaster situations. As you work through this chapter to meet the above objectives, there is some additional information that will be essential to consider and act upon at the scene of certain critical incidents.

One of the most common critical incidents for a First Responder may be motor vehicle accidents, especially if you are a police officer. You should be able to:

✔ State what conditions you must evaluate at the scene of a motor vehicle accident.

✔ Describe safety steps to take at a motor vehicle accident scene before you gain access to the patients.

✔ Describe how to stabilize a vehicle that is on its side.

✔ State how you would gain access to patients who are in a stabilized vehicle that is on its side.

✔ State how you would free patients pinned in the vehicle.

If your training agency provides old vehicles for practicing extrication skills, your instructor will teach you how to use simple tools to gain access to the patient. If so, you should be able to:

✔ Demonstrate the steps of evaluating and making the accident scene safe.

✔ Demonstrate how to stabilize an upright vehicle.

✔ Demonstrate how to stabilize an overturned vehicle.

✔ Demonstrate how to gain access to patients, using simple tools.

Many First Responders are firefighters who often discover, report, or arrive first at structure fires. Firefighters wearing appropriate protective gear may be assigned to find victims in the building and to care for patients brought from the building. You should be able to:

✔ Describe the basic ways to gain access to patients found in houses and buildings.

✔ List the rules of safety you should follow at a fire scene.

✔ State what you should do if electrical or gas hazards exist at the scene.

Hazardous materials training is a separate and special program. Many jurisdictions require all emergency services personnel to complete the "awareness" level of hazardous materials training before they may respond on any emergency call. For any emergency incident, you should be able to:

✔ State how to recognize a possible hazardous materials incident.

✔ Describe First Responder duties at hazardous materials incidents.

✔ List the types of information that must be gathered from and reported on a hazardous materials scene.

Many critical incidents will have multiple patients who require care. First Responders will have to determine whom to help first by quickly assessing who is hurt the worst. This process of determining first care is called "triage." As you learn about multiple-casualty incidents and how to triage, you should also be able to:

✔ Discuss how to set up and carry out triage for a simulated multiple-victim incident.

✔ Discuss how to assess patients of a multiple-victim incident.

✔ Create multiple-victim incident scenarios and practice triage operations and provide care to patients.

SAFETY

Your first consideration at any emergency scene is your own safety. To assure your safety, follow standard operating guidelines (SOGs), limit your actions to your training level, and use the proper equipment and the required number of trained persons for any task. There are always risks, but emergency services personnel must limit their risks and learn what risks they can control before acting. For example, you have no control over the chance that a drunk driver could crash into you as you provide care at an accident scene. But you do have control over the normal risks at such a scene. By using proper warning devices to divert traffic (for example, flares) and positioning your own car or response unit a proper distance from the scene, you minimize your risks. At any emergency scene, you must always:

1. *Evaluate the scene*—Before you approach the patient, make certain that you will be in no danger while you work on the patient. If there is a hazard, make sure you can control it before you approach. If you cannot control a hazard, wait for assistance.

2. *Wear proper protective gear*—Use the gear that is appropriate for the situation and that you are certified or qualified to wear. Examples include turn-out gear, hazmat suit, reflective vest, eye protection, gloves.

3. *Do only what you have been trained to do*—Legally and ethically you are limited by your training level. If you attempt to act beyond your training, you may injure yourself, cause harm to the patient, or add to the extent of the accident.

4. *Call the dispatcher for the appropriate assistance*—Describe the incident so that the needed personnel and equipment may respond.

MOTOR VEHICLE ACCIDENTS

PREPARING FOR THE CALL

First Responder responsibilities on motor vehicle accidents will vary depending on your agency and jurisdiction requirements, regulations, and standard operating procedures (SOPs) or standard operating guidelines (SOGs). Your first responsibility will always require that you be prepared to perform First Responder duties on any out-of-hospital emergency call. All emergency responses progress through several phases. These phases may vary depending on the level of care you provide. For First Responders, the phases of an out-of-hospital call include:

Phase 1 *Preparation:* Being prepared means having the proper training, tools, equipment, and personnel.
- Medical supplies—Make sure your unit is stocked with medical supplies such as airways, suctioning equipment, artificial ventilation devices (pocket face masks, bag-valve masks), basic wound-care supplies (dressings, bandages), and BSI equipment.
- Nonmedical supplies—Check for other necessary items such as personal safety equipment (helmets), flares, flashlights, fire extinguisher, blanket, simple tools (screwdrivers, hammer, spring-loaded punch), and area maps.

■ Equipment and supplies—Be sure to check that all special equipment is operating and on your unit, that any malfunctioning equipment is replaced and repaired, and that all supplies are restocked. Check the fluid levels of your vehicle (fuel, oil, transmission, windshield washer). It is also important to check the emergency equipment, including flashing lights, sirens, and radios, at the beginning of every shift or on some other daily basis.

■ Personnel—Assure that the appropriate number of personnel are on duty and will be able to respond with you or can be dispatched to assist you with your response if necessary.

Phase 2 *Dispatch:* Be familiar with your dispatch or communications system and what procedures you follow when dispatched. Note any information the dispatcher gives you about the call.

■ Most dispatch systems have a central dispatch or communications center with 24-hour access.

■ Dispatch centers are staffed with personnel trained to efficiently operate at the communications center and to dispatch the appropriate units. Many dispatch centers are training their personnel in "Emergency Medical Dispatch" programs so they may provide patient-care directions to the public over the telephone while emergency services personnel are responding.

■ Dispatchers will attempt to get as much information from the caller as possible and give responding emergency services personnel such information as the nature of the call, location of the incident and the patient, number of patients and severity of illness or injury, and any other special problems that responders might encounter at the scene.

Phase 3 *En route to the scene:* First Responder duties continue while en route and include more than finding the location on the map.

■ First, fasten your seatbelt and be sure you have personal protective equipment ready.

■ Contact dispatch and let them know you are en route.

■ Be sure you have the essential information on the call, such as location, hazards, and number of patients. Check back with dispatch if you need more information.

Phase 4 *Arrival at the scene:* Always approach alertly and cautiously, look for hazards, and position your unit where you have access to it but where it will not interfere with traffic flow. Activate emergency lights or flashers. Watch traffic. Do not become a victim.

■ Notify dispatch of your arrival. Since dispatch center can only communicate what they are given from the emergency caller, you may have to provide additional information, such as the following: actual location of the incident if it is different from what was given on dispatch; type of incident; need for additional resources (engine company, helicopter medevac, rescue squad); number of victims or an estimate if there are many; where and by what unit the patient is being transported; and appropriate patient information. Note that some departments are using cellular phones as a backup to radios.

■ Size up the scene to assure that it is safe and contains no hazards. Put on your personal protective equipment. Don reflective vests. If you wear dark clothing, other drivers may not see you. As you approach, look for the mechanism of injury on trauma scenes or determine if it is a medical incident. Determine if it is mass casualty and, if so, determine the approximate number of patients. Evaluate patients quickly to determine if they are high or low priority. Do you need to move patients immediately? Can it be done safely? Will you need more assistance? Let dispatch know.

Phase 5 *Transferring patients:* First Responders will help load, lift, and carry patients on appropriate devices.
- Assist in preparing the patient for transport.
- Assist in lifting and moving patients, using appropriate lifting and moving procedures.

Phase 6 *After the emergency:* The phases of out-of-hospital calls are cyclic. Once a call is finished, you will prepare for the next call.
- Clean and disinfect equipment, restock the unit with supplies, and refuel the unit.
- Complete paperwork and file reports.
- Notify dispatch that you are back in service.

THE SCENE

Once you ensure your own safety, your main duty at the scene of a critical incident is to provide patient care. At the scene of a motor vehicle accident, however, you may have other duties to perform before you can reach the patients to provide this care. Your responsibilities at the scene may include:
- Making the scene safe; assuring that no one else is hurt as they approach
- Evaluating the situation and calling dispatch for appropriate help
- Gaining access to patients
- Freeing trapped patients
- Evaluating patients and providing emergency care
- Moving patients who are in danger from fire, explosion, and other hazards
- Determining which patients can be moved so that you can reach and provide care for another more critically injured patient

Many First Responders are injured when they attempt to help vehicle accident victims. Usually, the First Responders are struck by another vehicle when they did not take initial steps to make the scene safe. Your first step is to secure an area around the scene so you can work in it safely.

First | Law enforcement officers and firefighters must follow their department's SOGs on vehicle accidents. However, if you are a First Responder without a special course in accident scene procedures, use the items listed here as guidelines or follow your department's protocols. Since each motor vehicle scene is unique, you will need to act as a professional, carefully observe the scene, and decide what actions to take to control the situation.

1. Pull your vehicle completely off the road at least 50 feet from the scene. Turn on your vehicle's emergency flashers. You may want to use your headlights to light up the scene. If so, be sure you angle your vehicle so you do not blind oncoming drivers.

2. Make certain that you have parked in a safe location. Look for fuel spills and fire. If you are downhill from the scene, fuel may run in your direction. Check the wind direction. Will the wind carry smoke or fire to where you have parked?

3. Turn off the engine and set the parking brake. If your jurisdiction or agency has SOGs for positioning your unit and using warning lights, follow those guidelines. If you turn off the unit, you cannot leave your warning lights on.

4. Set out emergency warning devices, such as flashing lights or flares, to warn others (see Scan 15-1). On high-speed roads, place one of these devices at least 250 feet from the scene. On low-speed roads, set one of these devices at least 100 feet from the scene. Add at least 25 feet to these measurements if the scene is on a curved road.

5. As you approach, check the scene again for safety. Is there fire, leaking fuel or gases, unstable vehicles, or downed electrical wires? If any of these conditions are present, make certain someone phones or radios for help. If a power line is down, get the nearest pole number so you may request that power be turned off. You may need the fire department and rescue squad at the scene. Some jurisdictions automatically dispatch these units for motor vehicle accidents.

6. As you approach, observe the scene for clues: How many potential patients can you see? Could someone have been thrown from a vehicle? Could someone have walked away from the scene? Do you see signs indicating that children were in the vehicle (bottles, toys, schoolbooks, car seats)? Are there signs that a pedestrian or bike rider was involved? Have someone alert dispatch and report the number of possible patients.

7. If the scene is safe, gain access to the patients, do your assessments, and begin care on those who appear to be most critical. (See the Triage section later in this chapter.)

Do not approach or attempt to gain access to patients if the scene is too dangerous. If you cannot control traffic, if electric lines are down, if there is fire at the scene, or if there are fuel or hazardous materials spills, you are in danger. Call dispatch for help for any of these conditions. If you are not trained to deal with fires, electricity, or hazardous materials, protect yourself and stay uphill and upwind from any spills.

First | A First Responder's first priority is personal safety. Your primary duty is to provide patient care at a safe scene. Do only what you have been trained to do.

THE CLOSED UPRIGHT VEHICLE

In most traffic accidents, the accident vehicles remain upright and are therefore safe to approach and easy to work in and around. Usually, the vehicles are stable, with little chance of rolling or sliding away from the at-rest position.

Always evaluate vehicle stability when you assess the scene. As you look for traffic hazards, electrical hazards, spilled fuel, and fire, also see if there is any chance that the vehicle(s) may roll away or flip over. Make sure vehicles are in PARK and the ignition is turned off if you have immediate access. You may find the following situations:

- **Hills or slight inclines**—The vehicle may have come to rest on a surface that slants enough to allow forward or backward roll. To keep the vehicle from rolling, place wheel chocks, spare tires, logs, rocks, or similar objects under one or more wheels (Figure 15.1).

- **Slippery surfaces**—Ice, snow, or oil can produce a slippery road surface. If available, sprinkle dirt, sand, ashes, or kitty litter, or place newspapers around the wheels, and chock the wheels to reduce the chances of slipping.

Note

Your jurisdiction or agency may have regulations about using bystanders at emergency scenes; if so, follow them. If you use bystanders, you must inform them of dangers and risks, or you will have other patients to care for if they are hurt. In addition, they may file a lawsuit to recover damages if they are injured.

Warning Devices

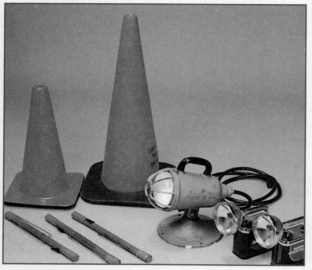

Use your vehicle's emergency flashers and set up emergency warning devices approved for highway use. For low visibility and night use, you must use flashing lights or flares.

WARNING: Keep the flare pointed away from your body. Watch out for spilled or leaking fuel, dry grass, and debris on the road surface. Remember, leaking fuel will flow downhill.

IGNITING FLARES

Use one hand to grasp the flare near its base and your other hand to pry off the plastic cap to expose the scratching surface. Pull off the cap to expose the igniter. Hold the flare in one hand and the cap in the other, keeping the scratching surface against the igniter. Use a sharp movement so that the igniter strikes against the scratching surface. Always move the flare away from your body.

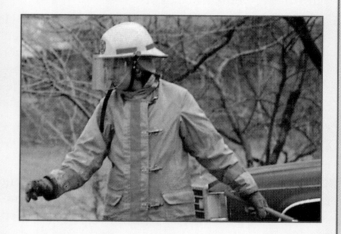

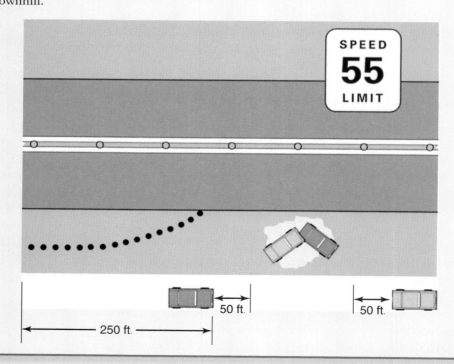

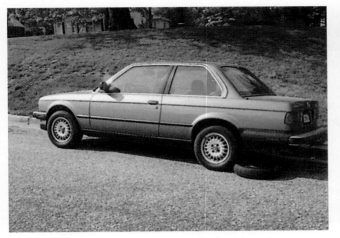
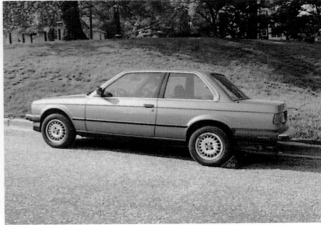

FIGURE 15.1
Stabilize the vehicle before beginning patient care.

- **Tilted vehicle**—Even upright vehicles may be tilted to one side by their position or by the terrain. Do *not* work beneath a tilted vehicle or on the downhill side of one. Chocking the wheels may prevent the vehicle from tilting over, but tying the vehicle in place is safer. If strong rope is available, tie lines to the frame of the car (not the bumper) in front and back or to both sides, then secure the lines to large trees or poles, guardrails, or heavier stable vehicles while waiting for fire-department units to arrive.
- **Stacked vehicles**—Part of one vehicle may be resting on top of another vehicle. There are several ways to stabilize the vehicles: chock the wheels of both vehicles; insert tires, lumber, blocks, or similar sturdy items between the road surface and the vehicles; use line or rope to tie and secure both vehicles.

 Never try to enter or work around a vehicle until you are certain that it is stable.

 Once you stabilize the vehicle, there are two access methods to use for reaching a patient: *simple access* and *complex access*. Simple access does not require equipment; complex access requires tools and special equipment, which also requires additional training. In most cases, you will approach an upright, stable vehicle and reach the patient by simple access. If the doors and windows are closed, there are four ways to gain access to the patients:

1. **Open the doors**—Many people drive without locking the doors. Check all the doors, including side and rear doors on vans and hatchbacks before trying another entry method. If all doors are locked, one of the occupants may be able to unlock a door. "Try before you pry."

2. **Enter through a window**—If doors are locked or jammed, gain access through a window. The patient may be able to roll down a window; if not, you will have to break a window. Directions for breaking windows will be given later in this section. When you begin using tools to reach patients, access becomes complex.

3. **Pry open the doors**—The doors on most cars made before 1967 can be pried open with a pry bar or jack handle. This method will not work for most cars made after this date. When it does work, the method is very time consuming. Prying open doors is not considered a First Responder skill. Access through windows is usually more practical.

4. **Cut through the metal**—The only other access when entry through doors and windows is not possible is cutting through vehicle roofs, trunks, and

REMEMBER:

Make certain that vehicles are stable before working around them.

doors. This entry method takes special tools that First Responders do not usually carry unless they are also members of the fire department. If you cannot gain access through a door or window, it may be possible to cut around the lock of a door using a sharp tool (chisel or strong screwdriver) and a hammer.

Keep in mind that speed is crucial when you need to reach patients in a vehicle. Precious time is lost if you have to return to your vehicle to retrieve tools. Take all tools with you as you approach a vehicle. Many simple tools will help you gain access to a vehicle including slotted and Phillips screwdrivers, chisels, hammers, pliers, wire, washers, and pry bars. Some First Responder tool kits include "slim jims" and spring-loaded punches. Access with tools and special equipment is considered complex because it takes time, planning, and sometimes special training; and it requires taking precautions to protect the patient.

Unlocking Vehicle Doors

Special commercial tools for unlocking doors may be part of your First Responder kit. You might be able to unlock doors of older vehicles by slipping a commercial tool between the window and the door. You also might be able to pry open the window with a screwdriver or pry bar and slip a wire coat hanger or a wire looped around a washer inside the window (Scan 15-2). Opening newer locks using these methods might be impossible, depending on the manufacturer. Some cars have a deadbolt system that cannot be unlocked with special tools; these types of locks are designed to unlock on impact and allow rescuers to gain access. If you cannot unlock or open a door, gain access through a window (see below).

Before you attempt to unlock a door, first make sure the vehicle cannot be opened by you from the outside or unlocked by an occupant on the inside. Check the doors for damage. A severely damaged door may not open easily even if you do unlock it. If all of the doors are damaged, be prepared to break glass and gain access through the window. Look in the windows to see if the car has buttons in the armrest. It will not be easy to unlock doors with this type of locking device. Vehicles with electric locks and windows cannot be unlocked if the battery is disabled.

Gaining Access Through Vehicle Windows

At the scene of an accident, most people consider breaking the windshield of a vehicle first if they cannot gain access through the doors. Unfortunately, this is the wrong approach. Windshields are made of laminated safety glass, which has great strength. Even when shattered, the glass will still cling to an inner plastic layer. All cars have laminated safety glass windshields. Many foreign cars have this type of glass in all the vehicle's windows.

Rear and side windows are usually made of tempered safety glass. When this glass is broken, there is no plastic layer to hold the pieces. Tempered safety glass will not shatter into sharp pieces or shards. Instead, this glass will shatter into small rounded pieces and will often drop straight down into the vehicle if you break it in a corner. The small glass pieces can cut, but the cuts are usually minor.

The risk of flying glass is reduced if you use a sharp tool (screwdriver or punch) and a hammer to tap the window until it breaks. To simply bash the center of the glass with a hammer will send pieces throughout the entire passenger compartment. If you apply adhesive-backed contact paper or duct tape to the window before breaking the glass, it will help prevent the glass from spraying the occupants.

*U*nlocking *V*ehicle *D*oors

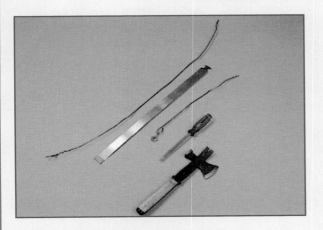

Various tools can be used to help unlock vehicle doors:

- ❑ wire hook (coat hanger)
- ❑ slim-jim (or similar device)
- ❑ wire and washer
- ❑ screwdriver
- ❑ flat pry bar

An oil dipstick or a keyhole saw may be used to help force up a locking button.

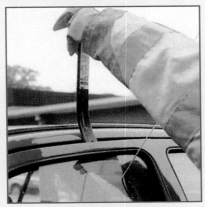

1. Framed windows. Pry frame away from vehicle body and insert wire hook.

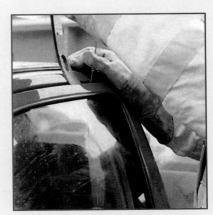

2. Snag the locking button and pull upward.

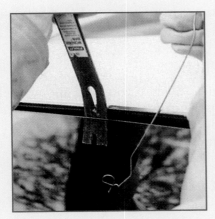

Unframed windows. Pry window and insert wire hook, screwdriver, keyhole saw, or dipstick to lift button.

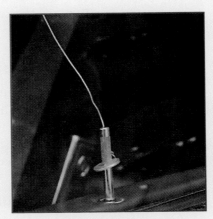

Thief-proof lock. Insert washer on wire and drop over shank. Pull up and allow washer to turn and grab.

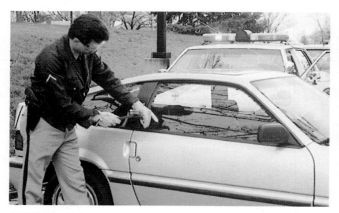

FIGURE 15.2
Protect yourself when breaking glass.

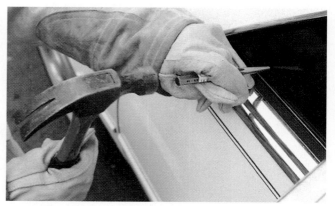

FIGURE 15.3
Use a sharp object positioned at a lower corner of the glass.

First | When gaining access through a vehicle window, you should:

1. Make certain the vehicle is stable. If possible, have the driver turn off the ignition.
2. Be sure that access through a door is not possible.
3. Protect yourself by wearing gloves and protecting your eyes with goggles, safety glasses, or a face shield (Figure 15.2). If you do not have gloves or eye protection, drape a coat, towel, or blanket over the glass before you attempt to break the window and position yourself so you can shield your face with your shoulder and upper arm.
4. If possible, select a window that is away from the patients. Use a sharp tool to break through a tempered safety glass window (a punch, Halligan tool, or the pike of a Pry-Axe or similar tool). *Begin in one of the lower corners, as close to the door as possible* (Figure 15.3). Lightly tap the tool with a hammer and increase the strength of each blow until the glass shatters.
5. After breaking the window, reach in and try to open the door. You may only have to unlock the door to open it. Often jammed doors that will not open from the outside will open from the inside.
6. Turn off the vehicle ignition, set the transmission in PARK, and set the parking brake.

THE OVERTURNED CLOSED VEHICLE

Do not try to right an overturned vehicle. Even if you have enough help to turn the vehicle upright, moving it can cause further injury to the occupants. Stabilize the overturned vehicle while waiting for fire department units and before you try to reach the occupants. Always look for fuel spills, battery acid, and other chemical hazards around an overturned vehicle.

THE VEHICLE ON ITS SIDE

First | If you find a vehicle on its side and have some simple equipment, take the following precautions to stabilize it. You should:

1. Stabilize the vehicle with tires, blocks, lumber, wheel chocks, rocks, or similar available materials. Place these items between the road surface

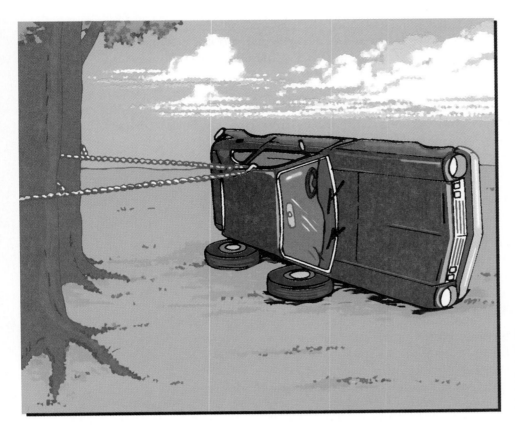

FIGURE 15.4
Stabilize the vehicle before
trying to gain access to the
patients. This requires special
training. Do only what you
have been trained to do.

and roof line. Note how this is done in Figure 15.4. Also place stabilizing items between the road surface and the lower wheels if the wheels are not resting on the road surface.

2. If the vehicle is still unstable, use strong rope or line to tie the vehicle to secure objects.

3. Attempt to gain access to occupants. Entry through a door is very dangerous since the door may be seven feet or more off the ground and your weight will move the vehicle as you climb on it. It will also be difficult to open the door with the vehicle on its side. Your first and more sensible entry point will be through a window. The rear window is the best approach to take. Never attempt access to a damaged interior through broken glass without adequate protective clothing and equipment.

4. If you open a door, tie it securely open. Do not use a prop. Props can slip or be knocked away, causing the door to slam on you or the occupants.

PATIENTS PINNED BENEATH VEHICLES

It usually is best to wait for the rescue squad to arrive in cases in which patients are pinned beneath a vehicle. Never place yourself in danger by reaching or crawling into the area where the patient is pinned. If it appears that the scene is too dangerous, First Responders can perform certain procedures to move the vehicle and free the patient, but this is often risky. Follow your department guidelines if you take any action.

A jack or pry bar and blocks can be used to raise a vehicle, which will enable rescuers to move the patient from beneath the vehicle. With enough help, you may be able to lift the vehicle off the patient. In any attempt to raise a vehicle off a pinned patient, others must shore up the vehicle as you raise it so that it will not slip or fall back onto the rescuers or the patient. Use blocks, tires, lumber, or similar sturdy items at the scene. Do not attempt to enter the space to remove the victim until the entire vehicle is stable.

*P*ATIENTS CAUGHT IN WRECKAGE

You may find patients with their arms, legs, or heads thrown through the window. Before trying to free them, you should:

1. Use dressing materials, towels, blankets, or clothing to protect the body part thrown through the window (Figure 15.5).
2. Use pliers, hammer claws, or a knife to carefully break or fold away glass around the patient.

When patients are trapped inside crushed vehicles, you must wait for special power tools and skilled rescue personnel. Often the trapped patient can be easily freed or disentangled from the wreck.

First | First Responders working on vehicles with occupants pinned inside will often be able to free some patients by:

- Simply removing wreckage from on top of and around the patient
- Carefully moving a seat forward or backward
- Carefully lifting out a back seat
- Removing a patient's shoe to free a foot, or cutting away clothing caught on wreckage
- Cutting seat belts (Be sure to properly support the patient during the cutting and after the tension has been released.)
  NOTE: In general, C-spine immobilizations should be applied by qualified personnel prior to performing these maneuvers that will cause the patient to move.
- Checking air bag deployment (Follow manufacturer and agency guidelines for working around vehicles with deployed and undeployed airbags; check the steering wheel beneath the deployed airbag for damage indicating that the patient might have struck it. Airbags may also activate in areas of the front seat passenger, and some more recent models have side airbags.)
  NOTE: Powders used to lubricate the airbag may irritate the skin. Wear personal protective equipment when working around vehicles with deployed airbags.

FIGURE 15.5
Protect the patient from injury while removing glass.

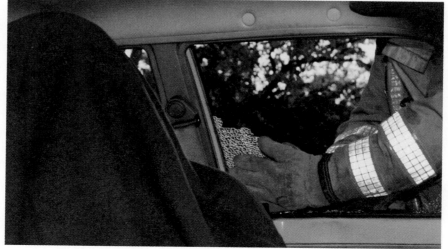

In any attempt to free patients from vehicles, you must consider the immediate need for quick access. If immediate access and patient movement is necessary to save a life, make every attempt to reach the patient. If the patient's life is not at risk but immediate movement will cause further injury, then leave the patient in place until more highly trained personnel respond to the scene. During the wait, talk to the patient to offer reassurance and explain why you are taking precautions. While you are talking to the patient, begin your initial patient assessment steps and provide oxygen while another First Responder stabilizes the head. If you must move the patient before EMTs arrive, make every attempt to maintain stabilization of the patient's spine during the move. Once EMTs and other emergency medical personnel arrive, report your patient assessment findings and provide them with any assistance they need, such as taking vital signs, controlling bleeding, gathering special equipment, or loading and lifting the patient.

BUILDINGS

FIRST RESPONDER RESPONSIBILITIES

Gaining access to a patient in a locked building may require special skills and tools outside the range of First Responder duties. There are many types of gates, doors, windows, and locks that restrict access to buildings. In addition to access problems, older buildings may have many hidden and unsuspected dangers; security devices will present special barriers, and guard dogs will limit or halt your actions until they are contained.

First Responders are not expected to know how to open or destroy locks or have all the tools needed for the variety of windows, doors, and gates found in buildings. Unless you are trained in fire and rescue operations, you are not expected to know how to enter and make your way safely around an empty or abandoned building. No one expects First Responders to go up against trained guard dogs.

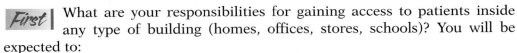 What are your responsibilities for gaining access to patients inside any type of building (homes, offices, stores, schools)? You will be expected to:

- Make certain that someone contacts dispatch
- Try opening and entering through doors first
- Try opening and entering through windows
- Look quickly for a key under mats or in mailboxes
- Call bystanders and neighbors to see if they have a key
- Break glass to unlock doors or windows

Follow your department's SOGs regarding notification of local law enforcement following "forcible" entry.

If you know or see that someone inside needs immediate care, do not try to gain access before calling for help. Your efforts to gain entry may fail, and you will need help as soon as possible. Call dispatch first so help is sent immediately.

ENTERING BUILDINGS

While waiting for help, try different entry points. Try to open a door. If the door is locked, try opening a few low windows on your way to finding a second door. If the second door is locked, break the glass in a window or a door and enter as quickly but as safely as possible. Do not attempt to break through doors or windows made of large sheets of tempered glass. This glass is very strong and it is flexible enough to bounce a hammer back into your face. Do *not* try climbing up walls or posts to reach a high window. Do *not* try to gain access to a window by walking across roofs.

 To break any window, you should:

1. Make certain that the patient is not lying near the other side of the glass.
2. Use a hammer or similar blunt object to strike the glass near one of its edges (Figure 15.6). A nightstick or an aluminum aircraft flashlight will break most window glass. If you do not have tools, throw a rock or similar solid object through the glass.
3. Carefully clear all glass from the frame and reach in to unlock the door or window.
4. Make certain that you are stepping onto a safe floor. Be sure that you do not have an unusual drop when entering. Take a moment to visually inspect the floor for damage or poke the floor for signs of weakness.

*H*AZARDS

Hazards are not just "hazardous materials" but any situation that puts you, patients, and bystanders in danger.

*F*IRE

Television and movies have led people to believe that they should enter burning buildings or run up to burning vehicles in order to save victims. This is a dangerous tactic. Those in the fire service are highly trained to do their jobs. They are given special equipment and use special strategies to fight fires, which minimizes risks to their safety. Fire fighting requires special training, protective clothing, the right equipment, and usually more than one firefighter.

If you are a member of the fire service, follow SOGs for rescuing victims from vehicle and structure fires. If you are in law enforcement and have special training in rescuing victims from vehicle and structure fires, do only what you have been trained to do. If you are a First Responder without fire fighting training, do not risk your life to approach a fire and provide care.

Motor vehicle accidents do not usually produce fire, and most medical and injury emergency calls to buildings do not involve fire. However, these events do occur, and you must be prepared to protect yourself. Your own safety is the

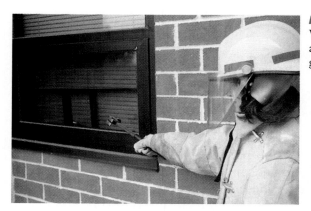

FIGURE 15.6
When doors and windows are locked, break glass to gain access to the locks.

first priority. The following rules should be followed by First Responders with no training or little experience at fighting fires:

- *Never* approach a vehicle that is in flames. Using blankets, sand, or a hand extinguisher is appropriate if you know how to evaluate the fire and the danger of explosion and if you have protective clothing and know how to attack a fire. If you do not know these things and do not have the necessary protection, stay clear. Make sure that dispatch knows there is a fire.
- *Never* attempt to enter a building that is obviously on fire or has smoke showing. Even a small fire can spread toxic fumes throughout the structure. If you enter, look and smell for signs of fire. Remember that fire could be hidden within the walls, floors, and ceilings.
- *Never* enter a smoky room or building or go through an area of dense smoke.
- *Never* attempt to enter a closed building or room giving off grayish yellow smoke. Opening a door to this building or room will cause a backdraft condition that immediately increases the intensity of the fire or causes an explosion.
- *Do not* work by yourself or enter a building unless others know that you are doing so. If you are injured or trapped, you are an unknown victim who may not be rescued.
- *Never* open a door that is hot to your touch. Always feel the top of the door before opening it (Figure 15.7). If it is hot, do not open the door. (*Note:* Doorknobs and handles also may be hot.) If the door is cool, open it slowly and cautiously and avoid standing in its path as you open it.
- *Never* use the elevator if there is a possibility of a fire in a building. The elevator shaft can act as a flue and pull flames, hot toxic gases, and smoke into the shaft. Also, the fire can cause an electrical failure, which could trap you in the elevator. Some elevators have heat-activated call buttons. The elevator may take you to the fire floor, open, and expose you to lethal heat or toxic gases.
- If you find yourself in smoke, stay close to the floor and crawl to safety (Figure 15.8). If possible, cover your mouth and nose with a cloth.

> **IMPORTANT:**
> If you do not have training in fire fighting, do not enter any building that is or may be on fire. If bystanders tell you there is a fire, do not enter, even if you do not see smoke or flames. Leave rescue and fire fighting to the fire service.

*G*AS

If you notice the odor of natural gas at any scene, move patients away from the area, keep bystanders away from the scene, and alert dispatchers so that they can activate other services and request that gas in the area be shut off or diverted.

FIGURE 15.7
If a door is hot, do not open it.

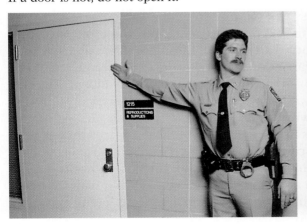

FIGURE 15.8
If trapped by fire or smoke, stay low and crawl to safety.

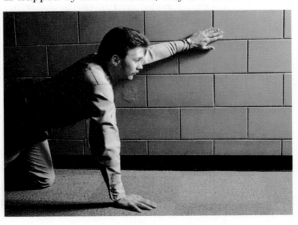

First | The smell of natural gas in a building is a signal for immediate action. Evacuate the building and call dispatch to report the odor of gas. If the gas is coming from a bottled source, do not try to turn off this source unless you have experience with this type of system. You can vent the area by opening windows and doors as you leave. *Do not* enter an area to rescue a patient. You must wear self-contained breathing apparatus (SCBA) and be trained to handle such emergencies. Remember that there is always a danger of fire or explosion from simple acts such as turning on or off a light switch, or even from the spark of an appliance kicking on. Play it safe and request the help you will need.

ELECTRICAL WIRES

First | If electrical wires are down at a scene and block your pathway to a patient, or if they are lying across a car, do *not* attempt a rescue. Never assume that the lines are dead or that a "dead" line will stay dead. Consider all downed lines as "live." Do not be fooled by the fact that lights are out in the surrounding area. Even if lights are off all around you, the wire blocking your path may be "live" or could be reenergized as you pass by. Call or have someone alert the dispatcher to call the power company and request that the power be turned off. Even if you believe the power has been turned off, it is still best to wait for rescue personnel to arrive.

If patients are in a car that is touching a downed wire or near a downed wire, tell them to stay in the vehicle and avoid touching any metal parts. If downed wires are touching the car and the patients have to leave the vehicle because of fire or other danger, you must tell them to jump clear of the car without touching it and the ground at the same time. If they touch both simultaneously, they will complete a circuit and may be electrocuted.

HAZARDOUS MATERIALS

There may be hazardous chemicals and other materials at the scene of an accident or a medical emergency. If so, do *not* attempt a rescue or perform patient care. No one should enter a hazardous materials area unless he or she is trained to do so, has the proper equipment, and is in radio or phone contact with hazardous materials experts.

The possibility of hazardous materials incidents exists at every industrial site and every farm, truck, train, ship, barge, and airplane accident. At such sites or incidents, assume that there are unsafe hazardous materials until their presence can be ruled out. When in doubt, stay clear.

First Responder Responsibilities

Your role as a First Responder in a hazardous materials situation is to first **protect yourself and others around the scene.** Set up a HOT (danger) zone and keep all people out of this area. Set up a COLD (safe) zone, which should be on the same level as and upwind from the hazardous materials accident. The safe zone must not be downhill or downwind from the scene or on a high point that may be exposed to vapors if the wind shifts. Avoid low spots, streams, drainage fields, sewers, and sewer openings where spills may flow and fumes may collect.

Contact dispatch with a description of the incident so you can get the appropriate help on the way immediately. Let the dispatcher know your position and stay on the line until you are told to disconnect. Ask and wait for information about the danger of the materials and for directions as to what you should do until the hazmat teams arrive. Make certain you give your name and call-back number.

If, for some reason, you cannot contact dispatch, call one of the following:

■ CHEM-TEL on its 24-hour toll-free number at 800-255-3924 (for the United States and Canada). For calls originating from other areas, call 813-070-0626.

■ **CHEMTREC** on its 24-hour toll-free number at 800-424-9300 (for the United States and Canada). For calls originating from other areas, call 703-527-3887.

When possible, provide the following information:

1. The nature and location of the problem. Can you estimate how long the scene has been dangerous? Are other possible hazardous materials near the scene?

2. The type of material: gas, liquid, or dry chemical, or a radioactive solid, liquid, or gas. Can you estimate how much material is at the scene?

3. The name or identification number of the material. Look for labels or placards that are visible from your safe point. Use binoculars to help in reading this information.

4. The name of the shipper or manufacturer. From a safe point or with binoculars, look for names on railroad cars, trucks, or containers. Ask bystanders, drivers, or railroad or factory personnel.

5. The type of container: Is the material in a railcar, truck, open storage, covered storage, or housed storage? Is the container still intact, or is liquid leaking, is gas escaping, or is a powder spilled? Report if the material is stable or if it is flaming, vaporizing, or blowing into the air.

6. The weather conditions. Rain and wind are major concerns because they will carry hazardous materials to and contaminate other locations.

7. An estimate of how many possible patients there are both in the HOT zone (closest to the spill) and around the HOT zone (in circles farther from the spill).

8. Other significant problems at the scene such as fire, crowds, and traffic.

You may not be able to obtain and pass on most of this information, but any information is important.

A major source of information at a hazardous materials scene is the standard materials placard required by the Department of Transportation (Figure 15.9). This placard is on the vehicle, tank, or railroad car. The numbers, symbols, and colors provide information about the material in the container. All emergency response units should carry the *North American Emergency*

CHEMTREC
the Chemical Transportation Emergency Center that provides immediate expert information to emergency personnel at the scene of a hazardous materials incident.

FIGURE 15.9
Hazardous materials placard.

Response Guidebook published by the United States Department of Transportation. Canada and Mexico also publish a guidebook.

Managing Patients

All contaminated victims must remain in the HOT zone until the hazmat team decontaminates them and brings them to the COLD zone for care by EMS personnel. If a victim of a hazardous materials incident leaves the HOT zone, you must first protect yourself from exposure. Victims may have chemicals on their bodies and clothing that could be harmful to you. If you have stayed in contact with the dispatcher, you can obtain information about safety procedures. Initial care includes flushing with water contaminated areas such as the skin, clothing, and eyes for at least 20 minutes, unless the material is dry lime. (Brush away excess dry lime first, then flush.) Remove contaminated clothing and jewelry as you flush the patient with water. Once the patient is flushed, use blankets to protect him from the environment and to maintain body temperature.

The victims may be able to wash themselves or you may wash the victim. Use a small diameter hose and make sure the victim stands in a large tub, small wading pool, or similar collection container so the contaminated rinse water does not run off into nearby sewers or streams. Perform wash operations uphill and upwind from the site if possible. Do not place yourself at risk. Do not provide mouth-to-mouth resuscitation on a contaminated victim. Use resuscitation devices with one-way valves so contaminants do not "blow back" into your mouth or face.

The best thing for you to do at a hazardous materials incident is to contact the experts (Figure 15.10) and remain in a COLD zone.

RADIATION ACCIDENTS

First | Stay clear of accidents involving radioactive materials. Your first duty is to protect yourself from exposure. Your next step should be to call for assistance from a safe area away from the scene.

> **REMEMBER:**
>
> At hazardous materials incidents, notify dispatch and stay in a COLD zone.

FIGURE 15.10
Special personnel and equipment are required at a hazardous materials incident.

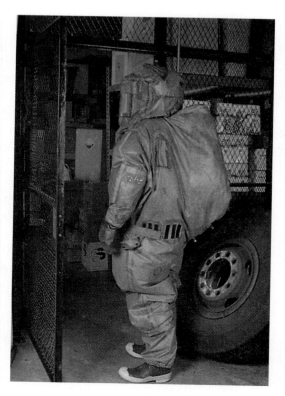

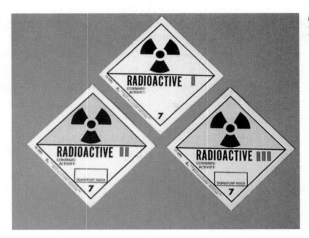

FIGURE 15.11
Radiation hazard labels.

Look for radiation hazard labels (Figure 15.11). Stay upwind from any containers having these labels. Follow the same basic rules as you would when dealing with any hazardous material. The greater the distance you are from the source and the more objects there are between you and the source (concrete, thick steel, earth banks, heavy vehicles), the safer you will be.

Patients may be exposed to radiation, contaminated by it, or both. An *exposed* patient is in the presence of radioactive material, but the material has not actually touched his clothing or body. Exposure to radiation may have been harmful to the patient, but the patient is not radioactive and cannot pass on the exposure to you. However, the source of the radiation exposure can be harmful to you; and if the patient is still in the area of the radiation source, you must wait until the hazmat team brings him to the safe area.

Patients are *contaminated* when they have come in contact with radiation sources, which may be gases, liquids, or particles. The radioactive materials may be on a patient's clothes, skin, or hair and will contaminate you when you touch the patient during assessment or care. The hazmat team will have to decontaminate the patient before you can provide care. Do not attempt to clean or care for radiation patients until they are in a safe area and are decontaminated.

TRIAGE

PRIORITIES

First | **Triage** is a process of sorting a number of patients into categories and ordering their treatment and transport based on the severity of their injuries and medical conditions. This process is used at the scene of multiple-victim accidents and disasters. When there are more victims than there are rescuers, triage assures that the most critical but still *salvageable* patients are cared for first. On many multiple-casualty incidents, there may be a delay before additional help will be on the scene. If the disaster is large enough or in a remote area, an hour or more may pass before there are enough rescuers present to render care for all the patients.

triage a method of sorting patients for care and transport based on the severity of their injuries or illnesses.

Triage is also used to determine the order of transport for patients. Patients who appear to have medical or trauma problems, such as heart attack, allergy shock, multiple injuries, and heat stroke must be transported quickly, while patients with minor fractures or illness are transported to the hospital later.

Since First Responders may be first on the scene, they must be able to triage patients and initiate care. When additional emergency services personnel arrive, First Responders pass on information, help complete the triage process, and help provide care to the worst patients first. You cannot begin to provide care to patients randomly. You must begin treating those people who have the highest priority based on their injuries. You will need to make brief notes on each patient while you are performing triage.

Some jurisdictions have their First Responders use triage tags (see Figure 15.12). Even if you do not carry these tags, you should be familiar with them in case you are called on to help when others are using triage tags. If you use triage tags, use one triage tag per patient and leave the tag attached to the patient so that others arriving at the scene can have immediate access to information. Do not delay the triage process in order to make elaborate notes.

The typical triage process does not allow for you to stop and provide interventions for each person in need of care, including patients who are in respiratory or cardiac arrest. If there are too many victims, you will have to complete triage before beginning care on anyone. The purpose of triage is to assess the patient's condition, determine the urgency of the patient's condition, and assign a treatment priority. To begin the triage process, you will perform an initial assessment that will include the following steps:

- Check airway. If it is not open, open it. If the patient responds or begins to breathe on his own, move on to the next patient.
- Check responsiveness. If the patient is unresponsive, check for breathing and pulse. If there is no breathing or no pulse, do not provide care for that patient. Move on to the next patient.
- Check pulse. If you feel a pulse, check for severe bleeding. If there is severe bleeding, quickly apply a pressure dressing and move on to the next patient.

FIGURE 15.12
An example of standard triage tags (the METTAG system).

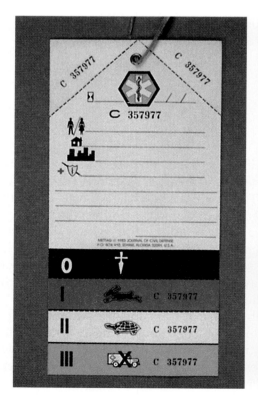
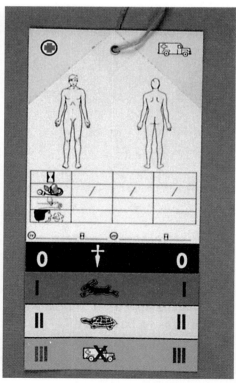

If the scene is unstable or dangerous in any way, begin to move people regardless of their injuries. Patients who are able to move and walk on their own can help you move other patients.

As more trained personnel arrive, they will take assigned positions and perform duties based on the jurisdiction's triage protocols. Those assigned to provide care will begin caring first for the patients tagged serious while you and others complete the triage process. Even when additional rescuers arrive, they may give a low priority of care to a patient in cardiac arrest (unwitnessed and possibly not able to be saved) because there are too many other patients who need lifesaving care.

If you are dispatched and respond to a multiple-casualty incident already operating under the direction of an Incident Commander at a command post, report to the Staging Officer if there is one, or to the command post. Identify yourself and your level of training, then follow the directions that the Staging Officer or Incident Commander gives you.

First | There are several triage systems, and each has slightly different injury classifications. Use the triage system and classifications that your jurisdiction has adopted.

The following is an example of a four-category triage:

- *Priority 1* (red tag)—Treatable life-threatening illness or injuries
    - Airway and breathing problems
    - Uncontrolled or severe bleeding
    - Altered mental status
    - Severe medical problems
    - Shock (hypoperfusion)
    - Severe burns

- *Priority 2* (yellow tag)—Serious but not life-threatening illness or injuries
    - Burns without airway problems
    - Major or multiple bone or joint injuries
    - Back injuries with or without spinal cord damage

- *Priority 3* (green tag)—"Walking wounded"
    - Minor musculoskeletal injuries (pain or stiffness, but able to move normally)
    - Minor soft-tissue injuries (minor lacerations, bruises)

    NOTE: In three-category triage systems, those who are dead or fatally injured are included as low priority and placed in Priority 3.

- *Priority 4* (sometimes called Priority O—gray or black tag) Dead or fatally injured
    - Exposed brain matter
    - Cardiac arrest (no pulse for over 20 minutes, except with cold-water drowning and extreme hypothermia)
    - Severed trunk
    - Decapitation
    - Incineration

    NOTE: Your system may not have a "deceased" category. Instead it might use a "probable death" category that includes obvious death, mortal wounds, and all injuries where death is considered to be certain under the conditions in which the rescue is taking place.

Many factors can change the patient's priority during the triage process. These factors include the type of incident, location, how quickly the patient can be assessed, weather conditions, number of patients, types of injuries, number of rescuers, availability of high-level trauma services, and limitations of the EMS system.

Another factor that affects triage is that patients do not always remain stable. You may have to update a patient's priority because his condition has worsened or improved. You also will have to modify care procedures if you are dealing with a large number of patients. For example, you may classify an unconscious person as your highest priority, then move on to triage the next patient. The next patient appears to have minor bleeding but after a quick check of vital signs, you decide the patient needs immediate care. You will go back to monitor the unconscious patient, but you cannot provide continuous monitoring while the other patient continues to bleed. Uncontrolled bleeding can fairly rapidly result in shock, so the patient will then need to be upgraded to the higher priority.

THE START PLAN

START plan a four-step simple triage and rapid treatment (care) program designed for use in multiple-casualty incidents. It is usually employed when additional help will be delayed.

A modified triage system often used is the **START plan** (Table 15-1). The term START stands for simple triage and rapid treatment. The first rescuers on the scene begin the triage process and quickly identify and separate those patients who are probably the least injured and classify them as "delayed." First rescuers will tag the dead and the nonsalvageable as "dead" and tag those patients who are most in need of care as "immediate." During the process of triage, the rescuers will take some basic actions to ensure an airway and control serious bleeding. The START plan sorts patients into four broad categories that are based on the need for treatment and the chances of survival under the circumstances of the disaster. Following are the four categories, or steps, of the START plan:

- **STEP ONE: Identify the "Walking Wounded" or Delayed Patients/Green Tag**—Rescuers direct all patients who can walk to go to an assigned area. These patients are considered to be in the delayed category. The rescuers move to the closest patients who cannot walk and continue the triage.

  Move the delayed patients to a designated area and assign someone to stay with them and keep them there. This individual keeps the walking wounded from wandering back into the triage and treatment areas, looking for friends and family, or trying to help. The individual assigned to this area should be instructed to make the walking wounded as comfortable as possible, keep them calm, establish a log of names or tag numbers, and relay information to them about the progress of the incident and status of their friends and family where appropriate. Some of the walking wounded may be able to help on the scene by performing simple rescue tasks that will aid emergency care providers in maintaining an airway or controlling bleeding. Once you have moved the walking wounded, you can attend to the remaining victims. Start from where you stand. Begin assessing patients systematically from where you are until you have reached every victim. Stop at each patient for only a minute to assess *breathing*, *circulation*, and *mental status*.

- **STEP TWO: Respiration Check**—Each patient who cannot walk is assessed for respirations. Open the airway and check for breathing. Patients who can walk can assist in keeping the airway open for an unconscious patient. If other patients cannot help, use items on the scene to

TABLE 15-1: Triage—the START Plan

IMMEDIATE	DELAYED	DEAD
Respirations above 30/minute	Walking wounded	No respirations
Respirations below 30/minute; no radial pulse	Respirations below 30/minute; radial pulse	
Adequate respirations and perfusion; unable to follow directions	Adequate respirations and perfusion; able to follow directions	

position the head and maintain the airway. Respiration is used to classify the patients as:

- Dead/nonsalvageable (tagged)—no respirations
- Immediate (tagged)—respirations above 30 per minute
- Delayed (no tag)—respirations below 30 per minute

All respiratory rates are estimates based on quick observation. No actual rates are determined.

■ **STEP THREE: Circulation Assessment**—Check the breathing patient's pulse, which will give an indication of the flow of blood through the vital organs. This is done on the basis of the presence or absence of a radial pulse. A radial pulse indicates a systolic blood pressure of at least 80 mmHg (American College of Surgeons standard). Any patient with a radial pulse is assumed to have adequate perfusion and is considered to be delayed but is not yet tagged. Any patient without a radial pulse is assumed to have inadequate perfusion and is tagged immediate. During this third step, if you find major bleeding, apply direct pressure, which can be maintained by the patient or another walking wounded patient. Elevate the legs of any patient without a radial pulse and keep him or her in this position with near-at-hand items.

■ **STEP FOUR: Mental Assessment**—If a patient with adequate respirations and perfusion can follow simple directions (for example, open or close the eyes), assume that the central nervous system is intact and give the patient a "normal mental status." This patient is tagged delayed. Any patient with adequate respirations and perfusion who cannot follow the simple direction is tagged immediate.

You may complete the fourth step during the assessments for respiration and perfusion. If necessary, it can be done as a separate step for certain patients.

PATIENT ASSESSMENT

It is critical to consider the mechanism of injury and the findings from the initial and focused assessments when you determine order of care for multiple-casualty incidents. Vital signs and significant signs of injury will help you determine priority and care. Relate patient signs to possible injuries or illness (Figure 15.13).

REMEMBER:

First Responder-level care is assessment-based. The rescuer typically provides a given set of care procedures for a category of injury or illness.

FIGURE 15.13
First Responders must be able to relate signs to specific injuries and illnesses.

First | As a First Responder, you must be able to apply the following information to the assessment and care of patients:

■ **Pulse** *(vital sign)*

– *Rapid, full:* fear, overexertion, heat stroke and advanced heat exhaustion, high blood pressure, early stages of internal bleeding

– *Rapid, thready:* shock, blood loss, developing heat exhaustion, diabetic coma, falling blood pressure

– *Slow, full:* stroke, skull fracture

– *No pulse:* carotid = cardiac arrest; distal = injury to the extremity (usually a fracture or dislocation) or shock with low blood pressure

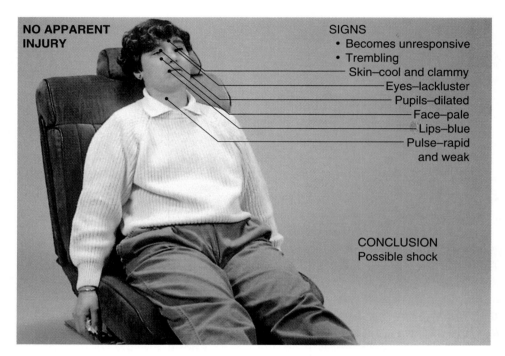

NO APPARENT INJURY

SIGNS
• Becomes unresponsive
• Trembling
Skin–cool and clammy
Eyes–lackluster
Pupils–dilated
Face–pale
Lips–blue
Pulse–rapid and weak

CONCLUSION
Possible shock

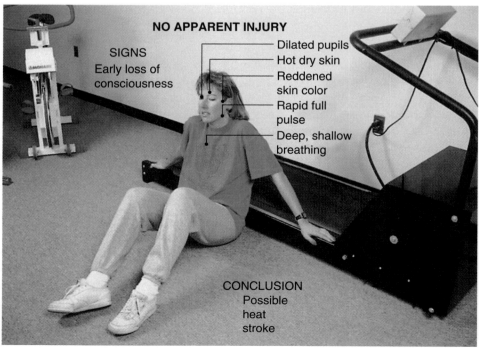

NO APPARENT INJURY

SIGNS
Early loss of consciousness

Dilated pupils
Hot dry skin
Reddened skin color
Rapid full pulse
Deep, shallow breathing

CONCLUSION
Possible heat stroke

- **Respiration** (*vital sign*)
  - *Rapid, shallow:* shock, heart problems, heat exhaustion, insulin shock, congestive heart failure
  - *Deep, gasping, labored:* airway obstruction, congestive heart failure, heart problems, lung disease, lung injury from excessive heat, chest injuries, diabetic coma
  - *Snoring:* stroke, fractured skull, drug or alcohol abuse, airway obstruction
  - *Stridor:* high-pitched sounds on inspiration
  - *Crowing:* atypical breathing sound indicating airway obstruction
  - *Gurgling:* liquid in the airway—for example, vomitus, blood, or normal secretions and inability to clear them—usually due to impaired mental status; airway obstruction; lung disease; lung damage due to excessive heat; fluids in lungs from pulmonary edema
  - *Coughing blood:* chest wound, rib fracture, internal injuries

- **Skin temperature** (*vital sign*)
  - *Cool, moist:* shock, bleeding, body losing heat, heat exhaustion
  - *Cool, dry:* exposure to cold
  - *Cool, clammy:* shock
  - *Hot, dry:* heat stroke, high fever, chemical (pesticide) exposure
  - *Hot, moist:* heat exhaustion or heat stroke (but heat stroke may be either sweaty or dry), infectious disease

- **Skin color** (*vital sign*)
  - *Red:* high blood pressure, heart attack, heat stroke, diabetic coma, minor burn, fever or infection, allergic reaction (anaphylaxis)
  - *White, pale, ashen:* shock, heart attack, excessive bleeding, heat exhaustion, fright, insulin shock
  - *Blue:* heart failure, airway obstruction, lung disease, certain poisonings, shock

- **Pupils of the eyes** (*vital sign*)
  - *Dilated, unresponsive to light:* cardiac arrest, unconsciousness, shock, bleeding, heat stroke, drugs (LSD, uppers)
  - *Constricted:* damage to the central nervous system, drugs (heroin, morphine, codeine)
  - *Unequal:* stroke, head injury—only useful in setting of profoundly altered mental status

- **Level of consciousness**
  - *Confusion:* fright, anxiety, illness, minor head injury, alcohol or drug abuse, mental illness, shock, epilepsy
  - *Stupor:* head injury, alcohol or drug abuse, stroke
  - *Brief unconsciousness:* head injury, fainting, epilepsy
  - *Coma:* stroke, allergy shock, head injury, poisoning, drug or alcohol abuse, diabetic coma, heat stroke or advanced heat exhaustion, shock, heart attack

- **Paralysis or loss of sensation**
    - *One side of body:* stroke, head injury
    - *Arms only:* spinal injury in neck
    - *Legs only:* spinal injury along back
    - *Arms and legs:* spinal injury in neck and possibly along back
    - *No pain, obvious injury:* spinal cord or brain damage, shock, hysteria, drug or alcohol abuse

You have learned about the significance of the injuries and how to provide care for patients with these signs and symptoms throughout your First Responder course. When you are faced with multiple casualties at critical incidents, be aware of your mental and physical stress levels. Critical incident stress debriefing (CISD) sessions or other qualified psychological support should be available after a disaster or unusual emergency incident to address the needs of rescuers who may have been influenced by the scene and the stress generated in providing emergency care (Figure 15.14).

HELICOPTER OPERATIONS/AIR MEDICAL TRANSPORT

Multiple-casualty incidents often require multiple resources, and helicopters are often used to transport the most critical patients. Most EMS systems use helicopters to transport critically ill or injured patients to specialty referral centers (trauma and hand centers, pediatric centers) or to evacuate patients from hard-to-reach or hazardous areas. Your instructor will tell you the circumstances that usually require a helicopter, often referred to as *medevac unit*, or medical evaluation unit. Check your local protocols for medevac procedures or contact your medical director on-line about patients who may need a medevac. Generally for helicopter transport, take the following steps:

Request the helicopter:

- If the patient needs to be transported to a specialty center that is more than a reasonable distance or drive time from the incident (check local protocols) *and* air transport will save time over ground transport.
- If the patient is a high-priority one who is trapped and extrication time will be prolonged.
- If the patient is in a remote area that cannot be reached by ground units or if ambulance access is blocked.

FIGURE 15.14
On the scene, personnel often don't realize they are under stress, and problems may surface after the event.

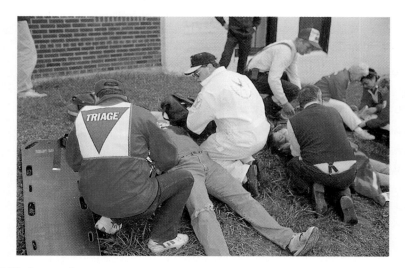

- If the air transport crew has a higher level of medical skills needed for patient care than ground crews.
- If the patient is a high-priority one with any of the following:
  – Shock
  – Chest or abdominal trauma with respiratory distress or shock
  – Serious mechanism of injury with altered vital signs
  – Penetrating injuries to any body cavity
  – Carbon monoxide poisoning
  – Heart attack
  – Amputation of limbs or digits (especially fingers)

Provide information to the helicopter:

- Your name, department name, call-back number or radio frequency
- Nature of the incident
- Exact location of the incident with landmarks and crossroads where possible, or latitudes and longitudes where known and appropriate
- Exact location of the landing zone

Set up the landing zone:

- Select a flat area that is clear of obstructions, such as utility poles and wires, radio towers, trees and shrubs. For daytime landings, the area should be at least 60 by 60 feet; for nighttime landings, 100 by 100 feet. (Check with your jurisdiction, as different aircraft have different landing requirements.) For large helicopters, double the landing area. (Check local protocols.) Pick up loose items that might blow into bystanders or into the helicopter's rotary blades.
- The landing area should be at least 50 feet away from the incident so rescuers are not hampered by noise and rotor wind. The patient can be packaged and placed in the ambulance and transported to the helicopter landing site.
- If the landing area must be a highway, stop traffic in both directions, even if the helicopter will land only on one side of the highway.
- Warn the crew of nearby obstructions, such as utility lines, radio towers, antennas, and trees.
- Mark the corner of the landing area with high-visibility objects: iridescent flags or tape by day; lights at night; flares for either day or night if there is no danger of fire. Never shine lights up to the helicopter at night. Bright lights directed toward the pilot take away his or her night vision, and make it harder for the pilot to see to land.
- Keep rescue crews and bystanders at least 200 feet away while the helicopter is landing.
- Do not approach the helicopter until the pilot signals you. Never approach from behind the helicopter where the pilot cannot see you and where the tail rotor is located. Always cross in front of the helicopter.
- Approach the unit in a crouch to avoid the dipping rotor blades. If the helicopter has to land on an incline, approach only from the downhill side.
- Secure loose items when approaching the helicopter so nothing will blow into the rotor blades.

Summary

As a First Responder, your first priority is your own safety, and your first duty is patient care. Before approaching a patient, make sure the scene is safe. Evaluate the scene of an auto accident by looking for hazards, such as traffic, fire, downed electrical lines, hazardous materials, and unstable vehicles. Also survey the scene for ejected or initially ambulatory patients.

Always make certain that an upright vehicle will not roll. Stabilize vehicles that are on inclines or slippery surfaces. If one vehicle is stacked on another or on its side, stabilize both before trying to reach patients. *Do not work in or around unstabilized vehicles or try to right overturned vehicles.*

Gain access to patients in a stabilized vehicle by trying doors first. If door access is not possible, attempt to gain access through a rear or side window. Break glass only after stabilizing the vehicle. Wear gloves and eye protection, or cover the glass and your face before breaking it. Break a window that is farthest from the patient.

Remove patients from vehicles only when there is danger or if lifesaving care is required. First Responders may not have the skills or tools to remove patients trapped under a vehicle. If you must free a pinned patient, use a jack or pry bars to lift the vehicle and, while lifting, place blocks to stabilize and shore up the vehicle.

When caring for a patient with a body part protruding through a window, cover the body part first, then break or fold the glass away before moving the patient.

Patients who are jammed or trapped in wreckage often can be freed by removing wreckage from around them, adjusting or removing seats, removing shoes, or cutting away clothing or seat belts.

The initial routes for gaining access to patients in buildings are doors, then windows. If you must break glass, protect yourself with gloves and goggles or cover the glass and your face. Be sure the patient is safe from flying glass and that you are stepping onto a safe floor.

At the scene of a fire, do *not* approach a burning vehicle or building unless you have the proper equipment and have been trained to assess the hazards and fight the fire. Do *not* enter a building that may be on fire. Do *not* try to go through smoke or potentially toxic gases. Do *not* attempt to enter a building or room that has any smoke coming from doors, windows, or vents. Do *not* open a door if it is hot. If caught in a burning building, stay low and crawl to safety.

Only trained personnel should shut off gas or electricity. If you smell natural gas, do *not* approach, but do alert dispatch. If there are electrical hazards, do *not* attempt a rescue. If electrical wires are touching a vehicle, have passengers stay in the vehicle and instruct them to avoid touching any metal object. If they must get out, warn them to jump clear without touching the vehicle and the ground at the same time.

If the scene contains hazardous or radioactive materials, stay in a safe area and call dispatch for help. Provide dispatch with essential information.

Triage is the sorting of patients based on the severity of their injuries and illnesses.

Triage systems vary by jurisdiction, but many will use a three- or four-category system. The categories are usually immediate (highest) priority, second (high) priority but a stable patient, delayed (low) priority, and sometimes a fourth category for the deceased or nonsalvageable (obvious death).

Patient assessment is important during triage. Vital signs and other key signs will help to determine the seriousness of the patient's injuries and to prioritize them properly.

An alternate triage system uses the **START plan**—a four-step simple triage and rapid treatment (care) program designed for use in multiple-casualty incidents.

Remember and Consider...

✔ If you came upon a situation in which a person was trapped in a vehicle or a building, what would you do first? Remember that the first thing to consider is your own personal safety. Are you equipped to handle a rescue on your own? If not, what kind of help is available for different types of rescue situations?

Check with your department and find out what emergency support personnel and equipment are available to be sent to assist First Responders on emergencies where people are trapped.

✔ What tools do you carry in your vehicle or on your unit? Are they simple tools that typically do not need a special training class to show you how to use them? Or are the tools more mechanical with special attachments that require training in order to use them properly? Regardless of the type of tool, will you know what to do with that tool when you need it to free a person from an entrapment situation?

Even simple tools are useless unless you know what to do with them or how to apply them effectively and safely in certain situations. If you have never actually removed a windshield with a putty knife, glazier's tool, or screwdriver, find out if your department can get an old junked vehicle so personnel can practice taking it apart. Work under the guidance and instruction of someone who has had training or experience in auto extrication so that you can learn the appropriate techniques properly.

Investigate...

Many response areas include a variety of building types in their residential, commercial, and industrial neighborhoods.

✔ Orient yourself and other department personnel to the different types of buildings in your response area by examining various neighborhoods and noting the type of building, what the normal entry points are, and what other entry points there may be. Consider how you would enter different buildings if you could not gain access to trapped victims by the normal entry point.

Firefighters work with local businesses and industries to preplan their fire attack and rescue operations in the event of a fire or other disaster. First Responders should do the same.

✔ Check with personnel at schools, stores, businesses, warehouses, and other commercial properties to find out where their first-aid room is, what medical personnel may be on duty and when, what is the closest access point to work areas, first-aid rooms, and offices or classrooms. Find out which areas will be hard to access if there is an emergency and what hazards may hinder your care of any personnel or students.

DETERMINING BLOOD PRESSURE

NOTE: It is recommended that you follow the American Heart Association (AHA) guidelines for determining blood pressure unless your state EMS system or local protocols recommend a different method.

In some localities, particularly those in which First Responders work in isolated areas, a special training program for determining blood pressure is included in the standard First Responder course. If this is not part of your course, do not try to train yourself in the use of the blood pressure cuff. Do only what you have been trained to do.

WHAT IS BLOOD PRESSURE?

Blood pressure is a measurement of the pressure of blood against the walls of the arteries. It is a vital sign. A blood pressure reading that is significantly above or below what is the normal range for a patient can be a valuable sign in determining what may be wrong (for example, shock). Repeated blood pressure measurements also help you monitor the patient's condition and check the patient's stability as you wait for the EMTs to arrive.

Blood pressure is determined by measuring the pressure changes in the arteries. The lower chamber on the left side of the heart (left ventricle) receives blood, **contracts,** and forces blood into the arteries to circulate throughout the body. The heart's contraction phase is called **systole.** When measured, the blood pumped into the system of arteries is called the **systolic** (sis-TOL-ik) blood pressure. It is affected by the force of the heart's pumping action, the resistance and elasticity of the arteries, blood volume (blood loss means lower pressure), blood thickness, and the amount of other fluids in the cells.

After the lower left chamber of the heart contracts, it **relaxes** and refills. This relaxation phase is called **diastole.** During diastole, the pressure in the arteries falls. When measured, this pressure is called the **diastolic** (di-as-TOL-ik) blood pressure.

Blood pressure is measured in specific units called millimeters of mercury (mmHg). These are the units on the blood pressure gauge. Since this system of

measurement is standard and known to the people receiving patient information from First Responders, you will not have to say "millimeters of mercury" after each reading. You will report the systolic pressure first and then the diastolic, as in 120 over 80 (120/80). The reading of 120/80 is considered a normal blood pressure reading, which represents the average blood pressure obtained from a large sampling of healthy adults. There is a wide range of "normal" for adults and children. Blood pressures are not usually measured in the field for children under 3 because it is difficult to get accurate measurements.

You will not know the normal blood pressure for a patient unless the person is alert, knows the information, and can tell you what it is. Blood pressure varies greatly among individuals; however, there is a general rule for estimating what a patient's blood pressure should be. This rule works for adults up to the age of 40. To estimate the systolic blood pressure of an adult male at rest, add his age to 100. To estimate the systolic blood pressure of an adult female at rest, add her age to 90.

Since you will not know the normal reading for a particular patient, you will take several readings in order to monitor the patient's status. One blood pressure reading is of little use. The first reading may be high because of the effects of stress produced by the emergency. After several readings, you will get a more accurate reading once you have started interventions and calmed the patient. An initial measurement may show that a patient has a blood pressure within normal range, but the condition may worsen. For example, a patient going into shock (hypoperfusion) may have a rapid pulse and a normal blood pressure reading when you first arrive at the scene. A few minutes later, the blood pressure may fall dramatically. Taking several readings while you are providing care is a way of monitoring patient status. Changes in blood pressure are significant and let you know that additional care is needed and transport is a priority.

A systolic blood pressure reading below 90 mmHg is serious in most adults. Some small adult females and small-build athletes may have a normal systolic blood pressure of 90 mmHg. But usually any systolic blood pressure measurement of 90 or less or a measurement that drops to 90/60 or below may be an indication that the patient is going into shock.

A reading above 150/90 is typically considered high blood pressure. But many patients will show a short-term initial rise in blood pressure at the emergency scene, usually due to anxiety, fear, and stress. You will need more than one reading to confirm high blood pressure. High blood pressure readings are typical in individuals who are obese or who have a history of high cholesterol. There are many other underlying medical conditions that cause high blood pressure that you will be unable to determine at the emergency scene. Several readings will help you determine patient status and guide your care and transport decisions.

Use the following general guidelines at the emergency scene. These guidelines are for your consideration in making assessment decisions:

Adults
- Systolic above 150—serious
- Systolic below 90—serious
- Diastolic above 90—serious
- Diastolic below 60—serious

Children: Ages 3 to 5
(Blood pressure is not taken in a child under 3 years of age.)
- Systolic above 120—serious
- Systolic below 70—serious
- Diastolic above 70—serious
- Diastolic below 50—serious

Children: Ages 6 to 14
- Systolic above 140—serious
- Systolic below 80—serious
- Diastolic above 70—serious
- Diastolic below 50—serious

NOTE: Ranges considered normal for children vary among physicians.

MEASURING BLOOD PRESSURE

NOTE: Photos are included in this appendix for demonstration purposes only. Protective gloves are normally worn by the rescuer for any patient intervention.

There are two common techniques used to measure blood pressure in emergency field situations. They are:

1. **Auscultation** (os-kul-TAY-shun)—using a blood pressure cuff and a stethoscope (Figure A1.1) to listen for characteristic sounds.
2. **Palpation**—using a blood pressure cuff and feeling the patient's radial pulse in the wrist or brachial pulse on the inner arm above the elbow.

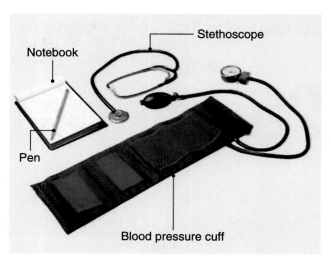

FIGURE A1.1
Blood pressure determination equipment.

DETERMINING BLOOD PRESSURE BY AUSCULTATION

To determine blood pressure using a blood pressure cuff and a stethoscope, you should:

1. Have the patient sitting or lying down (Figure A1.2). Cut away or remove clothing over the arm. Support the arm at the level of the heart. **WARNING:** Do *not* move the patient's arm if there is any possibility of spinal injury. Check to be sure the arm to be used has not been injured.

2. Select the correct-sized blood pressure cuff. Do not try to use an adult-sized cuff on a child. The cuff should be two-thirds the width of the upper arm.

3. Wrap the cuff around the patient's upper arm. The lower border of the cuff should be about 1 inch above the crease in the patient's elbow. The center of the bladder inside the cuff must be placed over the brachial artery in the upper arm (Figure A1.3).
NOTE: Some cuffs have a marker to tell you how to line up the cuff over the brachial artery. Know your equipment. Some cuffs have no markers, while others have inaccurate markers. The tubes entering the bladder in the cuff may not be in the correct location. The AHA recommends that you find the bladder center and line up the center of the bladder over the brachial artery.

4. Apply the cuff securely but not too tightly (Figure A1.4). You should be able to place one finger under the bottom edge of the cuff.

5. Place the ends of the stethoscope in your ears.

6. Use your fingertips to locate the brachial artery at the crease in the elbow.

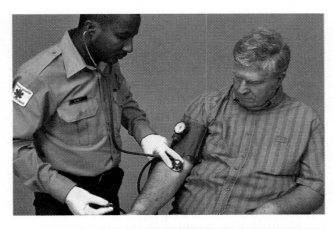

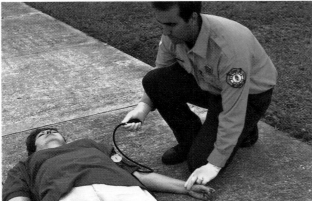

FIGURE A1.2
Positions for taking blood pressure.

7. Position the diaphragm or bell of the stethoscope over the brachial artery pulse site. Do not let the head of the stethoscope touch the cuff. If it touches the cuff, the stethoscope rubs against it during inflation and deflation. You will hear the rubbing sounds, which may cause you to record a false reading.

8. Close the bulb valve and inflate the cuff. As you do this, listen to the pulse sounds through the stethoscope. At a certain point, you will not be able to hear the pulse sounds.
   NOTE: The AHA preferred technique is to place your fingertips over the radial pulse as you inflate the cuff—explained below. When you can no longer feel the pulse, pump up the cuff pressure 30 more mmHg, place the stethoscope on the brachial artery, then slowly release the pressure as you listen for the systolic pressure sounds.

9. Keep inflating the cuff to a point 30 mmHg higher than the point where the pulse sounds stopped.

10. Open the bulb valve slowly to release pressure from the cuff. It should fall at a smooth rate of 2 to 3 mmHg per second.

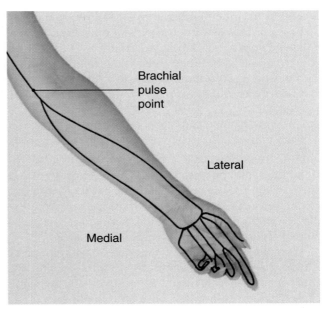

FIGURE A1.3
The brachial pulse point.

11. Listen carefully for and note the start of clicking or tapping sounds. This is the systolic pressure.

12. Let the cuff continue to deflate. Listen for and note when the clicking or tapping sounds fade (not when they stop). When the sound turns dull or soft, this is the diastolic pressure (Figure A1.5).
    NOTE: Some EMS systems have First Responders use the point where the sounds stop as the diastolic pressure.

13. Let the rest of the air out of the cuff quickly. If practical, leave the cuff in place so you can take additional readings.

14. Record the time, the arm used, the position of the patient (lying down, sitting), and the patient's pressure. Round off the readings to the next

FIGURE A1.4
Positioning the blood pressure cuff.

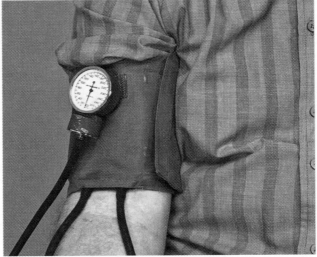

highest number. For example, 145 mmHg should be recorded as 146 mmHg. (The markings on the gauge are in even numbers. You may "see" the first sound in between two markings and want to record it as an odd number—145—but all blood pressure readings are in even numbers.)

Some people cannot find the brachial artery, or they cannot hear the pulse sounds when they inflate the cuff, but they can hear the sounds when they deflate the cuff. If you have this problem, use your fingertips to find the radial pulse in the wrist of the arm to which you have applied the cuff. Inflate the cuff until you can no longer feel the radial pulse. Continue to inflate the cuff to a point 30 mmHg higher than where the pulse stopped. The rest of the procedure is the same.

If you are not certain of a reading, be sure the cuff is totally deflated and wait 1 or 2 minutes and try again, or use the other arm. Should you try the same arm too soon, you may get false high readings.

Sometimes patients with high systolic readings have sounds that disappear as you deflate the cuff, only to reappear again. This can lead to both false systolic and diastolic readings as you record the high systolic reading and record the first disappearance of sound as the diastolic reading. If you continued to

FIGURE A1.5
Example of blood pressure sounds.

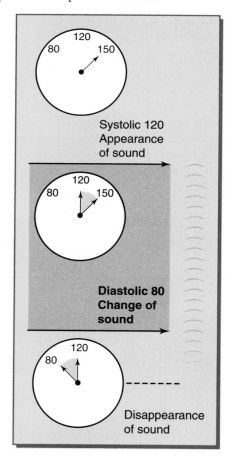

Systolic 120
Appearance of sound

Diastolic 80
Change of sound

Disappearance of sound

listen, you might find that sounds start up again about 20 mmHg lower. Whenever you have a high diastolic reading, wait 1 or 2 minutes and take a second reading and be sure to listen for sounds until all air is deflated from the cuff. On a subsequent reading, feel for the disappearance of the radial pulse as you inflate the cuff (this will ensure that you did not measure a false systolic pressure) and listen as you deflate the cuff down into the normal range and until all air is released from the cuff. Use the last fade of sound as the diastolic pressure.

See Scan A1-1 for a summary of determining blood pressure by auscultation.

DETERMINING BLOOD PRESSURE BY PALPATION

Using the palpation method (feeling the radial pulse) is not a very accurate method. It will provide you with one reading, an **approximate systolic pressure.** This method is used when there is too much noise around to use a stethoscope, or when there are too many patients for the number of rescuers at the scene. To determine blood pressure by palpation, place the cuff in the same position on the arm as you would for auscultation and:

1. Find the radial pulse on the arm with the cuff (Figure A1.6).
2. Close the valve and inflate the cuff until you can no longer feel the pulse.
3. Continue to inflate the cuff to a point 30 mmHg above the point where the pulse disappeared.
4. Slowly deflate the cuff and note the reading when you feel the pulse return.
5. Record the time, the arm used and the position of the patient, and the systolic pressure. Note that the reading was by palpation. If you give this information orally to someone, make sure they know the reading was by palpation, as in, "Blood pressure is 146 by palpation."

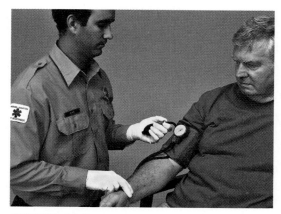

FIGURE A1.6
Measuring blood pressure by palpation.

Measuring Blood Pressure—Auscultation

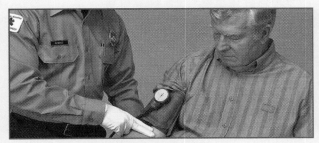

1. Position cuff and find pulse site.

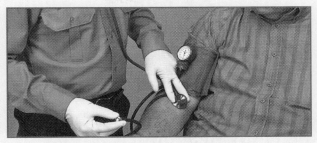

2. Set bell or diaphragm over pulse site.

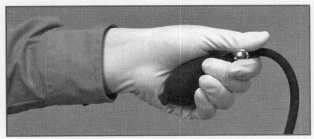

3. Close valve and inflate cuff.

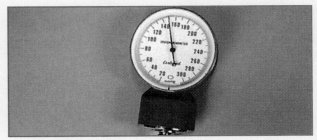

4. Listen for sound to disappear. Inflate 30 mmHg beyond this point.

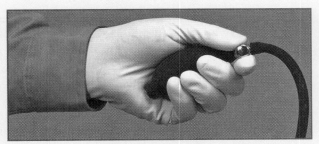

5. Open valve to deflate 2–3 mmHg/sec.

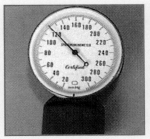

6. Listen for start of sound—systolic. Listen for sound to fade—diastolic.

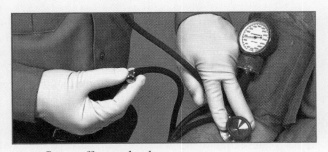

7. Deflate cuff completely.

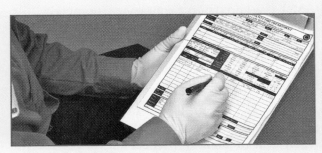

8. Record results.

APPENDIX 2

BREATHING AIDS AND OXYGEN THERAPY

THE FIRST RESPONDER'S ROLE

Some EMS systems do not train First Responders in the use of aids for breathing and oxygen therapy. But in many jurisdictions, supplemental training programs are offered to meet community needs. Learning how to use ventilation aids and how to administer oxygen may be part of your course or may be offered as a special supplement or continuing education program. Your jurisdiction may require this training especially if you are to perform your First Responder duties in an isolated area. You cannot train yourself to use oxygen administration equipment. Do only what you have been trained to do.

Basic life support is possible without equipment and should never be delayed while you locate, retrieve, and set up mechanical or other special devices. There is no doubt that the prompt and efficient use of certain pieces of equipment allows you to provide more effective emergency care for maintaining an open airway, assisting ventilations, and providing oxygen to the patient. But, the patient may suffer if you delay care, use faulty equipment, or use the wrong equipment.

New responsibilities come with the use of equipment in basic life support. You must:

- Be sure that the equipment is clean and operational before it will be needed at an emergency.
- Select the proper equipment for the patient.
- Monitor the patient more closely once you begin to use any device or delivery system.
- Make certain that the equipment is properly discarded, cleaned, refilled, replaced, or tested after its use.
- Practice and maintain the skills needed to use basic life-support equipment in order to provide efficient emergency care.

The administration of oxygen may require orders from a Medical Director in your jurisdiction. This is because **oxygen is a medication.** As a First Responder, you may be able to initiate the use of oxygen by radio communications with a medical facility, or you may be able to begin oxygen administration without oral orders in very specific situations because you are operating under direction of local protocols. You may only be allowed to work with certain devices or administer oxygen while assisting EMTs. Your instructor will give you the guidelines for your jurisdiction.

VENTILATION-ASSIST DEVICES

Chapter 6 describes the use of oropharyngeal and nasopharyngeal airways and the use of the pocket face mask with one-way valve and HEPA filter. These devices are used to assist in delivering ventilations. The bag-valve-mask ventilator is another device that is also used to assist with ventilations.

THE BAG-VALVE-MASK VENTILATOR

NOTE: Most EMS systems recommend that an oropharyngeal airway be inserted before attempting to ventilate the patient with a bag-valve-mask ventilator.

The bag-valve-mask ventilator is one of the most commonly used field devices for ventilating a nonbreathing patient. This handheld resuscitator is commonly called a bag-mask unit. Some EMS systems also use the unit to ventilate patients with shallow failing respirations (for example, in drug overdose). The bag-mask unit is available in sizes for infants, children, and adults. It also acts as an infection control barrier between you and your patient.

The bag-valve-mask unit delivers 21% oxygen to the patient when air from the atmosphere (room air) is squeezed through the unit to the patient's lungs. The unit can be connected to an oxygen supply source to enrich room air and deliver from 50% to nearly 100% oxygen. More will be said later about using oxygen sources with a bag-valve-mask unit.

REMEMBER: When providing mouth-to-mask ventilations, you are delivering 16% oxygen to the patient from your exhaled air. The bag-valve-mask unit will deliver 21% oxygen from the atmosphere and from 50% to up to nearly 100% oxygen from an oxygen delivery source.

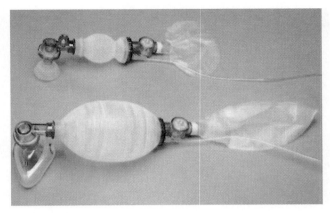

FIGURE A2.1
Disposable bag-valve-mask ventilator.

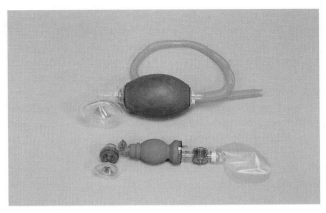

FIGURE A2.2
Pediatric and adult bag-valve-mask ventilators.

Many types of bag-valve-mask ventilators are available, and all have the same basic parts. There is a self-refilling bag, valves that control the flow of air, and a face mask to place on the patient's face. The face mask must have a transparent face piece so that the rescuer can see the patient's mouth in order to monitor for vomiting and to note lip color changes. There is also a standard 15/22 mm respiratory fitting, so a variety of respiratory equipment and face masks can be used with it. The bag-valve-mask unit must be made of material that can be easily cleaned and sterilized. Many EMS systems now use disposable units (Figure A2.1).

The principle behind the operation of the bag-valve-mask ventilator is simple. When you squeeze the bag, air is delivered to the patient's airway through a one-way, nonrebreathing valve. When you release the bag, air can flow from the patient's lungs out of another valve and into the atmosphere. The exhaled air does not go back into the bag. While the patient is exhaling, air from the atmosphere refills the bag and delivers a fresh air supply with the next squeeze.

The bag-valve-mask unit can be difficult to operate. This is especially true if you do not use it on a regular basis. You must practice to maintain your skill and effectiveness. If you are assigned a bag-valve-mask unit for use in the field, practice using it in the classroom until your skill technique is well developed. Some EMS systems have decided that skills for this device are poorly maintained, and thus they have selected the pocket face mask as the ventilation assist device for First Responders.

When using the bag-valve-mask ventilator as a single rescuer:

1. Position yourself at the patient's head and provide an open airway. Clear the airway if necessary.

2. Insert an oropharyngeal airway (see Chapter 6).

3. Use the correct mask size for the patient (Figure A2.2). Place the apex, or top, of the triangular mask over the bridge of the nose (between the eyebrows). Rest the base of the mask between the patient's lower lip and the projection of the chin.

4. Hold the mask firmly in position with (Figure A2.3):
   – The thumb holding the upper part of the mask
   – The index finger between the valve and the lower cushion
   – The third, fourth, and fifth fingers on the lower jaw, between the chin and ear

5. With your other hand, squeeze the bag fully once every 5 seconds and make sure the patient's chest rises.

6. Release pressure on the bag and let the patient passively exhale; the bag will refill from the atmosphere.

For trauma patients who must have their airway opened by the jaw-thrust maneuver, the two-rescuer method is more effective. The rescuer holding the mask in place can more easily perform the jaw-thrust maneuver while the other rescuer provides effective ventilations.

FIGURE A2.3
Hand positioning for using the bag-valve-mask ventilator.

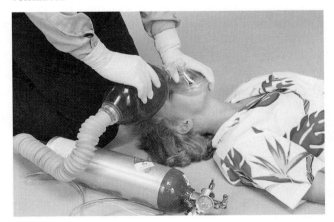

The bag-valve-mask unit can be used effectively during two-rescuer CPR by a skilled operator. The ventilator squeezes the bag on the compressor's fifth upstroke.

There are times when the bag-valve-mask unit will not deliver air to the patient's lungs. It is rare for the bag, valves, or mask to be the problem if you have kept the unit clean and in working order. Sometimes the problem is because of an airway obstruction that must be cleared. More often, the problem is caused by an improper seal between the patient's face and mask. If this occurs, you should reposition your fingers and check placement of the mask.

The most difficult part of operation is maintaining an adequate seal with the face mask in the one-person operation. For this reason, it is recommended that ventilating a patient with a bag-valve-mask unit should be done by two rescuers when they are available. One person uses two hands to maintain an airway (head-tilt, chin-lift or jaw-thrust maneuver as necessary) and a seal with the mask, while the other person squeezes the bag to ventilate the patient. Two-rescuer bag-valve-mask ventilation assures better airway management and ventilation.

To provide ventilations using the two-rescuer bag-valve-mask technique (Figure A2.4):

1. Position yourself so you can open the airway using the head-tilt, chin-lift or the jaw-thrust maneuver. Clear the airway with a finger sweep (adult) or suction and insert an oropharyngeal or nasopharyngeal airway if necessary.

2. Select the correct bag-valve-mask size for the patient (adult, child, or infant). Place the apex (top) of the mask over the bridge of the nose, then lower the mask over the mouth and upper chin. If the mask is the type that has a large, round cuff surrounding the ventilation port, center the port over the patient's mouth.

3. Kneel at the patient's head. For the chin-lift technique, place your thumbs over the top half of the mask, index and middle fingers over the bottom half, and your remaining fingers under the chin. For the jaw-thrust maneuver, place your thumbs over the nose portion of the mask, your index and middle fingers on the part of the mask that covers the mouth, and stretch your other fingers behind the jaw.

4. Use your ring and little fingers to bring the patient's jaw up to the mask and maintain the head-tilt, chin-lift; or to bring the jaw upward without tilting the head or neck for the jaw-thrust maneuver.

5. The second rescuer connects the bag to the mask (if not already done) and squeezes the bag with two hands, while you maintain a seal. The second rescuer squeezes the bag once every 5 seconds for an adult; once every 3 seconds for a child or an

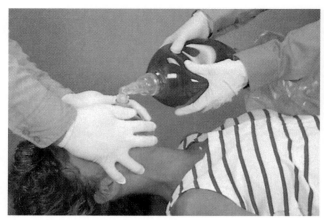

FIGURE A2.4
Two-rescuer bag-valve-mask technique.

infant. Watch for the patient's chest to rise as the bag is squeezed.

6. The second rescuer releases pressure on the bag, and the patient exhales passively. The bag refills from the oxygen source or from the atmospheric air.

OXYGEN THERAPY

THE IMPORTANCE OF OXYGEN

A patient may need oxygen for many reasons, including respiratory and cardiac arrest, shock, major blood loss (which reduces the number of red blood cells that carry oxygen), heart attack or heart failure, lung disease, injury to the lungs or the chest, airway obstruction, and stroke (the brain requires a constant supply of oxygen).

The 21% oxygen provided by the bag-valve mask is far more than the patient needs and is effective if the airway is open, the exchange surfaces of the lungs are working properly, there is enough oxygen available to be picked up by the blood, and the patient's heart and blood vessels are properly circulating blood to all the body tissues. When any one of these factors is missing or fails, a higher concentration of oxygen must be delivered to the patient so that the required amount reaches the body's tissues.

When performing CPR and using mouth-to-mask ventilations, your exhaled air only delivers 16% oxygen to the patient's lungs. This is enough to keep the patient alive. CPR is two-thirds less efficient than a healthy, beating heart circulating blood and oxygen. Ventilating by mouth-to-mask provides the patient with only the minimum oxygen required for short-term survival. By providing oxygen from a supply source, nearly 100% oxygen can reach the lungs. With more oxygen in the patient's blood, CPR efficiency is improved and the patient has a better chance for survival.

REMEMBER: *Oxygen is a medication.* Providing oxygen is a special responsibility that can be given only to someone trained in its use.

DISADVANTAGES OF OXYGEN THERAPY

There are certain hazards associated with oxygen administration including:

1. Oxygen used in emergency care is stored under **pressure** (2000 pounds per square inch [psi] or greater). If the tank is punctured or if a valve breaks off, the supply tank can become a missile.

2. Oxygen supports **combustion** and causes fire to burn more rapidly. Oxygen can saturate linens and clothing and cause them to ignite quickly.

3. Under pressure, **oxygen and oil do not mix.** When they come into contact with each other, there will be a severe reaction, which will cause an explosion. This can easily occur if you try to lubricate a delivery system or gauge with petroleum products.

4. Long-term use of high oxygen concentrations can result in **medical dangers.** These dangers include lung-tissue destruction (oxygen toxicity), lung collapse, eye damage in premature infants, and respiratory arrest in patients with *chronic obstructive pulmonary disease* (COPD), including emphysema, chronic bronchitis, and black lung. Except for the problems seen with COPD patients, these events are not typically field problems because of the short duration of administration.

Do not attempt to administer oxygen directly to newborn infants unless ordered to do so by a physician. When oxygen is required (difficult delivery, respiratory distress, very weak infant, premature birth, or other emergency), provide oxygen by blowing it into a foil tent formed over the infant's head, neck, and shoulders. If this is not practical, use the blow-by method by placing the mask near the side of the infant's mouth and nose.

For patients who have a history of chronic obstructive pulmonary disease (COPD), giving them too high a level of oxygen (above 28%) may cause these patients to go into respiratory arrest. In most cases, the patient will have to be in distress before this will happen. Most EMS system guidelines call for no more than 24% oxygen to be delivered initially to the COPD patient unless the patient is developing shock, has respiratory distress not related to COPD, or is already in respiratory arrest. Many times, though, the patient's respiratory distress is caused by another medical or trauma problem. In that situation, even if there is a history of COPD, provide a high level of oxygen.
REMEMBER: Never withhold the concentration of oxygen that is appropriate for the patient. If you are in doubt as to how much oxygen to deliver, radio or phone the hospital emergency department for advice.

EQUIPMENT AND SUPPLIES FOR OXYGEN THERAPY

An oxygen delivery system for the breathing patient includes a source (oxygen cylinder), pressure regulator, flowmeter, and a delivery device (face mask or cannula) (Figure A2.5). When possible, a humidifier should be added to provide moisture to the dry oxygen if the patient will be on the system for more than 30 minutes. (Some EMS systems will not allow the use of humidifiers because of improper storage and potential contamination.) The delivery system is the same for a nonbreathing patient, but a device must be added to allow the rescuer to force oxygen into the patient's lungs. This is known as a flow-restricted, oxygen-powered ventilation device. As a First Responder, you will probably use a bag-valve-mask ventilator connected to 100% oxygen when administering oxygen to the nonbreathing patient.

Oxygen Cylinders

When providing oxygen in the field, the standard source of oxygen is a seamless steel or lightweight alloy cylinder filled with oxygen under pressure. The pressure is equal to 2000 to 2200 pounds per square inch (psi). Cylinders come in various sizes, identified by letters. The smaller sizes practical for the First Responder include (Figure A2.6):

■ *D cylinder*—contains about 350 liters of oxygen
■ *E cylinder*—contains about 625 liters of oxygen

FIGURE A2.5
An oxygen delivery system.

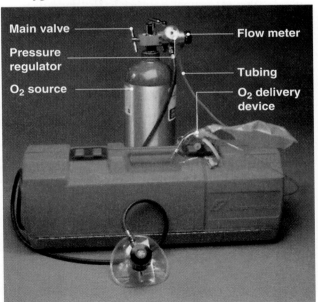

Main valve — Flow meter
Pressure regulator — Tubing
O₂ source — O₂ delivery device

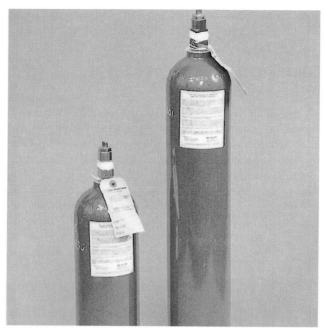

FIGURE A2.6
D cylinder (left); E cylinder (right).

You cannot tell if an oxygen cylinder is full, partially full, or empty by lifting or moving the cylinder. Part of your duty as a First Responder is to make certain that the oxygen cylinders are full and ready for use before they are needed for patient care. The length of time that you can use an oxygen cylinder depends on the pressure in the cylinder and the flow rate. The method of calculating cylinder duration is shown in Table A2-1. Oxygen cylinders should never be allowed to empty **below the safe residual level.** The safe residual level for an oxygen cylinder is determined when the pressure gauge reads 200 psi. At this point, you must switch to a fresh cylinder; below this point, there is not enough oxygen for proper delivery to the patient.

Safety is of prime importance when working with oxygen cylinders. You should:

■ *Never* allow a cylinder to drop or fall against any object. The cylinder must be well secured, preferably in an upright position. Never let a cylinder stand by itself.

■ *Never* allow smoking around oxygen equipment. Carry and use signs to clearly mark the area of oxygen use. The signs should read, "OXYGEN— NO SMOKING."

■ *Never* use oxygen equipment around open flames or sparks.

■ *Never* use grease or oil on devices that will be attached to an oxygen supply cylinder. Do *not* handle these devices when your hands are greasy.

■ *Never* put tape on the cylinder outlet or use tape to mark or label any oxygen cylinder or oxygen delivery equipment. The oxygen can react with the adhesive when it is torn from the cylinder and produce a fire.

■ *Never* try to move an oxygen cylinder by rolling it on its side or bottom.

■ *Never* store a cylinder near high heat or in a closed vehicle that is parked in the sun.

■ *Always* use the pressure gauges and regulators that are intended for use with oxygen and the equipment you are using.

■ *Always* ensure that valve seat inserts and gaskets are in good working order. This will help prevent dangerous leaks.

■ *Always* use medical-grade oxygen (USP). There are impurities in industrial-grade oxygen. The cylinder's label should state, "Oxygen USP."

■ *Always* fully open the valve of an oxygen cylinder; then close it half a turn when it is in use. This will serve as a safety measure in the event someone else thinks the valve is closed and tries to force it open.

TABLE A2-1: *D*URATION OF FLOW FORMULA

SIMPLE FORMULA
$\dfrac{\text{Gauge pressure in psi} - \text{residual pressure} \times \text{constant}}{\text{Flow rate in liters/minute}}$ = the safe duration of flow in minutes

RESIDUAL PRESSURE = 200 PSI CYLINDER CONSTANT

D = 0.16	G = 2.41
E = 0.28	H = 3.14
M = 1.56	K = 3.14

Determine the life of a D cylinder that has a pressure of 2000 psi and a flow rate of 10 liters/minute.

$$\frac{(2000 - 200) \times 0.16}{10} = \frac{288}{10} = 28.8 \text{ minutes}$$

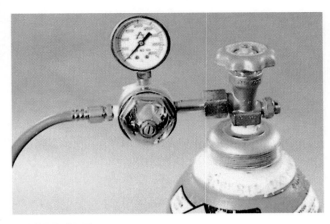

FIGURE A2.7
Single-stage regulator.

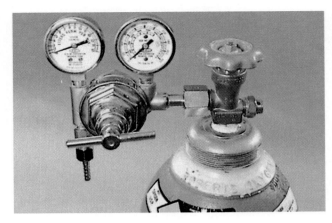

FIGURE A2.8
Two-stage regulator for D and E cylinders.

- *Always* store reserve oxygen cylinders in a cool, ventilated room as approved by your EMS system.
- *Always* have oxygen cylinders hydrostatically tested. This should be done **every 5 years** (3 years for aluminum cylinders). The date for retesting should be stamped on the cylinder.

Pressure Regulators

The safe working pressure for oxygen administration is 30 to 70 pounds per square inch (psi). The pressure in an oxygen cylinder is too high to be used directly from the cylinder, so a pressure regulator must be connected to the oxygen cylinder before it can be used to deliver oxygen to a patient.

On cylinders of the E size or smaller, a yoke assembly is used to secure the pressure regulator to the cylinder valve assembly. The yoke has pins that must mate with the corresponding holes found in the valve assembly. This is called a *pin-index safety system*. The position of the pins varies for different gases to prevent an oxygen delivery system from being connected to a cylinder containing another gas.

Cylinder pressure can be reduced in either one or two steps. For a one-step reduction, a single-stage pressure regulator is used (Figure A2.7). A two-step reduction requires a two-stage regulator (Figure A2.8). Most regulators used in emergency care are the single-stage type.

Before connecting the pressure regulator to an oxygen supply cylinder, *open the cylinder valve slightly* for just a second to clear dirt and dust out of the delivery port or threaded outlet. This is called "cracking" the cylinder valve. Part of the maintenance of the regulator includes cleaning the inlet filter. Checking the filter for damage and dirt will prevent damage to and contamination of the regulator.

Flowmeters

A flowmeter is connected to the pressure regulator to give the user control over the flow of oxygen in liters

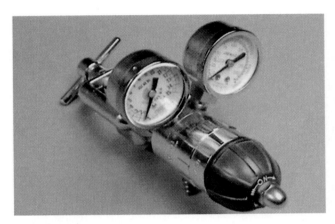

FIGURE A2.9
Bourdon gauge flowmeter (pressure gauge).

per minute. Three types of flowmeters are available. For emergency care in the field, the pressure-compensated flowmeter is considered superior to the bourdon gauge flowmeter; however, it is more delicate than the bourdon gauge and must be in an upright position for proper operation. For these reasons, most EMS systems employ the bourdon gauge for field use. The constant-flow selector valve is a new type of flowmeter that is gaining in popularity.

- *Bourdon gauge flowmeter* (Figure A2.9)—This flowmeter is a pressure gauge calibrated to indicate flow of gas in liters per minute. It is inaccurate at low flow rates and has been criticized for being unstable. This device will not compensate for back pressure. A partial obstruction (as from a kinked hose) will produce a reading higher than the actual flow. The gauge may read 4 liters per minute and be delivering only 1 liter per minute. False high readings also can be produced when the filter in the gauge becomes clogged. The bourdon gauge is fairly sturdy and will operate in any position.
- *Pressure compensated flowmeter* (Figure A2.10)— This is a gravity-dependent meter that must be in

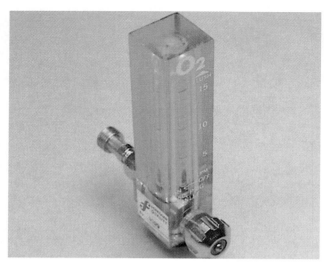

FIGURE A2.10
Pressure-compensated flowmeter.

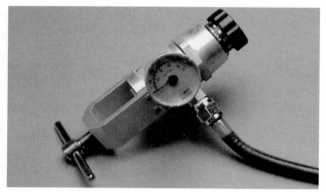

FIGURE A2.11
Constant flow selector valve.

an upright position to deliver accurate readings. It has an upright, calibrated glass tube containing a ball float. The float will rise and fall according to the amount of gas passing through the tube. Its readings indicate the actual flow of the gas at all times. This is true even when there is a partial obstruction to gas flow (as from a kinked delivery tube). Should the delivery tubing collapse, the ball will drop to indicate the lowered delivery rate.

■ *Constant-flow selector valve* (Figure A2.11)—This device has no gauge. It allows for the adjustment of flow in liters per minute in stepped increments (2, 4, 6, 8, . . . 15 liters per minute). When using this type of flowmeter, make certain that it is properly adjusted for the desired flow and monitor the meter to make certain that it stays properly adjusted. This type of meter should be tested for accuracy as recommended by the manufacturer.

Humidifiers

A humidifier is a nonbreakable jar of sterile water that can be attached to the flowmeter. As the dry oxygen from the cylinder passes through the water, it is mois-

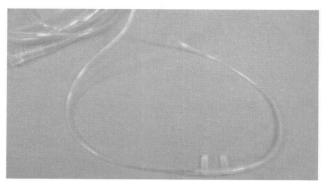

FIGURE A2.12
A loop-type nasal cannula.

turized and becomes more comfortable for the patient to breathe. Unhumidified oxygen delivered to a patient over a long period of time (usually more than 20 minutes) will dry out the mucous membranes in the airway and lungs. For the short period of time that the patient receives oxygen in the field, this is not usually a problem. A problem does arise, though, when humidifiers are not used appropriately. Too often, the task of changing them between patients is overlooked, or the device is opened but not used, which allows it to become contaminated over time. Because of this infection risk and the fact that they are not required for short transports, many EMS systems no longer use humidifiers.

Oxygen Delivery Devices: Breathing Patients

The *nasal cannula* and one type of face mask, the *nonrebreather*, are the main oxygen delivery devices used for the field administration of oxygen to breathing patients.

■ *Nasal cannula*—A nasal cannula delivers oxygen into the patient's nostrils by way of two small plastic prongs (Figure A2.12). Its efficiency is greatly reduced by nasal injuries, colds, and other types of nasal airway obstruction. In common use, a flow rate of 4 to 6 liters per minute will provide the patient with 36% to 44% oxygen. The relationship of oxygen concentration to liter per minute flow is:

– 1 liter/minute	24% oxygen
– 2 liters/minute	28% oxygen
– 3 liters/minute	32% oxygen
– 4 liters/minute	36% oxygen
– 5 liters/minute	40% oxygen
– 6 liters/minute	44% oxygen

For every 1 liter per minute increase in oxygen flow, you deliver a 4% increase in the concentration of oxygen.

At 4 liters per minute and above, the patient's breathing patterns may prevent the delivery of the stated percentages. At 5 liters per minute, rapid drying of the nasal membranes is possible. After 6 liters per minute, the device does not deliver any higher concentration of oxygen and may be uncomfortable for most patients.

NOTE: The Venturi mask is the delivery device of choice for COPD patients in a hospital setting; however, the nasal cannula is often used in field emergency care. Follow your local guidelines. The nasal cannula can be used for COPD patients if a flow rate no greater than 1 to 2 liters per minute is required by the patient's doctor or prescription or by local protocols. A higher concentration can be provided with a nonrebreather mask if the patient is still in distress after you have tried the nasal cannula. Some patients who need a higher concentration of oxygen from the nonrebreather mask cannot tolerate a mask on the face. In that case, use a nasal cannula set to a higher flow, but keep in mind that a flow rate of 6 liters per minute may be uncomfortable for the patient.

- *Nonrebreather mask*—This device is used to deliver high concentrations of oxygen (Table A2-2). Inflate the reservoir bag before placing the mask on the patient's face (Figure A2.13). This is done by using your finger to cover the exhaust portal or the connection between the mask and the reservoir. Care must be taken to ensure a proper seal with the patient's face. The reservoir must not deflate by more than one-third when the patient takes his deepest inspiration. You can maintain the volume in the bag by adjusting the oxygen flow. The patient's exhaled air does not return to the reservoir; it is vented through the one-way flaps or portholes on the mask. The minimum flow rate when using this mask is 8 liters per minute, but a higher flow (12–15 liters per minute) may be required.

*A*DMINISTERING OXYGEN

Scans A2-1 and A2-2 will take you step-by-step through the process of preparing the oxygen delivery system,

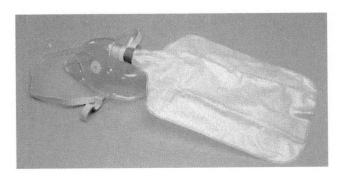

administering oxygen, and discontinuing the administration of oxygen.

Administration of Oxygen to a Nonbreathing Patient

The EMS-approved pocket face mask (see Chapter 6) with oxygen inlet and your own breath can be combined to deliver oxygen to a nonbreathing patient. The bag-valve-mask ventilator used alone or with 100% oxygen under pressure and the flow-restricted, oxygen-powered ventilation device with 100% oxygen under pressure can be used in ventilating the nonbreathing patient. The flow restricted, oxygen-powered ventilation device is considered an EMT-level device. You may receive training with this device so that you can assist EMTs.

NOTE: When using these devices, an oropharyngeal airway should be inserted (see Chapter 6).

WARNING: These devices can be used effectively for two-rescuer CPR. For one-rescuer CPR, these devices will not remain in place and keep a tight seal. You will have to place and seal the masks on these devices and open the airway each time you return to the ventilation position. This causes too great a delay between compressions and ventilations for one-rescuer CPR. The simplest device to use in one-rescuer CPR is the pocket face mask with oxygen inlet.

TABLE A2-2: *O*XYGEN DELIVERY DEVICES

OXYGEN DELIVERY DEVICE	FLOW RATE	% OXYGEN DELIVERED	SPECIAL USE
Nasal cannula	1 to 6 liters per minute	24% to 44%	Most medical and COPD patients at low concentrations
Nonrebreather mask	Start with 8 liters per minute, practical high is 12 liters per minute	80% to 95%	Good for severe non-COPD and shock patients. Provides high-oxygen concentrations

Preparing the Oxygen Delivery System

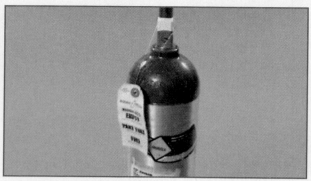

1. Select desired cylinder and check label for "Oxygen USP."

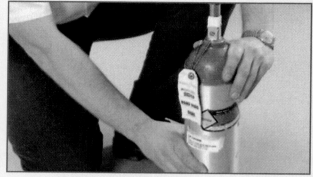

2. Place the cylinder in an upright position and stand to one side.

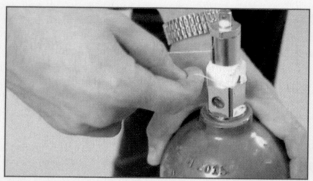

3. Remove the plastic wrapper or cap protecting the cylinder outlet.

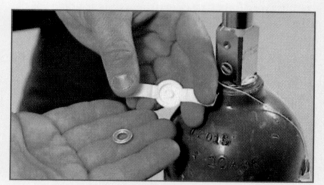

4. Keep the plastic washer that is used in some setups.

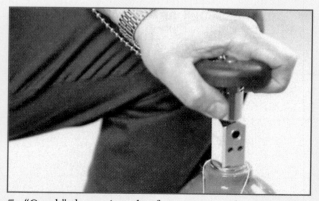

5. "Crack" the main valve for one second.

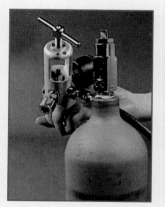 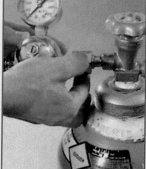

6. Select the correct pressure regulator and flowmeter.

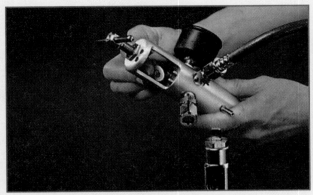

7. Place cylinder valve gasket on regulator oxygen port.

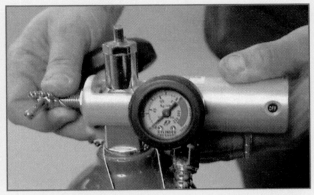

8. Make certain that the pressure regulator is closed.

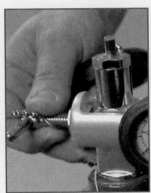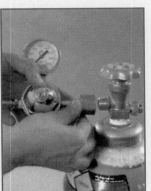

9. Align PIN or thread by hand.

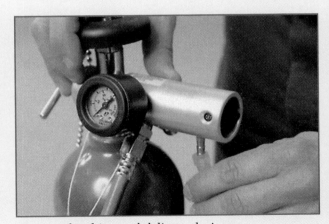

10. Tighten T-screw for PIN-index.

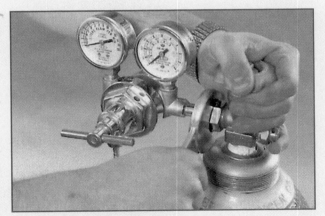

11. Tighten with a wrench for threaded system.

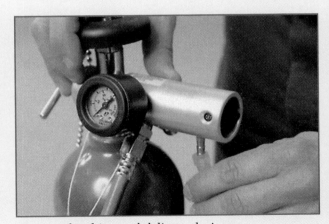

12. Attach tubing and delivery device.

Administering Oxygen

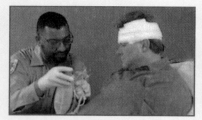

1. Explain the need for oxygen to patient.

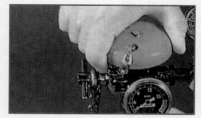

2. Open main valve and adjust flowmeter.

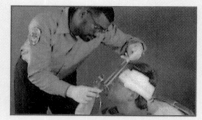

3. Position oxygen delivery device.

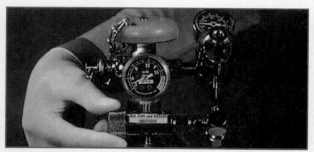

4. Adjust flowmeter.

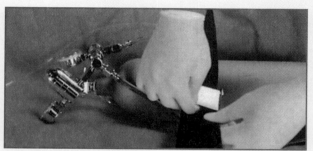

5. Secure during transfer.

Discontinuing Oxygen

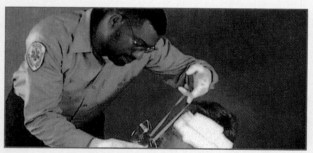

1. Remove the delivery device.

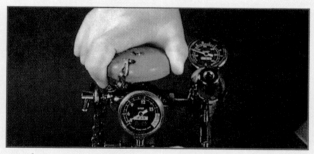

2. Close main valve.

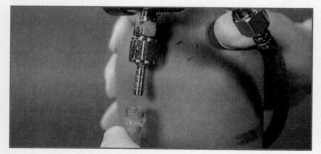

3. Remove delivery tubing.

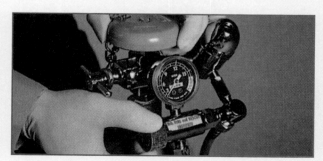

4. Bleed flowmeter.

Bag-Valve-Mask Ventilator and Oxygen Oxygen tubing is connected to the outlet of the flowmeter and the oxygen inlet of the bag-valve-mask unit to deliver 100% oxygen to the patient's airway at 15 liters per minute. Most bag-valve-mask units have an oxygen reservoir (long tube or bag) attached to the bag to increase the oxygen concentration delivered to the patient. Used without a reservoir, it will deliver approximately 50% oxygen; used with a reservoir, nearly 100%. Maintain an open airway, a tight mask-to-face seal, squeeze the bag to deliver oxygen, and release the bag to allow for a passive expiration. There is no need to remove the mask when the patient exhales.

This device can also be used to assist the breathing efforts of a patient who has failing respirations (as in a drug overdose).

The Flow-Restricted, Oxygen-Powered Ventilation Device A flow-restricted, oxygen-powered ventilation device (FROPVD) delivers oxygen through a regulator from a pressurized cylinder. By depressing a trigger on the mask, the First Responder can deliver artificial ventilations to the patient. This device is similar to the demand-valve resuscitator but with newer features that help to provide effective ventilation and help to safeguard the patient.

Standard features of this device include:

■ A peak flow rate of 100% oxygen delivered at up to 40 liters per minute
■ An inspiratory pressure relief valve that opens at approximately 60 cm of water pressure
■ An audible alarm that sounds when the relief valve is activated
■ A rugged design and construction
■ A trigger that enables the rescuer to use both hands to maintain a mask seal while activating the device
■ Easy and effective operation during both usual and extreme environmental conditions

To operate the FROPVD, follow the same procedures for placing and sealing the mask as you would for the bag-valve-mask unit. Press the trigger to deliver oxygen until the chest rises and repeat every 5 seconds. Release the trigger after the chest inflates and allow for passive exhalation. If the chest does not rise, reposition the head or reopen the airway, check for obstructions, reposition the mask, check for a seal, and try again. If the chest still does not rise, check for airway obstruction, assure you have a good mask-to-face seal, and assure you have opened the airway. If the chest still does not rise, consider an alternative ventilation device or procedure.

Monitor your patient carefully when using an FROPVD. High pressure caused by the device can force air into the esophagus and fill the stomach. Air distends the stomach, which presses into the lung cavity and reduces oxygen to the lungs. To avoid or correct this problem, carefully maintain and monitor airway, mask-to-face seal, and chest rise. Do *not* continue to provide air after chest rise—allow passive exhalation and reventilate.

If you suspect neck injury, have an assistant stabilize the patient's head or use your knees to prevent head movement. Bring the jaw to the mask without tilting the head or neck and trigger the mask to ventilate the patient.

WARNING: The flow-restricted, oxygen-powered ventilation device (FROPVD) should be used only on adults.

General Guidelines for Oxygen Dosages

The following dosages of oxygen are recommended according to the nature of the patient's problem. The standing orders for oxygen vary slightly in different EMS systems. Follow your local protocols.

NOTE: In the following scenarios, when the nonrebreather mask is recommended and you only have a nasal cannula or the patient will not tolerate the mask, provide oxygen by cannula at a rate of 6 liters per minute.

Trauma Provide oxygen by nonrebreather at 12–15 LPM to deliver 80% to 90% concentration (not necessary for minor scratches, scrapes and cuts, minor extremity injuries [finger or toe], strains, and sprains).

Childbirth Provide oxygen by nonrebreather at 12–15 LPM to deliver 80% to 90% concentration for the mother with predelivery bleeding, excessive postdelivery bleeding, breech birth, miscarriage or induced abortion that has excessive bleeding, ectopic pregnancy, and toxemia (eclampsia).

For the newborn, provide oxygen into a tent placed over the infant's head and shoulders or by mask and blow-by method to premature infants, difficult breech births, infants with bleeding from the umbilical cord, weak infants, or those with lasting blue color (cyanosis) other than hands and feet.

Environmental Emergencies Provide oxygen by nonrebreather at 12–15 LPM to deliver 80% to 90% concentration for the following:

■ Allergy (anaphylactic) shock
■ Burns
■ Drug overdose
■ Near-drowning
■ Poisoning
■ Scuba accidents

If the patient is not breathing, provide oxygen through the pocket face mask with oxygen inlet while performing mouth-to-mask ventilations or by bag-valve-mask ventilator attached to an oxygen cylinder. Use a reservoir with the bag-valve mask to provide nearly 100% oxygen concentration.

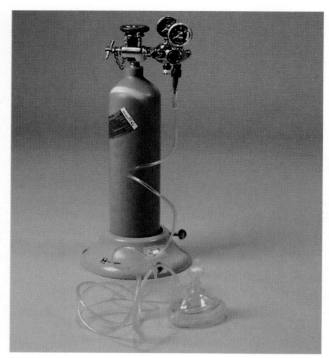

FIGURE A2.14
An EMS-approved pocket face mask with one-way valve set to deliver supplemental oxygen.

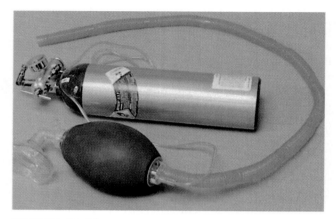

FIGURE A2.15
A bag-valve-mask ventilator connected to an oxygen supply.

Medical Emergencies Provide oxygen by non-rebreather at 12–15 LPM to deliver 80% to 90% concentration for the following:

■ Chest pain
■ Respiratory disorders and distress or trouble breathing
■ Diabetic emergencies
■ Patients recovering from seizure
■ Abdominal pain or distress

If the patient is not breathing, provide oxygen through the pocket face mask with oxygen inlet (Figure A2.14) while performing mouth-to-mask ventilations or by bag-valve-mask unit attached to an oxygen cylinder (Figure A2.15). Use a reservoir with the bag-valve mask to provide nearly 100% oxygen concentration.

APPENDIX 3

PHARMACOLOGY

NOTE: This appendix is designed to aid First Responders who are being trained to assist patients in taking specific prescribed medications of their own. This training is meant to be a part of a formal training program that is under the guidance and supervision of a Medical Director. Any provider level in the EMS system that gives or assists patients in taking their prescribed medications must follow either specific written protocols or oral medical direction. First Responders must not attempt to give any medication without medical direction.

INTRODUCTION

Pharmacology is the study of drugs, their origins, nature, chemistry, effects, and use. First Responders will assess and care for many patients whose histories include the medications they take, and whose problems may be caused by the effects of taking or of not taking those medications properly. This appendix lists and describes the few medications that First Responders may be carrying and the few prescribed medications that you may assist a patient in taking. It also discusses how to give or assist the patient in taking the medications and the effects of these medications on the patients.

REMEMBER: You may only give or assist in giving certain medications under the supervision of medical direction.

MEDICATIONS

There are typically six medications that EMTs and First Responders may be trained to use in the field. Three of the medications are used so commonly and may be carried by First Responders that we often do not even consider them medications. They are *oxygen*, *activated charcoal*, and *oral glucose*, which you may administer under specific conditions and circumstances. Activated charcoal and oral glucose are sold over the counter in pharmacies and are found in many households. The other three medications are those prescribed by a physician for patients and are usually found in the patients' homes. They are *prescribed inhalers*, *nitroglycerin*, and *epinephrine*, which you may be able to assist a patient in taking with the approval of medical direction only and under specific conditions and circumstances.

SIDE EFFECTS, INDICATIONS, AND CONTRAINDICATIONS

For every medication, there are side effects, indications, and contraindications. After a patient has taken any medication, you must monitor the patient to see how the drug affected him or her. If taken properly, medications will usually reverse the ill-effects of the medical condition; but if the medications are expired or the patient's condition is beyond the help of the drug, the medication will be ineffective. Medications sometimes have side effects. A *side effect* is any unwanted action or reaction of the drug other than the desired effect. Some effects are expected and predictable. Nitroglycerin will dilate vessels, not just in the heart, but throughout the body. It will cause a drop in blood pressure as the vascular system enlarges, and it will cause a headache as the vessels in the brain expand in limited skull space. You must watch for side effects and report them, especially before administering a second dose, which may cause life-threatening problems.

For each drug, there are indications for its use. These *indications* are specific signs or conditions for which it is appropriate to use the drug. For example, a patient with chest pain has the "indications" for using nitroglycerin; or, nitroglycerin is indicated for chest pain. Also, there are contraindications for each drug's use. These *contraindications* are specific signs or conditions for which it is *not* appropriate to use the drug. For example, a patient with chest pain but low blood pressure has the "contraindications" for nitroglycerin use since it dilates blood vessels and causes blood pressure to drop.

MEDICATIONS CARRIED ON THE FIRST RESPONDER UNIT

Activated Charcoal (Scan A3-1)

Activated charcoal is not the kind from the barbecue grill, but a powder prepared from charred wood and usually premixed with water, called a slurry, for use in the prehospital emergency situation. (Some brands require you to add the water.) Activated charcoal is used to treat a patient who swallowed a poison or who took an oral overdose of drugs or medications. When the patient drinks the activated charcoal slurry, it absorbs some of the poisonous substance or drug in the patient's stomach. The activated charcoal also helps prevent the poison or drug from being absorbed by the body.

Oral Glucose (Scan A3-2)

Glucose is a simple sugar, which is found in foods such as fruit, and is normally present in the blood. It is our chief source of energy and an all-purpose fuel for the body and brain. The brain is very sensitive to low levels of glucose and functions poorly without it. A patient with low glucose levels will have an altered mental status. Glucose levels can be raised by giving oral glucose, a form of glucose that comes in a gel and is packaged in different-sized tubes like toothpaste. It can be given to a patient with an altered mental status and a history of diabetes by placing it inside the mouth.

To administer oral glucose, apply some of the gel to a tongue depressor and spread it between the patient's cheek and gum. Continue to apply small doses until the tube is empty. This gum area is rich in blood vessels, which quickly absorb the glucose and carry it through the bloodstream to the brain. Once the level of glucose is elevated in the brain, the patient's condition usually begins to improve.

Oxygen (Figure A3.1)

You know that the atmosphere contains 21% oxygen. But pure 100% oxygen is used as a drug to treat patients who have low oxygen levels in their blood because of medical or traumatic conditions. Appendix 2 describes oxygen therapy and how to use the special adjuncts that help deliver oxygen to a patient. If your First Responder unit carries oxygen and oxygen delivery adjuncts, you must participate in a training program to learn how and when to use them properly. You must also practice your skills so you are able to provide appropriate care to patients who need oxygen. In addition, you must follow your jurisdiction's guidelines, protocols, and medical direction in order to administer oxygen.

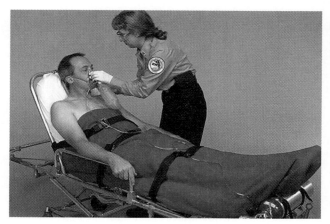

FIGURE A3.1
Oxygen is a powerful drug.

PRESCRIBED MEDICATIONS

Prescribed Inhalers (Scan A3-3)

Many patients have chronic respiratory diseases such as asthma, emphysema, or bronchitis that cause the airway passages in the lungs to narrow, or become constricted. Such patients usually carry a medication called a "bronchodilator" in an inhaler device. This medication enlarges, or dilates, the airway passages so the patient can breathe easier. The inhaler device holds the dilating medication in an aerosol form, which can be sprayed into the mouth and inhaled. You must have medical direction to help a patient self-administer this medication. You must also make sure that this medication belongs to the patient and was not lent to him by a well-meaning family member or friend with a similar problem. Checking for an expiration date is important since expired medication is not effective.

Nitroglycerin (Scan A3-4)

Nitroglycerin is a chemical that is well known as an explosive, but it also has medical uses. It dilates blood vessels and relieves certain types of pain, particularly the type caused by a heart condition called *angina pectoris*. Patients who have heart conditions that cause recurring chest pain or who have a history of heart attack may have a prescription for nitroglycerin, often called "nitro," and carry it with them. Nitroglycerin dilates, or enlarges, the constricted vessels in the heart muscle so it can receive blood and oxygen, which help ease the pain.

Often, First Responders will arrive at the scene to find out during the focused assessment that the patient with chest pain has taken a dose of nitroglycerin. Just as often, the patient with chest pain is carrying the medication and has not thought to take it. Patients can usually take up to three tablets—one every 5 minutes—

over a 15-minute period. You will need to consult medical direction to help administer nitroglycerin or to get permission to give more after the patient has taken the three doses. As with the inhaler, be sure to check that the nitroglycerin is actually the patient's medication and that it has not reached the expiration date. Sometimes the medication may not be effective because the patient has not stored it properly. If the patient still has pain after taking the maximum dose, arrange to transport. If the medication does not seem to be working, either it is defective or the patient's condition needs immediate in-hospital attention.

Epinephrine Auto-Injectors (Scan A3-5)

Many people have allergies and will react severely to certain foods, medicines, or the poisons of insect stings and snakebites. These reactions may be life-threatening as they cause the airway to become swollen and narrow or cause blood vessels to dilate, which appears as skin flushing and swelling. Epinephrine is a medication that can reverse these reactions. It relaxes the air passages so breathing becomes easier, and it constricts the enlarged blood vessels. Reactions to allergies can have a very sudden onset, and any reaction that causes breathing and circulation problems must be recognized and treated quickly. The patient must take his prescribed epinephrine immediately. Those patients who know of their allergies and expect severe reactions generally carry their prescription with them in a device called an auto-injector. This is a syringe with a spring-loaded needle that will release and inject epinephrine into a muscle when the patient presses it against his skin (usually in the thigh). If you need to assist the patient in taking epinephrine, first check to see if the injector is prescribed for that patient and get permission from medical direction. Also, check the expiration date.

REMEMBER: An expired medication will be ineffective and the patient must be transported to a hospital quickly.

RULES TO FOLLOW WHEN ADMINISTERING MEDICATIONS

Before you give any of the three medications you may carry, or before you assist a patient in taking any of the three prescribed medications, there are a few more things you need to know. First you will check the four "rights" that are rules for giving any medication. Often you will have to rely on the patient's word. Ask the following questions:

■ *Is this the right patient for this medication?* (As you read from the bottle, ask, "Is your name Henry Melvin?" If the patient doesn't have the labeled box or bottle, simply ask if this is his own medication. If he says yes, you may believe him.)

■ *Is this the right medication for this patient?* (The patient is having chest pain but hands you a bottle of penicillin; or the patient has strep throat and hands you a bottle of nitroglycerin.)

■ *Is this the right dose?* (The dosage is usually written on the label, but the patient doesn't always carry the original box or bottle the medication came in.)

■ *Is this the right route for taking the medication?* (Different types of medications, such as tablets, powders, sprays, gels, slurries, pastes, are given by different routes—swallowed by mouth, inhaled by mouth, dissolved under the tongue, injected into or absorbed through the skin.)

ROUTES FOR ADMINISTERING MEDICATIONS

The way a patient takes a medication has an effect on how quickly the medication enters the bloodstream and begins to relieve the medical condition. Medications are administered by the following routes:

■ Oral or swallowed, usually in some solid form (a tablet or pill), or in some liquid form (powder dissolved in or mixed with a liquid such as the activated charcoal slurry).

■ Intramuscular, or injected into a muscle, like the epinephrine auto-injector.

■ Sublingual, or dissolved under the tongue, like the nitroglycerin tablets.

■ Inhaled, or breathed into the lungs, from an inhaler or oxygen delivery device such as the medication given for chronic respiratory problems or the oxygen gas given for respiratory distress and for medical and trauma conditions.

■ Endotracheal, or sprayed into a tube inserted into the trachea (windpipe), so it can more directly reach the lungs and be absorbed quickly. (First Responders will not administer medication in this form.)

You can see there is a lot to know and understand about medications. Once you have become familiar with these medications and their effects, you will become more confident in giving the ones that you carry and that you can assist patients in taking if the medications are prescribed for them. Remember, you will give and assist with all medications only under medical direction.

Activated Charcoal

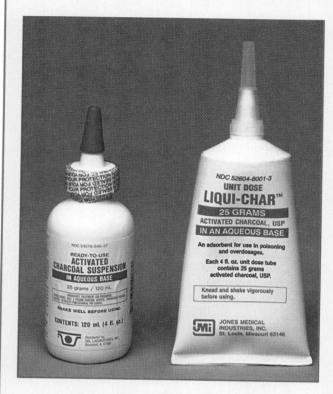

DOSAGE

1. Adults and children: 1 gram activated charcoal/kg of body weight
2. Usual adult dose: 25–50 grams
3. Usual pediatric dose: 12.5–25 grams

ADMINISTRATION

1. Consult medical direction.
2. Shake container *vigorously*.
3. Since medication looks like mud, patient may need to be persuaded to drink it. Providing a covered container and a straw will prevent the patient from seeing the medication and so may improve patient compliance.
4. If patient does not drink the medication right away, the charcoal will settle. Shake or stir it again before administering.
5. Record the name, dose, route, and time of administration of the medication.

ACTIONS

1. Activated charcoal binds to certain poisons and prevents them from being absorbed into the body.
2. Not all brands of activated charcoal are the same; some bind much more than others, so consult medical direction about the brand to use.

MEDICATION NAME

1. Generic: activated charcoal
2. Trade: SuperChar, InstaChar, Actidose, Liqui-Char, and others

INDICATIONS

Poisoning by mouth

CONTRAINDICATIONS

1. Altered mental status
2. Ingestion of acids or alkalis
3. Unable to swallow

MEDICATION FORM

1. Premixed in water, frequently available in plastic bottle containing 12.5 grams of activated charcoal
2. Powder—should be avoided in field

SIDE EFFECTS

1. Black stools
2. Some patients, particularly those who have ingested poisons that cause nausea, may vomit. If patient vomits, repeat the dose once.

REASSESSMENT STRATEGIES

Be prepared for the patient to vomit or further deteriorate.

Oral Glucose

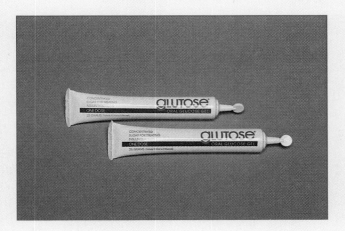

MEDICATION NAME

1. Generic: Glucose, oral
2. Trade: Glutose, Insta-glucose

INDICATIONS

Patients with altered mental status with a known history of diabetes mellitus

CONTRAINDICATIONS

1. Unconsciousness
2. Known diabetic who has not taken insulin for days
3. Unable to swallow

MEDICATION FORM

Gel, in toothpaste-type tubes

DOSAGE

One tube

ADMINISTRATION

1. Assure signs and symptoms of altered mental status with a known history of diabetes.
2. Assure patient is conscious.
3. Administer glucose.
    a. Place on tongue depressor between cheek and gum.
    b. Self-administered between cheek and gum.
4. Perform ongoing assessment.

ACTIONS

Increases blood sugar

SIDE EFFECTS

None when given properly. May be aspirated by the patient without a gag reflex.

REASSESSMENT STRATEGIES

If patient loses consciousness or seizes, remove tongue depressor from mouth.

Prescribed Inhaler

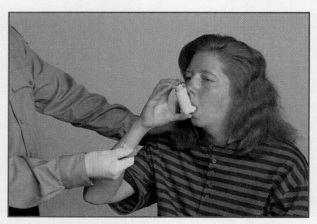

MEDICATION NAME

1. Generic: albuterol, isoetharine, metaprotarnol
2. Trade: Proventil, Ventolin, Bronkosol, Bronkometer, Alupent, Metaprel

INDICATIONS

Meets all of the following criteria:

1. Patient exhibits signs and symptoms of respiratory emergency.
2. Patient has physician-prescribed handheld inhaler.
3. Medical direction gives specific authorization to use.

CONTRAINDICATIONS

1. Patient is unable to use device (for example, not alert).
2. Inhaler is not prescribed for patient.
3. No permission has been given by medical direction.
4. Patient has already taken maximum prescribed dose prior to rescuer's arrival.

MEDICATION FORM

Handheld metered dose inhaler

DOSAGE

Number of inhalations based on medical direction's order or physician's order

ADMINISTRATION

1. Obtain order from medical direction either on-line or off-line.

2. Assure right patient, right medication, right dose, right route, patient alert enough to use inhaler.
3. Check expiration date of inhaler.
4. Check if patient has already taken any doses.
5. Assure inhaler is at room temperature or warmer.
6. Shake inhaler vigorously several times.
7. Have patient exhale deeply.
8. Have patient put her lips around the opening of the inhaler.
9. Have patient depress the handheld inhaler as she begins to inhale deeply.
10. Instruct patient to hold her breath for as long as she comfortably can so medication can be absorbed.
11. Allow patient to breathe a few times and repeat second dose if so ordered by medical direction.
12. If patient has a spacer device for use with her inhaler (device for attachment between inhaler and patient to allow for more effective use of medication), it should be used.
13. Put oxygen on patient.

ACTIONS

Beta agonist bronchodilator dilates bronchioles, reducing airway resistance.

SIDE EFFECTS

1. Increased pulse rate
2. Tremors
3. Nervousness

REASSESSMENT STRATEGIES

1. Gather vital signs.
2. Perform focused reassessment of chest and respiratory function.
3. Observe for deterioration of patient; if breathing becomes inadequate, provide artificial respirations.

Nitroglycerin

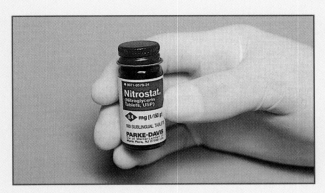

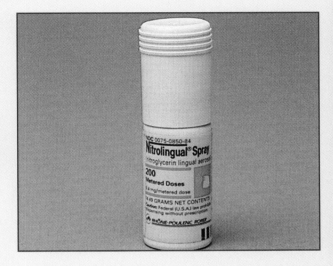

MEDICATION NAME

1. Generic: nitroglycerin
2. Trade: Nitrostat

INDICATIONS

All of the following conditions must be met:

1. The patient complains of chest pain.
2. The patient has a history of cardiac problems.
3. The patient's physician has prescribed nitroglycerin.
4. The systolic blood pressure is greater than 100 systolic.
5. Medical direction authorizes administration of the medication.

CONTRAINDICATIONS

1. The patient has hypotension (systolic blood pressure below 100).
2. The patient has a head injury.
3. The patient is an infant or a child.
4. The patient has already taken the maximum prescribed dose.

MEDICATION FORM

Tablet, sublingual (under-the-tongue) spray

DOSAGE

One dose, repeat in 3 to 5 minutes. If no relief, systolic blood pressure remains above 100, and if authorized by medical direction, up to a maximum of three doses.

ADMINISTRATION

1. Perform focused assessment for cardiac patient.
2. Take blood pressure. (Systolic pressure must be above 100.)
3. Contact medical direction if no standing orders.
4. Assure right medication, right patient, right dose, right route. Check expiration date.
5. Assure patient is alert.
6. Question patient on last dose taken and effects. Assure understanding of route of administration.
7. Ask patient to lift tongue and place tablet or spray dose under tongue (while you are wearing gloves) or have patient place tablet or spray under tongue.
8. Have patient keep mouth closed with tablet under tongue (without swallowing) until dissolved and absorbed.
9. Recheck blood pressure within 2 minutes.
10. Record administration, route, and time.
11. Perform reassessment.

ACTIONS

1. Relaxes blood vessels.
2. Decreases workload of heart.

SIDE EFFECTS

1. Hypotension (lowers blood pressure)
2. Headache
3. Pulse rate changes

REASSESSMENT STRATEGIES

1. Monitor blood pressure.
2. Ask patient about effect on pain relief.
3. Seek medical direction before readministering.
4. Record assessments.

Epinephrine Auto-Injector

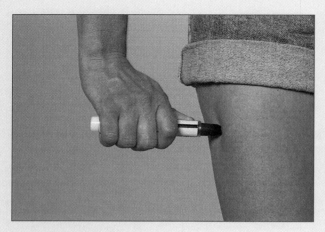

MEDICATION NAME

1. Generic: epinephrine
2. Trade: Adrenalin, Epi-Pen

INDICATIONS

Must meet the following three criteria:

1. Patient exhibits signs of a severe allergic reaction, including either respiratory distress or shock (hypoperfusion).
2. Medication is prescribed for this patient by a physician.
3. Medical direction authorizes use for this patient.

CONTRAINDICATIONS

No contraindications when used in a life-threatening situation

MEDICATION FORM

Liquid administered by an auto-injector—an automatically injectable needle-and-syringe system

DOSAGE

Adults—One adult auto-injector (0.3 mg)

Infant and child—One infant/child auto-injector (0.15 mg)

ADMINISTRATION

1. Obtain patient's prescribed auto-injector. Ensure:
   a. Prescription is written for the patient who is experiencing the severe allergic reaction
   b. Medication is not discolored (if visible)
2. Obtain order from medical direction, either on-line or off-line.
3. Remove cap from auto-injector.
4. Place tip of auto-injector against patient's thigh.
   a. Lateral portion of the thigh
   b. Midway between waist and knee
5. Push the injector firmly against the thigh until the injector activates.
6. Hold the injector in place until the medication is injected (at least 10 seconds).
7. Record activity and time.
8. Dispose of injector in biohazard container.

ACTIONS

1. Dilates the bronchioles
2. Constricts blood vessels

SIDE EFFECTS

1. Increased heart rate
2. Pallor
3. Dizziness
4. Chest pain
5. Headache
6. Nausea
7. Vomiting
8. Excitability, anxiety

REASSESSMENT STRATEGIES

1. Transport.
2. Continue focused assessment of airway, breathing, and circulatory status.

   If patient's condition continues to worsen (decreasing mental status, increasing breathing difficulty, decreasing blood pressure):

   a. Obtain medical direction for an additional dose of epinephrine.
   b. Treat for shock (hypoperfusion).
   c. Prepare to initiate basic life-support procedures (CPR, AED).

   If patient's condition improves, provide supportive care:

   a. Continue oxygen.
   b. Treat for shock (hypoperfusion).

APPENDIX 4

SWIMMING AND DIVING ACCIDENTS

NOTE: The amount of time spent on this subject in your First Responder course will depend upon the area in which you live and the length of your course. There are very few new procedures to learn about treating patients who have had swimming or diving accidents. Of key importance to you will be learning the types of injuries associated with water accidents and knowing the care skills used when the patient is a near-drowning victim. You also will have to know how to deal with the problems of water at the scene.

WARNING: Do *not* attempt a water rescue unless you have been trained to do so, you are a good swimmer, and others are on hand to help. *Never attempt a water rescue by yourself.* A personal flotation device (PFD) should be worn by all those involved in a water rescue. Except for shallow pools and open, shallow waters with uniform bottoms, the problems faced in water rescue are too great and too dangerous for the poor swimmer or untrained person to attempt. If not being able to help bothers you, take a course in water safety and rescue. Otherwise, you will probably become a victim yourself, rather than the person who rescues and provides care.

WARNING: Mouth-to-mask techniques and CPR are not practical while the patient is in the water. Follow your EMS system guidelines.

ACCIDENTS INVOLVING THE WATER

TYPES OF ACCIDENTS

Most people, when they think of water-related accidents, tend to think only of drowning. There is no doubt that drowning must be the number one consideration, even if the first problem faced by a person in the water is an injury or a medical emergency.

Injuries occur on, in, and near the water. Boating, waterskiing, and diving accidents produce airway obstructions, fractures, bleeding, and soft-tissue injuries. Other types of accidents, such as falls from bridges and motor vehicle accidents, also may involve the water. In these cases, the accident victims suffer injuries normally associated with the basic type of accident plus the effects of the water hazard (drowning, hypothermia, delayed care because of complicated rescue, and so on).

Sometimes, the accident or drowning may have been caused by a medical emergency that took place while the patient was in the water or on a boat. Knowing how the accident occurred may give clues to detecting the medical emergency. As with all aspects of First Responder care, considering the mechanism of injury or nature of illness and doing the patient assessment, complete with an interview, may be critical in deciding the procedures to be followed when caring for a patient.

Learn to associate the problems of drowning with scenes other than swimming pools and beaches. Remember, bathtub drownings do occur. Only a few inches of water are needed for an adult to drown. Even less is required for an infant.

As a First Responder, take particular care to look for the following when your patient is the victim of a water-related accident:

- **Airway obstruction**—This may be from water, foreign matter in the airway, or swollen airway tissues (often seen if the neck is injured in a dive). Spasms along the airway are common in cases of near-drowning.

- **Cardiac arrest**—This is usually related to respiratory arrest.

- **Signs of heart attack**—Through overexertion, the patient may have greater problems than the obvious near-drowning. Often, inexperienced rescuers are fooled into thinking that chest pains reported by the patient are due to muscle cramps produced during swimming or the panic of a near-drowning situation.

- **Injuries to the head and neck**—These are to be expected in boating, waterskiing, and diving accidents, but they also occur in cases of near-drowning.

- **Internal injuries**—While doing the patient assessment, be on the alert for fractures, soft-tissue injuries, and internal bleeding. The fact that the patient is suffering from internal bleeding is often missed during the first stages of care because of the concern for other problems associated with near-drowning. Constantly monitor patients for the signs and symptoms of shock (hypoperfusion).
- **Hypothermia**—The water does not have to be very cold and the length of stay in the water does not have to be very long for hypothermia to occur (see Chapter 10).

REACHING THE VICTIM

The U.S. Coast Guard, the American Red Cross, and the YMCA offer water safety and rescue courses. Unless you are a good swimmer and have been trained in water rescue, do *not* go into the water to save someone.

If the patient is responsive and close to shore or poolside, hold out an object to grab and **pull** the patient from the water. The best thing to use for such a rescue is rope (line). If none is available, use a branch, a fishing pole, an oar, a stick, or other such object. Keep in mind that a towel, a shirt, or an article of your own clothing may work quite well. In cases where there is no object near at hand or conditions are such that you may only have one opportunity to grab the person (for example, strong currents), lie down flat on your stomach and extend your arm or leg (not recommended for the nonswimmer). In all cases, make sure that your position is secure and that you will not be pulled into the water. This is critical if you are extending an arm or leg to the person.

Should the person be alert, but too far away to be pulled from the water, then you must carefully **throw** an object that will float. A personal flotation device (life jacket) or ring buoy (life preserver) is ideal, but these objects may not be at the scene. The best course of action is to throw anything that will float and to do this as soon as possible (Figure A4.1). Objects you

might use include inflated automobile tires, foam cushions, plastic jugs, logs, boards, plastic picnic containers, surfboards, flat boards, large balls, and plastic toys. Two empty, capped plastic milk jugs can keep an adult afloat for hours. It is best to tie rope to the objects so that they can be retrieved if they do not land near the patient. You may have to add some water to lightweight plastic jugs so that you can throw them the required distance.

Once you are sure that the person has a flotation device or floating object to hold on to, try to find a way to **tow** the patient to shore. Throw the patient a line or another flotation device attached to a line. Make sure that your own position is a safe one. If conditions are safe and you are a strong swimmer, wade no deeper than your waist if you must reduce the distance for throwing the line.

You may find that the near-drowning victim is too far from shore to allow for throwing and towing, or the victim may be unconscious and unable to respond to your efforts. In such cases, if there is a boat at the scene, you may be able to take the boat to the patient **(row)**. Do *not* go to the patient if you cannot swim. Even if you are a swimmer, you *must wear a personal flotation device* while you are in the boat. In cases where the patient is conscious, try to have the patient grab an oar or the stern (rear end) of the boat. Take great care in helping the person into the boat. This is a very tricky process in a canoe. Should the canoe or boat tip over, stay with the vessel, holding onto its bottom or side. It will almost certainly stay afloat.

If you take a boat out and find that the patient is unconscious, assume that the patient has neck or spinal injury. Care for the patient will be discussed later in this section.

In water rescue situations (Figure A4.2), begin by trying to **pull** the patient from the water. If this cannot be done, **throw** objects that will float and try to **tow** the patient from the water. Do *not* try to take a boat to the victim if you cannot swim. Wear a personal flotation device while in the boat. Unless you are a good swimmer and trained in water rescue and lifesaving, **do not swim to the patient.**

FIGURE A4.1
Throw the patient anything that will float.

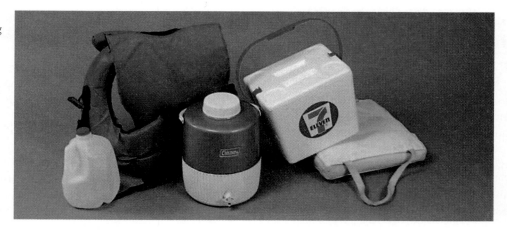

CARE FOR THE PATIENT

THE PATIENT WITHOUT NECK OR SPINAL INJURIES

REMINDER: In all cases of shallow water accidents, assume that the unconscious patient has neck and spinal injuries. If the patient can be removed quickly from the water using a cervical collar and spine board or if the patient is out of the water when you arrive, you should:

1. Start your initial assessment of the patient.
2. Provide mouth-to-mask resuscitation, if needed, as quickly as possible. Check for airway obstruction. Mouth-to-mask techniques are usually not practical when the patient is in the water. You may use the mouth-to-mouth procedure, but know that this might expose you to infectious agents. FOLLOW YOUR EMS GUIDELINES.
3. Once the patient is out of the water, provide CPR, if needed, as directed in Chapter 8. As in all such cases, make certain that someone alerts the EMS system dispatcher.
4. If the patient is breathing and has a pulse, check for bleeding and attempt to control any serious bleeding that you find.
5. If there is breathing and a pulse, cover the patient to conserve body heat and do a patient assessment. Be sure to put something under the patient to prevent heat loss. Uncover only those areas of the patient's body involved with your stage of the assessment. Care for any problems you may find.
6. If the patient can be moved, take him or her to a warm place. Do not allow the near-drowning patient to walk. Handle the patient *gently* at all times.
7. Provide care for shock and make certain that the EMS system dispatcher has been alerted.

You may find more resistance than expected to your efforts to provide breaths to someone with water in the airway. Apply more force, if necessary, once you are certain that no foreign objects are in the patient's airway. Watch the patient's chest rise and fall. Adjust your ventilations as needed to help prevent gastric distention. Remember, you must provide breaths to the patient's lungs as soon as possible.

Many times, a patient with water in the airway will also have water in the stomach. This may provide resistance to your efforts to resuscitate the patient. When this happens, you may find that some of the air from your breaths will go into the patient's stomach, even when you adjust your ventilations. Current American Heart Association and American Red Cross guidelines do *not* call for you to attempt to relieve water or

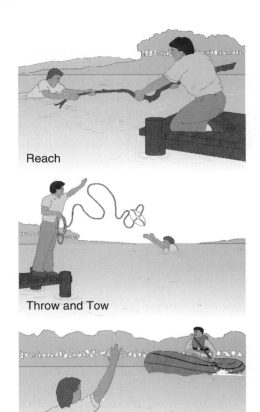

FIGURE A4.2
Pull the patient from the water, **throw** an object that will float, and try to **tow,** or, if necessary and you are properly equipped and trained, **row** to the patient.

air from the patient's stomach (unless immediate suctioning is available) due to the risk of driving material from the stomach and possibly obstructing the patient's airway. When gastric distention occurs, reposition the airway and continue with resuscitation, making sure the breaths are slow and full.

NOTE: Drowning victims who are resuscitated are very likely to vomit. Rescuers should be ready to clear the airway when this occurs.

Human beings have a reaction in cold water that is similar to other mammals. This reaction is called the **mammalian diving reflex.** When the face of a person or other mammal is submerged in cold water, the mammalian diving reflex slows down the body's metabolism, which results in a decrease in the oxygen consumption. At the same time, the reflex causes a redistribution of blood to more vital organs—the brain, heart, and lungs. The diving reflex is more pronounced in infants and children, and they may fare better in cold-water drowning than adults. Start CPR on all drowning victims as soon as they are pulled from the water and continue while en route to the hospital. Cases have been reported in which drowning victims, especially children, were revived and fully recovered after being in the water for longer than 30 minutes.

Never consider that a person has drowned; rather, consider the victim to be a near-drowning patient.

As a First Responder, you must be realistic when dealing with drownings. Many patients cannot be successfully resuscitated. The effects of water in the airway and the lack of oxygen to the brain may be too harsh for the body to endure. You may resuscitate some patients only to find out that they died within 48 hours due to pneumonia, lung damage, or brain damage. Even when you provide the best of care, some patients will die; however, you must give patients every opportunity for survival. You will not be able to tell which patient will survive. Provide resuscitation for all drowning victims.

Care for unconscious patients while they are still in the water is covered in the next section.

THE PATIENT WITH NECK OR SPINAL INJURIES

Injuries to the neck (cervical spine) and the rest of the spinal column occur during many water-related accidents. In First Responder care, you will not be expected to know how to use long spine boards and other floating, rigid devices for rescue situations. This does not mean that you cannot take certain actions to protect a patient's neck and spine during both rescue and care.

If a patient is unconscious, neck and spinal injuries may not be detected. In such a situation, assume that the patient has neck and spinal injuries and provide care accordingly. Whenever you assess a water-accident patient and find head injuries, assume there also are neck and spine injuries. Learn to quickly evaluate the patient for outward indications of possible neck and spinal injuries as described in Chapter 12. Remember, you will not have time to do a complete test for neck and spinal injuries for patients who are in the water. Likewise, a complete assessment will not be possible for any patient you find in respiratory or cardiac arrest.

In cases when a patient with possible neck and spinal injuries is conscious and you are in shallow, warm water, stabilize the patient until the EMS system responds with personnel trained to remove the patient from the water. Simply keep the patient floating in a face-up position while you support the back and stabilize the head and neck as shown in Scan A4-1. Seldom will this be the case. Too often, the water will be too cold or too deep, or there will be dangerous tides or currents. Often, the patient will need resuscitation and will have to be removed from the water as quickly as possible. Even though it may be difficult to stabilize a patient in such conditions, it is better to wait for trained, equipped rescue personnel to help remove a breathing patient from the water rather than risk injuring the patient's spine by doing it yourself.

Should you arrive at the scene and find the unconscious patient has already been removed from the water, have someone alert the EMS system dispatcher and begin your initial assessment. Provide life-support care as needed, using the jaw-thrust maneuver rather than the head-tilt, chin-lift maneuver. After breathing and circulation are ensured, and bleeding is cared for, do a patient assessment, providing care as needed. Keep the patient warm and provide care for shock. Unless absolutely necessary, do *not* move the patient if there is any chance of neck or spinal injuries.

If the patient is still in the water, do *not* attempt a rescue unless you are a good swimmer, are trained to do so, and have others on hand who can help you. Make certain that someone alerts the EMS system dispatcher. This should be done immediately. Do *not* wait until after the rescue is attempted. Valuable time will be lost should the rescue fail. Providing care for the possible spinal injury patient still in the water requires you to:

1. Turn the patient face up in the water. This should be done while you are in the water. Wear a personal flotation device. To turn the patient, you should:

   a. Position yourself at patient's side, as shown in Scan A4-1. Grasp the patient's arms midway between the elbow and shoulder and gently float them above the patient's head.

   b. Clasp the patient's arms firmly against his or her head to brace the neck and keep the head in line. Move forward in the water to bring the patient's body to the surface and in line.

   c. Rotate the patient toward you by pushing down on the near arm and pulling the far arm toward you, making sure you brace the patient's head firmly with his or her arms. Do *not* lift the patient.

   d. Once the patient is face up, maintain pressure on the patient's arms to brace the head.

   e. In shallow water, you can hold the patient's arms with one hand and support the hips with the other.

   f. In deeper water, continue to move toward shallow water where you can stand or can be supported by someone else.

2. If necessary, begin your initial assessment while the patient is still in the water. Do *not* delay the detection of respiratory arrest.

3. If needed, provide rescue breathing as soon as possible. Use the jaw-thrust maneuver to protect the patient's neck and spine. Check for airway obstruction. CPR and mouth-to-mask resuscitation will *not* be effective while the patient is in the water. Give priority to removing the patient from the water.

Water Rescue

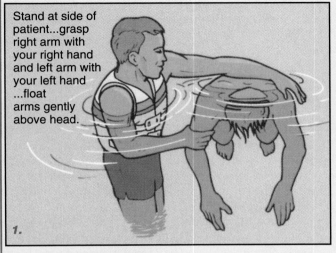

1. Stand at side of patient...grasp right arm with your right hand and left arm with your left hand ...float arms gently above head.

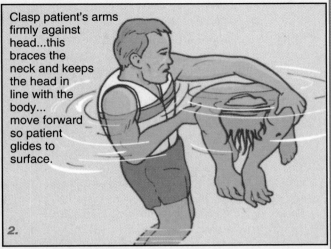

2. Clasp patient's arms firmly against head...this braces the neck and keeps the head in line with the body... move forward so patient glides to surface.

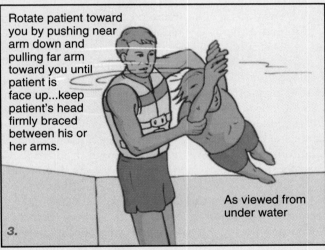

3. Rotate patient toward you by pushing near arm down and pulling far arm toward you until patient is face up...keep patient's head firmly braced between his or her arms.

As viewed from under water

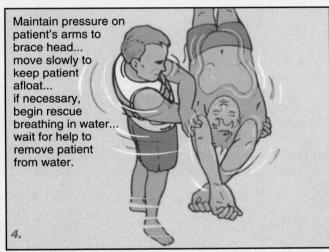

4. Maintain pressure on patient's arms to brace head... move slowly to keep patient afloat... if necessary, begin rescue breathing in water... wait for help to remove patient from water.

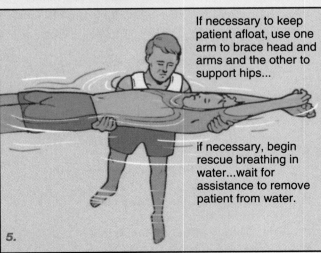

5. If necessary to keep patient afloat, use one arm to brace head and arms and the other to support hips...

if necessary, begin rescue breathing in water...wait for assistance to remove patient from water.

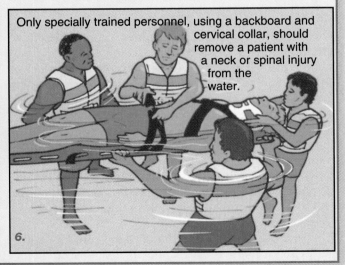

6. Only specially trained personnel, using a backboard and cervical collar, should remove a patient with a neck or spinal injury from the water.

Adapted from American Red Cross *Swimming and Diving*

4. If someone is there to help you, have him or her support the patient along the midline of the back while you provide support to the patient's head and neck. Use the method described in Chapter 12. Float the patient to shore and continue to provide back and neck support as shown in Scan A4-1. Wait for trained rescue personnel equipped with a backboard and cervical collar to remove the patient from the water.

   NOTE: You should attempt to remove the patient from the water yourself ONLY if trained rescue personnel will not arrive soon and the patient has no heartbeat. You must make every effort to maintain in-line stabilization of the patient's body. Support the patient's head and neck while those helping you lift the patient from the water.

5. Once the patient is out of the water, attempts at respiratory resuscitation can begin. Check for a pulse to see if CPR should be started. If you are by yourself, rowing a cardiac arrest patient to shore, delay CPR until you reach shore. You cannot row a boat and perform CPR. Also, CPR will be more effective on shore. In some cases, depending on the boat's stability and water conditions, you may be able to provide effective CPR in the boat until other rescuers arrive.

6. If the patient is breathing, check for and control all serious bleeding. Cover the patient to conserve body heat and perform a patient assessment, caring for any injuries you may find. Do *not* move the patient if there are any signs of possible neck or spinal injuries.

7. Give care for shock and make sure the EMS dispatcher has been alerted.

DIVING ACCIDENTS

DIVING BOARD ACCIDENTS

Each year, many people are injured as they attempt dives or enter the water from diving boards. These same injuries are seen in dives from poolsides, docks, boats, and the shore. A large number of such cases involve teenagers.

Most diving board accidents involve the head and neck. As a First Responder, you will also see injuries to the spine, hands, feet, and ribs occurring with great frequency. Any part of the body can be injured in these types of accidents, requiring complete assessment of all patients unless you are providing life-support measures. Remember, a medical emergency may have led to the diving accident.

Once the patient is out of the water, care for diving accident patients is the same as for any accident victim. Care provided in the water and in removing the patient from the water is the same as for any patient who may have neck and spine injuries. Remember, any unconscious or unresponsive patient is assumed to have possible neck and spinal injuries. If the patient is conscious, follow the procedures set down in Chapter 12 if you must deal with possible skull, neck, or spine injuries. Be sure to look for delayed reactions, particularly weakness, tingling sensations, or numbness in the limbs.

SCUBA DIVING ACCIDENTS

Scuba (self-contained underwater breathing apparatus) diving accidents have increased with the popularity of the sport and with inexperienced divers going into the water without the benefit of proper training. There are over two million people who scuba dive for sport or as part of their industrial or military employment. This number has been increasing at a rate of over 200,000 people each year.

Scuba diving accidents can produce body injuries or near-drownings. Medical problems can lead to scuba diving accidents. However, two special problems are seen in scuba diving accidents. They are gas bubbles in the diver's blood and the "bends."

Gas bubbles in the blood (**air embolism**) occur when gases leave a diver's injured lung and enter the bloodstream. This can occur for many reasons, though it is most often associated with divers who hold their breath because of inadequate training, equipment failure, underwater emergency, or when trying to conserve air during a long dive. Air embolism can develop in the automobile accident victim who is trapped below water, as he takes gulps of air from air bubbles held inside the vehicle.

Air embolism can develop in both shallow and deep waters. The onset is rapid, with signs of personality changes and distorted senses sometimes giving the impression of drunkenness. The patient may have convulsions and rapidly lapse into unconsciousness. There may be signs of air outside of the lungs being trapped in the chest cavity.

You should suspect possible air embolism when the scuba diving accident patient has any of the following signs or symptoms:

- Personality changes
- Distorted senses (blurred vision is most common)
- Chest pains
- Numbness and tingling sensations in the arms and/or legs
- Total body weakness, or weakness of one or more limbs
- Frothy blood in the mouth or nose
- Convulsions

WARNING: Do *not* assume air embolism without first considering possible head injury or stroke.

The "bends" are really part of what is called **decompression sickness.** Patients with decompression sickness usually are those individuals who have come up too quickly from a deep, prolonged dive. When they do this, nitrogen gas is trapped in their tissues and may find its way into the bloodstream. The onset of the bends is usually slow for scuba divers, taking from 1 to 48 hours to appear. Because of this delay, the patient interview and reports from the patient's family and friends may be your only clue to relate the patient's problems to a dive.

NOTE: Scuba divers increase the risk of decompression sickness if they fly within 12 hours of the dive.

The signs and symptoms of decompression sickness include:

- Fatigue
- Deep pain to the muscles and joints (the bends)
- Numbness or paralysis
- Choking, coughing, and/or labored breathing
- Chest pains
- Collapse that leads to unconsciousness
- Blotches on the skin (mottling). Sometimes, these rashes keep changing appearance.

If you think a patient has gas bubbles in the blood or decompression sickness due to a dive, be certain that the dispatcher is aware of the problem. The patient will need EMT transport to a medical facility as soon as possible. Dispatch may wish to direct the EMTs to take the patient to a special facility (hyperbaric trauma center) where a patient is exposed to oxygen under greatly increased pressure conditions. This procedure is done in a sealed (hyperbaric) chamber.

While waiting for the EMTs to arrive, treat for shock and constantly monitor the patient. Respiratory and cardiac arrest are possible. Positioning of the patient is critical in order to avoid gas bubbles in the blood damaging the brain (Figure A4.3). Place the patient on the *left side*. The patient may be placed in a slight head-down position, but for no more than 10 minutes and only if it can be maintained without impairing breathing or other resuscitative measures.

ACCIDENTS INVOLVING ICE

Ice rescues require special training. Unless you are trained specifically to work on ice, do not attempt a rescue. If you cannot swim, you have no business going out onto the ice. You may walk on an undetected thin spot, fall through the ice, and quickly drown. All rescuers who are on or at the edge of the ice must wear personal flotation devices.

The major problem faced in ice rescue is reaching the victim. Never walk out to the person or attempt to enter the water through a hole in the ice in order to find the victim. Never attempt an ice rescue by yourself unless you have some basic equipment, such as a personal flotation device and a ladder, and you are specifically trained in one-rescuer techniques. Never go onto ice that is rapidly breaking up. Your best course of action will be to work with others from a safe ice surface or the shore (Figure A4.4).

Throwing a line to the victim or reaching out with a stick or a pole is your first choice of action. If the victim is not holding onto the ice, but trying to keep afloat in open water, throw anything that will float. Should you have to go onto the ice to get the patient, it is strongly recommended that you have help. Pushing a long ladder out onto the ice and then crawling along this ladder is a very effective method of safe rescue, providing someone is holding the ladder from a safe position. If enough people are on hand, a human chain can be formed to reach the patient.

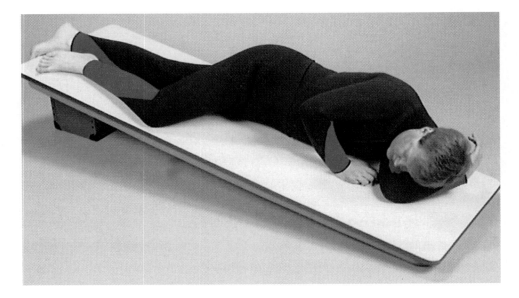

FIGURE A4.3
Position the patient after a scuba diving accident. He may be placed in a head-down tilt but for no more than 10 minutes.

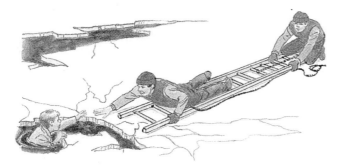

FIGURE A4.4
A safe ice rescue requires teamwork.

One of the few methods of ice rescue that can be tried by the single rescuer is the use of a light boat. This craft can be moved along the ice by riding inside of the boat and pushing the ice with your hands or with a stick or an oar. This is often a very slow and awkward method, but if the ice cracks, at least you are safe in a boat.

Expect to find injuries with any patient who has fallen through the ice. Broken leg bones are common. Hypothermia may be a problem and should always be considered. **Do not attempt to rewarm the severe hypothermia patient** (see Chapter 10).

Alert the EMS system dispatcher for all patients who have had accidents on ice or have been in cold water. There may be injuries that are difficult to detect and problems because of the cold that may be delayed.

ASSISTING THE EMTs

You may be the first on the scene of a water or an ice rescue and have the EMTs arrive during rescue or care. At other times, you may arrive at the scene after the EMTs. Some of the things you can do to help, if directed to do so, might be to:

- *Interview bystanders*—Information gained could indicate the number of victims, a hidden medical emergency, or the cause of the accident.
- *Crowd control*—Both the curiosity seeker and those wishing to help may come to the scene. Unless controlled, they may hinder rescue, fall into the water, or place too much weight on the ice surface.
- *Find additional help*—This is usual in cases of accidents involving ice.
- *Find items used in rescue*—You may have to look for a ladder or a boat.
- *Help provide care*—Two-rescuer CPR, positioning the patient, and splinting the patient may require your aid.
- *Helping with a spine board*—If you are a good swimmer and have been trained in water rescue, the EMTs may need you in the water. Remember, a spine board will float and will pop up very easily from below the surface of the water. If you are called upon to help place a spine board under a patient who is still in the water, make sure of your position so as not to slip, and keep a firm grip on the board. If you have any doubts as to what the EMTs want you to do, ask questions.

APPENDIX 5

MANAGING STRESS

ANOTHER SIDE OF PERSONAL SAFETY

The initial steps that First Responders take in the scene size-up are done to assure their own safety. It is essential that First Responders protect their own lives before trying to aid others. Sometimes, however, the threat is not something as obvious as a burning car or contaminated needle. First Responders often carry out their duties in situations that are visually dramatic and emotionally traumatic. They must care for patients with serious injuries and illnesses and help these individuals cope with the emotions associated with the emergency. Often, First Responders must depend on professional training that reduces or delays their own emotional reactions as assessments are made and care is provided. The scene and the various situations faced there by First Responders may delay responses we now know are essential to the provider's well-being. Many times, despite the First Responders' best efforts, people will suffer and some patients will die.

Such experiences are stressful and cause a range of reactions, some normal and some extreme. Though First Responders are trained to handle difficult situations, they are not untouched by what they see and do on the job. First Responders must find ways to cope with the stressors that come with the job. (A stressor is any factor that causes wear and tear on the body's physical or mental resources.) Those who do not can become depressed, suffer physical disorders, experience burnout, and as a result, have to leave the field permanently. Others may be able to battle the same events, but by following guidelines developed in EMS, fewer professionals are being lost to the stress of the job.

The jobs of police officers and firefighters are stressful. Admitting this fact to themselves does not make the people who work in these fields weak or cowardly. In fact, as professionals, First Responders have a duty to confront the psychological effects of the work they do. Ignoring stress does not make it go away. Instead, the stress may crop up in unexpected forms, such as insomnia, fatigue, irritability, high blood pressure, heart disease, alcohol use, or other disruptive responses.

This appendix will help you recognize the signs of stress in yourself and others and will suggest ways to reduce this stress and to help you and your fellow EMS professionals work together to recognize immediate and delayed reactions brought about when dealing with emergencies and providing First Responder-level care.

FIRST RESPONDERS AND STRESS

Almost everyone must face and deal with some type of stress daily, whether it's driving in traffic, coping with work and family problems or schedules, meeting school and office deadlines, or waiting to see the doctor for a physical. Surveys and research reports over the past two decades have revealed that 43% of all adults suffer adverse health effects from stress. As much as 90% of visits to primary care physicians are for stress-related complaints or disorders. The U.S. Surgeon General has said that stress is a factor in 80% of all nontraumatic deaths. Recent research confirms that stress contributes to cardiovascular disease, stroke, diabetes, cancer, arthritis, and gastrointestinal, skin, neurological, and emotional disorders.

For First Responders, stress is a concern for several reasons. Their jobs make intense physical and psychological demands on their emotional and physical well-being. Police officers, firefighters, and disaster response personnel must respond quickly to emergencies and react instantly to situations where lives are at risk. Their need to make instant decisions about patient care is quite a responsibility, and First Responders realize that making a mistake may mean a patient dies. Death is not the only fear associated with mistakes in providing care. An injury may be made more serious or pain can become more intense. What is delayed at the scene or done improperly may cause a problem that may become chronic for the patient or lead to loss of function and possibly the reduction of success in future care procedures.

TYPE A PERSONALITIES

Another reason for concern is that these high-pressure jobs often attract a certain kind of person. Some studies have found that many First Responders are what is commonly termed "Type A" personalities. These individuals are usually a mix of many traits that make them highly competitive, energetic, aggressive, self-sufficient, idealistic, detail- and action-oriented, compounded in complexity by trying to be perfectionists. Ironically, the very characteristics that may make good First Responders may also make them vulnerable to stress-related problems. Other studies have shown that personnel in the EMS system have higher rates of divorce, alcoholism, and suicide than the general population. Clearly, it is important for First Responders to recognize and defuse the sources of stress and to stay aware of changing views of the impact of stress.

Recently, many who held to the "Type A" personality designation are looking at a much more complex picture. The day-in and day-out exposure to stress-causing agents has been of primary focus. But what of a single event or exposure? We simply do not know how much it takes to produce what level of response and the duration of that response. No one should be able to easily adjust to the stress faced in First Responder-level activities. This simple statement means that all will face the need for making adjustments, working with others and working as a team to keep the level of emotional fitness at a level safe for the provider and optimum for the public. Professional growth depends on adjustment to the exposure to stressors that come with the job.

SOURCES OF STRESS

Sometimes a single terrible event can cause an overload of stress for First Responders.

- A minivan skids off an icy road and smashes into a concrete overpass. The First Responders on the scene find the driver and her two young children dead.
- As a fire crew enters a burning house, a wall collapses, killing a rookie firefighter.
- On a snowy evening, a commuter plane skids off an airport runway and bursts into flames. The number of seriously injured people temporarily overwhelms the fire and rescue crews at the scene.
- Horror may unfold as a trapped patient is consumed by fire.

Some of these examples are daily events when one views the entire country; others are extremes even for a national picture of emergency services. Any can happen to you as a First Responder trying to provide the care realistically expected by the public and of yourself. Understanding that which is realistic and possible to perform is difficult in a culture that shows fictional heroes doing tasks far beyond the ability of any professional. Realism, therefore, is an essential part of your training, requiring each individual to evaluate the limits within the EMS system care.

Each of these incidents is a likely scenario for what is called critical incident stress. Either at the time of the incident or after, First Responders may find themselves reacting unexpectedly. One First Responder may feel nausea and chest pain, another may become restless and have trouble making decisions or have loss of appetite and stomach pains, and yet another may become irritable and short-tempered with family and friends. The signs of stress are many and so varied that they might include any unexpected reaction.

Those who suffer from critical incident stress are not abnormal. Research shows that 85% of emergency personnel have experienced some type of temporary stress reaction. Most First Responders recover from acute stress reactions within days or in a few weeks, especially if they practice the stress-managing techniques we will describe in the next section. But while they are going through their stress reactions, their family and friends will become concerned. Often, a First Responder may feel that family and friends cannot understand what he or she is going through. Meanwhile, performance at work suffers because the First Responder has lost the concentration and energy that he or she needs and must be able to apply, as noted earlier, in a quick and precise manner. Coworkers should be looking for signs of stress and can begin helping their fellow First Responders manage by encouraging them to talk about their feelings. Pushing, demanding, teasing, or otherwise harassing someone to "get over it" may add to stress. An individual may have to work through several emotional and physical steps before recognizing and admitting that he or she has a problem and needs help. Encouraging the person to talk may be a first easy step to recognition and admission. On the other hand, ordering the individual to seek professional help may meet resistance and may not work. In not following orders, the individual might feel that he or she has failed and lose any inclination to seek help.

All professionals in EMS are affected by the demand of their jobs and the events to which they are exposed. Sometimes a period of rest is needed. With support and the correct, professional help, a stronger and more self-sufficient individual may develop.

A small percentage of First Responders do not rebound and return to normal after a traumatic event. They develop *post traumatic stress disorder* (PTSD). PTSD is a serious condition that is usually a result of an experience in a traumatic event that involved a real or threatened death or injury to the First Responder or the patient where the First Responder felt fear, helplessness, or horror. After the traumatic event, the First Responder may have flashbacks or nightmares (intrusions), may try to stay away from persons and places that are reminders of the event (avoidance), and may have an increased wariness and startle response (hyperarousal). If these symptoms are recognized, First Responders must seek professional help, or be urged by family, coworkers, and supervisors to do so, before their personal lives, health, and careers are affected. One form of professional help is available through critical incident stress debriefing (CISD), which is discussed in the next section. With appropriate help, First Responders can prevent stress disorders from developing and avoid anxiety and burnout.

Burnout

Stress problems can be triggered by a single traumatic incident, but some First Responders suffer from burnout, a reaction to cumulative stress or exposure to multiple traumatic incidents. First Responders are at special risk for burnout because of the demands and activities of their jobs. The signs of burnout include a loss of enthusiasm and energy, replaced by feelings of frustration, hopelessness, low self-esteem, isolation, inertia, and mistrust. Many factors contribute to burnout, such as multiple or back-to-back calls involving serious medical problems or trauma injuries and death, facing public hostility, struggling with bureaucratic obstacles, earning low pay, putting up with poor working conditions, and dealing with sexism.

Shift work, a disruption accepted by our society for generations, may be a significant source of problems, particularly when combined with other factors. This pattern of work is common in EMS and is found to be even more stressful now that so many families have both husbands and wives working, missing meals together and time shared with their children and with each other. Continuing education needs also strain schedules that add additional problems to those in EMS compared to people in families that have "typical" day schedules. Even meals that could be restful times, even for those dining by themselves, are too often replaced with coffee and donuts and high-fat fast foods, all consumed on the run. A healthier diet and lifestyle can help First Responders combat the stressors that are an unavoidable part of their job.

Both *short-term* and *long-term* stress are occupational hazards for First Responders. Fortunately, research in the past 15 years has found ways to reduce both kinds of stress. Newer variations and combinations of stress are being seen as people attempt to compensate for lost time and shared activities. Many individuals find that they suffer a crossover of job stress and "recreational stress" in attempts to participate to compensate for time lost with others or in a particular activity. The old saying of "work hard and play hard" may not be a useful expression for some, actually causing more difficulties by trying to solve a complex problem with too simple a solution.

Reducing Stress

Stress can affect both the personal life and on-the-job performance of First Responders. Reducing stress means that First Responders must look at both their personal and work lifestyles and make certain adjustments.

Lifestyle Changes

The new First Responder often feels that the job is exciting and challenging, and it is the fortunate First Responder who can keep that feeling throughout his or her career. Once First Responders recognize that their jobs can cause them stress, they can take steps to cope with their reactions to stressors. One reaction may be lifestyle, such as sleeping and eating habits and time spent in having fun, exercising, or relaxing. Try to create a healthier lifestyle. Reduce the intake of sugars, caffeine, and alcohol. Avoiding fatty foods can reduce cholesterol levels. Put aside time to exercise even if it is only for 20 minutes each day. Find excuses to take brief walks (to the mailbox, up and down flights of stairs, across the parking lot). These activities will, through time, lower blood pressure, reduce cholesterol, and as a result, minimize the risk of heart disease and stroke for many individuals. The vast majority of individuals show improved health when they give up sedentary lifestyles; however, a physician's guidance may be needed at first. Adding more stress to fit in an activity may show that the problem has more than one phase and all the phases may need adjustment. Thus, as noted earlier, help from the EMS system is essential to help avoid focusing on a limited aspect of the problem, being overwhelmed by solving too many problems, or causing a new problem while chasing down the solution to an old one.

Regular exercise helps reduce weight and lower blood pressure. In addition, aerobic exercise (brisk walking, jogging, bicycling, swimming) releases endorphins (a peptide produced by the nervous system and considered a natural pain reducing compound and tranquilizer) that may reduce stress. Some First Responders try other methods to relieve stress. Meditation, yoga, progressive muscle relaxation, and biofeedback can be effective, and so can simple deep breathing. There is also a technique called *self-control breathing approaches* (SCBA) that helps relax and relieve stress in some persons.

STRESS REDUCTION AT WORK

In the past decade, many employers have moved to help reduce stress on First Responders. The old attitude that police officers, firefighters, and other emergency personnel had to "tough out" their problems has given way to a recognition that both the day-to-day performance and long-term service of First Responders depend on managing stress-related problems.

Employers are becoming more aware that they must provide basic stress-reducing aids, such as:

- Setting up shifts to allow enough time for personnel to get a break from work demands and have time to relax with family and friends
- Making sure that First Responders get food and drinks at disaster scenes
- Allowing rotating assignments so that First Responders spend at least some time in less busy response areas.
- Tracking responses to assure that individuals do not respond to too many calls or too many traumas in a short time frame

Though individuals and employers are beginning to understand the effects of stress and are responding with changes in lifestyles and job requirements, First Responders will still face stressful situations and have normal reactions to them. These reactions may cause them to need or seek help. The professional help received from individuals who are specifically trained with EMS system daily stress and PTSD may be the most useful counseling that a First Responder can seek; however, family doctors, religious counselors, and psychologists and psychiatrists in general practice do have the background necessary to initiate care, screen the First Responder as to future needs, provide specific help, and where needed, redirect the First Responder to others who are specifically trained to care for a stress-related problem. The care required may be generic or may be a specific need seen immediately by a trained mental health professional.

Please keep in mind that you are a unique individual. Not only will there be differences in how you respond to stress and to the therapy recommended and received, but there are also the combined problems that may lead to different end results for two different people exposed to the same stress. Different backgrounds are enough to produce different reactions to stress and to stress therapy. Do not be surprised to find that you and a friend in EMS, both thinking that you have the same problem, may receive two different forms of therapy or that a group therapy session might have you realize that you are dealing with something that is unique for you to face, but not face alone.

CISD

One important stress management technique is Critical Incident Stress Debriefing, or CISD. First used in the 1970s, CISD brings together peer counselors and mental health professionals to help First Responders cope with their reactions to traumatic, or critical incidents, such as witnessing the death of a child or a coworker.

Usually, a jurisdiction will set up a multiagency CISD program that includes mental health professionals and police, fire, EMT, disaster relief, and similar personnel. Emergency personnel can be trained in peer counseling techniques, and individuals can participate in special training programs to become part of a CISD team.

Within 72 hours after a critical incident, the CISD team holds a group meeting, or "debriefing," for everyone present at the incident. The ground rules of the debriefing encourage open, honest discussion. The debriefing is not an investigation of the incident. Everything said at the debriefing is confidential, no one is forced to speak, and differences in rank are ignored. Often overlooked by the public as they read about CISD or experience coverage on the local media is the tremendous help that trust and sharing can build. Emergency services personnel are often seen by the public as independent members of law enforcement, fire service, rescue squads, or emergency medical response teams, yet, in part, they are all part of the chain of human resources that provide very special needs for the public during emergencies. Working as members of a very special team allows each division within EMS to cooperate to reduce stress and to help bring back those who in the past would have been lost to the physical and psychological effects of stress. Togetherness is EMS's strongest weapon against the stressful effects of doing the job. The debriefing often allows for this togetherness to build cooperation that gives strength to all involved.

At the debriefing, the facts of the incident are reviewed first. Then those present are asked to describe what their reaction was at the time and since the event. Later, the mental health professionals and CISD leaders ask questions and offer advice about how to recognize and cope with stress reactions. The CISD method works because it helps First Responders express their feelings to their peers in a nonthreatening atmosphere.

HANDLING STRESS

The techniques described in this appendix can help reduce job-related stress for First Responders. More importantly, though, First Responders must be aware of their reactions to stress and apply to themselves the concern they use to help others. If you see signs of stress in yourself or in your coworkers, do something about it. The "buddy system" extends beyond the procedures carried out at the emergency event to include stress management. The rule is simple. Keep a watch on your coworkers and allow them the privilege to do the same for you. As important as anything that is part of the EMS experience is to listen to those with whom you work and give value to any alert that you may be suffering from a stress-related problem. This may be something that builds over time, or it may be a single event of such magnitude that you are pushed over the line you have carefully developed for yourself at and after the emergency. You must develop a realistic view of what is done by those in EMS, whether you are a full-time First Responder working out of a specific squad or you are a law enforcement officer who utilizes your talents only in part or for specific phases of the emergency event. **NEVER** resent the difficult task someone faces trying to help you and others suffering stress-related problems. The beginning of teamwork does not come from their taking action, but from your reaction.

RESOURCES

There are many texts and journal articles that provide information on recognizing the signs and symptoms of stress and techniques for managing it. Following is a brief selection:

American Academy of Orthopedic Surgeons. (2000). *Managing Stress in Emergency Medical Services*. Boston: Jones & Bartlett Publishing.

Discusses types of stress and stress responses, describes CISD and burnout, and provides techniques for managing stress.

Asken, Michael J. (1993). *PsycheResponse*. New York: Brady.

Describes ways to build psychological skills for optimal First Responder performance.

Cline, Douglas. "Preventing Emotional Overload." *The Voice*, November 1999.

Discusses causes of stress, its many forms and effects on emergency care providers, its causes, and ways to help manage it.

Hafen, Brent Q. and Kathryn J. Frandsen (1991). *Psychological Emergencies and Crisis Intervention*. Englewood, CO.: Morton.

Includes chapters on burnout and stress reduction as well as material on handling psychiatric, drug, and sexual assault emergencies.

Limmer, Daniel, et al. *Emergency Care*, 9th ed. Upper Saddle River, NJ: Brady.

Presents essential information and skills necessary for the training of EMT-Basics.

Mitchell, Jeff and Grady Bray (1990). *Emergency Services Stress*. New York: Brady.

Gives detailed description of CISD and other stress-management techniques for individuals and agencies.

Mitchell, Jeffrey T. and George S. Everly (1994). *Human Elements Training for Emergency Services, Public Safety and Disaster Personnel*. Ellicott City, MD: Chevron Publishing Corporation.

Describes critical incident stress and the stress education strategy and provides guidelines for becoming a CISD instructor, instructional methodologies, and course outlines.

The following web sites provide stress-related information and links to other stress information resources:

- www.stress.org
- www.stress.org/problem.htm
- www.stresscure.com/hrn/facts.html
- www.trauma-pages.com/index.phtml
- www.uiuc.edu/departments/mckinley/ health-info/stress/copstrat.html
- www.algy.com/anxiety/relax.html

APPENDIX 6

*F*IRST RESPONDER ROLES AND RESPONSIBILITIES

Recall from Chapter 1 the section on Roles and Responsibilities of the First Responder. One of the most important roles was to take appropriate safety precautions. Once personal and scene safety are ensured, First Responders will begin to perform numerous patient-related duties. First Responders are a part of the EMS system, responding to emergencies, usually arriving first on the scene, providing initial care for patients, and working with other emergency care providers to assess, make care decisions, and transport. Each individual on an emergency scene works as a member of a team, whether performing as a First Responder, EMT, or paramedic. The team's actions and interactions are what makes the EMS system work effectively.

The following chart, *Actions and Interactions*, provides a matrix of how each level of emergency-care responder works together to perform the steps of scene safety, patient assessment care, and transport. You will find that you will work in one or several areas of the matrix as you arrive on the scene and begin assessment and care as a First Responder or with other emergency services units. This course of instruction will provide the knowledge, skills, and practice opportunities for performing the roles and responsibilities of a First Responder.

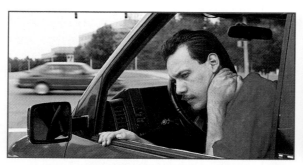
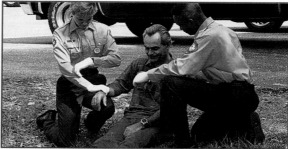
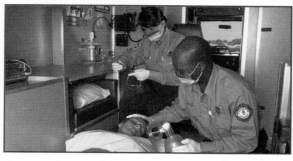
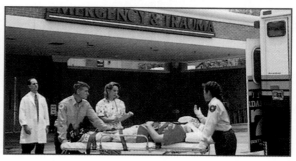

Team actions and interactions make the EMS system work effectively.

ROLES AND RESPONSIBILITIES

Phase	First Responder	EMT	Paramedic
Preparation (Green–Go)	Check unit; restock emergency care supplies; get dispatch information and respond to call	Check unit; restock emergency care supplies; get dispatch information and respond to call	Check unit; restock emergency care supplies; get dispatch information and respond to call
Size-up (Yellow–Caution)	Arrive; perform scene size-up Determine need for EMTs, paramedics, med-evac, rescue, specialty units Contact medical direction or communications as needed	Arrive; perform scene size-up Determine need for paramedics, med-evac, rescue, specialty units Contact medical direction or communications as needed	Arrive; perform scene size-up Determine need for med-evac, rescue, specialty units Contact medical direction or communications as needed
Initial Assessment (Orange–Alert)	Perform initial assessment; impression, AVPU, ABCs, priority	Perform initial assessment; impression, AVPU, ABCs, priority	Perform initial assessment; impression, AVPU, ABCs, priority
Assessment (Red–Action)	Perform rapid or focused assesssment; perform or assist EMTs, paramedics with assessment and history, vital signs, stabilization, splinting, medications per protocols and medical direction	Perform rapid or focused assesssment; assist paramedics with assessment and history, vital signs, stabilization, splinting, medications per protocols and medical direction	Perform rapid or focused assesssment; perform BLS and ALS procedures per protocols and medical direction
Care and Transport (Orange–Alert)	Transport or arrange for EMTs, paramedics, or med-evac to transport; report patient history, vital signs, nature of illness or mechanism of injury Monitor patient for change in status; notify EMTs or paramedics; change to higher or lower priority as needed	Transport or arrange for paramedics or med-evac to transport; report patient history, vital signs, nature of illness or mechanism of injury Monitor patient for change in status; notify paramedics; change to higher or lower priority as needed	Transport or arrange for med-evac to transport; report patient history, vital signs, nature of illness or mechanism of injury Monitor patient for change in status; change to higher or lower priority as needed
Detailed Exam and Ongoing Assessment (Yellow–Caution)	Perform detailed physical exam or assist EMTs or paramedics during transport Perform interventions (patient care) or assist EMTs or paramedics during assessment and transport Perform ongoing assessment or assist EMTs or paramedics en route	Perform detailed physical exam or assist paramedics during transport Perform interventions (patient care) or assist paramedics during assessment and transport Perform ongoing assessment or assist paramedics en route	Perform detailed physical exam during transport Perform interventions (patient care) during assessment and transport Perform ongoing assessment en route
Wrap-up, Report and Preparation (Green–Go)	Hand-off patient to ED; complete patient report; restock and return to service	Hand-off patient to ED; complete patient report; restock and return to service	Hand-off patient to ED; complete patient report; restock and return to service

GLOSSARY

A

Abandonment to leave a sick or an injured patient before equal or more highly trained EMS personnel can assume responsibility for care.

ABC method the sequence of operations required in cardiopulmonary resuscitation. *A* stands for airway, *B* stands for breathing, and *C* stands for circulation.

ABCs of emergency care these letters stand for the words *airway*, *breathing*, and *circulation* as they relate to the initial assessment.

Abdomen (AB-do-men) the region of the body between the diaphragm and pelvis.

Abdominal cavity the anterior body cavity that extends from the diaphragm to the region protected by the pelvic bones. It houses and protects the abdominal organs, glands, major blood vessels, and nerves.

Abdominal quadrants four divisions of the abdomen used to pinpoint the location of a pain or an injury; the right upper quadrant, the left upper quadrant, the right lower quadrant, and the left lower quadrant.

Abdominal thrusts manual thrusts that are delivered to the midline of the abdomen, between the xiphoid process and the navel, to create pressure to help expel an airway obstruction. See *manual thrusts*.

Abdominopelvic (ab-DOM-i-no-PEL-vik) the front (anterior) cavity below (inferior to) the diaphragm.

Abortion (ah-BOR-shun) spontaneous miscarriage or induced loss of the embryo or fetus. See *miscarriage*.

Abrasion (ab-RAY-zhun) a scratch.

Abscess (AB-ses) a contained or otherwise limited structure that collects the pus associated with tissue death and infection.

Acetone breath a sweet breath with a fruitlike odor. This is a sign of diabetic coma.

Achilles (ah-KEL-ez) tendon the common term for the tendon that connects the posterior leg muscles to the heel. The calcaneal (kal-KA-ne-al) tendon.

Acid being acidic, as opposed to being neutral or basic (alkaline). Associated with free hydrogen ions.

Acquired immune deficiency syndrome (AIDS) a contagious disease that is usually fatal, as it suppresses the immune system and allows infections and malignancies to invade the body. The infectious agent is HIV. This agent may be passed from person to person by sexual contact, blood transfusion, sharing needles, or across the placenta from mother to fetus (unborn child). The virus is found in blood, body fluids, and wastes. It is also associated with mucous membranes. Even though it is found in saliva, there is no clear evidence of the disease being transmitted in this substance.

Activated charcoal a very fine, treated powder of charcoal that is available in premixed form or ready to mix with water. When taken by mouth, it may absorb some forms of ingested poisons, thus preventing or reducing absorption by the patient's body.

Acute to have a rapid onset. Sometimes the term is used to mean *severe*.

Acute abdomen the sudden onset of severe abdominal pain. Abdominal distress related to one of many medical conditions or specific injury to the abdomen.

Acute myocardial infarction (AMI) (my-o-KARD-e-al in-FARK-shun) a heart attack. The sudden death of heart muscle due to oxygen starvation. Usually caused by a narrowing or blockage of one of the blood vessels (coronary arteries) supplying the heart muscle.

Advanced cardiac life support (ACLS) prehospital emergency care that involves the use of intravenous fluids, drug infusions, cardiac monitoring, defibrillation, intubations, and other advanced procedures. See *basic life support (BLS)*.

Afterbirth the placenta, part of the umbilical cord, and some tissues of the womb's lining that are delivered after the birth of the baby.

Agonal respirations sporadic noises from the patient's airway, without chest movement; these occur just prior to death.

AIDS See *acquired immune deficiency syndrome (AIDS)*.

Air embolism gas bubbles in the bloodstream.

Air sacs the microscopic parts of the lung where gas exchange takes place. The medical term is *alveoli* (al-VE-o-li).

Air splint See *inflatable splint*.

Airway the passageway for air from the nose and mouth to the exchange levels of the lungs. The term can also be used to mean artificial airways, such as an *oropharyngeal airway*.

Airway adjunct a device that is placed in the patient's mouth or nose to help maintain an open airway. Oral airway adjuncts may help to hold the tongue clear of the airway.

Alkali a substance that is basic, as opposed to being acid or neutral.

Allergen (AL-er-jin) any substance that can cause an allergic response.

Allergy shock See *anaphylactic shock*.

Alveoli (al-VE-o-li) See *air sacs*.

Amnesia the short- or long-term loss of memory. This loss usually has a sudden onset.

Amniotic sac the fluid-filled sac that surrounds the developing embryo and fetus. Also called *bag of water*s.

Amputation soft-tissue injury that involves the cutting or tearing off of a limb or one of its parts. Often, hard tissues are also injured.

Analgesic a pain reliever.

Anaphylactic (an-ah-fi-LAK-tik) shock the most severe type of allergic reaction, in which a person goes into shock when he comes into contact with a substance to which he is allergic. Also called *allergy shock*.

Anatomical position the standard reference position for the body in the study of anatomy. The body is standing erect, facing the observer. The arms are down at the sides, and the palms of the hands face forward.

Anatomy the study of body structure.

Anesthetic to be free of pain and feeling. Commonly used to mean a substance that will block pain or feeling.

Aneurysm (AN-u-RIZ-m) the dilated or weakened section of an arterial wall. A blood-filled sac formed by the localized dilation of an artery or a vein.

Angina pectoris (an-JI-nah PEK-to-ris) the chest pain often caused by an insufficient blood supply to the heart muscle. This is not a heart attack as defined by the average patient. Also *angina*.

Angulated fracture a fracture that causes a bone or joint to take on an unnatural shape or bend.

Angulation the angle formed above and below a break in a bone. The fracture changes the straight line of a bone into an angle.

Ankle bones the tarsals (TAR-sals).

Anterior the front of the body or body part. See *posterior*.

Antiseptic a substance that will stop the growth of or prevent the activities of germs (microorganisms).

Anus (A-nus) the outlet of the large intestine.

Aorta (a-OR-tah) the major artery that carries blood from the heart out to the body.

Apical pulse the pulse felt or heard over the apex (lower part where the heart forms a cone at the ventricles) of the heart.

Apnea (ap-NE-ah) absence of breathing.

Apoplexy (AP-o-plek-see) the loss of consciousness, movement, and awareness of sensation that is caused by a stroke (CVA).

Appendicular (ap-en-DIK-u-ler) **skeleton** bones and joints that form the upper and lower extremities. See *axial skeleton*.

Arm the body part from the shoulder to elbow.

Arrhythmia (ah-RITH-me-ah) disturbance of heart rate and rhythm. Sometimes the term *dysrhythmia* is used to mean the same thing.

Arterial bleeding the loss of bright red blood from an artery. The flow may be rapid, spurting as the heart beats. See *capillary bleeding* and *venous bleeding*.

Arteriole (ar-TE-re-ol) the smallest of the arteries that typically lead into *capillary beds*. See *venule*.

Arteriosclerosis (ar-TE-re-o-skle-RO-sis) "hardening of the arteries" caused by calcium deposits. See also *atherosclerosis*.

Artery any blood vessel that carries blood away from the heart.

Articulate to join together. To unite to form a joint.

Artificial breathing See *artificial respiration*.

Artificial respiration the process of forcing air or oxygen into the lungs of a patient who is in respiratory arrest or who does not have adequate breathing. Also called *artificial ventilation* and *artificial breathing*.

Artificial ventilation See *artificial respiration*.

Aseptic clean, free of particles of dirt and debris. This does not mean sterile.

Asphyxia (as-FIK-si-ah) suffocation resulting in the loss of consciousness caused by too little oxygen reaching the brain. The functions of the brain, heart, and lungs will cease.

Aspiration to inhale materials into the lungs. Often used to describe the breathing of vomitus.

Asthma (AS-mah) the condition in which the bronchioles constrict, causing a reduction of airflow and creating congestion. Air usually will enter to the level of the air sacs (alveoli), but it cannot be exhaled easily.

Asystole (a-SIS-to-le) when the heart stops beating. This is cardiac standstill.

Atherosclerosis (ATH-er-o-skle-RO-sis) the buildup of fatty deposits on the inner wall of an artery. This buildup is called plaque. If calcium is deposited in the plaque, the arterial wall will become hard and stiff. See *arteriosclerosis*.

Atrioventricular (a-tre-o-ven-TRIK-u-lar) or **AV node** node in the upper chamber of the heat where electrical wave is delayed and then transferred to the lower chambers of the heart.

Atrium (A-tree-um) a superior chamber of the heart. The heart has a right and a left atrium. Plural, *atria*.

Auscultation (os-kul-TAY-shun) listening to sounds that occur within the body.

Automated external defibrillator (AED) an electrical apparatus that can detect certain irregular heartbeats (fibrillations) and deliver a shock through the patient's chest. This shock may allow the heart to resume a normal pattern of beating. The AED does not "jump-start" a dead heart. See *defibrillation*.

AVPU a system for measuring patient level of responsiveness. The letters stand for alert, verbal response, painful response, unresponsive.

Avulsion (ah-VUL-shun) a soft-tissue injury in which flaps of skin are torn loose or torn off.

Axial (AK-se-al) **skeleton** bones and joints that form the center, or upright, axis of the body. It includes the skull, spine, breastbone, and ribs. See *appendicular skeleton*.

Axilla (ak-SIL-ah) the armpit.

Bag-valve-mask ventilator an aid for artificial ventilation. It has a face mask, a self-inflating bag, and a valve that allows the bag to refill while the patient exhales. It can be attached to an oxygen line.

Bandage any material that is used to hold a dressing in place.

Basic life support (BLS) the ABCs of emergency care. Those events related to the findings of the initial assessment. See *ABC method*.

Battle's sign discoloration behind the ear that suggests a fracture at the base of the skull.

Behavioral emergency a situation in which a patient exhibits abnormal behavior that is unacceptable or intolerable to the patient, family, or community.

Bilateral existing on both sides of the body.

Bile fluid formed in the liver and sent to the small intestine. It may be stored in the gallbladder. Bile has many functions, including changing the speed at which the intestine moves things along (intestinal motility) and helping to digest fatty foods.

Biological death when the brain cells die; this is usually within 10 minutes of respiratory arrest. See *clinical death*.

Bladder usually referring to the urinary bladder located in the pelvic cavity.

Blanch to become pale or to turn white.

Bleeding shock caused by the loss of blood or plasma. Also known as *hypovolemic* (HI-po-vo-LE-mic) *shock*.

Blood the formed elements (blood cells and platelets) and the fluids of the bloodstream that flow in the closed circulation that is pumped by the heart.

Blood pressure the pressure caused by blood exerting a force on the walls of blood vessels. Usually, arterial blood pressure is measured.

Blunt trauma an injury caused by an object that was not sharp enough to penetrate the skin.

Body fluid shock caused by the loss of body fluids, as in cases of severe vomiting or diarrhea. Also called *metabolic shock*.

Body mechanics the proper use of the body to facilitate lifting and moving and prevent injury.

Body substance isolation (BSI) a form of infection control based on the presumption that all body fluids are infectious. See *universal precautions*.

Bones the living tissues of the skeletal system that have a matrix of calcium (for hardness) and protein fibers (for limited flexibility). Bones provide attachment points for skeletal muscles, and in some cases bone marrow makes blood cells.

Bourdon (bor-DON) **gauge** a gauged flowmeter that indicates the flow of a gas in liters per minute.

Bowel the intestine.

Brachial (BRAY-ke-al) **artery pressure point** the pressure point in the upper arm that can be used to help control serious external bleeding from the upper limb.

Brachial (BRAY-ke-al) **pulse** the pulse found on the inside (medial) upper arm of the patient. This pulse is used to evaluate circulation during the initial assessment of an infant.

Bradycardia (bray-de-KAR-de-ah) an abnormal condition where the heart rate is slow. The pulse rate will be below 50 beats per minute.

Breastbone the sternum.

Breech birth a birth in which the buttocks or both legs of the baby are delivered first.

Bronchiole (BRONG-ke-ol) the small branches of the airway that carry air to and from the air sacs of the lungs.

Bronchus (BRON-kus) the portion of the airway connecting the trachea to the lungs. Plural, *bronchi*.

Bruise simple closed wound in which blood flows between soft tissues, causing a discoloration; a *contusion*.

Bulky dressing a thick, single dressing or a buildup of thin dressings used to help control profuse bleeding, stabilize impaled objects, or cover large open wounds.

Capillary a microscopic blood vessel that connects an artery to a vein; where exchange takes place between the bloodstream and the body tissues.

Capillary bleeding the slow oozing of blood from a capillary bed. See *arterial bleeding* and *venous bleeding*.

Capillary refill the return (refill) of capillaries after blood has been forced out by fingertip pressure applied by the rescuer to the patient's nail bed. Normal refill time is 2 seconds or less. This is an assessment technique for measuring distal circulation for pediatric patients.

Cardiac (KAR-de-ak) in reference to the heart.

Cardiac arrest when the heart stops beating. Also, the sudden end of effective circulation caused by erratic muscle activity in the lower chambers of the heart (ventricular fibrillation).

Cardiogenic (KAR-de-o-JEN-ik) **shock** See *heart shock*.

Cardiopulmonary resuscitation (KAR-de-o-PUL-mo-ner-e re-SUS-ci-TA-shun) **(CPR)** heart–lung resuscitation. Combined compression and breathing techniques that maintain circulation and breathing.

Carotid (kah-ROT-id) **pulse** the pulse that can be felt on each side of the neck.

Carpals (KAR-pals) the wrist bones.

Catheter a flexible tube passed through a body channel (such as the urethra or a blood vessel) to allow for drainage or the withdrawal of fluids.

Central nervous system (CNS) the brain and spinal cord.

Cerebrospinal (ser-e-bro-SPI-nal) **fluid (CSF)** the clear, watery fluid that helps to protect the brain and spinal cord.

Cerebrovascular accident (CVA) See *stroke*.

Cervical (SER-vi-kal) **spine** the neck bones.

Cervix (SUR-viks) the neck of the uterus; the lower portion of the uterus where it enters the vagina.

CHEMTREC the Chemical Transportation Emergency Center that provides immediate expert information to emergency personnel at the scene of a hazardous materials incident.

Chief complaint the reason EMS was called, usually in the patient's own words.

Child (AHA standard) 1 to 8 years of age.

Child abuse assault of an infant or a child that produces physical and/or emotional injuries. Sexual assault is included as a form of child abuse.

Chronic the opposite of acute. It can be used to mean long and drawn out or recurring.

Chronic obstructive pulmonary disease (COPD) a variety of lung problems related to disease of the airway passages or exchange levels. The patient will suffer difficulties in breathing.

Circulatory system the heart, blood vessels, and blood; system that moves blood, carrying oxygen and nutrients to the body's cells and removing wastes and carbon dioxide from these cells.

Clavicle (KLAV-i-kul) the collarbone.

Clinical death the moment when breathing and heart actions stop. See *biological death*.

Closed fracture a simple fracture where the skin is not broken by the fractured bones. The fracture site is not exposed to the outside world.

Closed injury an injury with no associated opening of the skin.

Closed wound an internal soft-tissue injury where the skin is not broken. Also *closed injury*.

Clot the formation composed of fibrin and entangled blood cells that acts to help stop the bleeding from a wound.

Coccyx (KOK-siks) the lowermost bones of the spinal column. They are fused into one bone in the adult.

Collarbone the clavicle (KLAV-i-kul).

Coma the state of complete unconsciousness. The depth of unconsciousness may vary.

Compensated shock when a patient's body is still able to maintain perfusion even though shock is developing. See *decompensated shock*, *hypoperfusion*, *perfusion*, and *shock*.

Concussion injury to the brain that results from a blow or impact from an object but does not cause an open head injury.

Confidentiality the privacy of patient information (except for medical reporting, medical records, and certain court subpoenas), including the details of the patient and the patient's behavior during the rendering of all aspects of care.

Congestive heart failure (CHF) the condition in which the heart cannot properly circulate the blood. This causes a backup of fluids in the lungs and other organs.

Consent oral or written permission from the patient to render care to the First Responder level. See *expressed consent* and *implied consent*.

Constant flow sector valve a meterless device that allows the user to adjust the flow of supplemental oxygen by selecting the flow in stepped increments (2, 4, 6, 8, . . . 15 liters per minute).

Constricting band used to restrict the flow of venom.

Contraction time the period of time a contraction of the womb lasts during labor. It is measured from the start of the uterus contracting until it releases. See *interval time*.

Contraindication any condition, sign, symptom, or existing treatment that makes a particular course of treatment or care procedure inadvisable.

Contusion (kun-TU-zhun) a bruise; a bruising of the brain caused by a force of a blow great enough to rupture blood vessels on the surface of or deep within the brain.

Convulsion uncontrolled skeletal muscle spasm, often violent.

COPD See *chronic obstructive pulmonary disease (COPD)*.

Core temperature the body temperature measured at a central point, such as within the rectum.

Cornea (KOR-ne-ah) the transparent tissue covering that lies over the top of the iris and the pupil of the eye.

Coronary artery disease the narrowing of one or more places in the coronary arteries brought about by atherosclerosis. Blockage (occlusion) will eventually occur in many cases.

CPR cardiopulmonary resuscitation.

CPR compression site the mid-breastbone (mid-sternal) point found by placing the hand approximately two finger widths above (superior to) the substernal notch. During CPR of adults and children, compressions are delivered to this site. For the infant, compressions are delivered with two or three fingertips placed one finger width below an imaginary line drawn directly between the nipples.

Cranial (KRAY-ne-al) **cavity** braincase of the skull that houses the brain and its specialized membranes.

Cranium (KRAY-ne-um) the bones that form the forehead and the floor, back, top, and upper sides of the skull.

Cravat a piece of cloth material that can be used to secure a dressing or splint.

Crepitus (KREP-i-tus) a grating noise or the sensation felt when broken bone ends rub together.

Critical incident stress debriefing (CISD) process in which teams of professional and peer counselors provide emotional and psychological support to EMS personnel who are or have been involved in a critical (highly stressful) incident.

Croup (kroop) acute respiratory condition found in infants and children, which is characterized by a barking type of cough or stridor.

Crowing an atypical sound made when a patient breathes. It usually indicates airway obstruction.

Crowning the bulging out of the vagina and eventual exposing of the baby's head during successive contractions of delivery. It is usually in reference to a normal head-first delivery.

Crush injury soft-tissue injury produced by crushing forces. Soft tissues and internal organs are crushed, and hard tissues are usually damaged.

Cut soft-tissue injury in which all the layers of skin are opened and the tissues immediately below the skin are damaged. Smooth cuts are incisions and jagged cuts are lacerations.

Cyanosis (si-ah-NO-sis) when the skin color changes to blue or gray because of too little oxygen in the blood.

Danger zone the area around a traffic accident or other emergency event in which special safety procedures must be followed. The size and type of zone is often dependent on the type of accident and environmental conditions.

DCAP-BTLS a study aid used to remember patient assessment factors. The letters stand for <u>d</u>eformities, <u>c</u>ontusions, <u>a</u>brasions, <u>p</u>unctures/penetrations, <u>b</u>urns, <u>t</u>enderness, <u>l</u>acerations, and <u>s</u>welling.

Decompensated shock takes place when the patient's body can no longer maintain perfusion as shock develops. Usually there is a pronounced fall in blood pressure. See *compensated shock*, *hypoperfusion*, *perfusion*, and *shock*.

Decompression sickness the "bends." In most cases, this involves scuba divers who have surfaced too rapidly. Nitrogen is trapped in body tissues and may find its way into the divers' bloodstreams.

Deep frostbite See *freezing*.

Defibrillation to apply an electric shock to a patient's heart in an attempt to disrupt a lethal rhythm and allow the heart to spontaneously reestablish a normal rhythm. This is done with a *defibrillator*. See *automated external defibrillator (AED)*.

Dehydration excessive loss of body water.

Delirium tremens (DTs) a severe, possibly life-threatening reaction related to alcohol withdrawal. The patient's hands tremble, hallucinations may be present, behavior may be unusual, and convulsions may occur.

Dermis (DER-mis) the inner (second) layer of the skin. It is the layer that is rich in blood vessels and nerves found below the epidermis.

Detailed physical exam an assessment used for unconscious patients or those who may be severely injured. The assessment is done more slowly than a rapid trauma assessment and includes a complete head-to-toe examination.

Diabetes (di-ah-BE-teez) usually refers to diabetes mellitus. This is the condition in which there is a decrease or absence of insulin produced by the pancreas. The glucose level of the blood will increase and the movement of this sugar into the cells will decrease as the insulin level falls. See *hyperglycemia* and *hypoglycemia*.

Diabetic coma severe hyperglycemia. The result of an inadequate insulin supply that leads to unconsciousness, coma, and eventually death unless treated.

Diaphragm (DI-ah-fram) the muscular structure that divides the chest cavity (thorax) from the abdominal cavity (abdominopelvic cavity). It is the major muscle used in breathing.

Diaphragmatic (DI-ah-FRAG-mat-ik) **breathing** weak and rapid respirations with little or no chest movement. There may be slight movement of the abdomen. The patient's attempt to breathe with the diaphragm alone.

Diastolic (di-as-TOL-ik) **blood pressure** the pressure exerted on the internal walls of the arteries when the heart is relaxing. See *systolic blood pressure*.

Digestive system system that stores and digests food, eliminates waste, and utilizes nutrients.

Dilation to enlarge, having expanded in diameter.

Direct pressure the quickest, most effective way to control most forms of external bleeding. Pressure is applied directly over the wound site.

Dislocation the pulling or pushing of a bone end partially or completely free of a joint.

Distal farther away from the torso. When used with the word *proximal* (closer to), *distal* means more distant from. See *proximal*.

Distal pulse a pulse measured at the distal end of an extremity. Usually, this is the radial pulse for the upper extremity and the dorsalis pedis pulse for the lower extremity. See *radial pulse* and *dorsalis pedis pulse*.

Distended inflated, stretched, or swollen.

Dorsalis pedis (dor-SAL-is PED-is) **pulse** a foot pulse. See *pedal pulse*.

Downer a depressant that will depress the central nervous system to relax the user.

Dressing any material used to cover a wound that will help control bleeding and reduce contamination.

Drowning death caused by water reaching the lungs and either causing lung tissue damage or spasms of the airway that prevent the inhalation of air. See *near-drowning*.

Duodenum (du-o-DE-num or du-OD-e-num) the first portion of the small intestine, connected to the stomach. It is more rigid than the other portions, causing it to suffer greater injury in accidents.

Duty to act requirement that First Responders in the police and paid fire service, at least while on duty, must provide care according to their department's standard operating procedures.

Dyspnea (disp-NE-ah) difficult or labored breathing.

Early or superficial local cooling minor damage to the skin surface related to cold exposure. Also called *frostnip*.

Eclampsia (e-KLAM-se-ah) a life-threatening complication of pregnancy that produces convulsions and may result in coma or death.

-ectomy (EK-toe-me) a word ending meaning surgical removal.

Edema (e-DE-mah) swelling due to the accumulation of fluids in the tissues.

Embolism (EM-bo-liz-m) movement and lodgement of a blood clot or foreign body (fat or air bubble) inside a blood vessel. The clot or foreign body is called an *embolus* (EM-bo-lus).

Emergency care the prehospital assessment and basic care for the sick or injured patient. The physical and emotional needs of the patient are considered and attended to during care.

Emergency medical services system the chain of human resources and services linked together to provide continuous emergency care from the prehospital scene, through transport, and at the medical facility.

Emergency medical technician (EMT) a professional-level provider of emergency care, trained above the level of the First Responder. This individual has received formal training equal to or greater than the standard DOT emergency medical technician training program and is state certified. The EMT-Basic classification.

Emergency move a patient move that is carried out quickly when the scene is hazardous, care of the patient requires repositioning, or you must reach another patient needing lifesaving care.

Emesis (EM-e-sis) vomiting.

Emotional emergency when a patient's behavior is not considered to be typical for the occasion. Often this behavior is not socially acceptable. The patient's emotions are strongly evident, interfering with his or her thoughts and behavior.

Emphysema (EM-fi-SEE-mah) a chronic disease in which the lungs suffer a progressive loss of elasticity. See *chronic obstructive pulmonary disease (COPD)*.

Endocrine (EN-do-krin) **system** the system that produces chemicals called *hormones*, which help regulate most body activities and functions.

Enhanced 911 service that allows for caller information (for example, phone number and address) to be received electronically.

Epidermis (ep-i-DER-mis) the outer layer of skin.

Epiglottis (EP-i-GLOT-is) a flap of cartilage and other tissues that is located above the voice box (larynx). It helps to close off the airway when a person swallows.

Epiglottitis (ep-ih-glot-I-tis) swelling of the epiglottis that can be caused by bacterial infection. It can obstruct the airway and can be potentially life-threatening.

Epilepsy (EP-i-lep-see) a medical disorder characterized by attacks of unconsciousness, with or without convulsions.

Epinephrine medicine used to treat severe allergic reactions; it relaxes the air passages so breathing becomes easier and constricts the enlarged blood vessels.

Episodic a medical problem that affects the patient at regular intervals.

Epistaxis (ep-e-STAK-sis) a nosebleed.

Esophagus (e-SOF-ah-gus) the muscular food tube leading from the throat to the stomach.

Evisceration (e-VIS-er-a-shun) usually applies to the intestine protruding through an incision or a wound.

Expiration the passive process of breathing out. See *inspiration*.

Expire to exhale air.

Expressed consent informed consent by a rational adult patient, usually in oral form, to accept emergency care.

External auditory canal the opening of the external ear and its pathway to the middle ear.

External chest compressions measured compressions performed during CPR at a set rate over the CPR compression site. These compressions are applied to help create circulation of the blood.

Extrication any actions that disentangle and free from entrapment.

Extruded when an organ, a bone, or a vessel is pushed out of position.

Fainting the simplest form of shock, occurring when the patient has a temporary, self-correcting loss of consciousness caused by a reduced supply of blood to the brain. Also called *psychogenic* (SI-ko-JEN-ic) *shock*.

Febrile feverish.

Femoral (FEM-o-ral) **artery** the main artery of the upper leg (thigh). It is a major pulse location and pressure point site.

Femoral (FEM-o-ral) **artery pressure point** the pressure point in the thigh that can be used to help control serious external bleeding from the lower limb.

Femur (FE-mer) the thigh bone.

Fetus (FE-tus) the developing unborn child. The fertilized egg is an embryo until the eighth week after fertilization, when it becomes a fetus.

Fibrillation uncoordinated contractions of the heart muscle (myocardium) that are produced from independent individual muscle fiber activity. The totally disorganized activity of heart muscle. See *ventricular fibrillation* and *defibrillation*.

Fibula (FIB-yo-lah) the lateral lower leg bone.

Finger bones the phalanges (fah-LAN-jez).

Finger sweeps a procedure used to clear the mouth of airway obstructions. The rescuer's gloved fingers are used to sweep and lift away objects, clots, and debris—but only when they are visible. Blind finger sweeps should not be used for pediatric patients.

First-degree burn a mild partial-thickness burn, involving only the outer layer of skin. See *superficial burn*.

First Responder a member of the EMS system who has been trained to render first care for a patient and to help EMTs at the emergency scene.

Flail chest the condition in which multiple rib fractures or the breastbone separating from the chest produce a loose segment of the chest wall. This segment will move in the opposite direction of the chest during breathing.

Flexion to lessen an angle of a joint. To bend, as in bending the knee or bending at the elbow.

Flowmeter a Bourdon, pressure-compensated, or constant flow selector valve device used to indicate supplemental oxygen flow in liters per minute.

Flow-restricted, oxygen-powered ventilation device (FROPVD) device that delivers oxygen through a regulator from a pressurized cylinder.

Focused assessment a patient assessment that includes the required physical exam, a patient history, and vital signs. Procedures differ for trauma and medical patients.

Focused history and physical exam this follows the initial assessment and can be modified as to the type of patient—trauma or medical. At the First Responder level, it includes for the seriously injured patient a rapid trauma assessment (or head-to-toe exam for unconscious patients), gathering vital signs, and obtaining a history. If injury is not serious, the physical exam can be focused on a specific area, often suggested by the patient. For medical patients, a history is followed by a focused physical exam and the gathering of vital signs.

Fontanelles areas in the infant skull where bones have not yet fused; soft spots.

Foot bones the metatarsals (meta-TAR-sals).

Forearm bones the ulna and radius.

Fracture any break, crack, split, chip, or crumbling of a bone.

Freezing an injury due to cold involving the skin and the layers below the skin. Deep structures such as bone and muscle may be involved. See *late or deep local cold injury*.

Frostbite localized cold injury. The skin is frozen, but the layers below it are still soft and have their normal bounce. See *freezing* and *late or deep local cold injury*.

Full-thickness burn a burn that damages all the layers of skin. Deep structures may also be burned. See *third-degree burn*.

Gag reflex a retching action, hacking, or vomiting that is induced when something touches a certain level of the patient's throat.

Gallbladder an organ attached to the lower back of the liver. It stores bile.

Gastric distention inflation of the stomach.

Gastro- (GAS-tro) used as a beginning of words in reference to the stomach.

Genitalia (jen-i-TA-le-ah) the external reproductive organs.

Genitourinary (jen-eh-to-U-reh-NER-e) **system** reproductive and urinary systems.

Glucose (GLU-kohs) a simple sugar that is the primary source of energy for the body's tissues.

Good Samaritan laws a series of state laws designed to protect certain care providers if they deliver the standard of care in good faith, to the level of their training, and to the best of their abilities.

Grand mal a severe epileptic seizure.

Gurgling an atypical sound of breathing made by patients having airway obstruction, lung disease, or lung injury due to heat.

H

Hallucinogen a mind-altering drug that acts on the central nervous system to excite the user or to distort his or her perception of the surroundings.

Hand bones the bones of the palm of the hand, known as the *metacarpals* (meta-KAR-pals).

Handoff the orderly transfer of the patient, patient information, and patient valuables to more highly trained personnel.

Hazardous materials incident the release of a harmful substance into the environment.

Head-tilt, chin-lift maneuver a procedure for use on patients who do not have neck or spinal injury. It opens the mouth, moves the tongue away from the throat, and provides for an open airway in most cases. See *jaw-thrust maneuver*.

Heart attack a general term used to indicate a failure of circulation to the heart muscle that damages or kills a portion of the heart.

Heart shock caused by the heart failing to pump enough blood to all parts of the body. Also known as *cardiogenic* (KAR-de-o-JEN-ik) *shock*.

Heat cramps typical layperson's term for muscle cramps in the lower limbs and abdomen associated with the loss of fluids and possibly salts while active in a hot environment. See *heat emergencies*.

Heat emergencies patients with moist, pale, normal-to-cool skin and hot, dry or moist skin due to exposure to excessive heat that leads to fluid and salt loss. The extreme case is the development of shock or the loss of the body's heat-regulating mechanisms.

Heat exhaustion prolonged exposure to heat, which creates moist, pale skin that may feel normal or cool to the touch. See *heat emergencies*.

Heat stroke prolonged exposure to heat, which creates dry or moist skin that may feel warm or hot to the touch. See *heat emergencies*.

Hematoma (hem-ah-TO-mah) the collection of blood under the skin or in tissues as a result of an injured blood vessel.

Hemorrhage (HEM-o-rej) internal or external bleeding.

Hemothorax (he-mo-THO-raks) the condition of blood and bloody fluids in the area between the lungs and the walls of the chest cavity.

HEPA in the EMS system, this refers to a high-efficiency particulate air filter, mask, or respirator.

Hepatitis a disease that inflames and damages the liver. It may be caused by infectious viral agents, which exist in several different forms. Some hepatitis viruses are very infectious and can lead to lifelong illness or death. It is a real danger for rescuers who fail to follow standard safety procedures.

Hip the joint made between the pelvis and the thigh bone (femur). Some people use this term to refer to the upper portion of the thigh bone.

Hives slightly elevated red or pale areas of the skin that may be produced as a reaction to certain foods, drugs, infections, or stress. Often there is an itching sensation associated with hives. See *wheal*.

Human immunodeficiency virus (HIV) virus that causes AIDS. See *acquired immune deficiency syndrome (AIDS)*.

Humerus (HU-mer-us) the upper arm bone.

Humidifier a device that is attached to a supplemental oxygen delivery system to add moisture to the dry oxygen coming from the cylinder.

Hyperextension the overextension of a limb or body part.

Hyperglycemia (hi-per-gli-SE-me-ah) the sugar (glucose) level increases in the blood and decreases in the tissue cells. The problem can be serious enough to produce a coma. See *diabetic coma*.

Hyperthermia (HI-per-THUR-me-ah) an increase in body core temperature above its normal temperature.

Hyperventilation uncontrolled rapid, deep breathing that is usually self-correcting. This may occur by itself or as a sign of a more serious problem.

Hypoglycemia (hi-po-gli-SE-me-ah) too little sugar in the blood. See *insulin shock*.

Hypoperfusion the failure of the body to provide adequate circulation to all its vital parts. The development of shock is actually the development of the state of hypoperfusion. See *compensated shock, decompensated shock, perfusion*, and *shock*.

Hypothermia a general cooling of the body. Severe forms can lead to death.

Hypovolemic (HI-po-vo-LE-mik) **shock** the state of shock that develops due to excessive loss of whole blood or plasma.

Hypoxia (hi-POK-se-ah) an inadequate supply of oxygen to the body tissues.

I

Ileum (IL-e-um) the upper portions of the pelvis that form the wings of the pelvis.

Iliac (IL-e-ak) **crest** the upper, curved boundary of the wings of the pelvis. See *ileum*.

Immobilize to fix or hold a body part in place in order to reduce or eliminate motion.

Implied consent a legal position that assumes that an unconscious or badly injured adult would consent to receiving emergency care. This form of consent may apply to other types of patients (for example, mentally ill).

Incident management system a system designed to allow EMS personnel to manage all phases of a multiple-casualty incident. It must include provisions for command at different stages, safety, assessment, care, and transport.

Incision a smooth cut produced by a sharp object.

Indication specific sign or condition for which it is appropriate to use a medication.

Infant (AHA standard) younger than 1 year of age.

Infarction (in-FARK-shun) localized tissue death due to the discontinuation of its blood supply. Sometimes used to mean a myocardial (heart muscle) infarction.

Infectious disease any disease produced by an infectious agent such as a bacterium or virus.

Inferior away from the head; usually compared with another structure that is closer to the head (for example, the lips are inferior to the nose). See *superior*.

Inflammation the pain, heat, redness, and swelling of tissues as they react to infection, irritation, or injury.

Inflatable splint a soft plastic splint that can be inflated with air to become rigid enough to help immobilize a fractured extremity.

Informed consent expressed consent given by a rational adult patient after being informed of the provider's training and what care procedures are to be done. Risks and options may have to be discussed.

Initial assessment the part of a patient assessment that is used to detect and immediately correct life-threatening problems that primarily involve the airway, breathing, and circulation.

Inspiration the process of breathing in. See *expiration*.

Inspire to inhale air

Insulin (IN-su-lin) a hormone produced in the pancreas that is needed to move sugar (glucose) from the blood into cells.

Insulin shock severe hypoglycemia. A state of shock usually caused by too high a level of insulin in the blood, producing a sudden drop in blood sugar.

Intercostal (in-ter-KOS-tal) **muscles** the muscles found between the ribs. These muscles contract during an inspiration, lifting the ribs. This helps to increase the volume of the chest (thoracic) cavity.

Interval time during labor, this term means the time from the start of one contraction until the beginning of the next. See *contraction time*.

Intravenous (IV) into a vein.

Iris the colored portion of the anterior eye. It adjusts the size of the pupil.

Ischium (IS-ke-em) the lower, posterior portions of the pelvis.

-itis (I-tis) a word ending used to mean inflammation.

Jaundice (JON-dis) the yellowing of the skin, usually associated with liver or bile apparatus (gallbladder and bile ducts) injury or disease.

Jaw-thrust maneuver a method of opening the airway without lifting the neck or tilting the head. See *head-tilt, chin-lift maneuver*.

Ketoacidosis (KE-to-as-i-DO-sis) a condition that occurs when a diabetic breaks down too many fats trying to obtain energy. Toxic ketone bodies form in the blood and the blood becomes acid.

Kidneys excretory organs located high in the back of the abdominal region. They are behind the abdominal cavity.

Kneecap the patella (pah-TEL-lah).

Labor the three stages of childbirth, including the beginning of contractions, delivery of the child, and delivery of the afterbirth (placenta, umbilical cord, and some of the lining tissues of the uterus).

Laceration a jagged cut with rough edges. See *cut*.

Laryngectomy (lar-in-JEK-to-me) the total or partial removal of the voice box (larynx). The patient is called a *neck breather* or a *laryngectomee*.

Larynx (LAR-inks) the airway between the throat and the windpipe. It contains the voice box.

Late or deep local cold injury tissue damage directly related to exposure to cold temperatures. Surface tissues are frozen (frostbite) and, in most cases, tissues below are also frozen (freezing or deep frostbite).

Lateral to the side, away from the midline of the body. See *medial*.

Ligament fibrous tissue that connects bone to bone.

Liter (LE-ter) the metric measurement of liquid volume that is equal to 1.057 quarts. One pint is almost equal to one-half liter. Also spelled *litre*.

Liver the largest gland in the body, having many functions. Located in the upper-right abdominal region, extending over to the central abdominal region.

Localized cold injury freezing or near freezing of a body part.

Log roll a procedure for moving a patient while keeping the patient's head, neck, and torso aligned (head and spine remain aligned). Two rescuers may be used, but at least four are recommended for the procedure.

Lumbar (LUM-bar) **spine** the five bones (vertebrae) of the lower back.

Lung shock caused by too little oxygen in the blood due to some sort of lung failure. Also called *respiratory shock*.

Major burn any full-thickness (third-degree) burn; a partial-thickness (second-degree) burn involving an entire body area or crucial area; a superficial (first-degree) burn that covers a large area; any burn to the face; or any burn that involves the respiratory system. See *minor burn*.

Mammalian diving reflex a reaction that occurs when a drowning person's face submerges in cold water. The cold water causes a slow heart rate, and blood flow is directed to the heart, lungs, and brain. Oxygen is diverted to the brain.

Mandible (MAN-di-bl) the lower jawbone.

Manual thrusts abdominal or chest thrusts provided to expel an object causing an airway obstruction.

Manual traction a stabilizing procedure that precedes the application of a rigid splint.

Mechanism of injury (MOI) a force or forces that may have caused injury. Consideration is given to the type of force, its intensity and direction, and the body part it affects.

Meconium staining amniotic fluid that has a green or brownish-yellow color due to fetal fecal contamination.

Medial toward the midline of the body. See *lateral*.

Medical patient one who has or describes symptoms of an illness.

Medical Practices Act requiring an individual to be licensed or certified in order to practice medicine or to provide certain levels of care.

Meninges (me-NIN-jez) the three membranes surrounding the brain and spinal cord.

Meningitis inflammation of the lining of the brain and spinal cord.

Metabolic shock See *body fluid shock*.

Metacarpals (meta-KAR-pals) hand bones.

Metatarsals (meta-TAR-sals) foot bones.

Midline an imaginary vertical line drawn down the center of the body, dividing it into right and left halves.

Minor burn a superficial or partial thickness burn (first- or second-degree) involving a small portion of the body with *no* damage to the respiratory system, face, hands, feet, groin, medial thigh, buttocks, or major joints. It does not circle or cover an entire body part. See *major burn*.

Minor's consent a form of implied consent used when a minor is seriously ill or injured and the parents or guardians cannot be reached quickly.

Miscarriage the natural loss of the embryo or fetus before the twenty-eighth week of pregnancy. Also called a spontaneous abortion.

Moves a general term used to describe any organized procedure that is employed to reposition or move a sick or an injured person from one location to another. See *emergency move* and *nonemergency move*.

Multiple-casualty incident (MCI) an EMS system term for any accident, disaster, or medical emergency that produces more than one patient.

Musculoskeletal system all the muscles, bones, joints, and related structures such as tendons and ligaments that enable the body and its parts to move and function.

Myocardium (mi-o-KAR-de-um) heart muscle. The cardiac muscle that makes up the walls of the heart.

Narcotic a class of drugs for the relief of pain that affects the central nervous system. Illicit use is to provide an intense state of relaxation.

Nasogastric (NA-zo-GAZ-trik) **tube (NG tube)** a flexible tube inserted through the nose to reach the stomach to allow drainage and/or feeding. Some patients under home care may have an NG tube. There are cases where this tube may be inserted in the field; however, this is *not* a First Responder-level procedure.

Nasopharyngeal (na-zo-fah-RIN-je-al) **airway** a flexible plastic tube that is lubricated and then inserted into a patient's nose down to the level of the nasopharynx (back of the throat) to allow for an open upper airway. Supplemental oxygen may be delivered through this tube.

Nature of illness (NOI) what is medically wrong with a patient.

Near-drowning when the process of drowning is stopped and is reversible. Vital signs may or may not be present; however, the patient can be resuscitated. Complications may still cause death at a later date (for example, pneumonia). See *drowning*.

Negligence at the First Responder level, negligence usually is a failure to provide the expected standard of care, leading to additional injury of the patient.

Neonate (AHA standard) newborn to 1 month of age.

Nervous system the system of brain, spinal cord, and nerves that governs sensation, movement, and thought.

Neurogenic (NU-ro-jen-ic) **shock** caused when the nervous system fails to control the diameter of the blood vessels. The vessels remain widely dilated, providing too great a volume to be filled by available blood. Also called *nerve shock*.

Nonemergency move a patient move that is carried out if there are other factors at the scene causing the patient to decline, you must reach other patients, part of the care required forces you to move the patient, or the patient insists on being moved.

Nonrebreather mask an oxygen delivery system mask that has an oxygen reservoir bag. This mask delivers a high concentration of oxygen and expels all of the patient's expired air.

Occlusion blockage. A blocked artery has an occlusion.

Occlusive dressing a dressing used to create an airtight seal or to close an open wound of a body cavity. Usually, it is made of plastic.

Off-line medical direction protocols developed by an EMS system that authorize rescuers to perform particular skills in certain situations without actually speaking to the Medical Director.

Ongoing assessment a process that may be initiated at the scene and continued through transport and patient transfer. It allows for reevaluation of the patient's condition and the effectiveness of care procedures. Often, First Responders may help the EMTs reassess vital signs.

On-line medical direction orders to perform a skill or administer care from the on-duty physician given by radio or phone to the rescuer.

Open fracture when a bone is broken and bone ends or fragments cut through the skin. Also called *compound fracture*. If a wound opens the fracture site to the outside world (for example, gunshot wound), the fracture is classified as an open fracture.

Open injury an injury with an associated opening of the skin.

Open wound an injury to the body in which the skin or its outer layers are opened. Also *open injury*.

Oral glucose a form of glucose that comes in a gel and is packaged in different-sized tubes like toothpaste. It can be given to a patient with an altered mental status and a history of diabetes by placing it inside the mouth.

Orbits refers to the orbits of the eyes, called the *eye sockets*.

Oropharyngeal (or-o-fah-RIN-je-al) **airway** a curved breathing tube inserted into the patient's mouth. It will hold the base of the tongue forward.

ℙ

Packaging part of the procedure of preparation for removal of the patient at an accident scene. It may involve applying splints and dressings, neck and spine immobilization, and stabilizing impaled objects.

Palpate to feel a part of the body as to palpate the abdomen or palpate a radial pulse. To use a blood pressure cuff while feeling the radial pulse in order to determine the approximate systolic blood pressure.

Pancreas (PAN-cre-as) the gland in the back of the upper portion of the abdominal cavity, behind the stomach. It produces insulin and digestive juices.

Paradoxical motion (movement) when a loose segment of an injured chest wall moves in the opposite direction to the rest of the wall during breathing movements. This is associated with *flail chest*.

Paralysis complete or partial loss of the ability to move a body part. Sensation in the area may also be lost.

Partial-thickness burn a second-degree burn in which the outer layer of skin is burned through and the second layer (dermis) is damaged. Another classification for this burn is a *second-degree burn*.

Patella (pah-TEL-ah) the kneecap.

Pathogen the organisms that cause infection, such as viruses and bacteria.

Patient assessment the gathering of information to determine the possible nature of the patient's illness or injury. It includes interviews and physical examination.

Pedal pulse a foot pulse.

Pelvic cavity the anterior body cavity surrounded by the bones of the pelvis.

Penetrating wound a puncture wound with only an entrance wound.

Perforating wound a puncture wound having an entrance wound and an exit wound.

Perfusion the constant flow of blood through the capillaries. See *hypoperfusion*.

Pericardium (per-e-KAR-de-um) the sac that surrounds the heart.

Perineum (per-i-NE-um) the region of the body located between the genitalia and the anus.

Peritoneum (per-i-to-NE-um) the membrane that lines the abdominal cavity.

Personal protective equipment (PPE) equipment such as eyewear, mask, gloves, gown, or turnout gear or helmet that protect the EMS worker from infection and/or from exposure to hazardous materials and the dangers of rescue operations. See *universal precautions*.

Petit mal the minor epileptic attack that is noted by a momentary loss of awareness, with no major convulsive seizures.

Phalanges (fah-LAN-jez) the bones of the toes and fingers.

Pharmacology the study of drugs, their origins, nature, chemistry, effects, and use.

Pharynx (FAR-inks) the throat.

Placenta (plah-SEN-tah) an organ of pregnancy that is composed of maternal and fetal tissues. Exchange between the circulatory systems of the mother and fetus can take place without the mixing of blood. It is the main component of afterbirth that must be delivered after the baby.

Plasma (PLAZ-mah) the fluid portion of the blood; the blood minus the blood cells and other structures.

Platelet (PLAT-let) element of the blood that releases factors needed to produce blood clots.

Pleura (PLOOR-ah) a double-membrane sac. The outer layer lines the chest wall, and the inner layer covers the outside of the lungs.

Pleural (PLOOR-al) **cavities** the right and left portions of the chest cavity (thorax) that contain the lungs and the pleura membranes.

Pneumatic anti-shock garment (PASG) garment similar to the air splint that can be used to control bleeding from the lower extremities by direct pressure.

Pneumothorax (NU-mo-THO-raks) the collection of air in the chest cavity to the outside of the lungs, caused by punctures to the chest wall or the lungs.

Pocket face mask a device used to help provide mouth-to-mouth ventilations. It has a chimney to allow the rescuer to provide breaths without touching the patient. A one-way valve is present in most models to prevent rescuer contact with the patient's blood and body fluids. A HEPA filter can also be inserted to prevent transmission of airborne pathogens. Some masks have an inlet for supplemental oxygen.

Position of function the natural position of a body part. For example, the natural position of the hand is slightly flexed.

Posterior the back of the body or body part. See *anterior*.

Premature baby a baby that is born before the thirty-seventh week (prior to the ninth month) of pregnancy; any baby with a birth weight of less than 5.5 pounds.

Prescribed inhaler a device that holds medication in an aerosol form, which can be sprayed into the mouth and inhaled in order to dilate (enlarge) the air passages of someone with a chronic respiratory disease, such as asthma.

Pressure regulator a device that is connected to an oxygen cylinder to reduce the cylinder pressure to a safe working level, thus providing a safe pressure for delivery to the patient.

Priapism (PRI-ah-pizm) persistent erection associated with spinal damage in the male patient.

Prolapsed cord umbilical cord that presents through the vaginal opening before the baby's head during delivery.

Prone lying face down.

Protocols a specific set of steps to be taken in different situations that are part of an EMS system's guidelines for safety, assessment, care, transport, and transfer. Protocols are developed by the EMS system's Medical Director.

Proximal closer to the torso. Used with *distal*, meaning away from. See *distal*.

PSD an abbreviation for p̲ainful, s̲wollen, d̲eformed extremity.

Psychogenic (SI-ko-JEN-ic) **shock** See *fainting*.

Pubic (PYOO-bik), **Pubis** (PYOO-bis) the middle, anterior region of the pelvis. The region associated with the external genitalia.

Pulmonary (PUL-mo-ner-e) applies to the lungs.

Pulmonary resuscitation (PUL-mo-ner-e re-SUS-ci-TAY-shun) to provide breaths to a patient in an attempt to artificially maintain lung function.

Pulse the alternate expansion and contraction of artery walls as the heart pumps blood.

Pulseless electrical activity (PEA) condition in which the electrical activity of the heart is within normal range, but the heart muscle is too weak and damaged to pump blood efficiently.

Puncture an open wound that tears through the skin and damages tissues in a straight line. See *penetrating wound* and *perforating wound*.

Radial pulse the wrist pulse. The site is the lateral wrist.

Radius the lateral forearm bone.

Rapid trauma assessment a quick but safely done survey of the patient as a modified head-to-toe exam. Both signs and symptoms are gathered. See *focused history* and *physical exam and patient assessment*.

Rectum (REK-tum) the lower portion of the large intestine, ending with the anus.

Red blood cells (RBCs) the circulating blood cells that carry oxygen to the tissues and return carbon dioxide to the lungs. The *erythrocytes* (e-RITH-ro-sites).

Referred pain the pain felt in a region of the body other than where the source or cause of the pain is located. For example, pain in the gallbladder may be felt over the right shoulder blade (scapula).

Reproductive system system that produces all structures and hormones needed for sexual reproduction.

Respiration the act of breathing; the exchange of oxygen and carbon dioxide that takes place in the lungs.

Respiratory arrest the cessation of breathing.

Respiratory distress any difficulty in breathing. Sometimes the problem is severe enough to require emergency care.

Respiratory shock See *lung shock*.

Respiratory system system that exchanges air to bring in oxygen and expel carbon dioxide. It includes the nose, mouth, structures in the throat, lungs, and associated muscles.

Resuscitation (re-SUS-eh-TA-shun) any effort to restore or provide normal heart and/or lung function artificially.

Rigid splint a stiff device made of a material with very little flexibility (such as metal, plastic, or wood) that is long enough to immobilize an extremity and the joints above and below the injury site.

Rule of nines a system used for estimating the amount of skin surface that is burned. The body is divided into 12 regions. Each of 11 regions equals 9% of the body surface and the genital section is classified as 1%.

Sacrum (SA-krum) the fused bones (vertebrae) of the lower back that are immediately inferior to the lumbar spine.

SAMPLE history a system of information gathering that allows the rescuer to ask questions about past or present medical or injury problems. The letters that direct the questioning stand for signs/symptoms, allergies, medications, pertinent past history, last oral intake, events leading to the injury or illness.

Sanitize a rigid standard of cleaning, often to the point of practical sterilization.

Scapula (SKAP-u-lah) the shoulder blade.

Scene size-up the first steps in rescuer safety and patient assessment. An assessment of the scene conditions, number of patients, mechanism of injury and/or nature of illness, and needed resources.

Sclera (SKLE-rah) the "whites" of the eyes.

Scope of practice set of responsibilities and ethical considerations that define the extent or limits of the care provider.

Scratches and scrapes the simplest forms of open wounds that damage the skin surface but do not break all the layers of skin. Collectively, these injuries are called abrasions.

Second-degree burn a partial-thickness burn. The outer layer of skin (epidermis) is burned through, and the second layer (dermis) is damaged. See *partial-thickness burn*.

Seizure in general, any event in the brain that causes uncontrolled muscle contractions (convulsions).

Septic shock caused by infection-producing poisons.

Septum a structure that divides two chambers, such as the septum in the nose that separates the two nostrils.

Shock the reaction of the body to the failure of the circulatory system to provide enough blood to all the vital organs of the body. The failure of perfusion. See *hypoperfusion* and *perfusion*.

Shoulder blade the scapula.

Side effect any unwanted action or reaction of a drug other than the desired effect.

Sign what you see, hear, feel, and smell in relation to the patient's illness or injury.

Sinoatrial (si-no-A-tre-al) **node** a small region of modified tissue in the heart that sends out electrical waves; also called the *pacemaker*.

Skeletal system all the bones and joints of the body. The skeletal system provides body support and organ protection, enables movement, and produces blood cells.

Sling a large triangular bandage or other cloth device that is applied as a soft splint to immobilize possible injuries to the shoulder girdle and upper extremity.

Soft splint a device, such as a sling and swathe or a pillow secured with cravats, that can be applied to immobilize a painful, swollen, deformed (PSD) extremity.

Soft tissues the tissues of the body that make up the skin, muscles, nerves, blood vessels, fatty tissues, and the cells that line and cover organs and glands. Bones, cartilage, and teeth are hard tissues.

Sphygmomanometer (SFIG-mo-mah-NOM-eh-ter) an instrument used to measure blood pressure, commonly called *blood pressure cuff*.

Spinal cavity the area within the spinal column that contains the spinal cord and its coverings, the meninges (me-NIN-jez).

Spleen an organ located to the left of the upper abdominal cavity behind the stomach. It stores blood and destroys old blood cells.

Splinting to apply a device that will immobilize a painful, swollen, deformed (PSD) extremity. See *soft splint* and *rigid splint*.

Sprain a partial or complete tearing of a ligament.

Stabilize to steady a body part in order to help reduce involuntary movement caused by pain or muscle spasm.

Standard of care the care expected based on the provider's training and experience, taking into account the conditions under which the care is rendered.

START plan a four-step simple triage and rapid treatment (care) program designed for use in multiple-casualty incidents. It is usually employed by the First Responder when additional help will be delayed.

Sterile free of all life-forms.

Sternum (STER-num) the breastbone.

Stethoscope an instrument used to amplify body sounds.

Stillborn infant that is born dead or dies shortly after birth.

Stoma (STO-mah) any permanent opening that has been surgically made; the opening in the neck of a neck breather.

Strain the overstretching or tearing of a muscle.

Stressor any factor that causes wear and tear on the body's physical or mental resources.

Stroke the blocking or bursting of a vessel that supplies blood to the brain. A portion of the brain is damaged or killed by this event. Also, *cerebrovascular accident (CVA)*.

Subcutaneous (SUB-ku-TA-ne-us) beneath the skin. It refers to the fats and connective tissues found immediately below the dermis.

Substernal notch referring to the area of the lower breastbone to which the ribs attach.

Sucking chest wound an open chest wound in which air is sucked through the wound opening and into the chest cavity each time the patient breathes.

Sudden infant death syndrome (SIDS) sudden unexplained death during sleep of an apparently healthy baby in his or her first year of life.

Superficial burn a first-degree burn involving only the outer layer of skin (epidermis). See *first-degree burn*.

Superficial frostbite See *frostbite*.

Superior toward the head (for example, the chest is superior to the abdomen). See *inferior*.

Supine lying flat on the back.

Swathe a large cravat, usually made of cloth, used to secure a sling or rigid splint and sling to the body. It may be used to hold an upper limb to the chest.

Sympathetic eye movement the coordinated movement of both eyes in the same direction. If one eye moves, the other eye will carry out the same movement.

Symptom what a patient tells about his injury or illness.

Syrup of ipecac (IP-e-kak) a compound used to induce vomiting in certain conscious poisoning patients. Its use must be approved by the EMS system medical advisory board and be directed by the poison control center or medical direction for each case unless otherwise stated in very special local protocols. Generally, it is considered to be a medication and is not used by civilian First Responders.

Systemic (sis-TEM-ik) referring to the entire body.

Systolic (sis-TOL-ik) **blood pressure** the force exerted on the artery walls when the heart is contracting. See *diastolic blood pressure*.

Tachycardia (tak-e-KAR-de-ah) rapid heartbeat, usually 100 or more beats per minute.

Tarsals (TAR-sals) the ankle bones.

Tendon fibrous tissue that connects muscle to bone.

Thigh bone the femur (FE-mur).

Third-degree burn a full-thickness burn involving all the layers of the skin. Muscle layers below the skin and bones may also be damaged. See *full-thickness burn*.

Thoracic (tho-RAS-ik) **cavity** the anterior body cavity that is above (superior to) the diaphragm; the thorax. It protects the heart and lungs. Also *chest cavity*.

Thorax (THO-raks) the chest.

Tibia (TIB-e-ah) the medial lower leg bone.

Toe bones the phalanges (fah-LAN-jez).

Tongue-jaw lift a procedure used to open the mouth of an unconscious patient. The rescuer grasps the tongue and lower jaw between thumb and fingers to move the tongue away from the back of the throat.

Tourniquet the last resort used to control bleeding from an extremity. A wide, flat band or belt is used to constrict blood vessels to help stop the flow of blood.

Trachea (TRAY-ke-ah) the windpipe.

Tracheostomy (TRA-ke-OS-to-me) a surgical opening made in the anterior neck that enters into the windpipe (trachea).

Traction a part of the action taken to pull gently along the length of the limb to stabilize a broken bone to prevent any additional injury. See *manual traction*.

Trauma physical injury caused by an external force. See *blunt trauma*.

Trauma patient one who has a physical injury caused by an external force.

Trendelenburg (trend-EL-un-berg) **position** a position in which the spine-stable patient's feet and legs are higher than the head and shoulders.

Triage a method of sorting patients for care and transport based on the severity of their injuries or illnesses.

Triangular bandage a piece of triangular cloth material about 50″ to 60″ long at its base and 36″ to 40″ long on each of its sides. It can be folded and used as a sling, a swathe, or a cravat.

Tuberculosis a lung infection that can be transmitted by airborne aerosolized droplets.

Tympanic (tim-PAN-ik) **membrane** the eardrum.

U

Ulna (UL-nah) the medial lower arm bone.

Umbilical (um-BIL-i-kal) **cord** the structure that connects the body of the fetus to the placenta.

Umbilicus (um-BIL-i-kus or um-bi-LIK-us) the navel.

Universal precautions recommendations from the Centers for Disease Control and Prevention for medical and emergency care personnel to wear latex or vinyl gloves, eye protection, masks, and gowns to avoid contact with the patient's blood, body fluids, wastes, and mucous membranes. Pocket face masks with one-way valves and HEPA filters or other approved methods of resuscitation are recommended to prevent infectious diseases resulting from resuscitative efforts.

Upper a stimulant that will affect the central nervous system to excite the user.

Urinary system system that removes chemical wastes from the blood and helps balance water and salt levels of the blood; it includes the bladder, ureters, and kidneys.

Uterus (U-ter-us) the womb; the muscular structure in which the fetus develops.

V

Vagina (vah-JI-nah) the birth canal.

Vascular referring to the blood vessels.

Vein any blood vessel that returns blood to the heart.

Venae cavae (VE-ne KA-ve) the superior and inferior vena cava. The two major veins that return blood from the body into the heart.

Venous bleeding the loss of blood from a vein. It is dark red to maroon in color. The bleeding is a steady flow and can be very heavy.

Ventilation supplying air to the lungs.

Ventral front of the body. See *anterior*.

Ventricle one of the two lower chambers of the heart. Ventricles pump blood from the heart.

Ventricular fibrillation the totally disorganized contractions of the myocardium of the lower heart chambers. See *defibrillation*.

Ventricular tachycardia (tak-e-KAR-de-ah) a very fast heart rate in the heart's lower chambers.

Venule (VEN-yul) typically the smallest of veins that begin at the end of capillary beds and return blood to the larger veins. See *arterioles* and *capillaries*.

Vertebra (VER-te-brah) each individual bone of the spinal column.

Vial of Life a program designed to aid emergency care personnel by having certain patients place information and medications in special vials in their refrigerators. A "Vial of Life" sticker is placed on the main outside door, closest window to the main door, or refrigerator door.

Viscera (VIS-er-ah) the internal organs. Usually refers to the abdominal organs.

Vital signs at the First Responder level, these include pulse, respiration, and relative skin temperature, color, and condition. Vital signs may also include blood pressure and pupil assessment.

Vitreous (VIT-re-us) **fluid** transparent, jellylike substance that fills the posterior cavity of the eye.

Volatile chemicals vaporizing chemicals that will cause excitement or produce a "high" when they are inhaled by the abuser.

Vulva (VUL-vah) the external female genitalia.

W

Wheal the localized collection of fluid under the skin that may be accompanied by itching and a change in skin coloration. A hive.

Wheeze a whistling breathing sound. This sound is often associated with asthma when air is trapped in the air sacs and cannot be expired easily.

White blood cells (WBCs) the blood cells that destroy microorganisms and produce antibodies to help fight off infection. The *leukocytes* (LU-co-sites).

Womb See *uterus*.

X

Xiphoid (ZI-foyd) **process** the inferior portion of the sternum.

Z

Zygomatic (zi-go-MAT-ik) **bone** the cheek bone. Also called the *malar* (MA-lar).